# STAYING ALIVE

# STAYING ALIVE

## Critical Perspectives on Health, Illness, and Health Care

Third Edition

Edited by
Toba Bryant, Dennis Raphael, and Marcia Rioux

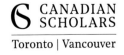

CANADIAN
SCHOLARS

Toronto | Vancouver

**Staying Alive: Critical Perspectives on Health, Illness, and Health Care, Third Edition**
Edited by Toba Bryant, Dennis Raphael, and Marcia Rioux

First published in 2019 by
**Canadian Scholars, an imprint of CSP Books Inc.**
425 Adelaide Street West, Suite 200
Toronto, Ontario
M5V 3C1

**www.canadianscholars.ca**

**Library and Archives Canada Cataloguing in Publication**

Title: Staying alive : critical perspectives on health, illness, and health care/edited by Toba Bryant,
    Dennis Raphael, and Marcia Rioux.
Names: Bryant, Toba, editor. | Raphael, Dennis, editor. | Rioux, Marcia H., editor.
Description: Third edition. | Includes index.
Identifiers: Canadiana (print) 20190172290 | Canadiana (ebook) 20190172339 |
    ISBN 9781773381305 (softcover) | ISBN 9781773381312 (PDF) |
    ISBN 9781773381329 (EPUB)
Subjects: LCSH: Social medicine—Canada. | LCSH: Medical care—Canada. |
    LCSH: Medical care. | LCGFT: Textbooks.
Classification: LCC RA418.3.C3 S68 2019 | DDC 362.1/0420971—dc23

Page layout by S4Carlisle Publishing Services
Cover design by Em Dash

19   20   21   22   23          5  4  3  2  1

Printed and bound in Ontario, Canada

Canadä

# Contents

*Foreword, by Gary Teeple*     *vii*
*Preface*     *xvi*


## PART I—PERSPECTIVES ON HEALTH, ILLNESS, AND HEALTH CARE

**Chapter 1**     Epidemiological Approaches to Population Health     4
*Stephen Bezruchka*

**Chapter 2**     Sociological Perspectives on Health and Health Care     38
*Ivy Lynn Bourgeault*

**Chapter 3**     Political Economy Perspectives on Health and Health Care     61
*Dennis Raphael and Toba Bryant*

**Chapter 4**     The Right to Health: Human Rights Approaches to Health     84
*Marcia Rioux*

**Chapter 5**     Researching Health: Knowledge Perspectives,
Methodologies, and Methods     113
*Toba Bryant, Dennis Raphael, and Marcia Rioux*


## PART II—SOCIAL DETERMINANTS OF HEALTH

**Chapter 6**     Social Determinants of Health     138
*Dennis Raphael*

**Chapter 7**     Social Class and Health Inequalities     171
*Ambreen Sayani*

**Chapter 8**     Shifting Vulnerabilities: Gender, Ethnicity/Race,
and Health Inequities in Canada     199
*Ann Pederson and Stefanie Machado*

**Chapter 9**     Politics, Public Policy, and Population Health     233
*Toba Bryant*

## PART III—CANADA'S HEALTHCARE SYSTEM

**Chapter 10**   Cracks in the Foundation: The Origins and Development of the
Canadian and American Healthcare Systems   261
*Georgina Feldberg, Robert Vipond, and Toba Bryant*

**Chapter 11**   Evolution of Healthcare Policy: Deconstructing Divergent
Approaches   281
*Mary E. Wiktorowicz and Michelle Wyndham-West*

**Chapter 12**   The Provision of Care: Professions, Politics, and Profit   311
*Ivy Lynn Bourgeault*


## PART IV—CRITICAL ISSUES IN HEALTH, ILLNESS, AND HEALTH CARE

**Chapter 13**   Women, Health, and Care   332
*Pat Armstrong*

**Chapter 14**   Constructing Disability and Illness   351
*Marcia Rioux and Tamara Daly*

**Chapter 15**   Pharmaceutical Policy: The Dance between Industry, Government,
and the Medical Profession   372
*Joel Lexchin*

**Chapter 16**   The Political Economy of Public Health: Public Health Concerns in
Canada, the U.S., U.K., Norway, and Sweden   394
*Dennis Raphael and Toba Bryant*

**Chapter 17**   Toward the Future: Current Themes in Health Research and Practice
in Canada   435
*Toba Bryant, Dennis Raphael, and Marcia Rioux*

*About the Contributors*   *444*
*Copyright Acknowledgements*   *448*
*Index*   *450*

# Foreword

This third edition of *Staying Alive* is not just welcome, but needed more than ever. First published almost 15 years ago, the book's contents, here updated, present a broad critical analysis of the social determinants of health and illness and the nature of care and treatment in contemporary society. In the first and second editions, the problems of health in industrial society were in full view, and the analyses of the authors were incisive, thought provoking, and hopeful. Since then, however, these problems have multiplied and become ever-more chronic and pervasive.

The trends of ill health are regularly mentioned in the mass media. Today, the two leading causes of death, cardiovascular diseases and cancer, are projected to continue to increase over the next generation. Chronic ailments, sometimes referred to as 21st-century diseases, include alcohol- and drug-related conditions, diabetes, asthma, Alzheimer's, dementia, multiple sclerosis, arthritis, and Parkinson's, among others; and they are on the rise. Mental conditions, deemed "disorders," including depression, addictions, and schizophrenia, along with a very long list of other debilitating mental states, are also increasing (World Health Organization [WHO], 2001a). These chronic illnesses are now the leading causes of disability, hospitalization, long-term use of prescribed pharmaceuticals, and a diminished quality of life (*Science Daily*, 2016; U.S. Department of Health and Human Services, 2018).

Such patterns of ill health are not restricted to adults or the elderly, but similar statistics characterize the health of children. Reports suggest dramatic and continuing rises in chronic childhood disorders since the 1990s—including cancer, arthritis, autism, ADHD, diabetes, asthma, food allergies, etc.—affecting somewhere between 25% and 50% of American children, depending on the study and definitions (Perera, 2018; Bethell et al., 2011). Not generally considered curable, chronic diseases become the subject of ongoing "management," that is, a life within the medical system. It is estimated that up to 50% or more of the world's population has one or more such chronic conditions (WHO, 2001b).

It is increasingly difficult to imagine a life free from illness. We now live on a planet where pollution harmful to health has spread to every continent and pervades the oceans, the atmosphere, soil, and fresh water sources. To mention a few frequently cited examples, we can point to micro-plastic pollution in our food chain that is spread through disintegrating plastic waste and many consumer products; toxic chemicals such as dioxins and PCBs that persist as micro-contaminants in air, water, and soil; herbicides and pesticides used in agriculture around the world that appear as residues throughout the food supply; radioactive waste that eludes permanent disposal everywhere and represents continuing widespread abuse of civilian safety and the environment across the world; and the use of depleted uranium munitions and other chemicals by U.S. forces that contaminate vast areas of former war zones. The International Atomic Energy Agency provides a long list of "nuclear and radiation accidents and incidents" and of nuclear weaponry long lost and forgotten. Oil extraction and refineries have left behind their marks of destruction for over 100 years (Ma, 2019; National Oceanic and Atmospheric Administration, 1992); and more recently, technologies for the "fracking" of gas and oil promise to pollute the surrounding ground water and soil for the foreseeable future.

These physical contaminants are not the only sources of poor mental and physical health; social and economic factors also play a significant role. Rates of morbidity and mortality have long been documented in the scientific literature to have a close relation to socio-economic inequality (Dasgupta, Beletsky, & Ciccarone, 2018; Pickett & Wilkinson, 2015; Townson, 1999). Work-related disease and injuries are not only physical but mental; a working life of taking orders, with little or no personal control, is not conducive to one's mental or physical health. In general, the greater the socio-economic inequality, the higher the rates of a host of physical and mental problems that come under the purview of the medical system.

It is frequently suggested that this state of affairs is the "price of industrialization" or that this is what "humans" are doing to the planet and, by extension, to ourselves. These are just two of many ways to rationalize the situation, but they suggest that the responsibility for ill health lies with the individual, and the remedy is to find recourse in the medical system (Potter, 2011). The medical system, however, despite some successes, has not been able to reverse the trends mentioned, and in many ways benefits from the growing pervasiveness of sickness. And individuals born to a system dedicated to profits rather than a clean environment and healthy population can hardly be expected to make "choices" that are not really there to make (Wohl, 1984). The pollution is planetary and increasing. To think that one can avoid or escape it does not correspond with the available evidence.

Rising rates of ill health are not the result of our behaviour as so many individuals. Planetary pollution, alienated work, and pervasive ill health are the consequences of a particular economic system. It is a system that addresses all of our needs indirectly by means of commodities, goods, and services for sale, for profit (Kassirer, 2005; Fuller, 1998; Griffith, Iliffe, & Rayner, 1987; Lexchin, 1984; Ehrenreich, 1970). And the producers of these commodities, corporations, compete with each other by producing them in the most cost-efficient way, without concern for the consumer or the planet. To do this, the costs of production manifest in the price are reduced to the lowest level possible, which means that some of the costs are not included—they appear as "externalities."

In the production process, toxic wastes of all sorts are released into the air, water, soil, and, it follows, our food chain, but are not counted in the price of commodities. At the end of their use, commodities themselves constitute waste and their disposal creates more pollutants, again not represented in the price. And during production and distribution, corporations attempt to extract the maximum amount of labour from workers, through demands for overtime work, low wages, unsafe working conditions, threats, and harassment, leading to the physical and mental exhaustion of the workers and personal and economic insecurity. These "externalities" of capitalist production, the unaccounted costs not found in the price, appear in disguised forms as planetary pollution, nature depleted and dying (Intergovernmental Panel on Climate Change, 2018), and the mental and physical ill health of humans (Hedegaard, 2018).

If this state of affairs is as obvious as the evidence would suggest and as global protests imply, why not change the way we address our needs, why not end production and distribution of commodities for profit, in order to reverse these trends? The answer is simply that corporate commodity production is the way human needs have come to be addressed the world over; it is the nature of capitalism and defended by the power of the state and corporate sector. The production of "externalities" and the exploitation of labour constitute the very foundations of the system.

Significant parts of the corporate sector are directly engaged in profiting from pollution and the destruction of nature, namely, the oil and gas producers; the auto companies; the military-industrial complex; chemical corporations; and the shipping, fishing, forestry, agricultural, and mining industries, among others. And as the destruction of nature and human health has increased, so has the healthcare industry grown. It is comprised of corporations in health insurance, pharmaceutical and medical equipment production, facility construction, and health-management firms, not to mention the institutions for producing doctors, nurses, and other trained medical staff, and hospitals and clinics to provide health services. The corporate sector benefits from both sides of production: It profits from the planetary pollution and ill health it produces, and then it profits from its attempts to address ill health. At both ends, the corporations produce "externalities" in the drive for cost efficiencies.

The pollution and damage, or "externalities," are largely left unaddressed by the corporate sector as too important as a source of profit to absorb; and so it falls to the state to "socialize" the costs in very limited ways through tax-based "clean-up" operations. And, in the industrial nations, part of the costs of ill health, an "externality," is "socialized" through so-called public health insurance and programs.

This paradox in the corporate sector goes a long way to account for the large number of inconsistencies that characterize the definition of health and the practice of health care in capitalist societies. These are among the very questions addressed in the chapters in this book.

First, the definition of health authoritatively given by the World Health Organization—the "state of complete physical, mental, and social well-being, and not merely the absence of disease or infirmity"—begs the question of what is "well-being." Does the definition imply that "well-being" can apply merely to individuals and not whole populations? Does the concept assume a world with an unpolluted environment, genuine democracy, and a benign labour market? The definition leaves us none the wiser about the meaning of health or the possibility of "well-being."

Second, because health and illness lie at the heart of a large, profitable, and complex industry, there is a conflict of interest over how they are defined. A healthy population, if possible, would not be a positive development for the health industry if it reduced its growth and profitability. For this reason, the definition of health, both mental and physical, has become the subject of contention. Witness the recent controversies over both the *Diagnostic and Statistical Manual of Mental Disorders* (DSM-5; Frances, 2013) and International Classification of Diseases (ICD-10) and their relation. The resultant damning question of what is "normal," raised in criticism of the increase of "disorders" in the DSM-5 for which treatment is recommended, points to the obvious: At what point is there no longer a "normal," that is, a concept of health? Another example of this conflict of interest is the 2017 lowering of the U.S. guidelines for the measure for blood pressure; the new guidelines will greatly expand the definition of hypertension to include over one-third of American adults (Husten, 2017).

Third, in this corporate paradox of both producing and "treating" the ill, the cause of ill health is concealed; it is not seen as the result of the "externalities" of corporate activity; it appears as if it were a matter of personal choice or bad luck, not systemic. Neither the illness nor the treatment can be seen as corporate driven because the cause and the "cure" are defined within the system, in terms presented by the system. And the ability to search for causes and cures outside the system is strongly discouraged (Angell, 2005; Barlow, 2002).

Fourth, the biomedical model continues to underlie formal medical research and practice across most of the world. It is a convenient "untruth" that fits the system well by assuming that illness is strictly a biological phenomenon belonging to the individual and treatable with select drugs and surgeries. Modern medical science has the distinction of studying and treating humans not as human beings, but rather as mere biological specimens, which humans cannot be. The human is nothing if not a social creation; the physical does not exist separately from the social; they are as one. It is not just that medical science misses part of its subject matter, however; it is that the part it addresses cannot be fully understood outside the part it misses, that is, the social determinants (Monynihan & Cassels, 2005; Sagan, 1987).

Fifth, lip service is often paid to the idea of preventative medicine, but the idea remains largely just that—an idea. If pervasive pollution, employment as following orders, and growing socio-economic inequality are the major sources of illness, then preventative medicine is not possible short of a transformation of the system. Illness and its "cures" are both products of the system (Doyal, 1979).

Sixth, health research and treatment are considered to be in the interests of human beings, but in reality the medical model of the human is the male of the species. Among the most damaging criticisms that can be made of the health system concerns its treatment of women. The list of practices and mal-practices that negatively affect women is long: the medicalization of pregnancy and maternity care, the attitudes toward abortion, the tragedies associated with birth control measures, the unnecessary surgeries, menstrual and menopausal health issues, and so on. A healthcare system biased in favour of one sex can make no claim to impartial diagnosis and treatment (Rowland, 1992; Corea, 1978).

Seventh, to become sick in this system, with its toxic food chain and stresses throughout, is not hard to do. But it is not a "role" being played to avoid responsibilities, as some have argued; it is for the most part empirically verifiable. The problem with being sick is what happens when the sick seek diagnosis and treatment. This is the moment that we are plunged into a world that is bureaucratic, institutionalized, and professionalized. Doctors, nurses, technicians, orderlies, secretaries, and administrators all have their roles to play, that is, they are guided by rules, regulations, procedures, and legal contracts and agreements that spell out their responsibilities and the limits to their jobs. It is only the sick who have no role—they are merely seeking a solution to their illness, but can only do it in an impersonalized world full of assumptions and of institutionalized behaviour: people "doing their jobs" within a system defined by corporate interest (York, 1987; Carter, 1958).

Eighth, health care in capitalist society was initially cast as a service in the marketplace; but the growth of mental and physical ill health in the 19th century, with the expansion of capital into every sphere of social reproduction, created a corresponding need for treatment. Because market principles kept medical care out of the reach of many strata in the working class, the struggle grew for "public" health provision, that is, state-sponsored medical services. This struggle for the right to health care was and remains a class struggle, making medical care a political issue, partially resolved by state-administered access and oversight rather than left to so-called market forces that benefited only the owners of the services and facilities and those who could afford treatment. The struggle reveals other paradoxes. Why in a supposed democracy does the working class have to fight for affordable medical care? Why, even in most publicly supplied medical systems, has the supply of drugs, equipment, and other medical necessaries been left in the hands of private corporations? Why, since the introduction of neo-liberal policies in the early 1980s, has much of the increased state spending on medical care gone to the private sector, in a surreptitious sell-off of what remains on the surface a state-administered medical system (Fuller, 1998)?

Ninth, whatever the health rights won by working people, state-sponsored medical care has never been quite what it seems. Although it benefits the working classes by providing them with various degrees and forms of "de-commodified" medical assistance, it remains subordinate to state direction, and so it is ultimately dependent on the vibrancy of the class struggle and the conditions of capital accumulation. Moreover, despite the benefits and the partial political rather than merely market basis to state sponsorship, the entire health industry remains defined by the political and economic system that gave rise to it. It follows that in capitalist countries the concepts of health, illness, and care are delimited by the boundaries of the capitalist mode of production (Griffith et al., 1987). That is, the human is defined largely as labour-power; the concept of health is rooted in notions of the ability to work; illness is broadly viewed as a physical condition that prevents work; and medical care emphasizes the physical reproduction of humans as labour-power and the consumption of "therapeutic" commodities.

Tenth, sickness and treatment in underdeveloped nations are not unrelated to the industrial world. The same causes or illnesses are to be found in both. The main difference is that in the latter, the working class has organized sufficiently to make demands for social reform, whereas, in the former colonial regimes, their legacies and ongoing repression by the state and corporations have meant that high levels of disease and disability and poor health care have to be endured because resistance has been suppressed. A two-year study by the Lancet Global Health Commission estimated that about 5 million deaths occur annually in "low- and middle income countries" due to poor quality health care or little or no access to care (Kruk et al., 2018).

An understanding of these paradoxes is necessary in order to challenge accepted paradigms about health and illness. But this understanding requires research methods that go beyond those of the mainstream that confine research and understanding within the boundaries of the system. One of the great strengths of *Staying Alive* is that it takes the reader/student outside these boundaries.

Another of its strengths is the examination of health care as a fought-for right in a social justice context. From this perspective, it would be a mistake to assume that the medical system is merely a normal part of systemic reproduction. In most industrial countries, the rights of citizens to state-supported medical care are not only a consequence of the need to reproduce and legitimize the system as a whole, but also the outcome of class struggle in the face of the inability of the market to address health-related issues adequately or, in some respects, at all.

In the industrial countries, there is a substantial commitment of national resources by the state that go far to de-commodify the practice of health care, that is, to keep it relatively free of market principles and practice. Arguably, it is accurate to say that all social legislation that benefits working people, including "socialized medicine," is a class victory of sorts and is the result of an implicit or explicit class struggle as its inspiration. But it must be remembered that so-called socialized medicine is state sponsored rather than genuinely socialized; the latter implies medical care as defined, organized, run, and critically assessed through the active participation of all people, without contradictory and self-serving interests at the heart of it.

That such victories are paradoxical cannot be an argument for not engaging in struggle for state-provided health care. The long and many-sided fights for state-sponsored medical care are important because these medical services do benefit working people; they are efficacious within limits; they prevent personal and family bankruptcies in the face of serious accidents, illness, or disease. If they are not fought for, the gains are gradually retrenched or even lost. Kept within a human rights discourse, however, the struggle itself is restricted to legal and structural boundaries set by the established powers; lawyers, politicians, officials, and experts prevail while the critical consciousness and participation of the classes concerned are undermined and de-politicized.

This book, through its critical perspectives, examines the questions raised here, among many others. In general, it is concerned with the numerous contradictions of health, illness, and care in a capitalist society, and how to understand them. An economic system whose principles and practices themselves lie at the heart of most medical problems is unlikely to be able to address them adequately or successfully. If the definitions of health, illness, and care are constructed as part of systemic social reproduction, they are likely to contain all the built-in assumptions, biases, and limitations of the system itself. The only real "cure" in this situation is prevention, but this cannot be admitted in a marketplace society without calling the whole system into question. For a critical understanding, it is necessary to step outside the confines of the system, and this is the position offered by the many authors in *Staying Alive*.

It could be argued that the health industry is not about human health any more than the automobile industry is about transportation. While the need for transport underlies auto manufacturing and highway construction, how the need is addressed is arguably the least efficient and most costly of all forms of transport, not to mention a common risk to life, to health, and a major contributor to ecological destruction. The need for health services similarly underlies the health industry, but how the need is addressed is more individual than social, more costly than necessary (given corporate involvement), more interest-based than health-centred, more "curative" than preventative, and in many ways hazardous to one's health. There is, for example, little demonstrable relation between expenditures for medical care and lower rates of morbidity and mortality; most major chronic illnesses stubbornly persist in the face of modern medical intervention; and thousands die each year of hospital errors and thousands more from adverse pharmaceutical drug reactions. It is difficult to see health as the first concern of the health system.

The book that follows, above all, provides us with critical methods to understand the health system, particularly in Canada, at this historical juncture. Hopefully, it will also lead to changes.

*Gary Teeple*
*Vancouver, May 2019*

## REFERENCES

Angell, M. (2005). *The truth about the drug companies: How they deceive us and what to do about it.* New York: Random House.

Barlow, M. (2002). *Profit is not the cure: A citizen's guide to saving medicare.* Toronto: McClelland & Stewart.

Bethell, C. D., Kogan, M. D., Strickland, B. B., Schor, E. L., Robertson, J., & Newacheck, P. W. (2011). A national and state profile of leading health problems and health care quality for US children: Key insurance disparities and across-state variations. *Academic Pediatrics, 1*(3), S22–S33. doi:10.1016/j.acap.2010.08.011

Carter, R. (1958). *The doctor business.* New York: Doubleday and Company.

Corea, G. (1978). *The hidden malpractice: How American medicine mistreats women.* New York: Jove Publications.

Dasgupta, N., Beletsky, L., & Ciccarone, D. (2018). Opioid crisis: No easy fix to its social and economic determinants. *American Journal of Public Health, 108*(2), 182–186. doi:10.2105/AJPH.2017.304187

Doyal, L. (1979). *The political economy of health.* London: Pluto Press.

Ehrenreich, B. J. (1970). *The American health empire: Power, profits, and politics.* New York: Vintage Books.

Frances, A. (2013). *Saving normal: An insider's revolt against out-of-control psychiatric diagnosis, DSM-5, big pharma, and the medicalization of ordinary life.* New York: HarperCollins.

Fuller, C. (1998). *Caring for profit: How corporations are taking over Canada's health care system.* Vancouver: New Star Books.

Griffith, B., Iliffe, S., & Rayner, G. (1987). *Banking on sickness: Commercial medicine in Britain and the USA.* London: Lawrence and Wishart.

Hedegaard, H., Curtin, S. C., & Warner, M. 2018. Suicide mortality in the United States, 1999–2017. *NCHS Data Brief 330.*

Husten, L. (2017). New blood pressure guideline sets lower 130/80 threshold. Retrieved from http://www.cardiobrief.org/2017/11/13/new-blood-pressure-guideline-sets-lower-13080-threshold/

Intergovernmental Panel on Climate Change (IPCC). (2018). *Special report: Climate warming.* Retrieved from https://www.ipcc.ch/

Kassirer, J. P. (2005). *On the take: How America's complicity with big business can endanger your health.* New York: Oxford University Press.

Kruk, M. E., Gage, A. D., Joseph, N. T., Danaei, G., Garcia-Saiso, S., & Salomon, J. S. (2018). Mortality due to low-quality health systems in the universal health coverage era: A systematic analysis of amenable deaths in 137 countries. *The Lancet, 392*(10160), 2203–2212. doi:10.1016/S0140-6736(18)31668-4

Lexchin, J. (1984). *The real pushers: A critical analysis of the Canadian drug industry.* Vancouver: New Star Books.

Ma, A. (2019, April 19). Nine years later, the BP oil spill's environmental mess isn't gone. *Mother Jones.* Retrieved from https://www.motherjones.com/environment/2019/04/deepwater-horizon-bp-oil-spill/

Monynihan, R., & Cassels, A. (2005). *Selling sickness: How the world's biggest pharmaceutical companies are turning us all into patients.* Vancouver: Greystone Books.

National Oceanic and Atmospheric Administration (NOAA). (1992). *HMRAD oil spill case histories 1967–1991.* Report no. HNRAD 92-11. Retrieved from https://web.archive.org/web/20100708011214/http://response.restoration.noaa.gov/book_shelf/26_spilldb.pdf

Pickett, K., & Wilkinson, R. G. (2015). Income inequality and health: A causal review. *Social Science and Medicine, 128*, 316–326. doi:10.1016/j.socscimed.2014.12.031

Perera, F. (2018). Pollution from fossil-fuel combustion is the leading environmental threat to global pediatric health and equity: Solutions exist. *International Journal of Environmental Research and Public Health, 15*(1), 16. https://doi.org/10.3390/ijerph15010016

Potter, W. (2011). *Deadly spin: An insurance company insider speaks out on how corporate PR is killing health care and deceiving Americans.* London: Bloomsbury.

Rowland, R. (1992). *Living laboratories: Women and reproductive technologies.* Bloomington, IN: Indiana University Press.

Sagan, L. A. (1987). *The health of nations.* New York: Basic Books.

*Science Daily.* (2016, October 25). More than 50% of Americans now have at least one chronic health condition, mental disorder or substance-use issue. Retrieved from https://www.sciencedaily.com/releases/2016/10/161025092655.htm

Singer, B. H., & Ryff, C. D. (Eds.). (2001). *New horizons in health: An integrative approach.* Washington, DC: National Academies Press.

Townson, M. (1999). *Health and wealth: How social and economic factors affect our well-being.* Toronto: Canadian Centre for Policy Alternatives.

U.S. Department of Health and Human Services. (2017). Health, United States 2017. Retrieved from https://www.cdc.gov/nchs/data/hus/hus17.pdf

World Health Organization. (2001a). Fact sheet on mental and neurological disorders. Retrieved from https://www.who.int/whr/2001/media_centre/press_release/en/

World Health Organization. (2001b). The global burden of chronic disease. *World Health Report 2001 press kit.* Retrieved from https://www.who.int/nutrition/topics/2_background/en/

Wohl, S. (1984). *The medical industrial complex.* New York: Random House.

York, G. (1987). *The high price of health: A patient's guide to the hazards of medical politics.* Toronto: James Lorimer and Co.

# Preface

Concerns about Canadians' health and Canada's healthcare system are now placed against the backdrop of increasing economic globalization and a shrinking Canadian welfare state. While the public is subjected to a daily onslaught of media stories about the causes and treatment of disease and the threats to the sustainability of the Canadian healthcare system, these issues are not being considered within these changing public policy environments. Traditionally, the study of health has been informed by a variety of narrow perspectives that, for too long, have been isolated from each other and from an explicit concern with these broader public policy issues. The very meaning of health, for instance, can no longer be defined as simply "the absence of disease," given what we now know about the complexity of social relations and human beings. The World Health Organization (WHO) defines health as a state of complete physical, mental, and social well-being and not merely the absence of disease or infirmity. The United Nations in its various Conventions sets the goal of health as working to ensure the highest attainable standard of health without discrimination. The way in which we conceptualize health from that perspective is impacted by various social and economic interests reflected in the chapters of this book.

Much of the isolation can be attributed to the nature of the disciplines that have evolved to ask and answer questions about health, illness, and the healthcare system. Epidemiology has been the primary tool wielded by the medical profession in quest of the causes of disease and illness. Its application, however, has been limited to a narrow scope, with little appreciation of the complex web of political, economic, and social factors that set the stage for the onset of disease and illness. The emerging field of social epidemiology is a favourable counterweight to this tradition.

Sociology has made major contributions to understanding the causes of illness and different groups' experiences of disease and illness by casting a wider net for the factors that explain health, illness, and the organization of health services. It has, however, been less concerned with identifying the forces that drive these different experiences of health and illness. Like epidemiology, there has been relatively little recognition of concepts and understandings into the sociology of health from the study of public policy and its implications for solving the problems that epidemiologists and sociologists identify.

More recently, however, two new perspectives have emerged that offer solutions to some of these problems. The political economy of health is explicitly concerned with the political and economic structures that shape citizens' experience of health and illness. It is specifically focused on understanding how the creation and distribution of resources influence the health and well-being of populations in general and specific groups in particular. The perspective has a strong commitment to identifying how these structures can be changed to promote health and well-being. The human rights perspective shares a concern with these broader issues, but places them within legal and ethical frameworks to monitor outcomes. The introduction of an explicit values and social justice dimension in discussions of health and healthcare issues constitutes a strong imperative for action.

*Staying Alive* was conceived with a view to bringing together these important yet usually isolated perspectives with the purpose of (1) identifying key issues in health, illness, and health care; (2) relating these to current policy environments; (3) identifying the complex origins of the problems identified; and (4) contributing in a meaningful way to their solution. Thus, we aim to put into action Marx's oft-quoted dictum: "The philosophers have attempted to understand the world in different ways; the point, however, is to change it."

The contributors are established authorities in their fields who have demonstrated a commitment to translate theory and empirical findings into action. Most contributors are sociologists, but all have been heavily influenced by sociological perspectives and insights. All of the contributors are concerned with public policy and its role in determining the degree of health and illness in society; the organization and distribution of political, economic, and social resources within society; and the organization, quality, accessibility, and delivery of healthcare services.

The focus of this third edition continues to be on the Canadian scene with relevant comparisons to the U.S. and other countries. It is organized in four parts. Part I provides an overview and critical review of four major health paradigms—the epidemiological, sociological, political economy, and human rights perspectives—and a chapter on research paradigms and methodologies. The basic assumptions of each paradigm are provided, as are overviews of recent activity and findings of those working within the area. The concluding chapter then makes links with varying research paradigms and methodologies. Part II explores the emerging field of the social determinants of health. There is a focus on social class, gender, and race as indicators of differential access to the economic and social resources available within a society. A unique contribution is the analysis of the role played by political ideology and public policy in shaping the distribution of these economic and social resources.

Part III focuses on the healthcare system. It provides a comparative history of the Canadian healthcare system, an overview of current attempts at reform, and a detailed analysis of the effects upon the system and its participants of recent trends toward privatization. Part IV considers critical issues in health and health care that illustrate some of the key themes of the volume: gender and its interaction with health and health care; the construction of illness and disability; health policy through the lens of pharmaceutical policy and the healthcare system; and public health concerns of varying national jurisdictions.

This volume was envisioned as being appropriate for courses on the sociology of health and illness, but its content is clearly relevant for both undergraduate and graduate courses in the health sciences, nursing, medicine, and other allied health professions. Its concern with public policy makes it appropriate for undergraduate and graduate studies in public policy. We welcome feedback concerning its usefulness in educating students and professionals engaged in promoting health, preventing illness, and planning and delivering healthcare services in Canada and elsewhere.

We acknowledge the continuing contributions to Canadians' health made by social welfare and health service providers, advocates, researchers, and policy analysts, whose ongoing efforts to promote the health and well-being of Canadians remain steadfast even in these difficult times.

*Toba Bryant*
*Dennis Raphael*
*Marcia Rioux*
*Toronto, January 2019*

# PART I

## PERSPECTIVES ON HEALTH, ILLNESS, AND HEALTH CARE

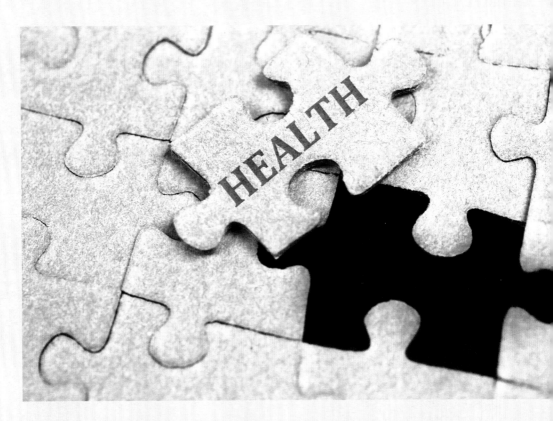

The study of health, illness, and health care is carried out within various conceptual frameworks. These perspectives, or paradigms, shape our understandings of health issues by identifying the broad dimensions or contexts within which these issues exist. These perspectives identify particular areas of concern, direct the research approaches we take to investigate these issues, and specify the appropriate means of addressing the problems that are identified. Each perspective has value for the study of health, illness, and health care in Canada. Each perspective also has a unique way of conceptualizing the manner in which these issues can and should be researched. Together, these perspectives provide a means of looking at health in a comprehensive way. Such an approach can lead to the development of innovative theory and enlightened practice.

The study of health issues has traditionally been dominated by two perspectives: the epidemiological and the sociological. Epidemiology is a branch of medicine that studies the causes, distribution, and control of disease in populations. Much of epidemiology is concerned with identifying individual risk factors that are precursors to disease and illness. In contrast, the sociological perspective has its roots in the social sciences and deals with a much wider range of health issues than the causes and distribution of disease. Society, how its organization affects health, and how individuals understand both society and health are the concerns of sociology.

The political economy and human rights perspectives are also presented. The political economy point of view examines the powerful political, economic, and social forces that shape our understanding of the world in general and health issues in particular. In Canada, the economic system and the beliefs associated with capitalism are prime determinants of both health and our understanding of health. The human rights perspective places issues of health and health care within ethical and legal frameworks that guide our expectations of what society considers fair and is obligated to offer its citizens. This view directs our attention to how society meets its commitments to a number of international agreements and commonly accepted ethical principles.

In Chapter 1, Stephen Bezruchka outlines the scope and methods of epidemiology. He provides a brief historical overview of the roots of epidemiology and describes how it is practiced today. Epidemiology has its origins in medicine and is primarily concerned with the origins of illness and disease. Bezruchka makes the distinction between studying health and illness at the cellular, organ, individual, and population level. While most of epidemiology is focused at the organ level—identifying the origins of illnesses that affect our bodily systems—there is increasing interest in how the organization of societies affects human health and well-being. He argues that the gap between rich and poor in a society may very well turn out to be the key factor in producing health.

In Chapter 2, Ivy Lynn Bourgeault provides an overview of sociological approaches to studying health, illness, and health care. Sociological approaches are concerned with human society and its structures and institutions as well as the social relations and experiences of its members. The major trends in sociological thinking about health—functionalism, conflict theory, and materialism, as well as symbolic interactionist and social constructionist approaches—are presented, as are the concerns of each approach. Bourgeault also recognizes the contributions of feminist, post-colonial, and post-structuralist perspectives. Sociological perspectives go well beyond the causes of disease and address the organization of society and how it affects the distribution of health among the population, the experience of illness, how people understand health and disease, and the organization of healthcare systems.

In Chapter 3, Dennis Raphael and Toba Bryant provide the key concepts that constitute a critical materialist approach to understanding how politics and economics shape health and healthcare systems in societies. By understanding the structure of society and how this structure determines the distribution of resources, differences in health among individuals within a society, as well as differences in health among societies, can be understood. They provide a model of how the organization of society—shaped by powerful interest groups—shapes health patterns in a society and the organization of healthcare systems. They demonstrate how a political economy approach can help us to understand why some nations are healthier than others and why Canada has a universal national healthcare system while the U.S. does not. The model also explains where there are such differences in outcomes amongst various groups in societies, including Canada.

In Chapter 4, Marcia Rioux outlines the basis of an ethical and legal approach to health and health care. The dimensions of a human rights approach to health are presented, and it is shown how these principles have been institutionalized in various international human rights agreements that define a right to health. These principles guarantee both the determinants of health—such as housing, income, employment, and security—as well as the right to receive health care when it is needed. She shows the implications of this approach for addressing current health issues of the day such as HIV/AIDS, reproductive health, mental health and disability, and access to health care. All of these and other issues have clear ethical and legal components.

In Chapter 5, Toba Bryant, Dennis Raphael, and Marcia Rioux provide an overview of the particular forms that research in health studies can take. The term "knowledge perspectives" is used to refer to the way researchers consider carrying out inquiries into health and healthcare issues. For some researchers, inquiry in health studies should be carried out in the same "scientific" way research occurs in the physical and life sciences. For others, humans' unique ability to interpret their world in different ways directs attention to studying these understandings. And for others, health studies is about examining the distribution of power and influence and whether these policies conform to human rights codes and ethical principles.

# CHAPTER 1

## Epidemiological Approaches to Population Health

*Stephen Bezruchka*

## INTRODUCTION

Epidemiology is the study of health and its determinants in specified populations, with the often unstated goal of improving health. The root word, "epidemic," derives its origin from a study of the causes of diseases. The word has been so used for over 125 years. Epidemiology as a discipline is mainly concerned with studying illness or disease, rather than health and well-being. This chapter traces the historical roots of epidemiology's evolution and its main concepts and discusses how the way it is practiced limits its potential to improve the health of populations. It considers what health means at various biological and social levels, including the sources of health in populations, and argues that the gap between rich and poor in a society is a key factor in producing health. The gap likely matters most in early life, somewhere between conception and age five. Political economic systems will be seen as the critical elements requiring change that will improve the health of populations. Comparisons of health between the United States and Canada provide a useful case study.

## EARLY EPIDEMIOLOGY

The origins of epidemiology and a classic example of its approach come from John Snow, who studied people who succumbed to cholera in London 150 years ago (Gordis, 1996). By plotting the incidence of death on maps, he discovered an association between deaths in various districts and the sources of drinking water. He went door to door, counting deaths and asking about those homes' water sources. He hypothesized that the scourge was spread by contaminated water from evacuations of infected people. Once these sources were identified, Snow removed the offending pumps' handles, even though he did not understand that it was a specific bacterium that spread the disease. Subsequently, deaths declined.

As Snow demonstrated, it's possible to improve health without understanding all the links between the causes and outcomes of disease. When Snow's study is discussed in standard textbooks, the action he undertook to control the epidemic is rarely mentioned. This lack of concern with improving health once the causes of disease are identified is all too common in the practice of epidemiology today. Asking what is the equivalent of the pump handle now is a very appropriate question. That is, what actions can have profoundly beneficial effects on health outcomes, even though the details of mechanisms of the action are not completely understood?

Epidemiologists mostly conduct studies and report results; action is not usually considered part of the discipline's domain. This reality can be equated with going to the doctor to find out what is wrong with you and then finding someone other than a physician (often a barber in medieval Europe) to provide treatment. We need a more positive and action-oriented approach to producing health.

Another health official during Snow's time, William Farr, the registrar-general in London, recognized that poverty was an important contributor to poor health (Farr, 2000). Others before and since have remarked on this. Veteran public health leader William Foege writes in *The Fears of the Rich, the Needs of the Poor: My Years at the CDC*, "The current corollary to slavery is poverty ... It is the single most important determinant of health" (2018, p. 230).

Public health typically posits that the factors responsible for poor health are behaviours and environmental exposures, many of which are associated with poverty. In this chapter, we develop the concept that there is something intrinsic about poverty or deprivation, both material and relative, that is itself unhealthy for humans. This approach is missing from many standard public health texts, as well as curricula in medical schools and specialty training programs. If studies demonstrate the critical importance of relative and absolute deprivation, but there is no action taken, we should wonder about the absence of an equivalent response to removing the pump handle.

Poverty is not a dichotomous relationship but a gradient, meaning that poorer people have poorer health. Although there is increasing recognition of the health impact of relative poverty at the individual, community, or country level, such understanding is still in very early stages among the public as well as among healthcare practitioners. Relative poverty should be considered as an illness and documented in the clinical record as a public health problem. It may be seen as an endemic issue, one that has a constant presence in a society. This recognition could lead to our treating poverty as a cause of illness, which could consist of some kind of cash transfer or other form of providing a sustainable income for inhabitants of a society.

## HEALTH DETERMINANTS DIFFER WITH THE LEVEL BEING CONSIDERED

Health can be considered at a cellular level, at the individual human level, and finally at the population level. A discussion of those approaches can help provide a perspective on how health can be produced within a society.

Consider a human being and ask of what an individual consists. In biology classes, we looked at cells under a microscope and saw small structures with nuclei and chromosomes in which DNA resided. There were also cell walls that contained proteins and energy sources. Cells come in many varieties: heart muscle cells, brain cells, lung cells, blood cells, and so on. As a medical student, I spent considerable time learning the different features of those cells and how to identify them.

In one sense, humans are nothing more than a community of different kinds of cells grouped together into various organ systems. These organs include our nervous system, which makes our limbs move when and how we want them to; our digestive system, which extracts and stores nutrients from food; our respiratory system, which extracts oxygen from the atmosphere to allow our cells to breathe; our cardiovascular system, which moves oxygen and energy to various parts of our body, and scavenges waste; our musculoskeletal system, which allows us to maintain our shape and move; and so on. Our bodies consist of cells arranged in these various communities, along with water and some other biochemical and structural material.

Suppose we isolate one of these cells, such as a heart muscle cell, and ask what that cell would need to be healthy. Cell biologists would say that a cell needs nutrients and oxygen. Glucose is the key nutrient or energy substance in our blood that powers cells. Oxygen is necessary, as well as a few trace elements. The same is true for other cells. If your heart cells do not get enough oxygen or glucose because of a faulty nutrient-delivery system, these cells die, and you will have a heart attack. The same is true for any cell in the body. If it is not nourished properly, the cell will not work as it should. Such cells will not be healthy, and premature death may occur. Later, we will review evidence suggesting that cells in poorer people are not as healthy as cells in those with higher incomes and status.

So the argument could be made that since human beings are but an assembly of cells that need oxygen and glucose plus some trace elements, then humans need those same things to be healthy. If cells benefit from oxygen and glucose, then the more food and oxygen we get, the better our health should be. But stuffing ourselves full of food is folly, as our increasing obesity rates demonstrate. Healthy adults breathing high concentrations of oxygen over long periods get lung disease, and babies breathing pure oxygen go blind. The lesson here: The logic of doing what is best for our component parts—our cells—and generalizing this prescription to the community of cells that comprise a human being may not be the best health advice for us as humans.

At the individual level—the community of cells that comprise each of us—our health is improved by following all the oft-preached do's and don'ts, such as eating healthy foods, exercising, not smoking, wearing a seat belt, using a condom, and getting a good night's sleep. That is good health advice for an individual human, but none of those recommendations make any sense to one of your cells. You cannot ask cells to exercise, to not smoke, to wear a seat belt, to get a good night's sleep, and so on. That isn't what cells can choose to do. There are no cellular-relevant versions of health advice for individuals.

What about other levels of organization such as communities, states/provinces, or nations? These locations contain populations of humans. Is it logical to assume that what is the best advice for individuals within that population—you and me—would be the best health advice for that group as a whole? Our health advisers tell us that we should exercise, eat properly, not smoke, wear seat belts, and use condoms, and expect that the population will be healthy. I suggest that approach makes the same mistake I pointed out in applying health advice for a cell to an individual human.

Looking at Japan's population suggests that there may be compelling reasons to re-think our health advice for populations, at least for rich countries. We have all learned how bad cigarette smoking is for our health. However, the Japanese have among the highest levels of smoking for rich nations, and they still lead the world in good health (Bezruchka et al., 2008). This startling observation shows how smoking, although harmful, can be secondary compared to other factors that affect a population's health. It suggests that there are population-level health-producing factors that have no individual-level counter-parts, just as health advice for individual cells doesn't work for individual peoples.

Epidemiologists and public health scholars are beginning to understand that if the social and economic factors in a society are right, then what individuals in that popula-tion do or don't do for their own health may not matter as much. They will be healthy as a by-product of the way the jurisdiction is organized, just as our cells are healthy if we do what's right for us as individuals. Societies can decide to organize society in such a way as to maximize the health of the population. The task of epidemiologists and others working for health is to make people aware of the critical importance of those factors. It is increasingly apparent that we need also to look for the equivalent of removing a pump handle in modern society.

## THE CAUSES OF THE CAUSES

There is an Indian tale—Clifford Geertz, the famous anthropologist, recounts hearing it as a story from India—about an Englishman who, having been told that the world rested on a platform on the back of an elephant, which rested in turn on the back of a turtle, asked what the turtle rested on. Another turtle. And that turtle? "Ah, Sahib, after that it is turtles all the way down."

In any discussion of disease and the causes of disease, we can look at the causes of the causes of the causes—that is, we need to go back to the source of the problem. The idea of an upstream or root cause approach that locates the source has been visually diagrammed by the Department of Health in Hawai'i in Figure 1.1.

Discovering the sources of health can be difficult, since a discussion of disease and its causes is often limited by various societal norms and understandings as to the appropriate way to identify and deal with a problem. The Department of Health in Hawai'i puts pol-itical context and governance at the source.

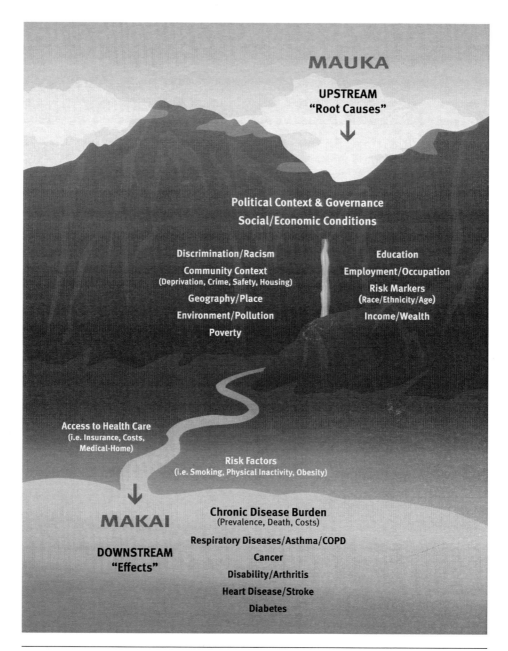

**Figure 1.1:** Root Causes and Downstream Effects

*Source:* Pobutsky, A., Bradbury, E., & Wong Tomiyasu, D. (2011). *Chronic disease disparities report 2011: Social determinants.* Honolulu: Hawai'i State Department of Health, Chronic Disease Management and Control Branch.

# POPULATION HEALTH EPIDEMIOLOGY

John Snow went door to door in what is called "shoe leather epidemiology" to collect information on water sources and deaths. Such observational data form the backbone of epidemiologic investigations. For a disease-focused approach, one needs to know whether someone has the disease and then obtain a variety of supplemental information to discern other factors that might be relevant. Imagine a study of lung cancer in a population where everyone smoked. It would be very difficult to identify smoking as a cause of lung cancer, since you could not compare the incidence of disease between smokers and non-smokers. The kinds of questions asked to study health in a population depend on a range of characteristics in that population. If you ask wrong or limited questions, or study the wrong population, you can be led astray, as suggested by the smoking and lung cancer example.

Today the term "social epidemiology" reflects the population or societal level of analysis, defined as the branch of epidemiology that studies the social distribution and social determinants of states of health. It looks at the way social, economic, and political structures and relationships influence health. Social determinants of health have been variously conceived as the conditions in which people are born, grow, live, work, and age. These circumstances are shaped by the distribution of money, power, and resources at local, national, and global levels. The social determinants of health are mostly responsible for health inequities—the unfair and avoidable differences in health status seen within and between countries.

Some advocate for a new discipline of political epidemiology that studies the impact of welfare regimes, political institutions, and specific policies on health and health equity. Recognizing the political determinants of health considers the political context as a determinant of "downstream" health outcomes, as graphically depicted by the Department of Health of Hawai'i.

Current concerns in social epidemiology relate to concepts of equity and equality. Health *inequalities* refer to differences in health status or in the distribution of health determinants between different population groups. These are often due to the unequal distribution of the social, economic, and political factors that produce health. Health *inequities* are those health inequalities that are unfair or unjust and can be remedied. A societal state of good health, health equity, is the absence of unfair and avoidable differences in health among population groups. Geoffrey Rose (1992) stated that "there is no known biological reason why every population should not be as healthy as the best." Accepting this idea requires societies to remove political obstacles to good health such as poverty and associated powerlessness. Such practices, once begun, may require generations to demonstrate results. In the United States, the weaker term "health disparity" is mostly used instead of "health inequality." "Disparity" connotes difference and lacks the moral underpinnings of "inequity."

One could ask why "turtles all the way down" is not the focus in epidemiology today. Epidemiologists have graduate training (usually in public health schools), and some work in public health departments. Many jobs for epidemiologists tend to have a narrow focus, and their projects are short term and focused on behavioural interventions. These foci may not be the most effective in producing health. Epidemiologic research is also done by private businesses or by federal agencies with close ties to private business. Despite the global economic collapse brought about by bankers in the U.S., credence is still given to the business model and so-called free markets in facilitating positive social and health change. The theme is often to create products, drugs, or instruments for a procedure or a communications campaign for individuals or their organs. The outcome is usually an action for individuals to take: Ask your doctor for this drug. Eat that food. Use this exercise appliance. Such a disease focus is severely limited in any ability to affect the factors that produce health in a population (Schwartz, Susser, & Susser, 1999).

Another factor limiting upstream efforts is typified by Upton Sinclair (1935), who wrote, "It is difficult to get a man to understand something, when his salary depends upon his not understanding it!" As an emergency physician, I was paid to diagnose and treat illness and injury, but not to ask why someone had that illness or injury. Most of us have limited areas of expertise and work on downstream issues where basic questions are not being asked.

Another explanation for the type of work done by epidemiologists relates to the emergence of powerful computers that allow analysis of complicated data on individual diseases. The focus on the individual and the ability to process vast amounts of data keep many researchers stuck in the study of individual health risks rather than social factors. This leads to a problem similar to studying lung cancer in a society where everyone smokes. Unless you look at people who are similar in important respects, you won't find what you are looking for. They must have similar incomes or education or wealth or status in society. In the jargon of epidemiology, you have to control for socio-economic status in a study, or you won't find an effect. Socio-economic status measures aspects of poverty, which has been stated to be the most important determinant of health. Controlling means that you factor out the importance of that variable in the analysis. Then you cannot ask questions about the variable. Hence socio-economic status, that is, level of poverty, must be very important in producing health. If it wasn't, then one wouldn't need to control for socio-economic status in studying other factors. How you frame the question profoundly impacts what answer you get.

Defining a disease can be very political (Illich, 1976). Homosexuality used to be labelled a disease in medical textbooks in the U.S., as it still is in some countries. On the other hand, in Canada and the United States same-sex marriages are now legal. Fibromyalgia and chronic fatigue syndrome are conditions that haven't yet appeared on the universally recognized disease stage but are termed "contested illnesses." Some suggest that relative poverty should be considered a disease, as its negative health effects are considerable.

A current global focus considers diseases and their disabilities at the population level by measuring Disability Adjusted Life Years, or DALYs, for various diseases. This approach leads to tallies of the global burden of disease. The Institute for Health Metrics and Evaluation, based in Seattle, has become the key organization aggregating and producing this information. This disease-oriented focus does not consider the social or political factors underlying their distribution,

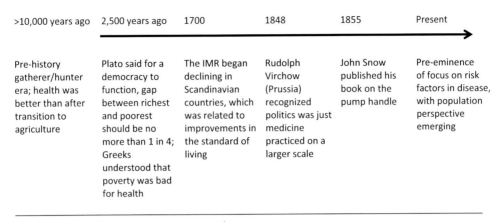

| >10,000 years ago | 2,500 years ago | 1700 | 1848 | 1855 | Present |
|---|---|---|---|---|---|
| Pre-history gatherer/hunter era; health was better than after transition to agriculture | Plato said for a democracy to function, gap between richest and poorest should be no more than 1 in 4; Greeks understood that poverty was bad for health | The IMR began declining in Scandinavian countries, which was related to improvements in the standard of living | Rudolph Virchow (Prussia) recognized politics was just medicine practiced on a larger scale | John Snow published his book on the pump handle | Pre-eminence of focus on risk factors in disease, with population perspective emerging |

**Figure 1.2:** Prehistoric to Present Timeline

instead focusing on the diseases that are a downstream manifestation of health. A disease focus may provide much useful information to guide health care in treating individuals, but this schema may not help produce health in populations (Evans, Barer, & Marmor, 1994).

## LEARNING FROM HEALTH DATA ON POPULATIONS

To understand what produces health in a population, we need to define health. The World Health Organization (WHO) states that "health is a state of complete physical, mental and social well-being and not merely the absence of disease or infirmity." A more measurable definition might be asking individuals how healthy they consider themselves on a scale from very unhealthy to very healthy. This is termed "self-assessed health" (SAH).

For a population, mortality measures allow for comparisons with others. Consider the average length of life (life expectancy) or the infant mortality rate (IMR). Out of 1,000 infants born, the IMR measures how many die in their first year of life. IMR is a more sensitive measure than others, since early life is so critical to adult health considered broadly. These rates can give us numbers, allowing us to ask what may maximize health. SAH measures mirror mortality measures when used in a culturally similar population and are often used to study factors affecting the health of populations that are not rooted in death rates.

To determine the life expectancy (LE) of a population, the dates of births and deaths are used to calculate age-specific death rates in a given year. The resulting table shows when those in a hypothetical population would die, demonstrating their expected average length of life. Life expectancies are computed for all countries recording vital events, births, and deaths, and estimated for other nations.

Other specific mortality measures include child or under-5 mortality, adult mortality (the probability of a 15-year-old dying before reach age 60), and maternal mortality ratio (number of maternal deaths per 100,000 live births). There are now many sources of these indicators to observe trends among nations.

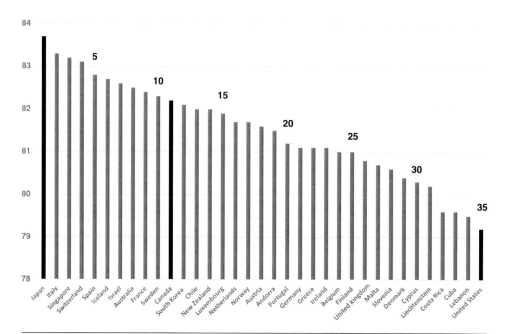

**Figure 1.3:** Health Olympics, 2015

*Source:* United Nations Development Program. (2016). *Human development report 2016: Human development for everyone.* Geneva: Author.

The United Nations' annual *Human Development Report* is a convenient data source. Consider health as an Olympic event, with life expectancy as the "race" with a clear finish line. The top 35 countries in this race are shown in Figure 1.3. For all data reported in 2016, estimating life expectancy for 2015, the LE range is from 83.7 years for Japan to 48.9 for Swaziland, the least healthy in a list of 189 countries.

We understand vital signs of individuals, our pulse, blood pressure, and temperature. If those numbers are far from what is considered normal, it may indicate the need to act quickly. If someone told me in the ER that a patient's blood pressure was 60/30 and had a pulse of 200, I'd be there in a heartbeat. If the blood pressure was 120/70 with a pulse of 60 and a temperature of 37°C, I could take my time. Why don't we look at vital signs for populations too?

To get a sense of what small LE differences mean, consider calculating life expectancy in the United States in 2001 with and without the 3,000 deaths of September 11. It would make only a 0.01 year difference for the country as a whole. New York City did this exercise for that jurisdiction alone and found a difference of 0.2 years for men and 0 for women.

Tiny differences in life expectancies can translate to huge inequities in death rates, however. The U.S. is undoubtedly the world's richest and most powerful country, with over a quarter of all billionaires and vast military might, yet it is far from being the healthiest. Canada is much healthier. Japan leads the world in most measures of health. The U.S.

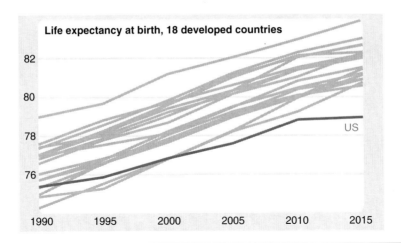

**Figure 1.4:** Rich Country Life Expectancy Trends, 1990–2015

*Source:* Ho, J. Y., and Hendi, A. S. (2018). Recent trends in life expectancy across high income countries: Retrospective observational study. *British Medical Journal, 362*(k2562). doi:10.1136/bmj.k2562

is 4.5 years behind Japan in life expectancy, which seems insignificant. But consider: if the U.S. could eliminate heart disease as a cause of death, its number one killer, accounting for one death in four, it still wouldn't be the healthiest country (Arias, Heron, & Tejada-Vera, 2013). The 4.5-year health gap is huge!

Seventy-five years ago, best estimates would put the U.S. in the top five countries for life expectancy. Japan would have been considerably below the 35th ranking enjoyed by the U.S. today, so there has been a profound deterioration in health in the U.S. compared to other countries. U.S. life expectancy has been declining absolutely since 2015, an unprecedented deterioration in health in this century. Figure 1.4 presents life expectancy trends for rich countries from 1990 to 2015, demonstrating how the United States has seen significant deterioration in rates of improvement and then in absolute numbers.

Life expectancy trends comparing Canada, Japan, and the U.S. from 1960 are revealing (Figure 1.5). Canada ranks 11th in the UN list of countries, with a life expectancy of 82.2. It was considerably higher in rank decades ago, although the absolute number of years was less. However, with American life expectancy decreasing recently as noted above, life expectancy elsewhere around the world keeps increasing.

In the "Health Olympics," Canada and the U.S. have more than changed places with Japan. Why? Consider health care. An easy measure is the per-capita expenditure. The U.S. spends about half of the world's healthcare budget, about U.S. $10,348 per person in 2016, comprising a sixth of its GDP, and almost 50% more than that spent by Canada. Underspending on health care is not the reason for the U.S. poor health.

Many mortality indicators other than life expectancy show similar shocking rates for the United States in comparison to other nations. There are no mortality indicators for

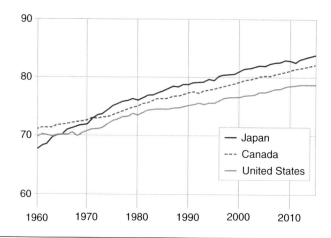

**Figure 1.5:** Canada, Japan, and United States Life Expectancy Trends, 1960–2015

*Source:* World Bank. (2015). https://www.google.com/publicdata/explore?ds=d5bncppjof8f9_&
ctype=l&strail=false&bcs=d&nselm=h&met_y=sp_dyn_le00_in&scale_y=lin&ind_y=
false&rdim=country&idim=country:CAN:JPN:USA&ifdim=country&hl=en&dl=en&ind=false

which the United States ranks in the top 30 nations, until examining survival at much older ages, such as the chance of dying after reaching age 75. Comparisons show that if the U.S. had the under-5 child mortality of Slovenia, which should be an attainable goal, over 40 fewer children would die every day in the United States. For female adult mortality, a 15-year old girl in Sri Lanka has a lower chance of dying before reaching age 60 than a U.S. girl. Similarly, for a 15-year old boy in Tunisia. Even more shameful is the 50% rise in maternal mortality in the United States over the last 15 years. This very rare event has only happened in eight nations. Canada is spared these humiliating results, ranking, for the most part, in the top 20 nations.

The embarrassing health status of the United States gets little attention in that country despite the undeniable evidence. In 2013, the Institute of Medicine there produced a report titled *U.S. Health in International Perspective: Shorter Lives, Poorer Health*. It highlighted that even the privileged few, who are white-skinned, earn substantial incomes, and practice all the health promoting behaviours, die younger than their counterparts in other rich nations. The report advised informing the public and looking at healthier nations to see what they do that could be of use in the U.S. Sadly, this advice has not been followed.

The U.S. is clearly not buying health with its healthcare dollars. We naturally assume that health and health care are synonymous, but they are not. In the United States, people speak of accessing health, paying for health, insuring health, and getting health when they are really speaking of health care in those phrases. We might ask: "Do you want health or health care?"

Similar analyses demonstrate that none of the usual factors explain why the U.S. is so unhealthy. Out of all the countries presented in Figure 1.3, Japanese men smoke the most, while the U.S. has the lowest prevalence of male smoking (World Health Organization, 2015). You could conclude that smoking is what makes Japan so healthy. Another interpretation is that although smoking is not good for your health, other factors are worse, and they supersede the bad effects of smoking. We must look beyond individual behaviours for understanding population health outcomes.

## Inequality in Society Is Bad for Your (Our) Health

Richard Wilkinson is an economic historian and epidemiologist who has been studying the health of countries for decades, trying to determine the factors related to their health. He has demonstrated that the usual factors do not offer satisfactory explanations. By 1986, he had found that the gap between the rich and poor in a country appeared to be correlated with the population's health. This was not something commonly recognized, but in 1992, his findings were published in the *British Medical Journal*. This paper helped spawn the study of population health today.

Wilkinson and Kate Pickett went on to create an index of health and social problems for 23 rich nations and looked at the impact of income inequality on this measure. The index comprised life expectancy, infant mortality rate, teenage births, obesity, mental illness, homicides, imprisonment rates, mistrust, social mobility, and education. The graph shows the remarkably clear association of the United States having the highest income gap and scoring very poorly on the indicators. Their bestselling book, *The Spirit Level: Why Greater Equality Makes Societies Stronger*, has had a profound impact on recognizing the importance of economic inequality on producing undesirable outcomes.

This relationship between income inequality and worse health and social problems is causal, using the accepted epidemiologic criteria for inferring causality (Pickett & Wilkinson, 2015). In the 40 years since the first study associating income inequality and mortality appeared, a scientific revolution has occurred. The concept has undergone fierce criticism, scrutiny, and now increasing acceptance. Social inequalities, such as income inequality, can be considered a fundamental cause of health inequities and lie near the source in the upstream metaphor.

Research has shown that this relationship is not found in small areas where people of similar economic means reside (Wilkinson & Pickett, 2009). The strength of the association can also depend on social spending policies that modify the effect of income, so that beneficial goods such as health care do not need to be purchased out of the paycheque. There are often lag effects when health impacts are seen some time after inequality changes. Context matters, such as in Canada where the association is not seen among new immigrants, but for long-term immigrants it approaches that seen in the Canadian-born (Auger, Hamel, Martinez, & Ross, 2012).

Explanations for the impact of income inequality on health rest on three observations. One is that there are diminishing returns for the effect of increasing income and increased health. The income health curve is concave downward; that is, additional income

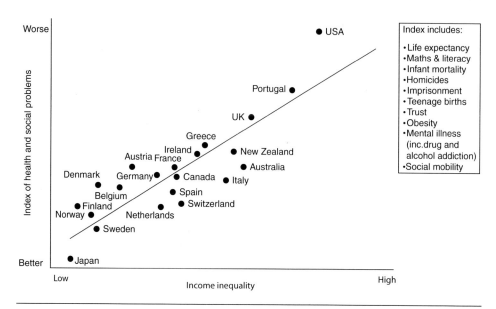

**Figure 1.6:** Health and Social Problems Related to Income Inequality

*Source:* Wilkinson, R. G., & Pickett, K. E. (2009). *The spirit level: Why more equal societies almost always do better.* London: Allen Lane.

results in very small health gains. Redistributing income from the very rich to the very poor results in an increase in average health.

A second mechanism relates to the psychosocial impacts of stress produced by social comparisons among and between economic classes in society. Stress has been termed the 21st-century tobacco. When people are aware of economic inequities or relative deprivation, they respond in various ways. Road rage is commonly experienced, and air rage has been observed in passenger planes that have first-class cabins. Mass shootings in the United States have been linked to county income inequality. The highest global level of opioid use is in the United States. It may be that the ten-fold increase in opioid mortality since 1980 demonstrates one way of trying to cope with the stress of inequality.

Finally, in what is termed a contextual effect of income inequality on health, with a large income gap in society, the rich pay directly for many services they receive. These include private education, concierge health care, security guards, and gated communities. They do not want to be taxed to pay for others to receive services that they pay for directly. Using their economic and political power, they push for further tax cuts for the rich, leading to less social spending for the rest of the population, a phenomenon termed "austerity." Fewer services are available to fill the gaps in income, health care, and other services. The $1.5 trillion-dollar tax cut passed in 2018 in the U.S. represents an example of this third contextual effect.

How is inequality measured? The most commonly used measure in rich countries is that of income differences, data that are collected regularly in the census and from other sources.

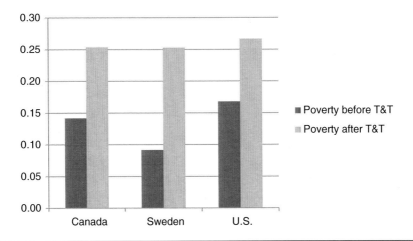

**Figure 1.7:** Poverty Rates Before and After Taxes and Transfers (T and T)

*Source:* Based on Bourgeault, I. L., Labonté, R., Packer, C., & Runnels, V. (Eds.). (2017). *Population health in Canada: Issues, research, and action* (Figure 24.1). Toronto: Canadian Scholars' Press.

Income is a flawed measure—especially at the country level—because there are a variety of behind-the-scenes redistribution mechanisms that mitigate the effects of differences. Using Organisation for Economic Co-operation and Development (OECD) data in 2015, through taxes, transfers, and other payments, Sweden reduced its poverty rate based on income over 63%, in comparison to about 44% for Canada and only 37% for the U.S. (author calculations from OECD, 2015). Some countries, such as Sweden, provide health care, education, and other benefits that people in countries like the U.S. must purchase directly.

There is a stronger relationship between income inequality and mortality in the United States than in Canada, which provides more social services that are not paid for by individuals directly. Besides universal health care in Canada, the government supports education, housing, transportation, and other social services (Ross et al., 2000; Sanmartin et al., 2003).

The geographic level at which income distribution is measured affects its association with health. In a small neighbourhood, most people are similar economically, so it would be unlikely that a small income gap there would be related to health. In the U.S., the relationship is seen at the city and state level throughout the country, but not at the county level within states. Other studies have demonstrated that even the rich in the United States are not as healthy as counterparts in Europe (Avendano, Glymour, Banks, & Mackenbach, 2009).

Epidemiologists speak of the ecological fallacy for population findings that may be misleading when applied to individuals (Berkman, Kawachi, & Glymour, 2014). For example, the finding that populations with more poverty have worse health than populations with less poverty implies that poorer people have poorer health. But this conclusion must be demonstrated by other means. It could reflect the opposite reality, for example, such as if it were the rich individuals that had worse health in a high-poverty population. However, numerous studies, including some using self-assessed health estimates, refute the ecological fallacy limitation: The poor are much more impacted by inequality than the rich. Nonetheless, even those who are economically advantaged would likely be healthier in a more equal society.

To summarize the findings, relative poverty is bad for your health. That is, being lower on the socio-economic ladder is a disadvantage in most measures of health. The steepness of the ladder or gradient reflects the severity of economic inequality, and a steeper gradient in more unequal societies is associated with worse health. The gap between the rich and poor in society represents how much the society cares for and shares with its members.

Canada has a better inequality profile than the U.S., but fares worse than do many European nations (see Chapters 6 and 9, this volume). A top CEO in the U.S. makes close to 500 times what an average worker does (Pizzigati, 2018). The figure used to be 20 times for Canada, although it is now higher. The rate used to be around 10 for Japan, but this has also risen today. Back in 1980, when the U.S. was considerably healthier compared to other countries, the pay gap was about 40 to 1. As Thomas Piketty (2014) points out in *Capital in the Twenty-First Century*, the phenomenal increases in top executive compensation in the United States represent something other than market forces at work.

## Role of Health Care in Producing Health

While universal health care is a human right and an important indicator of progress, the United States remains the only rich nation not taking this step. How important is health care in improving health and reducing health inequities? The best published study looking at the impact of healthcare services in advancing health was done in Winnipeg, Manitoba, by looking at mortality outcomes related to cuts in healthcare services (Roos, Brownell, & Menec, 2006). The more that was cut, the better the improvements in mortality. The study's last paragraph stated, "To conclude, a universal health care system is definitely the right policy tool for delivering care to those in need, and for this it must be respected and supported. However, investments in health care should never be confused with, or sold as, policies whose primary intent is to improve population health or to reduce inequalities in health. Claims to that effect are misleading at best, dangerous and highly wasteful at worst" (Roos et al., 2006, p. 125).

As many nations transitioned to universal health care, it was expected that the socio-economic gradient in health, namely poorer people having poorer health outcomes, would decline or perhaps disappear. That hasn't happened, which remains a concern, especially for European nations.

Medical care treats illnesses and injuries, but the lack of medical care is not the cause of illness and injury. To compound the issue, whenever medical care has been studied, it has been found to be a leading cause of death. One study in the U.S. (Makary & Daniel, 2016) suggested it was the third-leading cause of death.

Whereas health care definitely helps some, it harms others, and for populations, whenever it has been studied, there appears to be little or no net benefit for population mortality measures. Medical care can improve quality of life and health, but its impact is often limited. I write this as someone who was an emergency physician for 30 years: Consider medical services as necessary for a society, but not sufficient, to produce good health. Recognizing this is very difficult for most people.

Consider the argument presented earlier regarding the health of cells/organs, individuals, and populations. Does medical care treat individuals or populations? No, for the most part it treats cells and organs. You take aspirin to treat platelets, proton pump inhibitors to treat gastric mucosa cells, statins to treat hepatocytes, and sildenafil to treat smooth muscle cells in the corpora cavernosa. Surgery and coronary stenting work on organs. A different kind of political or upstream medicine is needed to treat populations. Rudolf Virchow, the founder of modern cellular pathology, stated in 1848 that "medicine is a social science and politics nothing more than medicine on a larger scale." This has been called public health's biggest idea.

Studies in rich nations have shown that a focus on primary as opposed to specialty care does influence health. In Europe, the strength of primary care system mitigates some of the adverse effect of income inequality on health (Detollenaere, Desmarest, Boeckxstaens, & Willems, 2018). Strong primary care can be defined as accessible services that provide a comprehensive scope, meeting the population's healthcare needs, coordinating care across different healthcare levels, and providing a continuous provider-patient relationship over time and different disease and illness episodes. With almost four times as many generalists as the U.S., Canada has a strong primary healthcare system.

What does produce health for a society are specific forms of social spending. Comparing social spending to healthcare expenditures among rich nations demonstrates that healthier nations privilege the former over the latter. Social expenditures have been shown to lead to better outcomes for infant mortality, life expectancy, and other measures of health (Bradley, Elkins, Herrin, & Elbel, 2011). In the U.S., states with higher expenditures on education, income support, transportation housing, and the environment have better outcomes compared to those that spend less.

## Basic Needs

Better caring and sharing in a society, along with less inequality, determines its health. Can we generalize this from what we know of rich countries? For the poorest nations, providing food, water, shelter, and basic needs for everyone takes priority. For countries with a low gross domestic product (GDP), a few hundred dollars up to $5,000 to $10,000 per person per year, life expectancy estimates tend to increase with increasing GDP (Wilkinson & Pickett, 2009). This seems to indicate that most are getting the basic necessities of life and living standards are improving. But economic growth, as measured by increasing per capita GDP, must be shared to be beneficial. A critical threshold relates more economic growth to further improvements in population health and other measures of

---

**Box 1.1:** What Produces Health in a Population

---

- Provision of basic needs (food, water, shelter, security)
- Provision of caring and sharing, especially in early life, which is typically measured by the distribution of wealth, resources, income, political power, and the status of women
- Access to basic healthcare services
- Cultural elements of reciprocity, social harmony, and vigilant sharing
- Focus on early life: early life lasts a lifetime

---

well-being. The threshold is reached at about $10,000 per capita GDP. Above that level, more economic growth does not by itself lead to longer lives, increases in happiness or well-being, or other measures of a good society. Once countries exceed that threshold, levels of inequality matter more in producing health.

Increasingly inequality is an upstream factor strongly related to infant and maternal health outcomes around the world. Income itself is difficult to measure in poorer countries, but inequality of household wealth, or assets, has been found to impact child health in low- and middle-income countries. Most low- and middle-income nations have not seen equitable economic growth to benefit their societies. Hunger and poverty remain common in both sub-Saharan Africa and South Asia. Yet, in 2010, India had more of the 10 richest people in the world than any other country.

What is needed is more global caring and sharing—providing the basics of food, water, and shelter—to address today's immense global inequities, as well as those within countries.

## Early Life Lasts a Lifetime

If we ask how much of our health as adults is determined during the first years of life, the answer is a great deal. Research shows that by age two or three, as much as half of our health as adults is already programmed. The first thousand days after conception matter the most for our health outcomes as adults—long before we make any conscious choices about behaviours to make us healthy. This perspective is known as the developmental origins of health and disease (DOHaD; Bezruchka, 2015).

How can such life-course issues be studied epidemiologically? Ideally, a cohort study would follow a group of people from conditions during their gestation until they died. Major challenges in such research include the need to follow people for longer than the lifespan of the investigator, as well as the huge costs involved. However, some countries have kept detailed records at birth for individuals who can be followed over time. Studies of these groups have found that in the trajectory from the womb to the tomb, the womb may be more important than the subsequent home as far as chronic diseases in adulthood are concerned. David Barker's (1998, 2012) initial studies on low birth weight affecting adult health, termed the fetal origins hypothesis, have spawned much understanding of the importance of early life conditions. The life history of a woman before she becomes pregnant also matters for the health of her baby, as much as or more than the prenatal period.

Significant stress during the mother's pregnancy can be linked to worse health later in a child's life. Research on this topic looks at surrogate markers, such as inflammation and other biological parameters in adulthood, to gauge later health outcomes. It has been found that susceptibility to lung cancer may depend on various conditions in the uterus, independent of smoking cigarettes. One source of such studies is the Helsinki birth cohort, a population for which birth data and long-term follow-up information were recorded from 1924 to 1944 (Barker, 2012).

Care during early life is immensely important for future development of the child. John Bowlby, studying orphans after the Second World War, demonstrated the importance of having a single caregiver present soon after birth and for the first year of a child's life. Such conditions were more likely to lead to secure attachment, meaning the infant felt more comfortable among strangers and in exploring surroundings. Better mental health, physical health, and healthy behaviours are more likely to result than when the newborn is unattended or cared for by several different individuals for much of the early part of their life, at least in Western societies.

Subsequent studies have demonstrated the impact of early life, especially conditions of poverty and socio-economic circumstances, on adult health. Societies that provide support for pregnant women and early life parenting, including economic support, have better health outcomes than countries that neglect that period. The United States stands with Papua-New Guinea as only two populous countries without a paid parental leave law.

Various forms of abuse or maltreatment in early life also cause great problems later in life. Adverse childhood experiences, or ACEs, are categorized as emotional, physical, and contact sexual abuse, as well as various forms of household dysfunction and neglect. The original studies followed people in San Diego enrolled in Kaiser, a health maintenance organization (Bezruchka, 2015). They found that higher ACE scores were associated with various forms of later impairments, unhealthy risk behaviours, chronic diseases, and early death. Such toxic stress in early life has permanent effects. Various forms of supportive care in later life can help but not eradicate that initial adversity.

ACEs are more common among those who are poorer and in more unequal U.S. states (Eckenrode, Smith, McCarthy, & Dineen, 2014; Halfon, Larson, Son, Lu, & Bethell, 2017). At present, there are few studies on this topic in Canada. The WHO is developing an international study to validate the concept in other parts of the world, which would include exposure to community, collective, and war violence. Many dysfunctions in adulthood, including criminal behaviours and recidivism, poor school performance, and various disabilities and chronic conditions have their origins in early life abuse.

Adverse childhood socio-economic circumstances add to the impact of ACEs. There is need to merge DOHaD material with ACEs to gain wider awareness.

Denmark is a country that serves as a case study of the complexities of the inequality-health relationships. It is the only more egalitarian and rich country that has relatively poor health outcomes, comparable to those of the United States. In 1994, the Danish government published a report mentioning that for the past two decades, life expectancy had been stagnating there, rather than growing as in all the other OECD nations (Bjerregaard & Hermann, 1994). Historically, life expectancies of both Danish men and women were far higher than in the United States in the 1970s, and close to those of Norway and Sweden. However, by 1990, they were equal for U.S. and Danish men, with U.S. women outliving Danish women.

The report noted that Danish women entered the labour market in large numbers during the period 1960–1968, which was earlier than women in other neighbouring countries such as Norway and Sweden, and that they typically began working when they had young children. Their jobs were mostly temporary, unskilled, and low-paying. In the 1970s and 1980s, many women were laid off and unemployment soared, especially in comparison to other nearby nations. Women's mortality increased as a result, while the welfare practices typical of other Scandinavian countries were not as comprehensive in Denmark. The resultant stresses led to high rates of women smoking, and later these women developed the highest lung cancer mortality of all European nations.

Adult mortality improvements stagnated from about 1970 to 1990, and child mortality from 1980 to 1990. Female adult mortality, which is the probability of a 15-year-old dying before reaching age 60, demonstrated rapid declines in Denmark after 1990, suggesting that the conditions producing worse outcomes have abated to some extent. Denmark has learned from the conditions producing health deprivation. Life expectancy is again increasing.

Bakah and Raphael (2017) reviewed the health paradox in Denmark and suggested that neo-liberal policies leading to high unemployment, wealth (not income) inequality, and the country's flexi-security policies were important antecedents to its health outcomes. Unlike other Scandinavian nations, the government is more invested in modifying personal behaviours rather than focusing on more upstream political policies.

## Biology of Inequality

Most of us go through life with a rudimentary understanding of biology and specific physiology and pathology. Our previous discussion of cells, organs, individuals, and populations leads us to consider what it would mean to have a biological explanation of health impacts on large human groups. Understanding proceeds from hypotheses that are tested by experiments and further refined and elaborated in different settings. Cells can be studied in cultures, and their components can be extracted and measured. Organs can be perfused in an artificial environment.

Experiments on populations are rarely carried out on humans for ethical reasons, but various natural experiments occur throughout history. Early life issues have been studied extensively in rats and sheep. Dog labs have been settings for much understanding of human physiology. Primate labs and alfresco experiments help understanding of our closer relatives.

But we do know quite a lot about inequality in human societies and its impact on health. Many aspects of the early environment matter tremendously in producing the health of offspring. Growth in the uterus is determined by many factors, and early child development has a profound effect on adult health. Stresses during pregnancy will affect the health of children and the adults they become. Generally, those lower in socio-economic positions in society have worse health outcomes that are independent of personal behaviours, to the extent that poverty in infancy can be considered a brain toxin, from which complete recovery is difficult (Bezruchka, 2015).

The social environment in early life is determined to a significant degree by the economic and political environment. The acute stress response, activated when one is faced with a threat or danger, allows energy to be mobilized and directed to the organs that will save one's life (Bezruchka, 2015). But chronic stress in pregnancy, such as that of economic insecurity, has a negative impact on the biological responsiveness of inflammatory cells that lasts through to adulthood. It's observable in adults in their 20s who appear to be otherwise healthy and predicts the development of more chronic illnesses as they age.

Cortisol and adrenaline are key effectors. Turning the fight-or-flight response on for a few minutes to get out of the path of a car has a marked survival benefit, but if it is turned on all the time—for example, when stuck in traffic and late for an appointment or worrying about being evicted or fearing a significant other will be violent at the next encounter—it may not have death-avoiding advantages. Overworking the stress system, a concept termed allostatic load, appears to be maladaptive and have lasting repercussions on the ability to mount a swift survival response when it is needed.

Those lower down the socio-economic ladder tend to be more affected by chronic stress in measured ways. This includes a greater likelihood of obesity, adult-onset diabetes, and cardiovascular disease. Mechanisms that produce chronic stress in society have received considerable research attention (Sapolsky, 2004). The production of cortisol from the adrenal gland, which is regulated by the hippocampus in the brain, is an important pathway leading to worse health when higher cortisol levels are sustained. Levels of cortisol in scalp hair provide a time-concentration integral of stress exposure. Increasing cortisol in recent hair growth is related to events such as a heart attack, and higher elevations afterwards have a worse prognosis. In addition to many individual studies, there are population data that demonstrate different stress responses (Kristenson et al., 1998).

At the same time, organs and bodies must continue with growth, tissue repair, and fighting potentially hazardous infectious invaders. Markers of the inflammatory response to infection and other illnesses suggest that those lower down the socio-economic hierarchy are working harder to combat contagion. They have higher allostatic loads measured by blood pressure, BMI, and various blood biomarkers such as cholesterol, and they also have worse health outcomes (Geronimus, Hicken, Keene, & Bound, 2006).

The nervous system turns out to be very plastic—that is, it is capable of remodelling depending on various social and environmental stimuli. It is the major conductor of the body's response to the physical, social, economic, and political environment. Mother Nurture facilitates Mother Nature, meaning that early life circumstances and both biological programming (before birth) and biological embedding (which relates to issues after birth) are heritable. Epigenetic mechanisms, which are heritable changes that are not due to alternations in the DNA, can transmit biology intergenerationally without genetic changes (Bezruchka, 2015).

Poorer people have poorer-functioning organs. This is easily demonstrated for the lungs by measuring how much individuals can blow out in one second (the medical term is FEV1). The lower someone is in the socio-economic hierarchy, the less air they can blow out. This observation is independent of the usual factors hypothesized to be responsible (Hegewald & Crapo, 2007). It's important to remember that the sociobiology described here does not imply that those lower down the hierarchy are inferior beings in the sense of Thomas Malthus. Rather, psychosocial and other mechanisms that are a *result of living in unequal societies* have profound and lasting biological effects on our health.

## NATURAL EXPERIMENTS IN POPULATION HEALTH EPIDEMIOLOGY

Just as John Snow could observe the decline in deaths from cholera after he removed the pump handle, which boosted his belief in the hypothesis that there was something in the water that caused the disease, we can be reassured by experiments that change the factors producing population health.

### Agriculture

There is ample evidence that human health was better before the advent of agriculture than after domestication of crops and animals began (Cohen, 1991). In early hunter-gatherer societies, vigilant sharing was a critical social value. They had few, if any, possessions, and

**Box 1.2:** Some Methods Used in Epidemiology

- Observational ecological studies
- Cohort studies
- Cross-sectional study
- Multi-level modelling (requiring powerful computers)

the key resource that was shared with everyone, whether they were related or not, was meat from an occasional big game kill. Given food, shelter, and safety sufficient to sustain health, everyone had the same level of resources. But with the development of agriculture, a food surplus could be produced. Some individuals proclaimed themselves lord or master and coerced others to produce food for them, build castles, and protect them. As a result, caring and sharing declined, exploitation of the weaker by the stronger became the norm, poverty appeared, diets changed, and food variety declined (Larsen, 1995, 2006). Famines began.

Living in close proximity to domestic animals also resulted in many infectious organisms jumping to new hosts to produce human disease. The nature of human relationships changed as exploitation began. Throughout recorded history until the 19th century, the health of human populations has been less than that of primitive societies.

Most of the increases in life expectancy beginning in the 19th century came from reductions in early life mortality. The more recent improvements in health affect older people and depend on forms of societal redistribution that favour poorer people, along with technological changes that have an impact on improved living standards. Much of the redistribution has been done by governments through taxation. Piketty (2014), in *Capital in the 21st Century*, presents a graph of tax revenues as a percentage of national income from 1870 to 2010 for Sweden, France, the United Kingdom, and the U.S. They were relatively stable until early last century, when Sweden rose to command the most tax revenue at almost 55% of income, and the U.S. plateaued at 30%. The Swedish government prioritizes social spending, which is considerably greater than in the U.S. They provide generous paid family leave and spend more government funds on the first year of life than in any subsequent year. In the United States, government funds go to remedial processes in later childhood that are less effective. Better health can result more from early life government policies favouring social justice directed at populations than from individual or non-governmental actions.

## Japan at the End of the Second World War

Japan became the healthiest country in the world in part because of economic policies resulting from the U.S. occupation of that country after the end of the Second World War (Bezruchka, Namekata, & Sistrom, 2008). The post-war "medicine" was administered by perhaps the world's greatest population health doctor, General Douglas MacArthur. It had three ingredients. The first was demilitarization: Japan was forbidden to have an army and had to resolve disputes peacefully, as specified in the constitution that MacArthur wrote. The second ingredient was democratization. Everyone got the vote, and labour unions obtained the right to organize and bargain collectively. A public health clause in the constitution required the government to do all it could to improve health. MacArthur legislated a maximum wage of 65,000 yen per year. The final ingredient was decentralization. The concentration of wealth and power that existed in pre-war Japan was broken up, and the most successful land-reform program in history was carried out.

With the dismantling of Japan's hierarchy, the resulting improvement in health was unequalled in any country in the world in history in a comparable period. Japan's health is better than that of many other nations with comparable income gaps. An important factor that allowed the "medicine" to work was the underlying culture of *wa*, or social harmony. Collectivist cultures with less inequality and a Confucian dynamism will have better health than more individualistic ones with greater social distance among society members that is accepted by the people (Hofstede & Hofstede, 2005).

We have already discussed Japan's good health status despite its having a high proportion of men smoking cigarettes. High prevalence of smoking is also found in many Western European nations that, nevertheless, have favourable mortality results. This is an example of the importance of context for behaviours and other health outcomes. One cohort study has compared civil service workers in the United Kingdom with those in France and examined early life circumstances affecting adult mortality outcomes. The patterning of health-related behaviours and association with the socio-economic gradient demonstrated that the steeper the gradient (as in the U.K. compared to France), the more smoking, physical inactivity, and diet impacted health, especially for those of lower socio-economic status. One recent study contrasted the impact of smoking on health in the United States with Finland. Death risks from smoking were 50% higher in U.S. women compared to those in Finland (Mehta et al., 2017). Such research challenges the concept that risk factors such as smoking are the same in different populations.

Japan represents a case study where rapidly decreasing inequality had profound good effects on population health. What happens when inequality increases rapidly?

## The Former Soviet Union

Countries of the former Soviet Union demonstrate what can happen when huge hierarchies are created overnight (Wilkinson, 2005). Russia was a very hierarchical society during the tsarist period and lagged about 25 life-expectancy years behind the U.S. in 1900. The centrally controlled, or command, economy in Russia dismantled the extreme wealth gap, and by 1960, the two countries had comparable female life expectancy. Health gains in Russia faltered in the 1970s and 1980s as its people felt deprived of the apparent wealth of the West, as depicted by outside media. Infant mortality began increasing in parts of the Soviet Union in the 1970s. This observation prompted Emmanual Todd (1976) to predict the collapse of the Soviet Union. With the dismantling of the former Soviet Union in 1991, fabulous wealth was created so that Russia now has the fourth-largest number of billionaires in the world (behind the U.S., China, and India), while 25 years ago it had none.

As the gap between rich and poor grew astronomically, health in Russia declined, something that had been unprecedented in the modern world (Parsons, 2014). Life expectancy in Russia had dropped about seven years for men and somewhat less for women. The decline then abated and reached pre-breakup levels, but the carnage has resulted in 20 million deaths that would not have occurred if health had remained at pre-dissolution levels. The gap between rich and poor in Russia today is greater than it was during the tsarist period.

---

**Box 1.3:** Health Care and the Public's Health

---

Whenever it has been studied, medical care is always one of the leading causes of death (Starfield, 2000). In studies of doctors' strikes, the common finding is that mortality does not increase. In fact, it tends to go down (Cunningham, Mitchell, Narayan, & Yusuf, 2008). The public believes that postmodernism doesn't apply to medical science. Perhaps half of what is believed to be true in medicine is not. Primary care may be the best part of medical care. Countries that have less of a specialist focus on healthcare services tend to have better health. Always ask: "Do you want health or health care?"

## Canada–U.S. Health Divergence

Canada is considerably healthier than the United States, although it is less wealthy and spends much less on medical care. Comparisons of the two nations' population health allow us to demonstrate the political situations that have created inequalities responsible for this difference. In the 1950s, life expectancies in the two nations were almost the same (Figure 1.5). Health in Canada then improved more rapidly than health in the United States. For working-age men today, for example, mortality rates in Canada are almost half of what they are in the United States.

Most American medical students are unaware of the extent to which health in the U.S. lags behind that of other wealthy countries (Agrawal et al., 2005). It is astonishing that citizens in the world's wealthiest and most powerful nation seem to accept dying much younger than they should. Remarkably, the U.S.'s inferior performance in many international comparative measures, such as teen birth rates, youth homicides, incarceration, child poverty, and poor educational performance, does not inspire their citizens' desire to do better. The United States was founded on a weak form of government, so individuals must rely on one another for support. The U.S.'s form of government was, by design, with its separation of powers and lack of a parliamentary system, not very responsive to the popular will (Kingdon, 1999).

Canada's government was more receptive to public opinion and engineered a social compact with more generous welfare provisions. Social expenditures have been higher in Canada and performance on many social indicators much better than in the U.S.

The United States undertook redistribution programs after the Great Depression to reduce the wealth of the richest 1% of Americans by 1975 to be roughly half of what it was in the Gilded Age. However, the rich and powerful have regained their wealth share through mechanisms such as limiting worker wage increases. The result has been requiring the citizenry to borrow their salaries from home equity and credit cards. The rich have also gained massive government support for their financial interests, and public welfare programs have been eroded. The result has been huge increases in inequality and the global economic collapse of 2008.

Canada, on the other hand, has continued to provide many social-welfare services as a part of government responsibility. These included low-cost education, subsidized housing, efficient public transportation systems, and universal medical care. Canada remained one of the world's healthiest nations until this century, when eroding government policies began to favour the rich. Income inequality increased in Canada in the 1990s, after which that trend levelled off and is now considerably below that of the United States. Canada stands in the middle of the collective–individual divide represented by Western Europe and the United States. Trends in the health differences between the U.S. and Canada in the coming years will depend to a large extent on how responsive governments are to the needs of their populations as they grapple with neo-liberal economic issues and their long-term global repercussions (Siddiqi, Kawachi, Keating, & Hertzman, 2013).

Racism remains a major barrier to achieving full health in Canada, the United States, and elsewhere. Indigenous populations almost always have higher mortality than settlers, and Aboriginal peoples in both Canada and the U.S. face stark health inequities. Race, which is essentially a social construct, leads to many forms of racism that have been given more critical attention in recent years. The negative effects of racism are likely programmed in early life. For example, black infant mortality rates are almost 2.5 times higher than that of whites in the United States, and black women have four times the maternal mortality of whites there. The stress of racism is likely a major contributing factor. Immigration has its own stresses that affect health. Minority Canadians, whether native-born or immigrants, have lower incomes and vastly lower wealth than whites, a trend that remains true for minorities globally. While Canada prides itself on fostering multiculturalism, systemic racism has yet to be fully addressed.

## Box 1.4: Power, Inequality, and the Physical Environment

Cross-sectional studies among U.S. states find that shared political power, less income inequality, strong environmental regulations, and better quality of the environment are associated with better health outcomes. Political power is measured by voting rates, tax fairness, Medicaid accessibility (meaning healthcare services for the more impoverished), and educational attainment (Boyce, Klemer, Templet, & Willis, 1999). Green space exposure in England has been linked to income inequality and mortality differences. Those living in greener environments have less inequality in health outcomes. Economic inequalities translate to less healthy physical environments, just as they do to disadvantaged social ones (Mitchell & Popham, 2008). Recovery in hospitals has been linked to a patient's window providing a bucolic view. This suggests that psychosocial factors team up with physical ones to produce health. Increasing economic growth above $5,000–$10,000 per capita increases the ecological footprint, indicating further strain on the environment, with no health benefits (Rainham, 2007).

The current global migrant and refugee crisis will continue to test governing systems as long as global inequality continues to increase. Populism is leading to strong-men leaders who garner popular support by trying to keep immigrants out and by suppressing dissent as well as creating conditions for an endless term in office. Rising inequality is the upstream factor as countries of birth determine economic prospects.

## CONCLUSIONS

Producing health in populations requires attention to the upstream determinants of health. To achieve population health, policies and practices that promote caring and sharing need to be operationalized and will need to transcend state boundaries. Such systems must prioritize early life.

A positive and action-oriented approach to producing health would be to publicize and act upon what is known regarding the poor health status of countries such as the U.S., which have large gaps between the rich and poor, relative to other rich countries. These gaps result from political policies that do not promote economic justice. Canadian policies that result in increases in the gap between rich and poor will move Canada toward U.S. outcomes. If Canadians want a healthier population, the government can take policy steps that further social and economic justice. The first step is to create awareness of what conditions produce health in populations, and then promote policies to ameliorate those conditions (Bezruchka, 2009).

## CRITICAL THINKING QUESTIONS

1.  What can you do personally to engage communities to help them understand population health issues concerned with histories of exploitation, current economic inequality, and adversity in early life to foster better health?
2.  A recent threat to Canada's social compact has eased, but voter turnout has declined from the levels seen in the 1960s. What can be done to maintain a well-functioning democracy that works for improving health?
3.  How can societies distinguish health and health care to foster understanding of the limited role of health care in producing health? Why is producing health so focused on changing individual behaviours?
4.  Given the importance of poverty, inequality, and racism in affected population health, how can one maintain a focus upstream while working at a downstream job?
5.  How does economic inequality affect you?

## FURTHER READINGS

Berkman, L. F., Kawachi, I., & Glymour, M. M. (Eds.). (2014). *Social epidemiology* (2nd ed.). New York: Oxford University Press.

A comprehensive look at the subject that requires some awareness of epidemiology but is well worth the effort.

Bourgeault, I. L., Labonté, R., Packer, C., & Runnels, V. (Eds.). (2017). *Population health in Canada: Issues, research, and action.* Toronto: Canadian Scholars' Press.
Diverse, hard-hitting material on key issues for Canada.

Bradbury, B., Corak, M., Waldfogel, J., & Washbrook, E. (2015). *Too many children left behind: The U.S. achievement gap in comparative perspective.* New York: Russell Sage Foundation.
An important look at early life differences among Australia, Canada, the United Kingdom, and the U.S. that considers the impact of various policies.

Burke Harris, N. (2018). *The deepest well: Healing the long-term effects of childhood adversity.* Boston: Houghton Mifflin.
A look at the health impact of adverse childhood experiences (ACEs).

Galea, S. (Ed.). (2007). *Macrosocial determinants of population health.* New York: Springer.
Diverse chapters present material on topics such as culture that are rarely discussed in population health.

Keating, D. P., & Hertzman, C. (Eds.). (1999). *Developmental health and the wealth of nations: Social, biological, and educational dynamics.* New York: Guilford Press.
A valuable perspective on the importance of early life.

Lundberg , O., Åberg, M., Yngwe, Stjärne, M. K., Björk, L., & Fritzell, J. (2008). *The Nordic experience: Welfare states and public health.* Stockholm: Centre for Health Equity Studies, Stockholm University/Karolinska Institutet.
The Scandinavian countries' road to health has not been discussed much here save for Denmark. There is a wealth of details on the Nordic approach. It can be downloaded at http://www.chess.su.se/polopoly_fs/1.54170.1321266667!/menu/standard/file/NEWS_Rapport_080819.pdf

Marmot, M. (2004). *Status syndrome: How our position on the social gradient affects longevity and health.* London: Bloomsbury.
A perspective from the pioneering social epidemiologist in England that communicates the results of many studies.

Pan-Canadian Health Inequalities Reporting Initiative. (2018). *Key health inequalities in Canada: A national portrait.* Ottawa: Public Health Agency of Canada.

This source presents a wealth of information on mortality and other health-related in-equalities in Canada that displays unfair differences in outcomes among immigrants and Indigenous people, depicting effects of residential concentration and the impact of deprivation, income, and education. Comparisons with other nations are made.

Ratcliff, K. S. (2017). *The social determinants of health: Looking upstream.* Cambridge: Polity Press.
A compelling look at the effects of the environment on health.

Schrecker, T., & Bambra, C. (2015). *How politics makes us sick: Neoliberal epidemics.* New York: Palgrave Macmillan.
Acknowledging the political determinants of health is the next big step that must be taken.

Szreter, S. (2005). *Health and wealth: Studies in history and policy.* Rochester, NY: University of Rochester Press.
A compendium of important research by a historian.

Wilkinson, R. G., & Pickett, K. E. (2009). *The spirit level: Why more equal societies almost always do better.* London: Allen Lane.
A paradigm-shifting book on how more equal societies do better for people and the planet.

Wilkinson, R. G., & Pickett, K. E. (2018). *The inner level: How more equal societies reduce stress, restore sanity and improve everybody's wellbeing.* London: Allen Lane.
A companion to *The Spirit Level*, this volume explores diverse psychosocial impacts of inequality. The authors start out stating this is not a self-help book but one to galvanize required changes in societies.

## RELEVANT WEBSITES

### Black Doll White Doll
https://www.youtube.com/watch?v=tkpUyB2xgTM
https://www.youtube.com/watch?v=QRZPw-9sJtQ
 A telling depiction of skin colour preferences in early life in both the USA (first) and Italy (second).

### Conference Board of Canada—How Canada Performs
https://www.conferenceboard.ca/hcp/
 Comparisons of health and inequality outcomes for Canada with nations and among Canadian provinces.

**Equality Trust**

https://www.equalitytrust.org.uk

Primarily focused on inequality in the United Kingdom, but very relevant for other parts of the world.

**Gapminder**

https://www.gapminder.org

A treasure trove of data, charts, and animations on inequalities around the world.

**Innocenti Research Group publications**

http://www.unicef-irc.org/

This branch of UNICEF presents a host of research compilations that includes report card comparisons of child indicators among rich nations. Search their publications and Publications Series for the Innocenti Report Card.

**Institute for Health Metrics and Evaluation**

http://www.healthdata.org/results/data-visualizations

A continually evolving treasure trove of data depicting trends and outcomes for various health and healthcare measures. With the mortality visualization, one can make comparisons of child and adult mortality for various countries and among regions within some countries.

**UCLA: John Snow**

http://www.ph.ucla.edu/epi/snow.html

A look at the profound influence this man has had on the subject of epidemiology.

**Population Health Forum**

http://depts.washington.edu/eqhlth/

The Population Health Forum's mission is to raise awareness and initiate dialogue about the ways in which political, economic, and social inequalities interact to affect the overall health status of our society. Ranking of countries in the health Olympics are depicted, as well as links to various studies, readings, and broadcasts.

**Primary Care Interventions in Poverty**

https://ocfp.on.ca/cpd/povertytool

An Ontario family medicine site that looks at what physicians can do about poverty.

**Public Health Agency of Canada**

https://www.canada.ca/en/public-health/services/health-promotion/population-health/what-determines-health/what-makes-canadians-healthy-unhealthy.html

Much useful material on determinants of health that stands in stark contrast to U.S. government information.

**Public Health Sudbury and Districts**

https://www.phsd.ca/health-topics-programs/health-equity/health-equity-resources

An example of a public health jurisdiction communicating the difference between health and health care.

**Raising of America**

http://www.raisingofamerica.org/

A documentary series looking at early life issues concerning the United States but with relevant, actionable material for the rest of the world.

**The Last Straw Board Game on the Social Determinants of Health**

http://www.thelaststraw.ca/

Designed by a McMaster University medical student and a University of Toronto graduate student, this board game provides an entertaining way to consider concepts in this chapter. Available in English, French, and Spanish.

## GLOSSARY

**Controlling for a factor:** Statistically adjusting in the analysis for a variable (factor) so that this factor has no impact on the outcome one is studying.

**Infant mortality rate:** The proportion of infants born that die in their first year of life, usually expressed per 1,000.

**Life expectancy:** The average number of years lived by a population if the age-specific mortality rates in place when the calculation was done continued until everyone had died.

**Population health:** A term that distinguishes what makes populations healthy as opposed to public health, which tends to mean a select group of interventions, such as immunizations, disease screening, prenatal care, and health education for behaviour change.

**Social determinants of health:** Variously defined as the conditions under which people are born, grow, live, work, and age. Determinants of health would add effects of health care.

## REFERENCES

Agrawal, J. R., Huebner, J., Hedgecock, J., Sehgal, A. R., Jung, P., & Simon, S. R. (2005). Medical students' knowledge of the U.S. health care system and their preferences for curricular change: A national survey. *Academic Medicine, 80*(5), 484–488.

Arias, E., Heron, M., & Tejada-Vera, B. (2013). United States life tables eliminating certain causes of death, 1999–2001. *National Vital Statistics Reports, 61*(9), 1–128.

Auger, N., Hamel, D., Martinez, J. R. M., & Ross, N. A. (2012). Mitigating effect of immigration on the relation between income inequality and mortality: A prospective study of 2 million Canadians. *Journal of Epidemiology and Community Health, 66*(6), e5. doi:10.1136/jech.2010.127977

Avendano, M., Glymour, M. M., Banks, J., & Mackenbach, J. P. (2009). Health disadvantage in U.S. adults aged 50 to 74 years: A comparison of the health of rich and poor Americans with that of Europeans. *American Journal of Public Health, 99*(3), 540–548. doi:10.2105/AJPH.2008.139469

Bakah, M., & Raphael, D. (2017). New hypotheses regarding the Danish health puzzle. *Scandinavian Journal of Public Health, 45*(8), 799–808. doi:10.1177/1403494817698889

Barker, D. J. P. (1998). *Mothers, babies, and health in later life* (2nd ed.). Edinburgh: Churchill Livingstone.

Barker, D. J. P. (2012). Developmental origins of chronic disease. *Public Health, 126*(3), 185–189. doi:10.1016/j.puhe.2011.11.014

Berkman, L. F., Kawachi, I., & Glymour, M. M. (Eds.). (2014). *Social epidemiology* (2nd ed.). New York: Oxford University Press.

Bezruchka, S. (2009). Promoting public understanding of population health. In S. J. Babones (Ed.), *Social inequality and public health* (pp. 201–214). Bristol, U.K.: Policy Press.

Bezruchka, S. (2015). Early life or early death: Support for child health lasts a lifetime. *International Journal of Child, Youth and Family Studies, 6*(2), 204–229.

Bezruchka, S., Namekata, T., & Sistrom, M. G. (2008). Interplay of politics and law to promote health: Improving economic equality and health: The case of postwar Japan. *American Journal of Public Health, 98*(4), 589–594. doi:10.2105/AJPH.2007.116012

Bjerregaard, P., & Hermann, N. (1994). *Lifetime in Denmark: Second report from the Life Expectancy Committee of the Ministry of Health, Denmark.* Copenhagen: Ministry of Health, The Life Expectancy Committee.

Boyce, J. K., Klemer, A. R., Templet, P. H., & Willis, C. E. (1999). Power distribution, the environment, and public health: A state-level analysis. *Ecological Economics, 29*(1), 127–140. doi:10.1016/S0921-8009(98)00056-1

Bradley, E. H., Elkins, B. R., Herrin, J., & Elbel, B. (2011). Health and social services expenditures: Associations with health outcomes. *British Medical Journal Quality & Safety, 20*(10), 826–831. doi:10.1136/bmjqs.2010.048363

Cohen, M. N. (1991). *Health and the rise of civilization.* New Haven, CT: Yale University Press.

Cunningham, S., Mitchell, K., Narayan, K. M., & Yusuf, S. (2008). Doctors' strikes and mortality: A review. *Social Science & Medicine, 67*(11): 1784–1788.

Detollenaere, J., Desmarest, A.-S., Boeckxstaens, P., & Willems, S. (2018). The link between income inequality and health in Europe, adding strength dimensions of primary care to the equation. *Social Science & Medicine, 201*, 103–110. doi:10.1016/j.socscimed.2018.01.041

Eckenrode, J., Smith, E. G., McCarthy, M. E., Dineen, M. (2014). Income inequality and child maltreatment in the United States. *Pediatrics, 133*(3), 454–461. doi:10.1542/peds.2013-1707

Evans, R. G., Barer, M. L., & Marmor, T. R. (Eds.). (1994). *Why are some people healthy and others not? The determinants of health of populations.* New York, NY: Aldine de Gruyter.

Farr, W. (2000). Vital statistics: Memorial volume of selections from the reports and writings. 1885. *Bulletin of the World Health Organization, 78*(1), 88–95.

Foege, W. H. (2018). *The fears of the rich, the needs of the poor: My years at the CDC.* Baltimore, MD: Johns Hopkins University Press.

Frakt, A. (2018). Medical mystery: Something happened to U.S. health spending after 1980. *New York Times.* Retrieved from https://mobile.nytimes.com/2018/05/14/upshot/medical-mystery-health-spending-1980.html

Geronimus, A. T., Hicken, M., Keene, D., & Bound, J. (2006). "Weathering" and age patterns of allostatic load scores among blacks and whites in the United States. *American Journal of Public Health, 96*(5), 8268–833.

Gordis, L. (1996). *Epidemiology.* Philadelphia, PA: Saunders.

Halfon, N., Larson, K., Son, J., Lu, M., & Bethell, C. (2017). Income inequality and the differential effect of adverse childhood experiences in US children. *Academic Pediatrics, 17*(7, Supplement), S70–S78. doi:10.1016/j.acap.2016.11.007

Hegewald, M. J., & Crapo, R. O. (2007). Socioeconomic status and lung function. *Chest, 132*(5), 1608–1614. doi:10.1378/chest.07-1405

Hofstede, G. H., & Hofstede, G. J. (2005). *Cultures and organizations: Software of the mind* (rev. 2nd ed.). New York: McGraw-Hill.

Illich, I. (1976). *Medical nemesis.* New York: Pantheon Books.

Kingdon, J. W. (1999). *America the unusual.* Belmont, CA: Wadsworth Publishing.

Kristenson, M., Orth-Gomér, K., Kucineskinë, Z., Bergdohl, B., Calkauskas, H., Balinkyniene, I., & Olsson, A. G. (1998). Attenuated cortisol response to a standardized stress test in Lithuanian versus Swedish men: The LiVicordia Study. *International Journal of Behavioral Medicine, 5*(1), 17–30. doi:10.1207/s15327558ijbm0501_2

Larsen, C. S. (1995). Biological changes in human populations with agriculture. *Annual Review of Anthropology 24*, 185–213. doi:10.1146/annurev.an.24.100195.001153

Larsen, C. S. (2006). The agricultural revolution as environmental catastrophe: Implications for health and lifestyle in the Holocene. *Quaternary International, 150*(1), 12–20. doi:10.1016/j.quaint.2006.01.004

Makary, M. A., & Daniel, M. (2016). Medical error—The third leading cause of death in the US. *British Medical Journal, 353*(i2139). doi:10.1136/bmj.i2139

Mehta, N., Elo, I., Stenholm, S., Aromaa, A., Heliövaara, M., & Koskinen, S. (2017). International differences in the risk of death from smoking and obesity: The case of the United States and Finland. *SSM - Population Health, 3*, 141–152. doi:10.1016/j.ssmph.2016.12.001

Mitchell, R., & Popham, F. (2008). Effect of exposure to natural environment on health inequalities: An observational population study. *The Lancet, 372*(9650), 1655–1660. doi:10.1016/S0140-6736(08)61689-X

Organisation for Economic Co-operation and Development. (2015). Income distribution and poverty. Dataset. Retrieved from http://stats.oecd.org/Index.aspx?DatasetCode=IDD

Parsons, M. A. (2014). *Dying unneeded : The cultural context of the Russian mortality crisis.* Nashville: Vanderbilt University Press.

Pickett, K. E., & Wilkinson, R. G. (2015). Income inequality and health: A causal review. *Social Science & Medicine, 128*, 316–326.

Piketty, T. (2014). *Capital in the twenty-first century.* Cambridge, MA: Belknap Press.

Pizzigati, S. (2018). *The case for a maximum wage.* Cambridge: Polity Press.

Pobutsky, A., Bradbury, E., & Tomiyasu, D. W. (2011). *Chronic disease disparities report 2011: Social determinants.* Honolulu: Hawai'i State Department of Health, Chronic Disease Management and Control Branch.

Rainham, D. (2007). Do differences in health make a difference? A review for health policymakers. *Health Policy 84*(2–3): 123–132.

Roos, N. P., Brownell, M., & Menec, V. (2006). Universal medical care and health inequalities: Right objectives, insufficient tools. In J. Heymann, C. Hertzman, M. L. Barer, & R. G. Evans (Eds.), *Healthier societies: From analysis to action* (pp. 107–131). New York: Oxford University Press.

Rose, G. A. (1992). *The strategy of preventive medicine.* New York: Oxford University Press.

Ross, N. A., Wolfson, M. C., Dunn, J. R., Berthlot, J. M., Kaplan, G. A., & Lynch, J. W. (2000). Relation between income inequality and mortality in Canada and in the United States: Cross-sectional assessment using census data and vital statistics. *British Medical Journal, 320*(7239), 898–902.

Sanmartin, C., Ross, N. A., Tremblay, S., Wolfson, M., Dunn, J. R., & Lynch, J. (2003). Labour market income inequality and mortality in North American metropolitan areas. *Journal of Epidemiology and Community Health, 57*(10), 792–797. doi:10.1136/jech.57.10.792

Sapolsky, R. M. (2004). *Why zebras don't get ulcers: The acclaimed guide to stress, stress-related diseases, and coping* (3rd ed.). New York: Henry Holt.

Schwartz, S., Susser, E., & Susser, M. (1999). A future for epidemiology. *Annual Review of Public Health, 20*(1), 15–33.

Siddiqi, A., Kawachi, I., Keating, D., & Hertzman, C. (2013). A comparative study of population health in the United States and Canada during the neoliberal era, 1980–2008. *International Journal of Health Services, 43*(2), 193–216. doi:10.2190/HS.43.2.b

Sinclair, U. (1935). *I, candidate for governor: And how I got licked.* New York: Farrar & Rinehart, Inc.

Starfield, B. (2000). Is U.S. health really the best in the world? *JAMA 284*(4): 483–485.

Todd, E. (1976). *La chute finale: Essais sur la décomposition de la sphère Soviétique.* Paris: R. Laffont.

United Nations Development Program (2016). *Human Development Report 2016: Human Development for Everyone.* New York: Author.

Vallgårda, S. (2001). Governing people's lives: Strategies for improving the health of the nations in England, Denmark, Norway and Sweden. *European Journal of Public Health, 11*(4), 386–392. doi:10.1093/eurpub/11.4.386

Vallgårda S. (2011). Addressing individual behaviours and living conditions: Four Nordic public health policies. *Scandinavian Journal of Public Health, 39*(6 suppl), 6–10. doi:10.1177/1403494810378922

Wilkinson, R. G. (2005). *The impact of inequality: How to make sick societies healthier.* New York: New Press.

Wilkinson, R. G., & Pickett, K. E. (2009). *The spirit level: Why more equal societies almost always do better.* London: Allen Lane.

World Health Organization. (2015). Prevalence of tobacco smoking. Geneva: World Health Organization. Retrieved from https://www.who.int/gho/tobacco/use/en/

# CHAPTER 2

## Sociological Perspectives on Health and Health Care

*Ivy Lynn Bourgeault*

## INTRODUCTION

Sociology is the systematic study of human society, including its social structures and institutions, as well as social relations and experiences. Ideally, it also involves studying the interactions among these various elements. Sociology offers a variety of means to understand the incidence and experience of illness and health within societies, as well as the social organization of the delivery of health care and differential access to healthcare resources. The specific application of sociology to the field of health, illness, and health care has been termed "medical sociology," although some prefer "sociology of health."

Medical sociology has its roots in public health and social medicine initiatives during the 19th century, but it grew into a separate field in the late 1940s and early 1950s, drawing mainly from currents within its parent discipline of sociology (Bloom, 2002). A key distinction made within this field—between *sociology in medicine* and the *sociology of medicine*—stems from these early roots. First explicitly articulated by Robert Straus (1957), sociological studies *in* medicine are oriented toward applying sociological theory or concepts toward a better understanding of health-related problems or creation of more informed public health policy. Sociological studies *of* medicine are oriented toward a better understanding of society or sociological concepts through the lens of health problems, medical settings, or the organization of health care. Some have argued that there is a trend from sociology *in* to the sociology *of* medicine and even more broadly to the sociology of health, fostered by the increasing institutionalization of sociology within universities (Coburn & Eakin, 1998; Cockerham & Ritchey, 1997). This reflects a movement away from a medically defined approach to one that is more theoretically oriented, deriving its inspiration— much like the rest of sociology—from the founding traditions of Durkheim, Weber, and Marx and, more recently, from feminist, anti-racist, and postmodernist scholars. While the distinction between sociology *in* and *of* is important to make, it is difficult to tease apart these orientations in practice because many medical sociologists are engaged both in advancing sociology through insights garnered from health and health care and in using their knowledge to create practical change.

In this chapter, I trace the historical evolution of sociological perspectives as applied to health from the grand theories of functionalism, conflict theory, and materialism to symbolic interactionist and social constructionist approaches that focus more specifically on the meaning and experience of health and illness in society. More recent developments in the sociology of health that build upon or react to these founding traditions—namely, feminism, anti-racism, and postmodernism—are also presented. Across all perspectives, I note in particular how each treats the role and experience of patients, or those who seek care, and the providers of that care. Providing an overview of this nature requires a fair degree of simplification of many intricate ideas in each of these literatures. At the end of this chapter, I thus suggest some key works from which the reader could gather more detailed accounts and expanded discussions.

# EVOLUTION OF SOCIOLOGICAL PERSPECTIVES ON HEALTH AND HEALTH CARE

## Structural Functionalism

Structural functionalism, or simply functionalism, is a theoretical orientation derived in large part from the work of Émile Durkheim (1858–1917). The Durkheimian tradition highlights the importance of studying social systems. It focuses on the interrelationships between individuals and groups within society and the way in which it is structured to function in order to maintain the society as a whole (Lachmann, 1991). This perspective is associated most closely with the work of A.R. Radcliffe-Brown, a British social anthropologist, who argued in the 1920s that the elements of society—that is, its social structure—have indispensable functions for one another such that the continued existence of the one element is dependent on that of the others and on society as whole.[1] The focus of inquiries in this field tends toward individual and group *roles* within society and how these are linked to the consensus-based functioning of society.

The application of structural functionalism to the field of medical sociology began with the introduction of *The Social System* (1951) by Talcott Parsons (1902–1979), who devoted considerable space in this text to the function of modern medical practice within society and the complementary roles of physicians and patients. His conceptualization of the *sick role* in particular became one of the most cited sociological concepts in the field (Matcha, 2000). Parsons (1951) described illness as a state of disturbance in the "normal" functioning of the total human individual, including both the state of the organism as a biological system and of the individual's personal and social adjustments (p. 431). Because of this dual impact—biological and social—the role of a sick person in society is defined as deviant both biologically and socially. Because of this deviant aspect, a new social role—the sick role—had to be defined. Being sick, therefore, constituted a social role with "institutionalised expectations and the corresponding sentiments and sanctions" (p. 436) in order for equilibrium, wellness, and a functioning society to be maintained. The four elements constituting this sick role include two rights or exemptions and two obligations (see Box 2.1).

To complement this sick role, the provider's role is to legitimate the condition, to treat the condition, and to make the person well again. In order to do so, physicians are granted privileged and extensive access to patients' bodies and their private lives. Keeping these powers in check are physicians' allegiance to a code of ethics and an altruistic orientation. Neither of these negates the controlling nature of medical practice, but from this perspective it is seen as functional and hence unproblematic.

Being more theoretical than empirical, Parsons's conceptualizations came under significant criticism for how they mask the variability in the temporary or legitimate nature of different illnesses, and the diversity in the actual behaviour of sick individuals and of their providers. Twaddle (1969), for example, claimed that there are multiple configurations of the sick role, of which Parsons's is but one. Mechanic and Volkart (1960) also noted how Parsons's description was most relevant to acute illnesses, and not the increasingly prevalent chronic illnesses and disabilities that would entail a permanent role status. With respect to the provider's role, Szasz and Hollender (1956) refined Parsons's work by elaborating different doctor–patient models arising from different types of illness. The first model—most akin to Parsons's sick role—matched patient passivity and physician assertiveness as the most common reaction to acute illness. The second was characterized by physician guidance and patient co-operation where a less acute illness was involved. The third model was characterized by physicians providing advice on a treatment plan that patients had most of the responsibility to implement; this latter case was most relevant for chronic illnesses and certain forms of disability.[2]

For the most part, these early criticisms were still based on the structural functional assumptions of a consensus-based society made up of interconnected social roles. What was called for were more possibilities of the various roles there could be. Broader criticisms, however, were levelled at the basic premises of this perspective—specifically, how society was not necessarily consensus-based and that the wielding of power was not

---

**Box 2.1:** The Sick Role

- The exemption from normal social role responsibilities
- The exemption from responsibility for their illness
- The state of being ill is itself undesirable and the person has the obligation to want to "get well" and return to a normal social role
- The sick person also has the obligation to seek technically competent help and comply with treatment regimens

*Source:* Adapted from Parsons, T. (1951). *The social system.* New York: The Free Press.

always functional but rather associated with several negative consequences. There is a clear middle-class bias in the assumptions in terms of access to professional services and the assumed unbiased nature of the provision of said services. This more critical focus is exemplified in two key strands of sociological theory—*interactionism* and *materialism.*

## Symbolic Interactionism and Social Constructionism[3]

The school of symbolic interactionist thought is derived from the thinking of Max Weber (1864–1920), where the focus is less on social institutions than on interactions between individuals and the meanings these create. The term was first coined by Herbert Blumer in 1937, drawing upon the work of George Herbert Mead (1863–1931), with whom he studied at the University of Chicago, and Charles Cooley (1864–1929). As he later described in a 1969 text, it involves the following key principles: (1) "human beings act towards things on the basis of the meanings that things have for them"; (2) these meanings "arise out of social interaction"; and (3) social action results from a "fitting together of individual lines of action" (Jary & Jary, 1991, p. 509). Stemming from these key principles, interactionists focus less on objective, macro-structural aspects of social systems than they do on the subjective aspects of social life and people as "pragmatic actors."[4]

One of the key symbolic interactionist theorists who contributed to the field of medical sociology is Canadian-born sociologist Erving Goffman (1922–1982). Because of his interest in how individuals develop their identity through the way in which others view them, he undertook an in-depth observational study of patients' subjective experience in mental institutions. In his book *Asylums*, he described how mental hospitals are "total institutions" in that they contain "a large number of like-situated individuals, cut off from the wider society for an appreciable period of time, [who] together lead an enclosed, formally administered round of life" (Goffman, 1961, p. xiii). Such institutions thereby control large parts of the lives of its inhabitants—including privacy—in a way that damages their individual self-image, replacing it with an institutionalized one. Patienthood becomes a total way of life for these people, and their behaviour is interpreted solely through the lens of their mental illness (Weitz, 1996).

In his later work *Stigma* (1963), Goffman examined what he refers to as the management of a spoiled identity. He describes three main forms of stigma: (1) abominations of the body in the form of physical deformities; (2) blemishes of character in the form of socially deviant behaviour; and (3) groups with minority status in society (Cockerham & Ritchey, 1997). A variant of symbolic interactionism, following along these studies by Goffman, is *labelling theory*, which posits that the impact of labelling a person as ill or deviant means that others will respond to them in accordance with that label, which is very difficult to shed. Labelling theory and Goffman's conceptualization of stigma led to a spate of studies on the stigmatizing features of various illnesses, from leprosy to epilepsy (Conrad & Schneider, 1980), as well as how stigma can change over time and vary significantly across cultures.

Other examinations from interactionist scholars on the subjective experience of people with illness include Everett Hughes (1971), who proposed the concept of *illness career*. Anselm Strauss and others (1984) similarly conceptualized the illness experience in terms of the work that needed to be accomplished both with respect to one's illness and everyday life:

> the various key problems facing the sick persons and their families involve them not only in a variety of different kinds of *work*—crisis work, symptom control work, regimen work—but in a host of other tasks that can for convenience be called comfort work, clinical safety work, the work of preparing for dying, the work of keeping marital relationships, and such. (Strauss et al., 1984, p. 18)

Other key themes from this literature are the importance of family relations, information awareness and sharing, how illness represents a *biographical disruption* (Bury, 1982) and involves the *reconstitution of the self* (Charmaz, 1987), and the management of regimens and uncertainty (Conrad, 1987).

Just as interactionists have delved into the subjective experience of people suffering from a variety of ailments, they have also examined the experience of healthcare providers. This began most notably with Becker and colleagues' (1961) treatment of medical socialization in *Boys in White*. In contrast to earlier functionalist perspectives on medical education—best exemplified by Robert Merton and his colleagues (1957) in *The Student Physician*, where medical training is oriented toward the mastery of skills and knowledge necessary for practice—Becker argued that medical socialization involves a process of "getting through." Any initial idealism that medical students have toward the practice of medicine quickly shifts to cynicism about their ability to cope with the vast knowledge they are expected to master. Canadian sociologists Jack Haas and William Shaffir (1977) referred to how medical students come to take on a *cloak of competence* as a form of impression management to convince others and themselves that they are sufficiently competent and confident to face the immense responsibilities of their privileged role.

A related school of thought that emerged out of symbolic interactionism is that of social constructionism. First described by Berger and Luckmann (1967) in the *The Social Construction of Reality*, they argued that "everyday knowledge is creatively produced by individuals and is oriented toward particular practical problems" (p. ii). Thus, social constructionists begin by taking as problematic the very issues that appear to be self-evident. "Facts," they argue, are created by way of social interactions and people's interpretations of these interactions. One of the most popular areas of focus within the social constructionist perspective addressed the social construction of illness, which paralleled a surge in criticisms against biomedicine in the 1970s. The specialty of psychiatry in particular came under intense scrutiny. According to this argument, disease entities do not exist in any objective sense, but are political accomplishments. That is, "disease" is a label that has been successfully applied to particular bodily processes. Thus, all medical "facts" are argued to be socially created products.

Further, medical knowledge is depicted as mediating social relations such that disease categories reinforce existing social structures. Irving Zola (1972) referred to this latter phenomenon as "medicine as an institution of social control." The means by which medicine has come to exert such control is by "'medicalizing' much of daily living and by making medicine and the labels 'healthy' and 'ill' relevant to an ever increasing part of human existence" (Zola, 1972, p. 487).[5] *Medicalization*, accordingly, is defined as the process by which a cluster of symptoms/life events/deviant behaviour comes to be medically defined as a disease (see Box 2.2). Once so defined, responsibility and control lie within the domain of medicine. Conrad and Schneider (1980) describe three levels by which this occurs: (1) at the conceptual level, where a medical vocabulary is used to define a problem; (2) at the institutional level, where medical personnel supervise treatment organizations or otherwise act as gatekeepers to state benefits; and (3) at the interactional level, where physicians actually treat patients' difficulties as medical problems.

Concepts emerging from the symbolic interactionist and social constructionist schools of thought have been very powerful both analytically and in terms of their impact on medical sociology. Many sociology scholars continue to study the illness experience and medicalization process (see discussion in section on feminism below). Conrad and Leiter (2004), for example, still find it a powerful tool to analyze such recent phenomena as erectile dysfunction and the "wonder drug" sildenafil. But as productive as these perspectives have been, they have come under criticism for their tendency to focus on the micro-level of analysis and inadequately acknowledge the importance of the macro context (perhaps more applicable for the social interactionists than the constructionists)

---

**Box 2.2:** The Process of Medicalization of Deviance

1. *behaviour is first defined as deviant* before the emergence of a medical definition
2. *prospecting*: the "discovery" of a medical conception of the disease/deviant behaviour is first announced in a medical journal
3. *claims-making*: both medical and non-medical interests engage in "claims-making" activities to promote the new medical designation
4. *legitimacy*: securing medical turf, which usually involves some type of appeal to the state for recognition of the medical designation
5. *institutionalization* of medical designation in an official medical and/or legal classification system and in the establishment of treatment organizations

*Source:* Adapted from Conrad, P., & Schneider, J. W. (1992). *Deviance and medicalization: From badness to sickness.* Philadelphia: Temple University Press.

and also for their more reflexive stance and elusive treatment of power. Because of these limitations, these theories are considered by some to be more descriptive than explanatory.

## Materialism

Sometimes referred to collectively as "conflict theory,"[6] a materialist perspective gives primacy to a macro- or structural level of analysis similar to the structural functionalists, but argues that society is based not on consensus but conflict. Social inequality is the primary focus of materialist scholars, who derive much of their inspiration from the works of Karl Marx (1818–1883). Marx argued that society is structured into two key social strata: those who own the *means of production* (land, labour, and capital)—*the capitalist class*—and those who do not—*the proletariat*. The capitalist class derives profit (or capital accumulation) from exploiting the labour power of the proletariat—that is, workers are paid less than the value of the product they produce. The pursuit of profit keeps wages low and increases the productivity of workers. Both have clear implications for health.

Vicente Navarro (1976, 1986) is one of the main contemporary theorists who have directly applied Marxist concepts to the study of health and health care. In his focus on the labour process under capitalism, he argued that there is a contradiction between the pursuit of profit and ensuring the safety of workers. That is, the capitalist mode of production actually produces disease (see Figure 2.1), what some have referred to as the *social production of disease* hypothesis. This could be directly in terms of physical, chemical, or biological pathogens at the workplace or in terms of the stress or risks of accidents as a result of the increasing intensification and fragmentation of work and alienation from the work process. He argued, for example, that "morbidity and mortality are higher among individuals doing routine types of work requiring low levels of skills than among individuals working in jobs that demand a large number of skills and which allow for some type of control over one's own work" (Navarro, 1986, p. 123).

The insights garnered from Navarro's expansion of Marxist concepts have been applied equally to the industrial labour force, as well as to certain segments of the health labour force. Barbara Ellen Smith (1987), for example, examined the social production of black lung disease, which miners contract in the workplace. She described:

> The instability of the industry frequently resulted in irregular work and a lowering of the piece rate, both of which forced miners to work faster and/or longer hours in an attempt to maintain their standard of living. The impact on health and safety conditions was almost invariably negative, as miners necessarily reduced non-productive, safety-oriented tasks, such as roof timbering, to a minimum. Working longer hours in mines where "towards quitting time [the air] becomes so foul that the miners' lamps will no longer burn" no doubt increased the respiratory disease risk. Moreover, a financially mandated speedup encouraged miners to re-enter their work areas as soon as possible after blasting the coal loose from the face, an operation that generated clouds of dust and powder smoke. (Smith, 1987, p. 345)

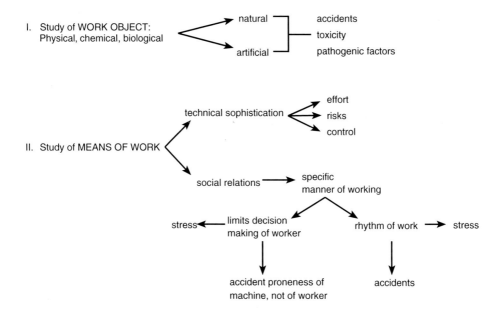

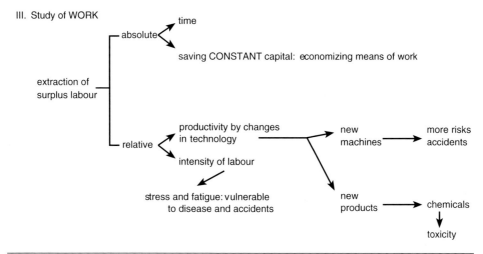

**Figure 2.1:** Navarro's Depiction of the Health Effects of the Labour Process in Capitalism

*Source:* Navarro, V. (1986). *Crisis, health, and medicine: A social critique* (p. 116). New York: Tavistock.

Canadian sociologists Novek, Yassi, and Spiegel (1990) made a similar argument in their examination of how the intensification of work in a Canadian meat-packing plant—a direct consequence of the increasing competitiveness in the market—resulted in a dramatic increase in the number and severity of accidents among workers. Workers within the healthcare system are not immune to these effects. Indeed, the work of Canadian sociologists Pat Armstrong and Hugh Armstrong (2010) and their colleagues is particularly instructive in this regard. They argued, for example, that the application of management strategies—derived in large part from the private for-profit sector—to the healthcare system in an effort to control escalating costs resulted in such work intensification that nurses referred to it as a "90-second minute" (Armstrong & Armstrong, 2010, p. 117).[7]

In addition to the negative health impacts of capitalist society on the labour process, the driving down of wages and general economic inequality have also been shown to influence health. Although not explicitly employing a Marxist perspective, many studies of social class differences in health status employ a materialist perspective in the spirit of Marx's arguments. One of the most famous is the 1982 *Black Report* on inequalities in health (Townsend, Davidson, & Whitehead, 1992), which addressed the persistence of class differences in health in Britain despite the supposed "equal access to health services" following the introduction of the National Health Service. In a summary of the report, Blane (1985) identified four possible explanations for the differences found (see Box 2.3).

Although the labour process of healthcare providers is influenced by the logic of capitalism as in any other form of work, materialist scholars note the unique situation that the medical profession holds. For example, although Navarro might agree that the profession

---

**Box 2.3:** Explanation of Social Class Differences in Health Status

---

1. *Measurement Artifact*:
   - The relationship between social class and health are inherent in the measures (particularly in the measurement of social class).
   - In actuality, this problem may result in an understating of class differences in health rather than an overstatement.
2. *Social Selection*:
   - Also known as the "drift hypothesis," this argues that health affects social mobility and therefore social class, so that those less healthy are less likely to achieve higher levels of social class.
   - Yes, this occurs, but it explains only a minor amount of the differences found and mainly for some diseases in childhood and later life (e.g., schizophrenia).
3. *Cultural/Behavioural*:
   - Gradients in health status are the result of social class differences in behaviours.
   - Yes, but behaviour cannot be separated from its context; moreover, behaviours are either intervening variables or indicators of structural influences on health.
4. *Materialist*:
   - Class differences in health are the result of social structural differences between the classes (poverty, poor housing, low educational attainment, and the level of business activity) and the competitive character of capitalism.

---

*Source:* Adapted from Blane, D. (1985). An assessment of the Black Report's explanation of health inequalities. *Sociology of Health and Illness, 7*(3), 423–445.

of medicine acts as an institution of social control, he argued that it is not the ultimate source of control. His argument in *Medicine Under Capitalism* was that "the system of medicine is determined primarily—although not exclusively—by the same forces that determine the overall social formation" (Navarro, 1976, p. vii), that being capitalism. Thus, the power of the medical profession is derivative of the dialectical relationship between capital and medicine specifically in terms of the *congruence* between the ideology of Western biomedicine and the logic of capitalism. The medical ideology of seeing illness in individualistic terms rather than in terms of social and environmental causes is consistent with the ideology of individualism in capitalist society.

The congruence of an individualizing focus on illness arose as a salient issue in Smith's (1987) examination of black lung disease. For example, she described how it was initially ignored by the medical profession as an "*ordinary* condition that need not cause worry" or in some extreme cases as a form of "malingering" or "compensationitis" (Smith, 1987, p. 345). When the cause of black lung came to be identified as respirable coal mine dust, the profession responded with the designation "coal workers' pneumoconiosis," but only for the most severe cases. She argued that:

> Medical science's understanding of black lung has not derived from observation unencumbered by a social and economic context, but has been profoundly shaped by that context; as a result, it has performed crucial political and ideological functions. In one era, it served to "normalize" and thereby mask the existence of disease altogether; in the more recent period, it has tended to minimize and individualize the problem. (Smith, 1987, p. 357)

Overall, studies that apply a materialist perspective have led to new and critical areas of medical sociology inquiry. But some consider Marxism to be a simplistic depiction of society (and it is important to stress that the description herein is a very simplified version of Marxist theory), and others criticize its usefulness in light of the fall of communism (cf. Turner, 1995) and the rise of global capital. Also, because of the macro nature of many of these arguments, they are difficult to test empirically, and some argue that data in this case are at best more suggestive than definitive. Many contemporary scholars, however, believe that the basic tenets of his arguments are reaffirmed in the highly stratified class structures in advanced global capitalism and in the relations between high- and low-income nations (cf. Jasso-Aguilar, Waitzkin, & Landwehr, 2004; Waitzkin, 1983). Other theoretical perspectives have grown out of or in response to, or otherwise borrowed from, the materialist perspective to examine other social cleavages in society, particularly feminism and anti-racism.

## Feminism

Whereas materialism is concerned with social inequity arising from the system of capitalism, feminism is concerned with gender inequalities arising from the system of *patriarchy*.

Although "patriarchy" has been used *descriptively* to denote the male-dominated nature of past and present societies, or a system of male privilege, it is also used *analytically* to denote an autonomous system of relations between men and women, comparable to an economic system of production such as capitalism (Fox, 1988). Thus, feminists argue that society is inherently gendered such that men and women have fundamentally different experiences and access to power, and that these differences are not natural but socially constructed. By extension, feminists have sought to understand society from the standpoint of women in light of its explicit absence from previous social discourse.

Feminists criticize the key theoretical perspectives outlined above—structural functionalism, symbolic interactionism, and conflict theory—for failing to adequately represent or otherwise take into consideration women's perspectives. A universal male perspective was often assumed by sociologists and social scientists, who were almost exclusively male. At the same time as criticizing these theoretical perspectives, feminists also draw upon and expand upon them with specific reference to the situation and experience of women. For example, some feminist sociologists draw heavily on symbolic interactionism, focusing on women's lived experience. Other feminist theories draw on elements of conflict theory—perhaps best exemplified by radical feminism's assumption that men and women are poised in adversarial positions, that men have power over women, and that society and its various social relationships can be best understood in terms of that situation (Eisenstein, 1983).[8] Thus, feminist studies look both at the micro- and macro-levels of analysis. Canadian feminist sociologist Dorothy Smith's (1993) *institutional ethnography* approach in particular offers us a way to examine the link between the lived experience and what she refers to as the relations of ruling not afforded in theoretical perspectives previously discussed.

Feminism has been a particularly influential perspective in medical sociology as more and more women enter the discipline. This is perhaps most evident in the spate of studies examining the medicalization of women's bodies and women's lives. This began with criticisms of the medicalization of pregnancy and childbirth, which helped foster an entire social movement toward normalizing birth and in some cases radicalizing it through the home birth movement (Ehrenreich & English, 1973; Oakley, 1984):

> we treat childbirth not as a natural event of great significance, but as an illness. We place the expectant mother in a hospital, otherwise assigned to the care of the ill, induce weakness and dependency in her by the use of drugs, straps and soon isolate her from her husband and other children just as we isolate the sick and the dying. … This classification of childbirth with illness has a great variety of repercussions all through our culture, some of which we are now attempting to correct. (F. D. MacGregor, as cited in McKinlay, 1972, p. 565)

With similar fervour, Frances McCrea (1983) teased apart the sexual politics involved in the medicalization of menopause. She described how menopause was "discovered" as a disease of deficiency in the late 1960s following the development of a synthetic form of estrogen. Estrogen-replacement therapy promised women that they could avoid the menopause completely and stay "feminine forever." McCrea describes four pervasive themes in the medical definitions of the menopause: "1) women's potential and function are biologically destined; 2) women's worth is determined by fecundity and attractiveness; 3) rejection of the feminine role will bring physical and emotional havoc; [and] 4) aging women are useless and repulsive" (1983, p. 111). Her primary argument, therefore, is that the "menopause as a disease" designation is intricately linked to women's role in society.

Another key focus of feminist medical sociological studies is regarding the predicament of female health workers. Pizurki and her colleagues (1987), for example, argued that one of the most notable features of the healthcare division of labour is its segregation by gender—both within and among professions—assigning a secondary status to women. The subordination of nursing in particular is problematized. In her historical examination of nursing work, Susan Reverby (1987) introduced the concept of the *caring dilemma*, which she described as the imposition upon nurses of a duty to care in a society that devalues the care that they provide both socially and financially. Caring is considered to be a natural extension of women's roles as wives and mothers and not an esoteric skill worthy of professional status. In *Professions and Patriarchy*, Anne Witz (1992) argued that there is nothing natural about the subordination of nurses, but rather it is directly related to the "differential access to the tactical means of achieving their aims in a patriarchal society within which male power is institutionalized" (p. 677).

Not only is the subordination of female health workers highlighted in the feminist medical sociology literature, but their exclusion is as well, most notably the decline of midwifery in North America (Biggs, 1983; Wertz & Wertz, 1979). These discussions created synergies with the literature problematizing the conceptualization of pregnancy and childbirth as an illness discussed above. For example, Ehrenreich and English (1973) argued that the medicalization of women's bodies—thereby promoting the notion of women's frailty—not only qualified them as natural patients, but also disqualified them as dependable healthcare practitioners. Many feminists specifically argued that patriarchal society's control over the reproduction process was oppressive (O'Brien, 1981), and many called for the legitimation of midwifery as a way for women to have more control over the birth process. That is, as reproductive choice and control became central concerns in the feminist movement, midwifery came to be seen as one component of reproductive choice and as a tool for the liberation of women (Rushing, 1993).

Thus, in many ways, feminist medical sociology has at least attempted to connect the social structural aspects of patriarchy to the lived experience of women as both providers and recipients of care more explicitly than other sociological perspectives applied to health, illness, and health care. In so doing, it has afforded particularly important insights to the field as a whole. But medical sociological studies from a feminist perspective have also suffered from some of the limitations of early feminist theory more broadly—namely, that it has tended to neglect the particular concerns of working-class women and women of colour. Patricia Hill Collins (1990), for example, argued that African-American women have a unique perspective to offer. More recently, feminists have begun to take up the challenge of these criticisms and have begun to analyze the ways that the effects of gender intersect with class and race for broader understandings of women's health and healthcare experiences.[9]

## Anti-racism and Post-colonialism

Another key social cleavage that causes us to look beyond the influence of class and gender is a focus on race and the process of racialization. Although many scholars who focus on the impact of race on health and health care have drawn from a conflict or materialist perspective, some have begun to develop theories addressing issues specific to the structure and experience of race, racism, and racialization. Anti-racism is one of these perspectives that attempts to uncover the particular structural determinants of racism within society (Dei, 1996).[10] Although we commonly consider racism to be an expression of individual prejudice, it is also structured into the very nature of our society. Thus, just as feminists have argued that social structures, ideology, and our everyday experiences are fundamentally gendered, anti-racism scholars argue that those experiences are also *racialized*. As Canadian race scholar Sheryl Nestel (1996/1997) summarizes:

> The term "racialized" is used … to signal that race is a historically and socially constructed category of differentiation and not in any way a "natural" one. "Racialization" then can be seen as a process through which racial significance comes to be conferred upon a wide range of human attributes. (p. 316)

The process of racializing groups results in unequal treatment (Dei, 1996).

A related perspective to the anti-racism school of thought is *post-colonialism*. The main problematic in post-colonial studies is the broader global and historical relations between societies that have been colonized and the colonizers or settlers. The link to anti-racism is due to the fact that the sizable majority of colonized societies are also societies of peoples disproportionately of colour. In fact, post-colonial scholars argue that the concept of race was particularly tied to the colonial and imperial expansion activities of Western European powers in the 17th century (Castagna & Dei, 2000), which distanced the colonizer from the colonized and in essence created Indigenous peoples as "the other." Post-colonial studies, therefore, attempt to increase knowledge about "the other," giving them voice and understanding the effects of displacement.

Anti-racism and post-colonialism perspectives are relative newcomers in the field of medical sociology in comparison to the others discussed here, so their full impact on the field has yet to be determined. Whether explicitly drawing from an anti-racism perspective—as it has come to be defined—or not, there have been an increasing number of studies of race differences in health status and inquiries focusing on the racialized experiences of both recipients and providers of care. This is clearly exemplified in studies of the health status of First Nations peoples in Canada and the decimation of their traditional health practices and systems of care following European contact (cf. Frideres, 1994; Wotherspoon, 1994). Specifically, First Nations people are consistently found to have lower life expectancy, higher infant mortality, and higher mortality rates in general, especially at early ages. Causes of death and illness patterns for First Nations peoples reflect those associated with poverty and inadequate standards of living, but systemic and structured racism is the ultimate cause of these social and economic circumstances. The recommendations of the Truth and Reconciliation Commission of Canada (2015) locate the cause of these disparities as a direct result of previous Canadian government policies of systemic cultural genocide through enforced residential school attendance.

Colonization has also had an impact on local systems of care. Specifically, some of the "exports" that Europeans brought to the "colonies" were training programs in Western medicine and nursing. This enabled the establishment of healthcare systems modelled after the settler societies. But the "Third World" debt crisis has more recently led to the decimation of these fledgling healthcare systems and massive migrations of local healthcare professionals to high-income countries. Ishi (1987), for example, outlines that some of the key factors explaining migration patterns include the demands of the service economy in high-income countries; their cultural, political, military, and economic hegemony over low-income countries; and immigrants' experience of uncertainty over their futures in their native land. He continues to describe how high-income countries benefit from hiring immigrant professional labour both economically (in terms of labour) and politically (in terms of a country's apparent attractiveness). Once in their new countries, immigrant healthcare providers, particularly those of colour, experience both implicit and explicit forms of racism in terms of barriers to access in practising their profession (Bourgeault, 2008; Nestel, 1996/1997) and status of position (cf. Calliste, 1996).

## Postmodernism

Postmodernism, which is alternately referred to by some as *post-structuralism*, is a theoretical perspective developed largely out of French philosophical thought often associated with the works of Jacques Derrida, Jean Baudrillard, and most notably Michel Foucault. Whereas materialists, some feminist theorists, and anti-racist scholars encourage us to look more critically at macro-structural conditions of society, postmodernists critique any attempt to create macro theories of society. They argue instead for the importance of subjectivism and microsociological analysis and, consistent with symbolic interactionism and social constructionism, stress cultural relativism and a plurality of viewpoints.[11] In line with this argument, these scholars stress that there is no "Truth" that can be uncovered or known—only different knowledges that can vary tremendously over time.

In a series of books—*Madness and Civilization* (1971), *The Birth of the Clinic* (1973), *Discipline and Punish* (1977), and *The History of Sexuality* (1979)—Foucault traced the historical changes in societal attitudes toward punishment, mental illness, and sexuality, stressing the disciplinary nature of knowledge and power (which he referred to as *pouvoir/ savoir* to denote that they were one and the same).[12] What is particularly applicable to medical sociology from Foucault's work is his focus on how medical knowledge and discourse have been used to control the body through various systems of surveillance in the supposed broader interests of society (Cockerham & Ritchey, 1997), what Turner (1992) coined "the government of the body." Bryan Turner states:

> [T]he works of Foucault ha[ve] radical implications for medical sociology. We can no longer regard "diseases" as natural events in the world which occur outside the language with which they are described. A disease entity is the product of medical discourses which in turn reflect the dominant mode of thinking … within society. For example, homosexuality was regarded as a sin under Christian therapy, as a behavioural disorder by early psychology and as merely sexual preference by contemporary medicine. (1995, p. 11)

Intricately connected with the increasing *governance* of the body is the focus of the medical profession. For example, in *The Birth of the Clinic*, Foucault described how medicine shifted its view of the body from patients' descriptions of their maladies toward direct clinical observations and physical examinations, or what he referred to as the "clinical gaze." Access to this kind of "scientific" knowledge of the body gave physicians considerable power to define health and illness and, by extension, measures of moral regulation and social control (Turner, 1995). Terence Johnson (1995) has also extended Foucault's notion of governmentality by describing how the medical profession has become constitutive of the state and, because of this institutionalization of expertise, is involved in the government of citizens.

A more focused analysis of the body is thus what a postmodernist perspective can bring to medical sociology—something that many authors argue has been heretofore inadequately addressed and is, in fact, considered potentially threatening (Armstrong, 1983). Turner (1995) states that "an adequate medical sociology would require a sociology of the body, since it is only by developing a notion of social embodiment that we can begin adequately to criticise the conventional divisions between mind and body, individual and society" (p. 3). Indeed, a postmodernist perspective has permeated other perspectives described here, most notably feminism. It is anticipated that through this lens, a more thorough understanding of the medicalization and regulation of women's bodies can be afforded.

In spite of the opportunities that postmodernism entails for medical sociology, others have cautioned about its limitations. For example, it is not clear how or where the space for resistance to insidious regulation and governance can occur—as indeed it has (Turner, 1995). Materialists also criticize that such a relativist position only obscures the relationship between discourse and the materialist conditions of society in the social constructionist phenomenon.[13]

# CONCLUSIONS

To conclude this brief overview of the key sociological perspectives on health, illness, and health care, it is important to stress how more recent theory has been built upon earlier theories by both expanding upon and in many cases critiquing their assumptions. Studies of the illness experience and medicalization were in part a response to Parsons's sick role concept and provided a more diverse foil to his portrayal. Materialism and conflict theory were also in direct contrast to the consensus-based assumption of functionalism, just as postmodernism later emerged as critical of materialism. This dynamic debate has been the way the discipline has moved forward.

It is also important to garner from this review that the point should not be to debate which level of analysis—macro or micro—is most important as both are, and, furthermore, both are intricately connected. That is, medical sociology is strongest when it is cognizant of the importance of all levels of analysis. As Coburn and Eakin noted in their review of Canadian medical sociology:

> Much of what sociology is all about as an intellectual enterprise concerns the tension between human actions and social structural constraints and opportunities. The discipline is thus characterized by dichotomy: human agency versus social structure; voluntarism versus determinism; "micro" versus "macro" level phenomena. Yet common to all of these positions is the view that phenomena involving human action, including that regarding health and health care, is the product of social interrelationships. (1998, p. 84)

The key approach to take is one that is critical of common and often unquestioned assumptions of how society is, and ought to be, and in doing so, focuses on the centrality of power.

## CRITICAL THINKING QUESTIONS

1. What are some events outside of medical sociology that may have influenced the particular trajectory of perspectives outlined here?
2. What is the difference between the social production and the social construction of disease? Are these two perspectives mutually exclusive?
3. How might we best reconcile micro perspectives on illness experience with macro perspectives on structural influences on health and illness?
4. What are some key questions about the social and structural nature of health, illness, and health care that remain to be uncovered in new, emerging perspectives?
5. Which approach(es) is particularly relevant for understanding health in Canada today?

## FURTHER READINGS

### Books

Bourgeault, I. L., Bouchard, L., & Benoit, C. (Eds.). (2013). Special issue of *Healthcare Policy* on Sociological Insights on Inequities in Health and Healthcare (vol. 9).
This is a special issue of *Healthcare Policy* containing some of the key articles from the 2012 Canadian Society for the Sociology of Health conference.

Bourgeault, I. L., Labonté, R., Packer, C., & Runnels, V. (Eds.). (2017). *Population health in Canada: A reader*. Toronto: Canadian Scholars Press.
This edited collection contains some of the key research undertaken by the Population Health Improvement Research Network.

Collyer, F. (Ed.). (2015). *The Palgrave handbook of social theory on health and medicine*. Basingstoke, U.K.: Palgrave Macmillan.
This is an edited collection on the key social theories as applied to health.

Scambler, G. (Ed.). (1987). *Sociological theory and medical sociology*. New York: Tavistock.
This classic links medical sociology and mainstream sociology, and stimulates other social scientists to do the same.

Wade, T., Bourgeault, I. L., &Neiterman, E. (2016). *Social dimensions of health and health care*. Toronto: Pearson.
This text covers the key debates in the sociology of health as it pertains to the Canadian context.

### Journals

*Health Sociology Review* is an international peer-reviewed journal that publishes high-quality conceptual and empirical research in the sociology of health, illness, and medicine.

*International Journal of Health Services* is a peer-reviewed journal that contains articles on health and social policy, political economy and sociology, history and philosophy, and ethics and law in the areas of health and well-being.

*Journal of Health and Social Behavior* is a medical sociology journal that publishes empirical and theoretical articles that apply sociological concepts and methods to the understanding of health and illness and the organization of medicine and health care.

*Social Science and Medicine* provides an international and interdisciplinary forum for the dissemination of social science research on health.

*Sociology of Health and Illness* is an international journal that publishes sociological articles on all aspects of health, illness, medicine, and health care.

## RELEVANT WEBSITES

### American Sociology Association, Medical Sociology Section

http://www.asanet.org/communities/sections/sites/medical-sociology

The Medical Sociology Section, one of the ASA's largest sections, brings together social and behavioural scientists from a variety of backgrounds who share an interest in the social contexts of health, illness, and health care.

### Australian Sociological Association, Sociology of Health Thematic Group

https://tasa.org.au/thematic-groups/groups/health/

The aims of the Sociology of Health Thematic Group are to support social and sociological research on health and medical issues; encourage and facilitate contact among academics and others researching in the field; encourage submission of papers to TASA conferences and HSR; provide an avenue for researchers to have draft papers informally reviewed by members; and encourage postgraduate interest in the field of the sociology of health.

### British Sociological Association, Medical Sociology Group (MedSoc)

https://www.britsoc.co.uk/groups/medical-sociology-groups

The BSA MedSoc Group promotes scholarship and communication in the field of the sociology of health and illness in the U.K. The group is one of the largest and most active study groups of the BSA.

### Canadian Society for the Sociology of Health/Société Canadienne de Sociologie de la Santé

http://www.cssh-scss.ca/

The Canadian Society for the Sociology of Health/Société Canadienne de Sociologie de la Santé is a nascent organization dedicated to the promotion of the sociological study of health, illness, and healthcare issues in Canada in both official languages.

### SocioSite

http://www.sociosite.net/topics/health.php

The SocioSite is a project based at the Faculty of Social Sciences at the University of Amsterdam. It presents high-quality resources, texts, and information that are important for the international sociological scene. It links students of sociology to many interesting, sociologically relevant locations in cyberspace.

## GLOSSARY

**Anti-racism:** An analytical perspective that attempts to uncover the structural determinants of racism within society.

**Congruence thesis:** A theory that argues the power of the medical profession is derivative from capital due in large part to the congruence between the individualistic focus of Western biomedicine and the ideology of individualism in capitalist society.

**Governance:** The way that medical knowledge and discourse have been used to control or regulate the body through various systems of surveillance.

**Medicalization:** The process by which a cluster of symptoms, life events, and deviant behaviour comes to be defined, medically, as a disease.

**Patriarchy:** Denotes an autonomous system of relations between men and women, comparable to an economic system of production.

## NOTES

1. Encyclopedia Britannica. (2019). A. R. Radcliffe-Brown. Retrieved from https://www.britannica.com/biography/A-R-Radcliffe-Brown
2. Hughes, J. (1994). The doctor-patient relationship: A review. *Organization and Information at the Bed-Side.* Doctoral dissertation, University of Michigan. Retrieved from www.changesurfer.com/Hlth/DPReview.html
3. I would like to thank Dorothy Pawluch for her insightful comments on this section.
4. McClelland, K. (2000, February 21). Symbolic interactionism. Retrieved from http://web.grinnell.edu/courses/soc/s00/soc111-01/IntroTheories/Symbolic.html
5. It is important to point out that, in some instances, groups who suffer from a particular ailment seek medical distinction; this has been argued to be the case for alcoholism.
6. This term could also be used to denote studies of power from a Weberian perspective (Cockerham & Ritchey, 1997).
7. For an expanded discussion of this, see Chapter 12, this volume. See also Brannon (1994) on the intensification of care and the reorganization of the nursing labour force in the U.S.
8. Hunter, A. D. Conflict: Marxism, radical feminism, and sociology. *The Radical Feminist Perspective in (and/or on) the Field of Sociology: A Metatheorietical Excursion.* Retrieved from http://home.earthlink.net/~ahunter/RFvSoc/conflict.html
9. McClelland, K. (2000, February 24). Other current theories. Retrieved from http://web.grinnell.edu/courses/soc/s00/soc111-01/IntroTheories/Other.html
10. See also Bolaria and Li (1988), and Dei, Karumanchery, and Karumanchery-Luik (2004).
11. Revise Sociology. (2017). Retrieved from https://revisesociology.com/2017/08/05/postmodernism-introduction-sociology/
12. McClelland, 2000.
13. Revise Sociology. (2017). Retrieved from https://revisesociology.com/2017/08/05/postmodernism-introduction-sociology/

## REFERENCES

Armstrong, D. (1983). *Political anatomy of the body: Medical knowledge in Britain in the twentieth century.* Cambridge: Cambridge University Press.

Armstrong, P., & Armstrong, H. (2010). *Wasting away: The undermining of Canadian health care* (2nd ed.). Toronto: Oxford University Press.

Becker, H. S., Hughes, E. C., Geer, B., & Strauss, A. L. (1961). *Boys in white: Student culture in medical school.* Chicago: University of Chicago Press.

Berger, P., & Luckmann, T. (1967). *The social construction of reality: A treatise in the sociology of knowledge.* Garden City, NY: Doubleday.

Biggs, C. L. (1983). The case of the missing midwives: A history of midwifery in Ontario from 1795–1900. *Ontario History, 75*(1), 21–35.

Blane, D. (1985). An assessment of the Black Report's "explanation of health inequalities." *Sociology of Health and Illness, 7*(3), 423–445. doi:10.1111/1467-9566.ep10832355

Bloom, S. W. (2002). *The word as scalpel: A history of medical sociology.* New York: Oxford University Press.

Bolaria, B. S., & Li, P. S. (1988). Theories and policies of racial discrimination. In B. S. Bolaria & P. S. Li (Eds.), *Racial oppression in Canada* (2nd ed., pp. 27–40). Aurora, ON: Garamond Press.

Bourgeault, I. L. (2008). On the move: The migration of health care providers into and out of Canada. In B. S. Bolaria & H. Dickinson (Eds.), *Health, illness, and health care in Canada* (rev. 4th ed., pp. 76–98). Toronto: Nelson Education.

Brannon, R. L. (1994). *Intensifying care: The hospital industry, professionalization, and the reorganization of the nursing labor process.* New York: Baywood.

Bury, M. (1982). Chronic illness as biographical disruption. *Sociology of Health and Illness, 4*(2), 167–182. doi:10.1111/1467-9566.ep11339939

Calliste, A. (1996). Antiracism organizing and resistance in nursing: African Canadian women. *Canadian Review of Sociology and Anthropology, 33*(3), 361–390.

Castagna, M., & Dei, G. S. (2000). An historical overview of the application of the race concept in social practice. In A. Calliste & G. S. Dei (Eds.), *Anti-racist feminism: Critical race and gender studies* (pp. 19–38). Halifax: Fernwood.

Charmaz, K. (1987). Struggling for a self: Identity levels of the chronically ill. The experience and management of chronic illness. In J. A. Roth & P. Conrad (Eds.), *Research in the sociology of health care* (vol. 6, pp. 283–321). Greenwich, CT: JAI Press.

Coburn, D., & Eakin, J. (1998). The sociology of health in Canada. In D. Coburn, C. D'Arcy, & G. Torrance (Eds.), *Health and Canadian society: Sociological perspectives* (3rd ed., pp. 619–634). Toronto: University of Toronto Press.

Cockerham, W. C., & Ritchey, F. J. (1997). *Dictionary of medical sociology.* Westport, CT: Greenwood Press.

Collins, P. H. (1990). *Black feminist thought: Knowledge, consciousness, and the politics of empowerment.* New York: Routledge.

Conrad, P. (1987). The experience of illness: Recent and new directions. The experience and management of chronic illness. In J. A. Roth and P. Conrad (Eds.), *Research in the sociology of health care* (vol. 6). Greenwich, CT: JAI Press.

Conrad, P., & Leiter, V. (2004). Medicalization, markets, and consumers. *Journal of Health and Social Behaviour, 45*(Suppl. 1), 158–176.

Conrad, P., & Schneider, J. W. (1980). A theoretical statement on the medicalization of deviance. In P. Conrad & J. W. Schneider (Eds.), *Deviance and medicalization: From badness to sickness* (pp. 261–276). St. Louis: C.V. Mosby.

Conrad, P., & Schneider, J. W. (1992). *Deviance and medicalization: From badness to sickness* (Expanded ed.). Philadelphia: Temple University Press.

Dei, G. J. S. (1996). Critical perspectives in antiracism: An introduction. *Canadian Review of Sociology and Anthropology, 33*(3), 247–267. doi:10.1111/j.1755-618X.1996.tb02452.x

Dei, G. J. S., Karumanchery, L. L., & Karumanchery-Luik, N. (2004). *Playing the race card: Exposing white power and privilege.* New York: Peter Lang.

Ehrenreich, B., & English, D. (1973). *Witches, midwives, and nurses: A history of women healers.* New York: Feminist Press.

Eisenstein, H. (1983). *Contemporary feminist thought.* Boston: G.K. Hall & Co.

Foucault, M. (1971). *Madness and civilization.* New York: Pantheon Books.

Foucault, M. (1973). *The birth of the clinic.* New York: Pantheon Books.

Foucault, M. (1977). *Discipline and punish.* New York: Pantheon Books.

Foucault, M. (1979). *The history of sexuality. Volume 1: An introduction.* Harmondsworth, U.K.: Penguin.

Fox, B. (1988). Conceptualizing "patriarchy." *Canadian Review of Sociology and Anthropology, 25*(2), 163–181.

Frideres, J. S. (1994). Racism and health: The case of the native people. In B. S. Bolaria & H. Dickinson (Eds.), *Health, illness, and health care in Canada* (2nd ed., pp. 202–220). Toronto: Harcourt Brace Jovanovich.

Goffman, E. (1961). *Asylums: Essays on the social situation of mental patients and other inmates.* Garden City, NY: Anchor.

Goffman, E. (1963). *Stigma: Notes on the management of spoiled identity.* Englewood Cliffs, NJ: Prentice Hall.

Haas, J., & Shaffir, W. (1977). The professionalization of medical students: Developing competence and a cloak of competence. *Symbolic Interaction, 1*(1), 71–88. doi:10.1525/si.1977.1.1.71

Hughes, E. C. (1971). *The sociological eye: Selected papers on institutions and race.* Chicago: Aldine-Atherton.

Ishi, T. (1987). Class conflict, the state, and linkage: The international migration of nurses from the Philippines. *Berkeley Journal of Sociology, 32*(1), 281–312.

Jary, D., & Jary, J. (1991). *The HarperCollins dictionary of sociology.* New York: HarperCollins.

Jasso-Aguilar, R., Waitzkin, H., & Landwehr, A. (2004). Multinational corporations and health care in the United States and Latin America strategies, actions, and effects. *Journal of Health and Social Behavior, 45*(Suppl.), 136–157.

Johnson, T. J. (1995). Governmentality and the institutionalization of expertise. In T. Johnson, G. Larkin, & M. Saks (Eds.), *Health professions and the state in Europe* (pp. 7–24). London: Routledge.

Lachmann, R. (1991). *The encyclopedic dictionary of sociology* (4th ed.). Guilford, CT: The Dushkin Publishing Group.

Matcha, D. A. (2000). *Medical sociology*. Boston: Allyn and Bacon.

McCrea, F. B. (1983). The politics of menopause: The "discovery" of a deficiency disease. *Social Problems, 31*(1), 111–123. doi:10.2307/800413

McKinlay, J. B. (1972). The sick role—Illness and pregnancy. *Social Science and Medicine, 6*(5), 561–572. doi:10.1016/0037-7856(72)90072-8

Mechanic, D., & Volkart, E. H. (1960). Illness behavior and medical diagnosis. *Journal of Health and Human Behavior, 1*(2), 86–94. doi:10.2307/2949006

Merton, R. K., Reader, G. G., & Kendall, P. L. (Eds.). (1957). *The student-physician: Introductory studies in the sociology of medical education*. Boston: Harvard University Press.

Navarro, V. (1976). *Medicine under capitalism*. New York: Prodist.

Navarro, V. (1986). *Crisis, health, and medicine: A social critique*. London: Tavistock.

Nestel, S. (1996/1997). "A new profession to the white population in Canada": Ontario midwifery and the politics of race. *Health and Canadian Society, 4*(2), 315–341.

Novek, J., Yassi, A., & Spiegel, J. (1990). Mechanization, the labor process, and injury risks in the Canadian meat packing industry. *International Journal of Health Services, 20*(2), 281–296. doi:10.2190/UJQ4-XXKC-072N-LKJL

Oakley, A. (1984). *The captured womb: A history of the medical care of pregnant women*. Oxford: Basil Blackwell.

O'Brien, M. (1981). *The politics of reproduction*. Boston: Routledge and Kegan Paul.

Parsons, T. (1951). *The social system*. New York: The Free Press.

Pizurki, H., Mejia, A., Butter, I., & Ewart, L. (1987). *Women as providers of health care*. Geneva: World Health Organization.

Reverby, S. (1987). *Ordered to care: The dilemma of American nursing, 1850–1945*. Cambridge: Cambridge University Press.

Rushing, B. (1993). Ideology in the re-emergence of North American midwifery. *Work and Occupations, 20*(1), 46–67.

Smith, B. E. (1981). Black lung: The social production of disease. *International Journal of Health Services, 11*(3), 343–359. doi:10.2190/LMPT-4G1J-15VQ-KWEK

Smith, B. E. (1987). *Digging our own graves: Coal miners and the struggle over black lung disease*. Philadelphia: Temple University Press.

Smith, D. E. (1993). *Texts, facts, and femininity: Exploring the relations of ruling*. London: Routledge.

Straus, R. (1957). The nature and status of medical sociology. *American Sociological Review, 22*(2), 200–204. doi:10.2307/2088858

Strauss, A. L., Corbin, J., Fagerhaugh, S., Glaser, B. G., Maines, D., Suczek, C., & Wiener, C. L. (1984). *Chronic illness and the quality of life* (2nd ed.). St. Louis: Mosby.

Szasz, T. S, & Hollender, M. H. (1956). A contribution of the philosophy of medicine: The basic models of the doctor–patient relationship. *Archives of Internal Medicine, 97*(5), 585–592. doi:10.1001/archinte.1956.00250230079008

Townsend, P., Davidson, N., & Whitehead, M. (Eds.). (1992). *Inequalities in health: The Black Report and the health divide*. New York: Penguin.

Truth and Reconciliation Commission of Canada (TRC). (2015). *Truth and Reconciliation Commission of Canada: Calls to action.* Winnipeg: Author.

Turner, B. S. (1992). *Regulating bodies: Essays in medical sociology.* London: Routledge.

Turner, B. S. (1995). *Medical power and social knowledge* (2nd ed.). Newbury Park, CA: Sage.

Twaddle, A. C. (1969). Health decisions and sick role variations: An exploration. *Journal of Health and Social Behavior, 10*(2), 105–115. doi:10.2307/2948358

Waitzkin, H. (1983). *The second sickness: Contradictions of capitalist health care.* New York: The Free Press.

Weitz, R. (1996). *The sociology of health, illness, and health care: A critical approach.* Belmont, CA: Wadsworth Publishing Company.

Wertz, R. W., & Wertz, D. C. (1979). *Lying-in: A history of childbirth in America.* New York: Schocken Books. doi:10.1177/0038038590024004007

Witz, A. (1990). Patriarchy and professions: The gendered politics of occupational closure. *Sociology, 24*(4), 675–690.

Witz, A. (1992). *Professions and patriarchy.* New York: Routledge.

Wotherspoon, T. (1994). Colonization, self-determination, and the health of Canada's First Nations peoples. In B. S. Bolaria & R. Bolaria (Eds.), *Racial minorities, medicine, and health* (pp. 247–267). Halifax: Fernwood.

Zola, I. K. (1972). Medicine as an institution of social control: The medicalization of society. *The Sociology Review, 20*(4), 487–504. doi:10.1111/j.1467-954X.1972.tb00220.x

# CHAPTER 3

## Political Economy Perspectives on Health and Health Care

*Dennis Raphael and Toba Bryant*

## INTRODUCTION

Political economy models of health and health care are concerned with how political ideology and the power and influence of different sectors in a society operate through economic and political systems to create public policy that distributes the resources necessary for health. Central to this perspective is the idea that politics and economics are intrinsically related and together shape the health of societal members, as well as the organization and delivery of healthcare services. Political economy models derive from the disciplines of sociology and political science and have proven to be very useful in understanding health and healthcare issues in Canada and other nations. Since these models look at the nature of society and how the broad contours of society shape health and health care, they require moving well beyond the usual health preoccupations of body organs and so-called healthy behaviours.

As applied to understanding health, a political economy approach draws a direct link between political and economic systems and the public policies that shape the health of the overall population and the health of specific groups occupying specific social locations such as social class, gender, age, and race, among other characteristics. These systems and public policies also shape the form of the healthcare system in a nation.

There are a variety of political economy models, and this chapter considers the insights that a critical materialist approach offers. This framework is *critical* in that it is concerned with uncovering less obvious societal structures and processes that shape public policy and public understandings of important issues such as health and health care. It is *materialist* in that it is concerned with the production and distribution of concrete resources such as income, employment, housing, and food, and how these living and working conditions shape health, as well as the understandings that people hold concerning these processes. Finally, it is concerned with the politics and economics of the society and how these structures and processes are influenced by sectors of society that differ in power and influence. These concepts, uncovering as they do the structures and processes that shape the distribution of resources, are especially relevant when considering issues of health and health care.

Since this approach sees public policies that shape health policies as resulting from the relative balance of power and influence among competing societal sectors, it is concerned with identifying the interests held by different sectors and how these may be actualized by governing authorities. For example, the business and corporate sector in Canada is concerned with making profits and rather less concerned with providing health-supporting wages and benefits to its workers. In contrast, the labour sector is concerned with providing higher wages and benefits to workers. Finally, the civil society sector is concerned with promoting a co-operative society that provides its members with both their basic needs and the opportunity for flourishing as human beings. In Canada, these sectors have had different power and influence at different times and for different issues.

The balance of power and influence among these three sectors will shape the kinds of public policies that governing authorities legislate. Some policies may be health promoting, while others may threaten health. Since this is the case, improving health involves acting upon these societal dynamics. The health of Canadians is directly influenced by the public policies that result from these structures and processes in two main ways. The first pathway is through public policy that shapes the living and working conditions of Canadians. These are the primary determinants of health and illness. The second pathway is through public policies that organize and deliver healthcare services. Since jurisdictions differ in how their economic and political systems operate, it is not surprising there are differences among these jurisdictions in the health of people and the healthcare systems that serve them.

Figure 3.1 provides a model of the structures and processes that shape health and healthcare systems identified by a critical materialist political economy approach. In the following sections, we describe each component and its importance for understanding health and health care. We begin with the most abstract features of the model at the top and then work our way down. The purpose is to provide means of understanding what contributions a political economy perspective can make in understanding health and health care. It also provides means of improving the health of populations and the operation of healthcare systems.

## POWER AND INFLUENCE OF SOCIETAL SECTORS

At the top of Figure 3.1 are the three key sectors that influence the entire public policy process in a nation. A sector is a group of people who share common interests and work to shape society to meet their desires and needs. The *business and corporate sector* is centrally placed as it has the greatest potential power and influence in capitalist societies—and all wealthy developed nations are capitalist—to shape aspects of economic and political systems, public policy-making, and the quality and distribution of the factors that shape health.

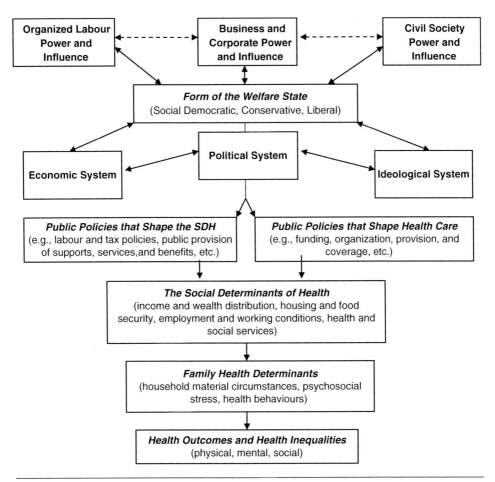

**Figure 3.1:** Depiction of Pathways by Which the Key Concepts of a Political Economy Approach Explain Health Outcomes across Different Jurisdictions

The business and corporate sector are the people whose interests are aligned with making profits through operation of the capitalist or so-called free-enterprise system. They include the owners and managers of corporations and other large businesses. They also include the owners and managers of smaller businesses who have come to believe that their interests are aligned with the larger corporate sector. The goal of this sector is to maximize the returns of the owners and investors in companies. This usually involves having governments play a smaller role in managing the economy and reducing programs and supports to the citizenry. It also calls for reducing corporate taxes and taxes on the wealthy as well as controlling wages and the provision of benefits to workers.

As an example of how powerful this sector is, consider how difficult it is to raise the wages of workers to levels that will move all above the poverty line. Many poor people in Canada are employed, but very low minimum wages preclude them from achieving health-promoting income levels and benefits (Jackson & Thomas, 2017). In contrast, in many developed nations where the corporate and business sector is less powerful, being employed guarantees exit out of poverty (Raphael, 2011a). The corporate and business sector in Canada has also been very successful in reducing taxes on the wealthy and powerful and reducing government programs (Langille, 2016). This is less apparent in most other developed nations.

In nations such as Canada where this sector is especially influential, there is usually rather little concern for how these processes may affect the health and well-being of societal members (Raphael, 2014). As discussed in later sections, this is less the case in other nations where the power and influence of the corporate and business sector are curbed either through the power of other societal sectors or through the business and corporate sector working together with these other sectors to moderate their profit-making activities.

The business and corporate sector has the power and influence to shape public policy through its control of the economic system. It possesses various levers of power—primarily its ability to move and invest money—that shape how governments develop and implement public policies that distribute economic and social resources that shape health. In regard to these public policies, the business and corporate sector usually favours less governmental provision of social and economic security and advocates for weakened government management of employment practices, and fewer support programs and benefits, all of which results in less redistribution of income and wealth (Langille, 2016; Macarov, 2003). Its call for lower taxes—especially for the corporate and business sector and the wealthy—weakens governmental ability to provide benefit and supports that provide economic and social security to the population (Menahem, 2010).

Langille (2016) provides a good overview of how the business and corporate sector has advocated for and been successful in having governments create public policy that inequitably distributes economic and social resources across members of Canadian society. He identifies these actors as business associations, conservative think tanks, citizen front institutions, and conservative lobbyists that influence governmental authorities and shape public opinion.

> The driving forces shaping our social determinants of health have been the owners and managers of major transnational enterprises—the men who have defined our corporate culture and wielded an enormous influence over public policy. Their main instrument has been macroeconomic policy, which they have used to set constraints on the role and scope of government. They have pushed for Canadian governments to adopt a free market or neo-liberal approach to macroeconomic policy. (Langille, 2016, p. 305)

Details of how this influence has led to particular forms of public policy are presented in the following sections. These policies have led to growing income inequality, lessening economic and social security for many Canadians, and threats to the sustainability of our healthcare and social services systems.

The organized labour sector includes labour unions and citizens who are members of these unions. This sector usually supports greater redistribution of income and wealth from the rich to others through higher taxation on the business and corporate sector and the wealthy, stronger government management of the workplace, and greater provision by governing authorities of supports and benefits (Peters, 2012). It gains power and influence through the percentage of the population that belong to trade unions and alliances with governing parties of the left (Brady, 2009; Bryant, 2016; Swank, 2010).

When the labour sector has more influence, public policies are created that equalize the power imbalances between employers and employees. This happens at the macro-level, where governments are pressured to create equity-related public policies, such as more progressive income taxes, and mandate that workplaces provide fairer wages and greater benefits. When the labour sector has less power and influence, economic and social security enhancing public policies become less likely and workplaces and their employment become more precarious with lower wages and benefits.

The civil society sector consists of all of the agencies, groups, and organizations that try to shape public policy for various causes, such as the environment, reducing poverty, providing child care, and other programs and services. It also includes citizens who desire that the government operate in certain ways, such as providing fairer taxation policies or helping to provide employment training and other opportunities to members of society. It gains power and influence from its ability to influence public opinion and shape public policy through networks of agencies, organizations, and other non-governmental institutions (Brady, 2009). And of course, the citizenry itself has influence through its ability to elect representatives to governments.

The balance of power among sectors differs among nations, with resulting impacts on the distribution of the factors that shape health and the nature of the healthcare system (Raphael, 2014). This analysis helps explain why, in some nations, citizens are provided with comprehensive health care that covers prescription medicines, rehabilitation, and dental care for children (Olsen, 2010). These same nations are likely to provide universal and affordable child care, free or very low tuition at post-secondary institutions, and employment for most that provides wages that are well above the poverty line and numerous benefits. And if employment is lost, they provide support and job retraining until employment is gained (Raphael, 2011a). If employment is unavailable or the person cannot work due to illness or disability, supports and benefits adequate for maintaining health are provided. This package of benefits and supports by which a nation provides economic and social security to its citizens has been termed the welfare state.

Figure 3.2 shows different distributions of labour union membership across different wealthy developed nations. Nations with a higher proportion of their members belonging to unions tend to have governing authorities implementing public policies that equitably distribute economic and social resources. As discussed below, the Nordic nations have

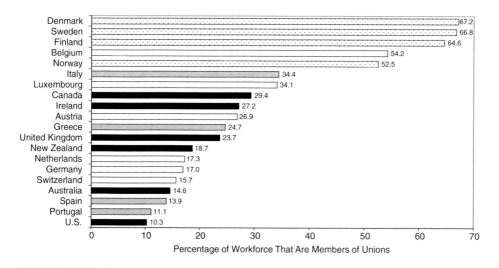

**Figure 3.2:** Union Density among Selected OECD Nations, 2015–2016

*Legend:* Dark = Liberal; Unshaded = Conservative; Grey = Latin; and Dotted = Social Democratic Welfare States
*Source:* Adapted from Organisation for Economic Cooperation and Development. (2018). Union density. Retrieved from https://stats.oecd.org/Index.aspx?DataSetCode=TUD#

higher proportions of workers belonging to unions. In contrast, the Anglo-Saxon nations, including Canada, have lower rates. These differences are related to a wide range of differences in public policies, reflecting different balances of power and influence amongst these sectors across nations. These national differences lead to different forms of what is called the welfare state.

# THE WELFARE STATE AND ITS DIFFERENT FORMS

Wealthy developed nations differ widely as to the extent that they meet the essential needs of their citizenry. While all nations provide universal education through the elementary and secondary levels and all, except the U.S., provide health care, some provide economic and social security as a right of citizenship, while others do not. Box 3.1 describes the essential aspects of a welfare state, but there are wide differences in the depth of the welfare state across nations. As we will see, Canada has one of the less-developed forms of the welfare state, a result of its historical traditions and the imbalance of power between societal sectors.

The welfare state has also been defined as "a capitalist society in which the State has intervened in the form of social policies, programs, standards, and regulations in order to mitigate class conflict and to provide for, answer, or accommodate certain social needs for which the capitalist mode of production in itself has no solution or makes no provision" (Teeple, 2000, p. 15). In both definitions, the welfare state acts to provide societal members with various forms of economic and social security, which are clearly related to the health of the population.

**Box 3.1:** What Is a Welfare State?

A welfare state is a nation in which organized power is used to modify the play of market forces in at least three directions: first, by guaranteeing individuals and families a minimum income irrespective of the market value of their work or property; second, by narrowing the extent of insecurity by enabling individuals and families to meet certain social contingencies (e.g., sickness, old age, and unemployment) that lead otherwise to individual and family crises; and third, by ensuring that all citizens without distinction of status or class are offered the best standards available in relation to a certain agreed range of social services.

*Source:* Briggs, A. (1961). The welfare state in historical perspective. *European Journal of Sociology,* 2(2), 251–258.

The welfare state was a significant development in most developed political economies following the Second World War. In policy studies, the welfare state refers to a set of social reforms—such as public pensions, public health care, employment insurance, and social assistance—implemented by governments to provide citizens with various supports and benefits. These reforms are important because such policies have been shown to be important predictors of the overall health of a population (Bryant, 2016).

The source of the Canadian welfare state as we know it today can be found in the insecurities and experiences of Canadians during the Depression and the Second World War (Teeple, 2000). Rather than seeing the advent of the advanced welfare state as a reasoned governmental response to perceived citizen need, it has been argued that in Canada it was actually a governmental concession to the significant and sustained calls for reforms by citizens and the labour movement (Teeple, 2000). This represented a period where the labour and civil society sectors' power and influence were more able to shape the making of public policy than is the present situation.

As a result, working families and individuals won some security against the unbridled operation of the economic system. A key guiding principle behind the welfare state is that the provision of public programs and services is an entitlement of citizenship rather than a commodity requiring purchase by earned income. These various programs and services enabled people to maintain a decent standard of living that was not totally dependent on their ability to earn market income. In essence, many programs and services came to be decommodified—that is, not subject to purchase in the open marketplace—a key concept in understanding the form and function of the welfare state in nations such as Canada.

In Canada, the welfare state also redistributes economic resources from high-income earners to low-income earners (Teeple, 2006). As one example, the healthcare system is funded by general revenues received from citizens. High-income earners pay greater taxes in both absolute (dollars) and relative (tax rates) amounts (Murphy, Roberts, & Wolfson, 2007). Higher-income earners, however, are less likely to become ill and make use of the healthcare system (Tjepkema, Wilkins, & Long, 2013). Thus, the public healthcare system is a very effective means of assuring healthcare provision to citizens, as well as a means of economic redistribution.

Yet, despite the presence of a welfare state in all developed capitalist nations, there are profound differences in what these welfare states look like in different nations. These reflect differences in the balance of power between the business and corporate, labour, and the civil society sectors. Three forms of the welfare state have been identified in developed nations (Esping-Andersen, 1990). These are the social democratic, conservative, and liberal. One form of the welfare state—the liberal—represents the situation where the corporate and business sector dominates public policy-making. Canada falls within this cluster of welfare states. The others represent a more balanced situation amongst these societal sectors.

Esping-Andersen's political economy model conceives ideas and institutions—and the public policy that flows from these—as evolving from societal arrangements influenced by historical traditions. The central features of welfare regimes are their extent of social stratification, decommodification, and the relative role of the state, market, and family in providing economic and social security to the population. Importantly, the state's role is influenced by class mobilization, in that the loyalties of the working and middle classes determine the forms by which these systems operate. These differing patterns of loyalties have contributed to the formation and maintenance of these welfare state regimes.

## The Social Democratic Welfare State

The social democratic welfare state (e.g., Denmark, Finland, Norway, and Sweden) has been strongly influenced by social democratic ideology and politics. Its concern with equality outlines a key role for the state in addressing inequality and providing the population with various forms of economic and social security (Saint-Arnaud & Bernard, 2003). Its provision of programs and supports on a universal basis is consistent with its goal of reducing social stratification and decommodifying the necessities of life. In essence, the social democratic welfare state strives to provide the means by which one can live a decent life independent of employment market involvement.

These social democratic welfare states emphasize universal welfare rights and provide generous benefits and entitlements. Their political and social history is one of political dominance by social democratic parties of the left, a result of political organization initially of industrial workers and farmers, and later the middle class. Through universal provision of a range of benefits, these regimes have been able to secure the loyalties of a significant proportion of the population. Two Canadian health researchers have described their public policies as *Scandinavian Common Sense: Policies to Tackle Social Inequalities in Health* (Côté & Raynauilt, 2015). The healthcare systems are comprehensive and usually run by governments. They cover areas such as pharmaceuticals and children's dental care in addition to primary and secondary healthcare services.

## The Conservative Welfare State

The conservative welfare state (e.g., Belgium, France, Germany, and the Netherlands) is distinguished by its concern with maintaining stability (Saint-Arnaud & Bernard, 2003). Historically, governance was by Christian democratic parties that maintained many aspects of social stratification, a moderate degree of decommodification of societal resources, and an important role for the family in providing economic and social support. The Church played a significant role in its development. An underdeveloped form of the conservative welfare state—the Latin (e.g., Greece, Italy, Portugal, and Spain)—has been added to Esping-Anderson's three regimes by Saint-Arnaud and Bernard (2003).

Conservative welfare states also offer generous benefits but provide these based on social insurance plans associated with employment status, with primary emphasis on male wage earners (Esping-Andersen, 1990). Their political and social history is one of traditional Church concerns with supporting citizens combined with traditional approaches toward maintaining status differences and adherence to authority. These tendencies sometimes manifest in corporatist approaches (e.g., Germany) where business interests are major influences, or in statist approaches (e.g., France) where the state plays a key role in provision of citizen security (Pontusson, 2005).

In these nations, the corporate and business sector acts in collaboration with the labour sector and state to maintain levels of income and social programs that maintain human dignity and well-being. In practicalities, the conservative welfare state looks very similar to the social democratic welfare state in terms of quality of life and overall health (Pontusson, 2005). Their healthcare systems are also similarly comprehensive, although they may be financed and delivered through non-profit private organizations and insurance agencies.

## The Liberal Welfare State

Finally, the emphasis of the liberal welfare state (e.g., Australia, Canada, the United Kingdom, and the United States) is on liberty and is dominated by the market and ruled by generally pro-business political parties (Saint-Arnaud & Bernard, 2003). Little attempt is made to reduce social stratification, and its degree of decommodification is the lowest. There is little state intervention in the operation of the economic system.

Liberal welfare states provide modest benefits, and the state usually steps in with assistance only when the market fails to meet citizens' most basic needs. Their political and social history is one of dominance by business interests that has led the population to give its loyalty to the economic system rather than the state as a means of providing economic and social security. These liberal welfare states are the least developed in terms of provision of citizen economic and social security. A key feature is their use of means-tested

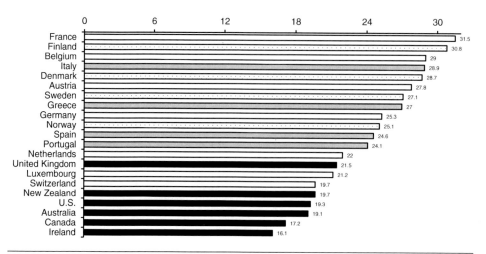

**Figure 3.3:** Total Public Social Expenditures as Percentage of GDP, Selected OECD Nations, 2015–2016

*Legend:* Dark = Liberal; Unshaded = Conservative; Grey = Latin; and Dotted = Social Democratic Welfare States.
*Source:* Adapted from Organisation for Economic Cooperation and Development. (2019). Social spending (indicator). doi: 10.1787/7497563b-en

benefits that are targeted only to the least well-off. Their healthcare systems are likely to be two-tiered, offering both public and private systems alongside each other. Coverage may be less than that offered by the social democratic and conservative welfare states. Liberal welfare states' healthcare systems are more subject to privatization and profit-making as well. This is the case in Canada (Whiteside, 2015).

Figure 3.3 shows differences in total public social expenditures as percentage of gross domestic product (the total size of the economy) for developed nations based on their form of the welfare state. These public expenditures are primarily in the form of supports and benefits provided to the population such as health care, pensions, employment training, education, and family and child benefits. What is most obvious is the very low level of expenditures among nations identified as liberal welfare states; Canada is the second-lowest spender.

## STRATIFICATION, DECOMMODIFICATION, AND THE ROLE OF THE STATE, FAMILY, AND MARKET

Three key differences among these forms of the welfare state are the extent of stratification, decommodification, and the role of the state in providing societal members with economic and social resources. Each is described below. Generally, the social democratic welfare state provides the most equitable profile regarding these factors; the liberal welfare state, the least.

*Stratification* refers to institutionalized differences among society members and is usually defined in terms of wealth and income, education and, in the political economy literature, power and influence (Scott, 2014). Stratification can refer to differences that result from membership by social class, access to wages, benefits and supports, and most importantly, ability to shape public policy. Welfare states are both a result of levels of stratification as well as means of maintaining these status differences. Provision of universal services that decommodify the necessities for health—most common in social democratic and least common in liberal welfare states—is another means of managing stratification (Menahem, 2010).

Stratification leads to social inequality, which is differences that are "consequential for the lives they lead, most particularly for the rights or opportunities they exercise and the rewards or privileges they enjoy" (Grabb, 2007, p. 1). Social inequality creates health inequities. One type of social inequality, income differences, is an important theme in health inequalities research.

*Decommodification* refers to the ability of people to have a decent quality of life independent of involvement in the paid employment market, or what Esping-Andersen (1990, 1994) terms the "cash nexus." In addition to replacement income associated with retirement, sickness and disability, and unemployment, important aspects of daily life that can be commodified or decommodified are child care; employment training; elementary, secondary, and post-secondary education; dental care; and health and social services, among others (Menahem, 2010).

*Roles of the state, family, and market* in providing economic and social security differ in welfare states (Saint-Arnaud & Bernard, 2003). The social democratic welfare state sees a strong state role, the conservative provides family-directed benefits based on earnings, and the liberal emphasizes market involvement. State involvement is most effective for the provision of economic and social security and more equitable distribution of the social determinants of health.

*Class/power mobilization* refers to the ability of classes or groups of citizens to attain the power to move a state toward public policy approaches that benefit them (Esping-Andersen, 1990). In the social democratic nations, working-class interests combined with those of farmers to produce the inclusive and universalist welfare state (Esping-Andersen, 1985). In contrast, the lack of working-class power in the liberal welfare state sees public policy dominated by the corporate and business sector. These mobilization processes are enhanced or reduced by degree of unionization, voter preferences, and self-perceived class/group loyalty. The conservative welfare state sees elite preferences for stability translated into strong supports for families through social insurance schemes. Esping-Andersen's distinction between social democratic, conservative, and liberal welfare states helps explain differences in what their economic, political, and ideological systems look like.

# ECONOMIC, POLITICAL, AND IDEOLOGICAL SYSTEMS

The political economy approach directs attention to the structures and processes of economic and political systems and the ideas that societal members have about these systems and the nature of the society.

## Economic System

The economic system both creates and distributes economic resources among the population. Since all economic systems in wealthy developed nations are capitalist, market principles—of which profit-making is paramount—have the potential to drive their operations (Coburn, 2010). Some of the main features associated with the market process that impact health are wage structures, benefits available through work, working conditions, and vacation time, among others (Jackson & Thomas, 2017).

It has long been recognized, however, that without state intervention in the operation of the market economy, the distribution of economic resources becomes skewed in favour of the wealthy and powerful (Macarov, 2003). In addition, some structures and processes necessary for societal functioning may not be made available at all by the economic system. The welfare state arose because the economic system itself is not capable of dealing with provision of basic societal resources such as education, health care, housing, and other programs and services that provide citizens with resources necessary for well-being (Teeple, 2000).

What are some of the influences upon how the market economy operates and distributes economic resources among the population? As noted, the business and corporate sectors, the organized labour sector, and civil society influence the political system that can manage the economic system through public policy-making (see below). The business and corporate sector has power and influence over the economic and political systems through its control of many economic levers, such as its ability to move and invest capital (Brooks & Miljan, 2003).

The organized labour sector usually supports greater redistribution of economic resources through higher taxation on the business and corporate sector, stronger government management of aspects of the workplace such as wages and benefits, and greater provision of supports and benefits through government programs funded by taxes (Navarro, 2004). The civil society sector gains power and influence over the economic system from its ability to influence public opinion and shape public policy through networks of agencies, organizations, and other non-governmental institutions (Brady, 2009).

## Political System

The political system consists of the organization of the state and its collection of laws and regulations. The political structure can intervene in the operation of the economic system by enacting laws and regulations that affect employment practices and by having governments provide supports and services to the citizenry through programs and benefits. These supports, benefits, and services come from the enactment of corporate and personal taxes, which are usually progressive in that greater proportions of taxes accrue from those with higher incomes. There are many specific areas where state activity impacts upon the social determinants of health. Working through the making of public policy, these areas include income and income distribution, employment and job insecurity, working conditions, housing and food security, and the availability of health and social services, among others (Mikkonen & Raphael, 2010). These social determinants of health directly affect the living conditions—and health—of individuals.

## Ideological System

Finally, the means by which economic and political systems distribute resources are usually justified by dominant discourses on the nature of society and the different roles that the state, market, and family should play in providing economic and social security. These different discourses usually involve dichotomies such as socialism versus liberalism, social justice versus economic justice, and communal versus individual responsibility for well-being.

The socialism versus liberalism dichotomy is well described by Wiktorowicz and Wyndham-West in Chapter 11. They point out that liberalism emphasizes personal freedom whereby individuals can pursue their own interests free of coercion by government. Governments should intervene only to assure the free market distributes basic resources. In contrast, socialism distrusts the results provided by the market economy and emphasizes that assets should be collectively owned, with the benefits of the economic system distributed equitably across the population. In essence, liberalism is concerned with equality of opportunity, while socialism is concerned with equality of result. Canada and other liberal welfare states tend toward liberalism, European nations toward socialism.

The social justice versus economic justice dichotomy is concerned with whether there is an inherent right for everyone to receive the benefits available in a society or whether individuals are entitled to only those earned through their participation in the market economy (Hofrichter, 2003). Not surprisingly, this dichotomy is related to the liberalism versus socialism dichotomy. The business sector usually espouses the economic justice view, while the labour sector and frequently the civil society sector favour the social justice view. Again, Canada and other liberal welfare states tend toward the economic justice approach, while European nations lean toward the social justice view.

Related to both of these dichotomies is the issue of broad concepts of society and how these lead to action and change in a society. Stone (2011) contrasts individualized (market) versus communal (polis) approaches. In the market conception of society, the emphasis is on the individual, and the primary motivation for action is self-interest. Society is inherently competitive, and the source of change is the exchange of material goods through the market economy.

By contrast, in the polis view of society the focus is on the community, and there is a strong role for public interest in addition to self-interest. While there is competition among individuals, there is also co-operation in the pursuit of common goals. The building blocks of social action are groups and organizations. The building blocks of change are ideas and alliances rather than material exchanges among individuals. Finally, the polis model sees the pursuit of the public interest as a source of change.

More recently, analysis had been made of the impact of neo-liberalism as a societal doctrine that shapes the distribution of resources. Neo-liberalism is an ideology that believes that governments should withdraw from managing the economy, thereby ceding more power and influence to the business and corporate sector (Schrecker & Bambra, 2015). This has been seen as leading to the skewing of the distribution of the social determinants of health and threatening the health of citizens in general and children in particular. Box 3.2 provides the essential aspects of neo-liberalism.

The ideological system is especially important because it shapes the means by which the population comes to understand these issues. If the general public is convinced of the validity of neo-liberal arguments about the primacy of the marketplace over the state, then little can be expected to come from public policies that will manage the economy in the service of promoting equitable distributions of economic and social resources. Ideological beliefs of the public are therefore important determinants of whether a jurisdiction comes to address the social determinants of health through public policy action. These ways of thinking about society and the responsibilities for providing citizens with economic and social security come together with the operation of the political and economic systems to shape the making of public policy.

---

**Box 3.2:** Key Tenets of Neo-liberalism

---

1. Markets are the most efficient allocators of resources in production and distribution and should therefore be the primary institution of society.
2. Societies are composed of autonomous individuals (producers and consumers) motivated chiefly by material or economic considerations; concern about others is less paramount.
3. Competition is the major market vehicle for innovations, suggesting little or no management of economy by the state.
4. "There is no such thing as society" was Margaret Thatcher's summary of how she approached being prime minister of the United Kingdom during the thrust of neo-liberal policy-making.

---

*Source:* Adapted from Coburn, D. (2000). Income inequality, social cohesion and the health status of populations: The role of neo-liberalism. *Social Science & Medicine, 51*(1), 135–146.

# PUBLIC POLICY

The term *social policy* is usually used to refer to issues that have direct relevance to social welfare, such as social assistance, child and family policy, and housing policy, but the factors that shape health and health care are affected by a wide range of other public policies that include labour and employment, revenue, and tax policies, among others. These public policy activities are courses of action or inaction taken by public authorities—usually governments—to address a given problem or set of problems (Bryant, 2016). Governments constantly make decisions about a wide range of issues, such as national defence and the organization and delivery of health, social, and other services. The decisions that are the special concern here determine how economic and social resources are distributed among the population.

Governments influence this distribution by establishing taxation levels, the nature and quality of benefits—whether these benefits are universal or targeted—and how employment agreements are negotiated. Governments are also responsible for establishing housing policies, maintaining transportation systems, enacting labour regulations and laws, and providing training related to employment and education.

Table 3.1 shows the interconnections between public policy issues and the social determinants of health. These social determinants of health are considered in greater detail below and in Chapter 6. They are important since they are the best predictors of whether individuals stay healthy or become ill. These public policy decisions that provide equitable or inequitable distribution of the social determinants of health do not exist in a vacuum.

# SOCIAL DETERMINANTS OF HEALTH

Social determinants of health are the specific economic and social conditions that shape the health of individuals, communities, and jurisdictions as a whole (Mikkonen & Raphael, 2010). Canadian researchers have outlined 16 of these: disability, early life, education, employment and working conditions, food security, gender, geography, health services, housing, immigrant status, income and income distribution, Indigenous ancestry, race, social exclusion, social safety net, and unemployment and employment insecurity (Raphael, 2016). Social determinants such as Indigenous ancestry, disability status, gender, and race can be thought of as social locations that do not by themselves lead to differing health outcomes, but interact with societal conditions to create particular health outcomes.

An emphasis upon societal conditions as determinants of health contrasts with the traditional health sciences and public health focus upon biomedical and behavioural risk factors. Since a social determinants of health approach sees the mainsprings of health as being how a society organizes and distributes economic and social resources, it directs attention to economic and social policies as means of improving it. It also requires consideration of the political, economic, and social forces that shape their distribution amongst the population.

**Table 3.1:** Social Determinants of Health and Their Public Policy Antecedents

| | |
|---|---|
| *Early life* | Wages that provide adequate income inside the workforce, or assistance that does so for those unable to work; affordable, quality child care and early education; affordable housing options; and responsive social and health services |
| *Education* | Support for adult literacy initiatives, adequate public education spending, tuition policy that improves access to post-secondary education |
| *Employment and working conditions* | Training and retraining programs (active labour policy), support for working conditions and collective bargaining, enforcing labour legislation and work-place regulations, increasing worker input into workplace environments |
| *Food security* | Developing adequate income and poverty-reduction policies, promoting healthy food policy, providing affordable housing and child care |
| *Health services* | Managing resources more effectively; providing integrated, comprehensive, accessible, responsive, and timely care |
| *Housing* | Providing adequate income and affordable housing, reasonable rental controls and housing supplements, and social housing for those in need |
| *Income and its distribution* | Fair taxation policy, adequate minimum wages and social assistance levels that support health, facilitating collective bargaining |
| *Social exclusion* | Developing and enforcing anti-discrimination laws, providing ESL and job training, approving foreign credentials, supporting other health determinants for newcomers |
| *Social safety net* | Providing economic and program supports to families and citizens comparable with those provided in other wealthy developed nations |
| *Unemployment and job security* | Strengthening active labour policy, providing adequate replacement job insecurity benefits, provisions for part-time benefits and advancement into secure employment |

## FAMILIAL HEALTH DETERMINANTS

Families' living and working conditions differ within and across jurisdictions. The most obvious manifestations of these differences—important because they predict health outcomes—are familial material circumstances, psychosocial factors, including stress experienced by families and coping mechanisms, and health-related behaviours (Benzeval, Dilnot, Judge, & Taylor, 2001).

Material circumstances refer to the concrete exposures to health-strengthening and health-threatening conditions that are associated with income and wealth. Income and wealth are important as these provide access to a wide range of material goods such as housing, food, and learning and recreational opportunities, among others. In addition, since income and wealth are associated with spatial segregation, differences manifest in quality of neighbourhoods and the opportunities for education and recreation associated with these neighbourhoods. The amount of crime and threat is also associated with material circumstances (Raphael, 2011b). These material exposures can have both immediate and long-lasting effects upon children's health.

In response to these material circumstances, families experience differences in a number of psychosocial variables such as stress, sense of efficacy and control, and self-identity. These come to shape parents' and children's health in both the present and future (Lynch, Kaplan, & Salonen, 1997). Psychological health-related effects may also result from early experience. A general non-adaptive reaction to stress may be established during early childhood as well as a general sense of hopelessness and lack of control, both of which are important determinants of health (Irwin, Siddiqui, & Hertzman, 2007).

The third aspect is how experience of varying circumstances and the levels of stress associated with these circumstances lead to the adoption of health-supporting or health-threatening behaviours. In the latter case, these behaviours can be seen as coping responses to adverse life circumstances. Numerous Canadian studies show that those living in conditions of low income, unemployment or precarious employment, poor-quality housing, and food insecurity are more likely to take up risk-related behaviours such as smoking, excessive alcohol consumption, and lack of physical activity (Frohlich & Poland, 2007). Similarly, adoption of carbohydrate-dense diets and weight gain are also seen as means of coping with difficult circumstances (Wilkinson, 1996).

## HEALTH AND HEALTH INEQUALITIES

Health is usually considered in terms of physical, mental, and social well-being. Physical health includes measures of mortality at any given age and mortality prior to age 75, and measures of morbidity such as the presence of various diseases or the occurrence of injury. It can also include functional health or health-related behaviours such as diet or physical activity. Mental health includes measures of psychological functioning and coping mechanisms as well as the presence of disorders. Social health includes measures of school performance and academic achievement, and quality of peer relationships, as well as involvement in delinquency and crime.

Health outcomes are strongly shaped by the components presented in Figure 3.1. Figure 3.4 shows differences in infant mortality rates among nations grouped by form of the welfare state. The infant mortality rate represents the proportion of children being born alive but dying within one year. It is felt to be a very sensitive measure of the overall health of the population (Human Development Reports, 2016). Of special note are the poor standings of nations identified as liberal welfare states.

Chapters 6–9 provide details of these associations as well as means of responding to them. Each analysis is informed in part by the political economy approach provided in this chapter. Figure 3.1 suggestions that intervention at each and any level can improve health, but intervention at the higher levels is more likely to be more effective, albeit more difficult.

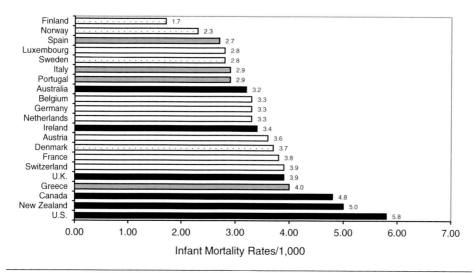

**Figure 3.4:** Infant Mortality Rates among Selected OECD Nations, 2015/16

*Legend:* Dark = Liberal; Unshaded = Conservative; Grey = Latin; and Dotted = Social Democratic Welfare States.
*Source:* Adapted from Organisation for Economic Cooperation and Development. (2019). Infant mortality rates (indicator). doi: 10.1787/83dea506-en

## IMPLICATIONS

Attempts to improve health and reduce health inequalities can benefit from the insights provided by a political economy approach. The approach specifies that health is shaped by a range of societal structures and processes that act to distribute the social determinants of health. These structures and processes create specific forms of public policy that provide individuals with the economic and social conditions necessary for health. These public policy areas include income and wealth distribution, employment security and working conditions, features supporting early child development, food and housing security, and the provision of health and social services.

Each jurisdiction will see a differing balance of power and influence among the business and corporate, labour, and civil society sectors. These differences in power and influence have a profound influence upon the direction that public policy will take. Ultimately, these differences in power—and the resultant distribution of the social determinants of children's health—are shaped by the politics of a nation. As well intentioned as efforts will be to work directly to influence public policy and strengthen specific social determinants of health through community action and direct service delivery, these efforts may have limited effects.

Instead, the political economy approach argues that the key goal should be to shape the politics of a nation in the direction of supporting health. This will require controlling the influence of the business and corporate sector and strengthening the organized labour and civil society sectors. It will also involve support of, and election of, political parties whose positions are consistent with such an approach. Ultimately, the promotion of health requires engagement in the political process with the goal of reordering a society's economic and political systems such that they provide the conditions necessary for health.

## CRITICAL THINKING QUESTIONS

1.  What has been said in the media about the health status of Canadians or about health inequalities in Canada? How do these statements align with some of the concepts presented in this chapter?
2.  What are the differences and similarities between a political science view and the traditional healthy lifestyles approach?
3.  What kinds of political and economic policies do you think would help Canadians improve their average levels of well-being?
4.  Are the media biased regarding their reporting of political, economic, and health issues and the way these are related? In what way and why?
5.  Could you now offer an alternative "political economy" view to key issues or events described and analyzed in the newspaper or on television news?

## FURTHER READINGS

Coburn, D. (2004). Beyond the income inequality hypothesis: Globalization, neo-liberalism, and health inequalities. *Social Science and Medicine, 58*(1), 41–56.
This article reports on a political economy approach to understanding health inequalities in terms of the impact of neo-liberalism on public policy.

Navarro, V., & Muntaner, C. (2016). *The financial and economic crises and their impact on health and social well-being.* New York: Routledge.
This volume provides a timely collection of the most germane studies and commentaries on the complex links between recent changes in national economies, welfare regimes, social inequalities, and population health.

Panitch, L., & Leys, C. (2009). *Morbid symptoms: Health under capitalism.* Toronto: The Merlin Press.
*Morbid Symptoms* sees health as a major field of political economy, one that focuses on the struggle between commercial forces seeking to make it into a field of profit and popular forces fighting to keep it—or make it—a public service with equal access for all.

Raphael, D. (2015). Beyond policy analysis: The raw politics behind opposition to healthy public policy. *Health Promotion International, 30*(2), 380–396.

This article examines how power and politics shape the distribution of key determinants of health in different nations. The business and corporate sector in Canada is identified as opposing public policies that would promote the health of Canadians as these would potentially reduce their profits.

Schrecker, T., & Bambra, C. (2015). *How politics makes us sick: Neoliberal epidemics.* Basingstoke, U.K.: Palgrave Macmillan.

The authors argue that the insecurity, austerity, and inequality that result from neo-liberal (or "market fundamentalist") policies are hazardous to our health, asserting that these neo-liberal epidemics require a political cure.

## RELEVANT WEBSITES

### The People's Health Movement (PHM)

http://phmovement.org/

The PHM is a global network bringing together grassroots health activists, civil society organizations, and academic institutions from around the world. Guided by the People's Charter for Health, PHM works on various programs and activities and is committed to comprehensive primary health care and addressing the social, environmental, and economic determinants of health.

### Luxembourg Income Studies Project

https://www.lisdatacenter.org/

This site describes the Luxembourg Income Studies Project, the most thorough examination of income and other inequalities. The most useful part is listed under "Working Papers," in which hundreds of papers on topics related to welfare state dynamics and income inequality are available for download.

### Organisation for Economic Co-operation and Development (OECD)

www.oecd.org

Clicking on "Health" in the Topics index brings up numerous publications related to health and welfare state issues. There are downloadable files of selected data from some of the OECD Health Data series issued annually.

### The Political Economy of Health—International People's Health University

https://www.iphu.org/en/polecon

In trying to understand how the global economy works (and how it affects health), the discipline of political economy seeks to locate economic analyses within a political environment and seeks to understand the interplay between politics and economics. This website provides an introductory course to this area.

**World Health Organization (WHO)**

http://www.who.int/gho/publications/world_health_statistics/2018/en/

Available on this site are copies of the *World Health Statistics*, published annually by the World Health Organization, as well as many other studies related to poverty and health.

## GLOSSARY

**Corporate power:** This is the placing of corporate owners, directors, and top executives in a dominant position in economic decision-making, including over the flow of initiatives that shapes the future. It places workers, communities, and governments in a position of dependence that requires following the dictates of these members of the corporate elite (Carroll & Sapinski, 2018).

**Decommodification:** Commodification means the production of goods or services for sale in the marketplace. Decommodification regarding welfare state issues means the degree to which individuals can live a reasonable life without relying on market wages. Can older people or the unemployed—that is, those not earning a market wage—live a reasonable life?

**Historical materialism:** This concept means that people's ideas are a product of their social existence rather than their social existence being the result of their consciousness. Related to this is the hypothesis that history can be viewed as a succession of differing modes of production—differing mechanisms for producing the means of existence and of reproducing human beings and society. Capitalism emerged from feudalism, and, in turn, capitalism is expected to be succeeded by another mode of production.

**Social position:** A person's position or socio-economic status is usually measured in terms of educational level, occupational status, income, or some combination of these. There are no real social relationships among people at different levels, and there is no necessary antagonism among those lower or higher. From our perspective, class factors (classes determined by their relationship to the means of production) determine socio-economic status (SES) differences. A focus on SES is thus not necessarily wrong, just simply radically incomplete.

**Welfare state:** Welfare regimes refer to the different ways in which different nations or societies provide for the well-being of their citizens or compensate for the failures of markets to do so. Social democratic welfare regimes tend to provide more resources and on a more universalistic basis than do liberal welfare regimes, which tend to target welfare measures to the poor and to provide fewer benefits to those less eligible for such benefits. The conservative-corporatist-familist regime provides benefits as an advantage of working or relies on the family to provide support.

# REFERENCES

Benzeval, M., Dilnot, A., Judge, K., & Taylor, J. (2001). Income and health over the lifecourse: Evidence and policy implications. In H. Graham (Ed.), *Understanding health inequalities* (pp. 96–112). Buckingham, U.K.: Open University Press.

Brady, D. (2009). *Rich democracies, poor people: How politics explain poverty.* New York: Oxford University Press.

Brooks, S., & Miljan, L. (2003). Theories of public policy. In S. Brooks & L. Miljan (Eds.), *Public policy in Canada: An introduction* (4th ed., pp. 22–49). Toronto: Oxford University Press.

Bryant, T. (2016). *Health policy in Canada* (2nd ed.). Toronto: Canadian Scholars' Press.

Carroll, W. K., & Sapinski, J. P. (2018). *Organizing the 1%: How corporate power works.* Halifax: Fernwood.

Coburn, D. (2010). Health and health care: A political economy perspective. In T. Bryant, D. Raphael, & M. Rioux (Eds.), *Staying alive: Critical perspectives on health, illness, and health care* (2nd ed., pp. 65–92). Toronto: Canadian Scholars' Press.

Côté, D., & Raynauilt, M.-F. (2015). *Scandinavian common sense: Policies to tackle social inequalities in health.* Montreal: Baraka Books.

Esping-Andersen, G. (1985). *Politics against markets: The social democratic road to power.* Princeton, NJ: Princeton University Press.

Esping-Andersen, G. (1990). *The three worlds of welfare capitalism.* Princeton, NJ: Princeton University Press.

Esping-Andersen, G. (1999). *Social foundations of post-industrial economies.* New York: Oxford University Press.

Frohlich, K., & Poland, B. (2007). Points of intervention in health promotion practice. In M. O'Neill, A. Pederson, S. Dupere, & I. Rootman (Eds.), *Health promotion in Canada: Critical perspectives* (2nd ed., pp. 46–60). Toronto: Canadian Scholars' Press.

Grabb, E. G. (2007). *Theories of social inequality* (5th ed.). Toronto: Nelson.

Hofrichter, R. (2003). The politics of health inequities: Contested terrain. In R. Hofrichter (Ed.), *Health and social justice: Politics, ideology, and inequity in the distribution of disease* (pp. 1–56). San Francisco: Jossey-Bass.

Human Development Reports. (2016). Mortality rate, infant (per 1,000 live births). Retrieved from http://hdr.undp.org/en/indicators/57206

Irwin, K. G., Siddiqui, A., & Hertzman, C. (2007). *Early child development: A powerful equalizer.* Geneva: World Health Organization.

Jackson, A., & Thomas, M. P. (2017). *Work and labour in Canada: Critical issues* (3rd ed.). Toronto: Canadian Scholars' Press.

Langille, D. (2016). Follow the money: How business and politics define our health. In D. Raphael (Ed.), *Social determinants of health: Canadian perspectives* (3rd ed., pp. 470–490). Toronto: Canadian Scholars' Press.

Lynch, J. W., Kaplan, G. A., & Salonen, J. T. (1997). Why do poor people behave poorly? Variation in adult health behaviours and psychosocial characteristics by stages of the socioeconomic lifecourse. *Social Science and Medicine, 44*(6), 809–819.

Macarov, D. (2003). *What the market does to people: Privatization, globalization, and poverty.* Atlanta, GA: Clarity Press.

Menahem, G. (2010). How can the decommodified security ratio assess social protection systems? *Working Paper No. 529.* Syracuse, NY: Luxembourg Income Study.

Mikkonen, J., & Raphael, D. (2010). *Social determinants of health: The Canadian facts.* Retrieved from http:/thecanadianfacts.org

Murphy, B., Roberts, P., & Wolfson, M. (2007). High income Canadians. *Perspectives on Labour and Income, 8*(12), 1–3.

Navarro, V. (Ed.) (2004). *The political and social contexts of health.* Amityville, NY: Baywood Press.

Olsen, G. (2010). *Power and inequality: A comparative introduction.* Toronto: Oxford University Press.

Peters, J. (2012). Free markets, and the decline of unions and good jobs. In J. Peters (Ed.), *Boom, bust and crisis: Labour, corporate power and politics in Canada* (pp. 16–54). Halifax: Fernwood.

Pontusson, J. (2005). *Inequality and prosperity: Social Europe versus liberal America.* Ithaca, NY: Cornell University Press.

Raphael, D. (2011a). The political economy of health promotion: Part 2, national provision of the prerequisites of health. *Health Promotion International, 28*(1), 112–132.

Raphael, D. (2011b). Poverty and health. In D. Raphael (Ed.), *Poverty and policy in Canada: Implications for health and quality of life* (2nd ed., pp. 223–264). Toronto: Canadian Scholars' Press.

Raphael, D. (2014). Beyond policy analysis: the raw politics behind opposition to healthy public policy. *Health Promotion International, 30*(2), 380–396.

Raphael, D. (Ed.) (2016). *Social determinants of health: Canadian perspectives* (3rd ed.). Toronto: Canadian Scholars' Press.

Saint-Arnaud, S., & Bernard, P. (2003). Convergence or resilience? A hierarchial cluster analysis of the welfare regimes in advanced countries. *Current Sociology, 51*(5), 499–527.

Schrecker, T., & Bambra, C. (2015). *How politics makes us sick: Neoliberal epidemics.* Basingstoke, U.K.: Palgrave Macmillan.

Scott, J. (2014). *Stratification and power: Structures of class, status and command.* Hoboken, NJ: John Wiley & Sons.

Stone, D. (2011). *Policy paradox: The art of political decision making* (3rd ed.). New York: W. W. Norton & Company.

Swank, D. (2010). Globalization. In F. G. Castles, S. Leibfried, J. Lewis, H. Obinger, & C. Pierson (Eds.), *The Oxford handbook of the welfare state* (pp. 318–330). Oxford: Oxford University Press.

Teeple, G. (2000). *Globalization and the decline of social reform: Into the twenty-first century.* Aurora, ON: Garamond Press.

Teeple, G. (2006). Foreword. In D. Raphael, T. Bryant, & M. Rioux (Eds.), *Staying alive: Critical perspectives on health, illness, and health care* (pp. 1–4). Toronto: Canadian Scholars' Press.

Tjepkema, M., Wilkins, R., & Long, A. (2013). Cause-specific mortality by income adequacy in Canada: A 16-year follow-up study. *Health Reports, 24*(7), 14–22.

Whiteside, H. (2015). *Purchase for profit: Public-private partnerships and Canada's public health care system* (Vol. 50). Toronto: University of Toronto Press.

Wilkinson, R. (1996). *Unhealthy societies: The afflictions of inequality.* New York: Routledge.

# CHAPTER 4

## The Right to Health: Human Rights Approaches to Health

*Marcia Rioux*[1]

## INTRODUCTION

> A table, which distances them from the litigants, the "third party" that is the judges. ... Now this idea that there are people who are neutral in relation to others, that they can make judgments about them on the basis of ideas of justice which have absolute validity, and that their decisions must be acted upon, I believe that all this is far removed from and quite foreign to the very idea of modern justice. (Foucault, 1980, p. 8)

How many people must feel like they are in front of such judges every time they need health care or every time they feel the influences of societies that do not provide justice in the context of the right to health? For people who are concerned with health, where judgments are the nature of the business for healthcare providers, for hospital administrators, for social policy-makers and analysts, for economists, for scientists, and for individuals, the who, how, and why of judgments are important. Judgments are made about which diseases take precedence in research, which determinants of health are addressed, about who will be vulnerable to ill health, and about which populations and individuals have access to treatment, to suggest just a few.

A recent development in understanding health is to contextualize it from the perspective of human rights—that is, to put it in the framework of justice as a way to approach it. "Health is influenced by a variety of social, economic and environmental factors, and not just by access to health care. ... The extensive empirical literature on social determinants of health—and inequalities in health—has yet to be matched by an appreciation of the normative underpinnings of health equity ..." (Anand, Peter, & Sen, 2004, p. 2). Moreover, health equity expresses a commitment of public health to social justice (Anand et al., 2004). A rights-based approach to health means using human rights as a framework for health development. It means making principles of human rights integral to the design, implementation, and evaluation of policies and programs. And it means assessing the human rights implications of health policy, programs, and legislation.

---

**Box 4.1:** Human Rights Principles

---

- Universal inherence
- Inalienability
- Inherent self-worth of each individual
- Autonomy and self-determination
- Equality for all
- Preservation of freedom of individual through social support

A human rights and social justice approach enables the use of various categories of rights and recognizes how rights have to be a concern in thinking about approaches to health and social policy that enhance, rather than diminish, the well-being of all people. These include political and civil rights, such as the right to life, freedom of opinion, a fair trial, and protection from torture and violence. These rights are the most common concern of nations, particularly in the North and West. Human rights also include economic, social, and cultural rights, such as the right to work, social protection, an adequate standard of living, the highest possible standards of physical and mental health, education, and enjoyment of the benefits of cultural freedom and scientific progress. Finally, human rights include the right of nations to development, economic autonomy, and security of their citizens.

Health, then, is not a condition that is set apart from issues of social justice, social values, or citizenship. Health is affected by cultural norms and practices; international, national, and regional laws; and individual and societal values. Health is connected to international agreements relating to human rights. It is linked to the national constitutional and legal protection of individuals.[2] These guarantees are intrinsic to the defence of equal access to treatment and an equal right to well-being. Notions of economic efficiency (Deber, 1999) and evidence-based quality of practice cannot be relied upon to provide a basic guarantee to good health, and even democratic political mandates and ethical standards do not do so. Even hospital ethics committees and self-regulating professions cannot guarantee equality in health, nor do they necessarily see that as their role. While an ethics committee will make sure that valid consent is assured for all patients in a hospital, they are not in a position to ensure that drug protocols that are not used in that hospital become available to patients. Medical care and healthcare decisions cannot be isolated from our basic social contract as though medical ethics and laws are a mysterious, exclusive domain comprehensible only to professional practitioners. Instead, it is necessary to apply existing rules of non-discrimination and human rights to health policy decisions, as we are in fact required to do by human rights policy, standards, and ethics.

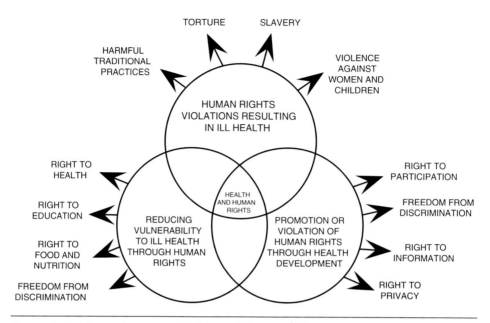

**Figure 4.1:** Linkages between Health and Human Rights

*Source:* World Health Organization. (2002). *Health and human rights.* Health and Human Rights Publication Series (1, p. 8). Geneva: Author.

## A SOCIAL IMPERATIVE

Using a human rights perspective is a means to making equitable health outcomes a social imperative. It would be naive to suggest that such an approach could provide a clear map through the minefields of decision-making, but it does give us a single standard against which we can measure our health priorities at the international level, the national level, and in individual treatment decisions. For example, it does hold us to a norm of non-discrimination in the provision of healthcare services so that a person with an income of less than $20,000 is not less likely to get a heart bypass than someone with an income of over $100,000.

What are the building blocks of health and human rights? The right to "the highest attainable standard of health" was first articulated in the World Health Organization (WHO) constitution, which was adopted by the World Health Conference in 1946 (WHO, 1948). It was reiterated in the 1978 *Declaration of Alma Atal*,[3] the United Nations' *International Covenant on Economic, Social, and Cultural Rights*[4] (ICESCR; UN General Assembly, 1966), which has been ratified by 145 countries and is the most authoritative international instrument. In 2000, the committee for that covenant adopted a General Comment on the right to health (UN Committee on Economic, Social, and Cultural Rights, 2000), clarifying[5] the meaning of this right. Most important, the General Comment recognized the relationship of the right to health to other rights, including the right to food, housing, work, education, participation, the enjoyment of the benefits of scientific progress and its application, life, non-discrimination, equality, the prohibition against torture, privacy, access to information, and freedom of association, assembly, and movement. It recognized that the right to health was dependent on these and other rights. In other words, the right to health is more than access to health care and applies equally to other social determinants of health. The General Comment further set out four criteria for evaluating the right to health: availability, accessibility, acceptability, and quality. As of January 2018, 166 countries have ratified the ICESCR (UN Office of the High Commissioner for Human Rights [OHCHR], 2018). Furthermore, every state has ratified at least one international treaty recognizing the right to health or some element of that right (UN OHCHR 2009). According to Eleanor Kinney (2000), 109 countries have recognized a right to health in their constitutions. Most states of the world have committed to protecting the right to health through international declarations and domestic policy and legislation. In 1992, the United Nations Commission on Human Rights created the mandate of a special rapporteur to ensure the right of every person to the highest attainable standard of physical and mental health.

---

**Box 4.2:** Selected International Instruments Incorporating a Right to Health

---

*Universal Declaration of Human Rights* (1948)
Article 25 (1): "Everyone has a right to a standard of living adequate for the health of himself and his family, including food, clothing, housing and medical care and necessary social services."

*International Convention on the Elimination of All Forms of Racial Discrimination* (1963)
Article 5 (e) (iv): States undertake to prohibit and eliminate racial discrimination and equality before the law, in respect to "The right to public health, medical care, social security, and social services."

*International Covenant on Economic, Social and Cultural Rights* (1966)
Article 12(1): States Parties recognize "the rights of everyone to the enjoyment of the highest attainable standard of physical and mental health."
    Article 12(2): Illustrates the breadth of areas that needed to be addressed and other human rights that have to be addressed "to achieve the full realization of this right."

*Convention on the Elimination of All Forms of Discrimination against Women* (1979)
Article 12(1): States Parties "shall take all appropriate measures to eliminate discrimination against women in the field of health care in order to ensure, on a basis of equality of men and women, access to health care services, including those related to family planning."

*Convention on the Right of the Child* (1989)

Article 24(1): "States Parties recognize the right of the child to the enjoyment of the highest attainable standard of health and to facilities for the treatment of illness and rehabilitation of health. States Parties shall strive to ensure that no child is deprived of his or her right to access to such health care services."

*Convention on the Protection of the Rights of All Migrant Workers and Members of Their Families* (1990)

Article 28: "Migrant workers and members of their families shall have the right to receive any medical care that is urgently required for the preservation of their life or the avoidance of irreparable harm to their health on the basis of equality of treatment with nationals of the State concerned. Such emergency medical care shall not be refused them by reason of any irregularity with regard to stay or employment."

Article 43(e): "Migrant workers shall enjoy equality of treatment with nationals of the State of employment in relation to: (e) Access to social and health services, provided that the requirements for participation in the respective schemes are met."

Article 45(c): "Members of the families of migrant workers shall, in the State of employment, enjoy equality of treatment with nationals of that State in relation to: (c) Access to social and health services, provided that requirements for participation in the respective schemes are met."

*Convention on the Rights of Persons with Disabilities* (2006)

Article 25: "States Parties recognize that persons with disabilities have the right to the enjoyment of the highest attainable standard of health without discrimination on the basis of disability. States Parties shall take all appropriate measures to ensure access for persons with disabilities to health services that are gender-sensitive, including health-related rehabilitation."

*United Nations Declaration on the Rights of Indigenous Peoples* (2007)

Article 17.2: "States shall in consultation and cooperation with indigenous peoples take specific measures to protect indigenous children from economic exploitation and from performing any work that is likely to be hazardous or to interfere with the child's education, or to be harmful to the child's health or physical, mental, spiritual, moral or social development, taking into account their special vulnerability and the importance of education for their empowerment."

Article 21.1: "Indigenous peoples have the right, without discrimination, to the improvement of their economic and social conditions, including, inter alia, in the areas of education, employment, vocational training and retraining, housing, sanitation, health and social security."

Article 23: "Indigenous peoples have the right to determine and develop priorities and strategies for exercising their right to development. In particular, indigenous peoples have the right to be actively involved in developing and determining health, housing and other economic and social programmes affecting them and, as far as possible, to administer such programmes through their own institutions."

Article 24.1: "Indigenous peoples have the right to their traditional medicines and to maintain their health practices, including the conservation of their vital medicinal plants, animals and minerals. Indigenous individuals also have the right to access, without any discrimination, to all social and health services."

Article 24.2: "Indigenous individuals have an equal right to the enjoyment of the highest attainable standard of physical and mental health. States shall take the necessary steps with a view to achieving progressively the full realization of this right."

Article 29.3: "States shall also take effective measures to ensure, as needed, that programmes for monitoring, maintaining and restoring the health of indigenous peoples, as developed and implemented by the peoples affected by such materials, are duly implemented."

*United Nations Declaration of the High-level Dialogue on International Migration and Development* (2013)
Article 13: "Express the commitment to protect the human rights of migrant children, given their vulnerability, particularly unaccompanied migrant children, and to provide for their health, education and psychosocial development, ensuring that the best interests of the child are a primary consideration in policies of integration, return and family reunification."

---

**Box 4.3:** Key Aspects of the Right to Health

---

- The right to health is an inclusive right.
- The right to health contains freedoms.
- The right to health contains entitlements.
- Health services, goods, and facilities must be provided to all without any discrimination.
- All services, goods, and facilities must be available, accessible, acceptable, affordable, and of good quality.

---

*Source:* United Nations Office of the High Commissioner for Human Rights. (2009). *Fact sheet no. 31: The right to health.* Geneva: Author.

The Committee on Economic, Social, and Cultural Rights, which monitors the ICESCR, has included the following as underlying determinants of health: safe drinking water and adequate sanitation, safe food, adequate nutrition and housing, healthy working and environmental conditions, health-related education and information, and gender equality.

The freedoms that are protected with the recognition of a right to health include notions of freedom from non-consensual medical treatment, including such practices as medical experiments and research; forced sterilization; torture; and cruel, inhumane, and degrading treatment or punishment. The entitlements that are guaranteed within a notion of the right to health include the right to health protection; access to basic health services; access to needed medicines; prevention and control of diseases; maternal, child, and reproductive health; access to health education and information; and participation in health decision-making at the state and local level.

The provision of health services and facilities without discrimination is a key human rights principle and underlies the right to health. Finally, all services must be available, accessible, acceptable, affordable, and of good quality. Availability includes adequate public health (including sanitation and safe drinking water) and healthcare facilities (including hospitals and clinics), as well as sufficient trained personnel and essential unexpired drugs. Under accessibility are the four categories of non-discrimination, physical accessibility, economic accessibility, and information accessibility. Acceptability means that health care is provided with attention to criteria of medical ethics, cultural sensitivity, gender and life cycle needs, and confidentiality. Health facilities and goods and services are expected to be scientifically and medically appropriate and of good quality.

Taken together, these international instruments outline a normative standard for the right to health. Most states have national constitutions that incorporate the key principles of respect for human rights, and many states have signed regional and international standards and treaties that specify the particular human rights they protect. The right to health is a comprehensive right extending to timely, affordable, and appropriate health care and to the basic determinants of health, including safe and potable water and adequate nutrition, healthy occupational and environmental conditions, and access to health-related information and education. It is also the right to the enjoyment of a variety of facilities, goods, and services necessary for the realization of the highest standard of health. And, finally, the facilities, goods and services, and the underlying social determinants of health have to be available, accessible, acceptable, and of good quality.

## DIFFERENTIAL ACCESS TO HEALTH AND WELL-BEING

The right to health cannot be viewed in isolation. It is closely related to the enjoyment of other human rights, including non-discrimination and equality, which are fundamental human rights principles and critical components of the right to health. Human rights are interdependent, indivisible, and interrelated. Links between one right and another can impact the realization of both rights. For example, there is a link between the right to health and the right to education, which can be found in the higher health status of those with higher education levels and higher inclusive education levels. A disproportional degree of compromised health is borne by those who are marginalized and vulnerable in society.

> It is one of the greatest of contemporary social injustices that people who live in the most disadvantaged circumstances have more illnesses, more disability and shorter lives than those who are more affluent. (Benzeval, Judge, & Whitehead, 1995, p. xxi)

This is a result of a number of factors that can include direct discrimination, as has been the case when individuals with disabilities are not given the same priority for organ transplants. In other cases, people's well-being is compromised due to their environment and living conditions. Examples include living in institutional settings, not uncommon among people with intellectual disabilities and seniors, in which their basic health needs are not met, or when people live in urban slums in which their access to good health is restricted by the lack of clean drinking water.

More often even than direct discrimination are the instances of indirect or covert discrimination faced by people who are marginalized, and the failure of governments and others in positions of power to put in place policies and programs that would address the inequalities in health and illness. These are conditions that may be both national and international. For example, governments' failure to monitor national industries so that they meet at least the minimum legal environmental standard in their home country when they are operating in developing countries is an omission that leads to inequity in health and disease patterns. Similarly, government failures to address income inequities results in differential patterns of disease based on socio-economic status.[6]

The *Declaration on the Elimination of the Violence against Women* (UN General Assembly, 1993) recognizes the link between violence against women and the historically unequal power relations between men and women.

With respect to health and health care, it is now generally recognized that the prohibition of discrimination includes:

> ... any discrimination in access to health care and the underlying determinants of health, as well as to means and entitlements for their procurement, on the grounds of race, colour, sex, language, religion, political or other opinion, property, birth, physical or mental disability, health status (including HIV/AIDS), sexual orientation, civil, political, social or other status, which has the intention or effect of nullifying or impairing the equal enjoyment or exercise of the right to health. (UN Committee on Economic, Social, and Cultural Rights, 2000)

The impact of discrimination is increased when an individual faces more than one source of discrimination. One example is presented in *Moore v. British Columbia (Education)*, [2012] 3 SCR 360, in which a student diagnosed with dyslexia and learning disabilities was not being accommodated within the public school system. The case went to the Supreme Court of Canada, which found that there were no alternatives for students with dyslexia and accommodations were not provided.

There are many examples of systemic discrimination in health. A precedent-setting case in Canada helps to underline the way in which systemic discrimination can occur. In October 1997, the Canadian Supreme Court, in *Eldridge v. British Columbia*, held that the legislation governing healthcare services and hospitals in the province was discriminatory because, in the case of the three deaf applicants, it neither included sign-language interpreter services as an insured service, nor required hospitals to provide sign-language interpreter services. The Court also held that the government had violated the equality provisions of the Canadian *Charter of Rights and Freedoms* in its implementation of the provincial medical services plan. The Court argued that in order for deaf people to receive the benefit of medical services, they required communication with their doctors. Interpreters were not an ancillary service but an integral part of medical care. In providing a benefit scheme, the state was obliged to provide the benefit in a non-discriminatory manner. "Failure to provide interpreters meant that deaf people would receive an inferior quality of health care to hearing persons" (Mosoff & Grant, 1999, p. 42).

This decision is important for a number of reasons. First, it is the Court's holding that "once the state provides a benefit, it is obliged to do so in a non-discriminatory manner" (*Eldridge v. British Columbia*, Ministry of Health (1997) 3 SCR 624). Second, it clarifies the interpretation of equality protected under the *Charter*. The denial of equality in *Eldridge* arose from the government's failure to take action (rather than the imposition of a burden). The discrimination arose from the adverse effects of a public benefit scheme that failed to provide the same level of health service (adverse impact discrimination) for everyone. The Court held that:

> To argue that governments should be entitled to provide benefits to the general population without ensuring that disadvantaged members of society have the resources to take full advantage of those benefits bespeaks a thin and impoverished vision of S 15(1). It is belied, more importantly, by the thrust of this Court's equality jurisprudence. (*Eldridge v. British Columbia*, Ministry of Health (1997) 3 SCR 624)

The principle held by the Court in this case is that the government has an obligation to remedy inequality notwithstanding that the health benefit scheme appeared neutral and the remedy meant that the government had to spend money. The third issue of importance is the Court's ruling that effective communication is an indispensable component of the delivery of a medical service. The Court recognized the systemic nature of the discrimination faced by people with disabilities in the health system and recognized that discrimination cannot be redressed without changes to the definition of the health services that a government provides (Degener, 1995).

## APPLYING THE RIGHT TO HEALTH TO SPECIFIC GROUPS

For individuals to have access to the highest attainable standard of health, states have to provide access to health care and services and living conditions that are not discriminatory or that differentiate particular groups in way that disadvantages some groups. It is not simply a matter of providing equal access to health care and other social determinants of health but providing those in a way that results in equal outcome (Rioux, 2003). For those who are particularly vulnerable to reduced health status as a consequence of their circumstances, whether biomedical or social or political, states have to provide affirmative measures to address these situations. The following section looks at the particular health circumstances and health rights of groups that are socially excluded. In these cases, the importance of affirmative action as fundamental to addressing their health outcomes are considered.

## DISABILITY AND THE RIGHT TO HEALTH

The UN *Convention on the Rights of Persons with Disabilities* (CRPD) was formally opened for signature and ratification in March 2007. More than 15% of the world population has disabilities, and 80 million of them live in low-income countries (WHO, 2011). Most disabled people are poor and have little or no access to basic services, including acute health services, rehabilitation, and other primary health services. There are a number of articles of the Convention that specifically address the health of people with disabilities, including Article 9 (access to medical facilities), Article 15 (freedom from torture or cruel, inhumane, or degrading treatment or punishment), Article 16 (freedom from exploitation, violence, and abuse), Article 20 (personal mobility), Article 22 (respect for privacy), Article 23 (respect for home and family), Article 25 (health), and Article 27 (habilitation and rehabilitation). Many of the other articles also impact health either directly or indirectly as they impact the social determinants of health and are interdependent factors.

The right to health for people with disabilities is often infringed because of their limited access to health services. They are commonly unable to take advantage of available

**Box 4.4:** Food for Thought

Should one deny medical care to a person solely on the grounds of their disability?

medical services because of assumptions by others about their quality of life and whether it is beneficial to them or to others to provide limited medical and health benefits that others receive. Such is the example of Terry Urquhart, a young man with Down syndrome, being denied a place on a waiting list for a lung transplant. It was purported by the hospital that because he apparently lacked "satisfactory intelligence" (Lock, 1995)—that is, because he had Down syndrome—he would not benefit as much from a transplant as someone without a disability, so the hospital staff argued solely on the basis of his disability that he should not be placed on the list. Triaging is not uncommon in medical care, and widely held prejudices against people with disabilities and other marginal statuses often result in discrimination in access to the benefits of medical treatment. Health needs of people with disabilities are regularly limited to curing or improving their impairments, rather than improving their health. The reported incidences of selective non-treatment of people with disabilities suggest that medical standards are differentially applied, a practice that infringes the right to health and rehabilitation. People with disabilities are also particularly vulnerable to standards of living that affect health: poverty, poor housing, unemployment, lack of services, and literacy.

The *Principles for the Protection of Persons with Mental Illness and the Improvement of Mental Health Care* address issues related to the right to health in principles 6–14 and 22 (UN General Assembly, 1991). These principles cover confidentiality; the role of the community and culture; standards of care, treatment, medication, consent to treatment; notice of rights, rights, and conditions in mental health facilities; and resources for mental health facilities.[7] The Mental Health Commission of Canada (2018) released a report highlighting the need for a performance measurement framework focused on mental health and addiction, an initiative driven by the increasing international recognition of the detrimental effects of mental illness on individuals and communities.

The Committee on Economic, Social, and Cultural Rights (CESCR) General Comment no. 5 (1994) on people with disabilities holds that the same level of medical care within the same medical system for those with disabilities and those without disabilities is a key element of the right to health. The UN Economic and Social Council (ECOSOC) interprets Article 12 of the ICESCR as a guarantee "to have access to, and to benefit from, those medical and social services … which enable persons with disabilities to become independent, prevent further disabilities and support social integration." The paragraph continues:

> Similarly, such persons should be provided with rehabilitation services which would enable them to reach and sustain their optimum level of independence and functioning. All such services should be provided in such a way that the persons concerned are able to maintain full respect for their rights and dignity. (UN Committee on Economic, Social, and Cultural Rights, 1994, para. 34)

The Mental Health Care Principles, the UN *Convention on the Rights of Persons with Disabilities*, and the ECOSOC approach to the right to health in the context of disability

---

**Box 4.5:** International Instruments Recognizing a Right to Health

---

**Regional Instruments Recognizing a Right to Health**
*European Social Charter* (1961)
*African Charter on Human and Peoples' Rights* (1981)
*Additional Protocol to the American Convention on Human Rights in the Area of Economic, Social and Cultural Rights* (1988)
*The World Health Report: Health Systems Financing: The Path to Universal Coverage* (2010)

**Other United Nations Affirmations on the Right to Health**
*Vienna Declaration and Programme of Action* (1993)
*Commission on Human Rights proclaimed the right to health* (2000)

**Special Rapporteur Reports on the Right to Health**
*Realization of Health* (2013)
*Right to Enjoyment of Physical and Mental Health* (2015)
*Equity, Non-Discrimination and Equality in Millennium Development Goals* (2016)
*Mental Health* (2017)
*Corruption in Health Sector* (2017)
*Health and Confinement* (2018)

---

are important because they recognize the social determinants of health—that is, determinants of health that originate from the exercise of other rights, including self-determination and control over one's own lifestyle and surroundings, human dignity, inclusion and active participation in the community, and non-discrimination. This connection between health status and the exercise of rights has significant implications for people with disabilities.

The ICESCR's General Comment no. 14 on the right to health lays out the core obligations and elements of the right: "availability, accessibility, acceptability and quality" (UN Committee on Economic, Social, and Cultural Rights, 2000, para. 12). Non-discrimination is a key element of accessibility, and the ICESCR highlights the accessibility needs of vulnerable groups, including people with disabilities. It stresses "the need to ensure that not only the public health sector but also private providers of health services and facilities comply with the principle of non-discrimination in relation to persons with disabilities." Both physical and mental disabilities are specifically included as prohibited grounds for discrimination (UN Committee on Economic, Social, and Cultural Rights, 2000, para. 14). Furthermore, persons with disabilities should be provided with "the same range, quality and standard of free or affordable health care and programmes as provided to other persons" (CRPD, art. 25, 26).

The UN's *Convention on the Elimination of All Forms of Discrimination against Women*'s (CEDAW) General Recommendation no. 24 on women and health[8] refers to the need to give special attention to the health needs and rights of women who belong to vulnerable and disadvantaged groups, including women with physical or mental disabilities (UN General Assembly, 1979, para. 6). The CRPD emphasizes in Articles 5 and 6 the particular vulnerabilities of women and children with disabilities, recognizing that women and children experience similar health conditions in different ways than men and adults. It also recognizes that both women and children have increased/higher prevalence of certain health conditions, for example, for women related to childbirth and pregnancy and also significant issues related to violence and abuse.

The General Recommendation of CEDAW also refers specifically to the needs of women with disabilities:

> Women with disabilities, of all ages, often have difficulty with physical access to health services. Women with mental disabilities are particularly vulnerable, while there is limited understanding, in general, of the broad range of risks to mental health to which women are disproportionately susceptible as a result of gender discrimination, violence, poverty, armed conflict, dislocation and other forms of social deprivation. States parties should take appropriate measures to ensure that health services are sensitive to the needs of women with disabilities and are respectful of their human rights and dignity. (UN General Assembly, 1979, para. 14)

The United Nations *Declaration on the Rights of Indigenous Peoples* (UNDRIP), adopted by the General Assembly on Thursday September 13, 2007, outlines international human rights of Indigenous persons. Indigenous persons around the world are subject to inequalities of health care and are frequently denied the right to health. This is largely a result of poor living conditions, forced displacement, and armed conflict. Statistically, Indigenous persons are more likely to experience disability and ill health, primarily a result of social determinants of health such as access to education, food, and shelter. The right to health for Indigenous persons articulated in UNDRIP also acknowledges the right to traditional medicine and health practices, suggesting Indigenous persons must participate in the implementation of health services that affect Indigenous persons and populations.

The United Nations Committee on the Rights of the Child (CRC) has issued General Comment no. 4 on adolescent health and development. The committee requires states to "adopt special measures to ensure the physical, sexual and mental integrity of adolescents with disabilities, who are particularly vulnerable to abuse and neglect" (UN Committee on the Rights of the Child, 2003, para. 12). The committee notes that systematic collection of data is necessary to monitor the right to health, including data on adolescents with disabilities (UN Committee on the Rights of the Child, 2003, para. 13). The committee reaffirms that those adolescents with mental and/or physical disabilities "have an equal right to the highest attainable standard of physical and mental health." This obligates states parties to:

> (a) Ensure that health facilities, goods and services are available and accessible to all adolescents with disabilities and that these facilities and services promote their self-reliance and their active participation in the community; (b) ensure that the necessary equipment and personal support are available to enable them to move around, participate and communicate; (c) pay specific attention to the special needs relating to the sexuality of adolescents with disabilities; and (d) remove barriers that hinder adolescents with disabilities in realizing their rights. (UN Committee on the Rights of the Child, 2003, para. 35)

There are some particular rights that need to be protected for people with disabilities. These include[9] the quality and accessibility of services as well as the availability of a range of services, particularly rights related to:

- Free and informed consent; prevention of unwanted medical and related interventions and corrective surgeries from being imposed on people with disabilities
- Protection of the privacy of health and rehabilitation information
- Participation in legislative and policy development, as well as in the planning, delivery, and evaluation of health and rehabilitation services

Finally, and perhaps most importantly, the "highest attainable standard of health" for people with disabilities is related to the recognition that they are entitled to the same human rights, citizenship, and social inclusion as others. The presumption in public health and in the biomedical sciences that the goal of health policies is to reduce illness, death, *and disability* is to fundamentally deny the nature of disability as a social condition and to stigmatize people with disabilities in a way that drives an irresolvable wedge between health and disability.

Defining disability as a contingent part of ill health is, in itself, the most fundamental barrier to the right to health for people with disabilities.

## REPRODUCTION AND THE RIGHT TO HEALTH

Reproductive health refers to people being able to have satisfying and safe sexual expression and to make decisions about whether and when they want to reproduce. It is an area of health that is fraught with an overlay of norms and values about sexuality, responsibility, and prejudice. It involves the enjoyment of sexuality and choice in pregnancy; protection against abuse, coercion, and harassment; and safety from sexually transmitted diseases. Two international conferences in the 1990s focused attention on the promotion and protection of human rights in reproductive and sexual health. The *Convention on the*

*Elimination of All Forms of Discrimination against Women* (1979) also specifically mentioned women's rights related to reproductive planning.

In the *Programme of Action* developed at the International Conference on Population and Development in Cairo in 1994 (UN Department of Economic, Social Information, and Policy Analysis, 1995) and subsequently at the International Conference on Women in Beijing in 1995, reproductive health was defined in the context of the World Health Organization's definition of health as a "state of complete physical, mental and social well-being and not merely the absence of disease or infirmity in all matters relating to the reproductive system and to its functions and processes" (UN Department of Public Information, 1996, para. 94).

The *Programme of Action* laid out the way in which reproductive rights are incorporated in the scope of human rights:

> These rights rest on the recognition of the basic right of all couples and individuals to decide freely and responsibly the number, spacing and timing of their children, and to have the information and means to do so; and the right to attain the highest level of sexual and reproductive health. It also includes their right to make decisions concerning reproduction free of discrimination, coercion and violence, as expressed in human rights documents. (UN Department of Economic, Social Information, and Policy Analysis, 1995, para. 7.3)

How are these rights expressed? An individual's right to free choice in decisions concerning their body and their reproductive options has been at the forefront of the reproductive rights movement. Some specific human rights that can contribute to reproductive and sexual health and well-being include rights relating to: life, survival, security, and sexuality; reproductive self-determination and free choice of maternity; health and the benefits of scientific progress; non-discrimination and due respect for difference; and information, education, and decision-making (Cook, Dickens, & Fathalla, 2003).

In practice, these rights have been protected by courts (Cook & Dickens, 2003; Cook, Dickens, & Fathalla, 2003, p. 159–161, 164, 170, 187–209; Cook, Dickens, Ngwena, & Plata, 2001) in cases involving rights to basic services necessary for reproductive and sexual health (rights to life, survival, security, and sexuality). These would include such examples as one's right to go through pregnancy and childbirth safely and protection of the confidentiality of people seeking reproductive health services.

Reproductive rights are an area of health in which examples of inequity are widespread. Not only is this inequity found between genders in reproductive rights, but also it is clear that there are significant inequities among countries. In particular, the differential is evident between high-income countries and low-income countries, and between countries in which the rights of women are respected and in those in which they are not. One's ability to control one's own fertility and safety from sexually transmitted communicable diseases is of particular concern for inequities and the contravention of human rights.

"Inability of individuals, and particularly of women, in developing countries to regulate and control their fertility is not only affecting the health of the people immediately concerned, but has implications for global stability and for the balance between population and natural resources and between people and environment, and is a violation of women's human rights" (Cook, Dickens, & Fathalla, 2003, p. 13).

## HIV/AIDS AND THE RIGHT TO HEALTH

The transmission of communicable diseases is another important and pressing issue in ensuring the right to health on an international basis (UN Office of the High Commissioner for Human Rights, 1998). Some 40 million people around the world now live with HIV/AIDS, and thousands die every day (WHO, 2017). It is estimated that treatment reaches fewer than 5% of those affected. As access to health care is one of the fundamental instruments of the right to health, it is of particular concern. People who are not receiving drugs are those in low-income countries and marginalized populations in high-income countries. For many people in low-income countries, the cost of treatment remains intolerably high. This type of discrimination is a human rights violation[10] that is a barrier both to prevention efforts and access to treatment and care.

The United Nations issued comprehensive, detailed, and specific guidelines in 1998 based on the recognition that there is a fundamental relationship between human rights and the HIV/AIDS epidemic. The guidelines have three broad and interrelated approaches:

> … improvement of governmental capacity for acknowledging the government's responsibility for multisectoral coordination and accountability; widespread reform of laws and legal support services, with a focus on anti-discrimination, protection of public health, and improvement of the status of women, children and marginalized groups; and support for increased private sector and community participation in the response to HIV/AIDS … (Cohen, 2002, p. 5)

An important issue here, as with reproductive health and disability, is how to understand and address the social determinants of vulnerability. Another issue is how to address the discrimination resulting from the subordination of women and girls; hostility toward gay, lesbian, bisexual, and transgender and Two-Spirit people; the subordination of Indigenous peoples; prisoners' dependency on others to prevent the spread of disease in prisons; and a disproportionate emphasis on controlling drug use and sex work through criminal and public health law.

This coercive use of law, added to demands to curtail the conventional notion of confidentiality of medical testing, makes clear the ease with which people's human rights can be disregarded in the area of public health. It exposes the fundamental importance of using human rights as a framework if people are to realize their health and well-being.

Increasingly, since 1988, there have been efforts to "add and integrate a societal dimension with the previous individually centered, risk-reduction approach" (Mann, 1999b, p. 218). The conventional notion that disease is a dynamic event taking place in a static environment as the basis for education and services has been challenged as the answer to the HIV/AIDS epidemic. Risk reduction is not sufficient to control the pandemic (Coates, Richter, and Caceres, 2008; Mann, 1999b).

In this context, access to information about the transmission of HIV/AIDS is important as a means to prevent transmission; adequate medical care and treatment, nutrition, shelter, and income are necessary to reduce the susceptibility of people with HIV/AIDS to ill health and disease; people with HIV/AIDS have to be engaged in the design and implementation of prevention programs and support services; and the stigma associated with HIV/AIDS, which results in discrimination in the workplace, housing, immigration, and access to health and social services, has to be addressed.

These conditions are similar to those that apply in cases of other marginalized populations and result in the inability to exercise the right to health. The enforcement of basic human rights—as outlined in international human rights treaties and instruments as well as in national law—is broad enough to address these pressing issues in health.

## HEALTH RESEARCH AND THE RIGHT TO HEALTH

The expenditures on health research, which result in the vast majority of health research and development being spent on health problems that affect only a small proportion of the world's population, have significant right-to-health implications. The World Health Organization calls these the "neglected diseases,"[11] which it says affect more than one billion people worldwide. First, "neglected diseases are hidden diseases as they affect almost exclusively extremely poor populations living in remote areas beyond the reach of health services" (Beyrer et al., 2007). Their low mortality despite high morbidity places them near the bottom of mortality tables and, in the past, they have received low priority (Kindhauser, 2003, p. 6).

Second, they are also neglected because, confined to poor populations, there has been a lack of financial incentives to develop drugs and vaccines for markets that cannot pay. And, third, they are neglected because even where effective and low-cost drugs are available, the inability to pay results in little or no demand for them. In other words, there is no effective market and no effective financial incentive for health research and development for new drugs, vaccines, or other medical interventions.[12] For example, it is estimated that a staggering 3.9 billion people are at risk of infection with dengue viruses (Brady et al., 2012; WHO, 2018). Article 2 of the ICESCR states that signatories have a responsibility "to take steps ... through international assistance and co-operation ... with a view to achieving progressively the full realization of the rights recognized in the present Covenant."

However, international support for such epidemics is hindered by the protection of trade relationships with countries such as the United States. Such relationships and trade agreements have taken precedence over the need for safe, low-cost, effective medications in low-income countries (Lexchin, 2013).

## IMPACT OF GLOBALIZATION AND THE RIGHT TO HEALTH

Globalization and the flow of capital have created new types of human rights issues for health (Fidler, 2000), many of which have been ignored until recently. The flow of capital can create new employment opportunities in some areas, but the consequence of those new jobs may be conditions that are harmful to the health of the people who work in those jobs or who live in proximity. For example, child labour is well documented in some parts of the majority world (i.e., India, China, and other areas where the majority of the world's population live) and clearly is hazardous to the health of children; environmental hazards may also be a consequence of some types of industry that are in areas where people's right to health is already compromised by poverty, poor nutrition, and unsanitary conditions generally.

A further impact of globalization is its potential to contribute to the spread of disease and pandemics because of people's increased mobility; this was evidenced with the pattern of transmission of severe acute respiratory syndrome (SARS). SARS moved from country to country, airport to airport, and town to town non-contiguously. The failure to see the right to health in its international context can lead to unintended consequences.

Globalization can lead to worldwide marketing of harmful substances. Fast foods, tobacco, and alcohol are examples of such marketing. In some cases, it has been suggested that as the market for tobacco has decreased in high-income countries, promotion of cigarettes has increased in the majority world. The right to health information has arguably been contravened with the marketing of fast foods both in high-income countries and evidently in the majority world. In these cases, relatively low-cost, overprocessed, high-calorie, and minimum-nutrition foods are made available in heavily marketed outlets, appealing in many cases to children and people with limited incomes. The impact of consuming these foods is not made clear to the consumer, nor are the environmental influences of the type of packaging divulged to the consumer.

Increasingly, those engaged with globalization are big business, biomedical research firms, pharmaceutical companies, health management organizations, and health insurance companies. They are non-government and multinational, the consequence of which is that legal control is limited and international human rights law is not very effective (Ahmadiani & Nikfar, 2016). Gostin and Taylor (2009) argue that "health hazards posed by contemporary globalization on human health [result in an urgent need] to facilitate effective multilateral cooperation in advancing the health of populations equitably" (p. 53). They provide a definition of the field of global health law as a basis for moving in this direction.

# MONITORING THE RIGHT TO HEALTH

The UN Special Rapporteur on the Right to Health (UN Economic and Social Council, 2003, p. 7) recommends the following categories of right to health indicators: structural indicators, process indicators, and outcome indicators. He includes in structural indicators those structures, systems, and mechanisms that are necessary to the realization of the right. By way of example, he includes constitutions and policies that incorporate the right to health, lists of essential medicines, and national pharmaceutical policies. Process indicators in this schema measure the degree to which "activities that are necessary to attain certain health objectives are carried out, and the progress of those indicators over time. They monitor, as it were, effort, not outcome" (UN General Assembly 2003, p. 9).

Some examples of process indicators would be the number of times a person sees a skilled health professional during a time of medical need; the number of available healthcare facilities available per population needing them; numbers of people with a particular condition receiving the needed drugs (e.g., people with HIV/AIDS receiving anti-retroviral combination therapy). Finally, outcome indicators measure the results achieved by health-related policies. This would include examples of measures such as maternal mortality rate; perinatal deaths per number of births; number of teens with HIV/AIDS; disease patterns disaggregated by income level, and so on. These outcome indicators are influenced by the wide variety of interrelated factors that affect health status.

Paul Hunt, the UN Special Rapporteur on Health from 2002 to 2008, proposed that a clear distinction needs to be made between health good practices and the right to health good practices. He identified an initial set of criteria for this distinction and has

---

**Box 4.6:** Health Good Practice → Right to Health Good Practice

---

Three criteria needed:
1. demonstrably enhances an individual's or group's enjoyment of one or more elements of the right to health, e.g., by:
   • improving access to essential medicines
   • enhancing quality of the workplace environment
   • reducing discriminatory health practices
   • improving participation of all in health policy-making
   • strengthening right to health accountability mechanisms, etc.
2. pays attention to vulnerable groups, including those living in poverty
3. in process and outcome, the good practice is consistent with the enjoyment of all rights

---

*Source:* UN General Assembly. (2003). *Human rights situations: Human rights situations and reports of Special Rapporteurs and Representatives,* 58th Session, October 10, UN Doc. A/58/427, p. 13.

challenged others to examine the adequacy of those criteria (Hunt, 2003a, 2003b). Thus, he has opened the debate for recognizing that a new framework on the right to health requires a new taxonomy and new criteria to enable the measure of compliance with a human rights approach to health nationally and under international norms and standards.

Special Rapporteur Hunt (2003a) proposed the following as categories for taxonomy to classify initiatives:

- The *availability* of health facilities, goods, and services with the jurisdiction
- The *accessibility without discrimination* in law or fact of health facilities, goods, and services
- The *physical accessibility* of health facilities, goods, and services
- The *economic accessibility* of health facilities, goods, and services
- The *accessibility* of health information
- The *cultural acceptability* of health facilities, goods, and services
- The *quality* of health facilities, goods, and services
- The *active and informed participation* of individuals and groups, especially the vulnerable and disadvantaged, including those living in poverty, in relation to health policies, programs, and projects
- The right to health *monitoring and accountability* mechanisms that are effective, transparent, and accessible

These provide a way to monitor good right to health practice at the national and international level and to measure the degree to which states are in compliance with human rights standards in their policies and programs. The realization of human rights as an indicator of well-being may prove to be more useful than traditional health status indicators (Mann, 1999a). It is necessary to collect statistics and information to foster a culture of accountability and to ultimately realize human rights (UN Development Programme, 2000, p. 10).

## RIGHTS-BASED MONITORING

Monitoring is essential to the exercise of rights. And having input from those whose rights are being protected is a key to understanding what to monitor. Rights are not abstract ideas but are found within the fabric of everyday life, meaning that we need to understand what the idea of the highest attainable standard of health means for people. Having that knowledge, it is possible to understand the outcome of right to health and also the means and compromises needed to enable that to be achieved. A holistic monitoring approach, including both systemic monitoring (monitoring laws, policies, and programs, and individual monitoring [monitoring the individual experience]) provides legitimacy and an evidence base to examine health rights in the context of human rights. Disability Rights Promotion International (DRPI) uses such a participatory approach, including various research methodologies and instruments that have been tried and tested in many countries around the world (Rioux, Pinto, & Parekh, 2015). DRPI is a collaborative human rights project working to establish an international monitoring system for disability rights, including the right to health. Monitoring, including the research questions and method of communication and interviewing, engages people with disabilities themselves (Rioux, Pinto, & Parekh, 2015).

Participatory monitoring involves identifying actual violations at an individual and communal level, examining the violation in relation to one's human rights as assured through human rights treaties, identifying the focus of monitoring, including the monitoring questions, organizing information around the identified issue, and finally collecting and critically examining the information through the various focus areas (Rioux, Pinto, & Parekh, 2015). It is important to put in place holistic monitoring to measure the level of implementation of rights and to provide evidence-based knowledge to understand progressive realization of the right to health.

## CONCLUSIONS

Globalization has led to greater recognition of health as an issue of human rights. States and courts are increasingly bringing health within the ambit of social, economic, cultural, political, and civil rights. This has had real effect. For example, the Supreme Court of Canada has interpreted state neglect of an individual's basic health needs as a denial of the right of security of the person, and the Court has argued the right to non-discrimination as a reason to ensure equitable access to health care. The recognition that controlling HIV/AIDS through criminal and public health law is not as effective as looking at health promotion strategies is an example of the effect of a human rights approach. Each legal precedent and public policy of this nature is an important step forward.

Human rights are another way to understand the problem of poor health status globally, regionally, and locally. They provide a lens by which to decide how to address health and well-being. It is a move away from translating data describing risk and distribution of health conditions being defined primarily or exclusively in individual terms to uncovering the societal dimensions that influence and constrain individual behaviour.

A sustainable human rights framework for health recognizes, at a minimum, that health is a result of social, legal, and economic status, and that a broad set of factors contribute to exclusion and the loss of human rights, which in turn lead to poor health status. It underscores that respect for diversity contributes to well-being. It recognizes that people must be supported in exercising their rights, and that people need a sense of fairness and participation in their communities and societies to reach the highest attainable standard of health. A human rights framework forces governments to address health disparities and holds governments accountable for the societal barriers to good health.

There is still a long way to go, but some progress in recognizing health as a human right is being made. Martin Luther King, Jr., the leader of another great movement for social justice, once said, "The arc of history is long, but it always bends towards justice." The urgency felt by those marginalized outside the boundaries of justice is palpable. But as they push, we can see the direction in which the arc is bending.

## CRITICAL THINKING QUESTIONS

1.  What is meant by a rights-based approach to health?
2.  The United Nations has claimed that health is an issue of human rights. Reframing health as a rights issue rather than an issue of social development changes its context. Why has it taken so long for this to happen? What are the particular circumstances surrounding health that have acted as barriers to this recognition?
3.  Why is it not enough simply to provide more and better medical services for marginalized groups if the goal is to improve health?
4.  How would you explain the differences in health between the rich and poor countries?
5.  If you could rewrite the *United Nations Declaration on the Human Rights*, what clauses would you add that are not there?
6.  If you could rewrite the United Nations Sustainable Development Goal (SDG) Goal #3 on health, what indicators would you add? How would you change the current indicators?

## FURTHER READINGS

Anand, S., Peter, F., & Sen, A. (Eds.). (2004). *Public health, ethics, and equity.* Oxford: Oxford University Press.
This book explores the foundations of health equity from the perspectives of philosophers, anthropologists, economists, and public health experts. It is organized around five major themes: (1) health equity; (2) health, society, and justice; (3) responsibility for health and health care; (4) ethical and measurement problems in health evaluation; and (5) equity and conflicting perspectives on health evaluation.

Cook, R. J., Dickens, B. M., & Fathalla, M. F. (2003). *Reproductive health and human rights: Integrating medicine, ethics, and law.* Oxford: Oxford University Press.
This book explores a unique and important area of study within the umbrella of health and human rights. It provides the different perspectives of medicine, ethics, and law toward human reproduction as a way of understanding how human rights values can interact to improve reproductive and sexual health.

Mann, J. M., Gruskin, S., Grodin, M. S., & Annas, G. J. (Eds.). (1999). *Health and human rights: A reader.* New York: Routledge.
This is an essential work in this field. The authors argue that public health, ethics, and human rights are integrally connected and motivated by the value of human well-being.

Human rights violations adversely affect the community's health, coercive health policies violate human rights, and the two fields are mutually reinforcing.

Office of the High Commissioner for Human Rights. (1998). *Basic human rights instruments*. Geneva: Author.
This is a compilation of the texts of the seven major international human rights treaties and the *Universal Declaration of Human Rights*.

Quinn, G., & Degener, T. (Eds.). (2002). *Human rights and disability: The current use and future potential of United Nations Human Rights Instruments in the context of disability*. Geneva: Office of the High Commission for Human Rights. Retrieved from http://193.194.138.190/disability/study.htm
A comprehensive guide to the literature on disability and human rights, this book covers the shift from traditional medical and charity models of disability to a human rights perspective, carefully documenting the evolution and the way in which international instruments of human rights can be applied to disability.

## RELEVANT WEBSITES

### Canadian HIV/AIDS Legal Network
www.aidslaw.ca
    The Canadian HIV/AIDS Legal Network is a national, community-based, charitable organization working in the area of policy and legal issues raised by HIV/AIDS. It was formed in November 1992 and has over 250 members across Canada and internationally. The website provides a wealth of information on current policies and links to other websites, policy documents, and information on international action.

### Disability Rights Promotion International (DRPI)
www.yorku.ca/drpi
    DRPI is a collaborative human rights project working to establish an international monitoring system for disability rights. The site provides detailed information about the ongoing monitoring in the areas of individual violation focus, system focus—including legislative frameworks, disability case law, and government policies and programs—and media focus.

### United Nations Office of the High Commissioner for Human Rights
www.ohchr.org/english
    The High Commissioner is the principal UN official with responsibility for human rights. This site provides both general information about the High Commissioner's Office, as well as details about the most recent meetings and activities of the commission.

**United Nations Special Rapporteur on Health**

https://www.ohchr.org/en/issues/health/pages/srrighthealthindex.aspx

This site provides the mandate of the UN Special Rapporteur on Health and also links to a number of sites about current activities and special initiatives on health within the framework of the UN Office of the High Commissioner for Human Rights.

**United Nations Treaty Body Database**

https://tbinternet.ohchr.org/SitePages/Home.aspx

This makes available all international treaties and treaty body documents for easy reference.

**World Health Organization (WHO)**

www.who.int/hhr/news/en

This site follows the specific issues of World Health Organization on health and human rights. It provides international news, activities, information resources, databases, and key instruments, and provides updates on health emergencies around the world.

## GLOSSARY

**Biotechnology:** The official definition of biotechnology (European Federation of Bio-technology, 1996) is "the integration of natural sciences and engineering sciences in order to achieve the application of organisms, cells, parts thereof and molecular analogues for products and services." In non-technical terms, it is the use of biological processes to solve problems or make useful products.

**Ethics:** The study of human conduct from the perspective of moral principles, which incorporate the body of obligations and duties that a particular society requires of its members. The field of ethics, sometimes called moral philosophy, involves understanding concepts of right and wrong behaviour.

**Globalization:** The international interaction and influence of people, businesses, and governments.

**Health:** A "state of complete physical, mental and social well-being, and not merely the absence of disease or infirmity" (WHO, 1946). The enjoyment of the highest attainable standard of health is one of the fundamental rights of every human being and is inseparable from the enjoyment of other human rights such as the right to food, housing, adequate income, education, participation, privacy, freedom from torture, and freedom from discrimination.

**Health equity:** A term that contextualizes health from a social justice perspective. It is a commitment of public health to social justice and is the absence of systemic disparities in health among groups with different levels of social advantage or disadvantage.

**Non-discrimination:** A term that describes a situation in which no different or unequal treatment has occurred on a categorical basis that is unjust. The principle of
non-discrimination requires that all rights be guaranteed to everyone without distinction, exclusion, or restriction based on disability or based on race, colour, sex, language, religion, political or other opinion, national or social origin, property, birth,
age, or any other status.

## NOTES

1.  I would like to recognize the contribution of Sukaina Dada, a doctoral student in
    Critical Disablity Studies, for her assistance with updating this chapter.
2.  In Canada, there is a constitutional commitment to reasonable, equal access to
    essential services, and equitable taxation and equality before and under the law.
    This commitment is the basis for all equality rights in Canada, and these constitutional
    guarantees are intrinsic to the defence of equal access to treatment and an equal right
    to well-being.
3.  The Declaration called on national governments to ensure the availability of the
    essentials of primary health care, including: education concerning health problems and
    the methods for preventing and controlling them; promotion of food supply and proper
    nutrition; adequate supply of safe water and basic sanitation; child and maternal
    health care, including family planning; immunization against major infectious diseases;
    prevention and control of locally endemic diseases; appropriate treatment of common
    diseases and injuries; and provision of essential drugs.
4.  International human rights treaties are binding on governments that ratify them. Two
    central UN treaties are the UN *International Covenant on Civil and Political Rights*
    (1966) and the UN *International Covenant on Economic, Social, and Cultural Rights*
    (1966). The most important Declarations are non-binding, although in many cases, the
    norms and standards laid out in them reflect principles that are binding in customary
    international law.
5.  General Comments in UN instruments clarify the nature and content of individual rights
    and the obligations of the states that have ratified the treaty.
6.  See Dennis Raphael's work in this volume.
7.  The Rules relevant to social and cultural rights are Rules 2, 3, 5, 6, 10, and 11.
8.  See also the next section of this chapter on reproductive health.
9.  Articles 25 and 26 of the UN *Convention on the Rights of Persons with Disabilities Draft
    Comprehensive and Integral International Convention on the Protection and Promotion of
    the Rights and Dignity of Persons with Disabilities* identify key human rights issues related
    to the health and rehabilitation of people with disabilities, as well as these areas.
10. The UN Declaration on HIV/AIDS emphasizes that the full realization of human rights
    and fundamental freedoms for all, including the right to the highest attainable standard
    of health, is an essential element of the global response to the HIV/AIDS pandemic.

The WHO passed the Trade-Related Aspects of Intellectual Property Rights (TRIPS) agreement to promote public health and to promote access to medicines for all. For further discussion of the TRIPS agreement, see Cohen (2002).

11. The WHO includes in this category of diseases: onchocerciasis, leprosy, guinea worm disease, lymphatic filariasis, schistosomiasis and soil-transmitted helminthiasis, African trypanosomiasis, human rabies, dengue and dengue hemorrhagic fever, leishmaniasis, and buruli ulcer (WHO, 2002).

12. For a more comprehensive discussion of the implications of international drug policy, see Joel Lexchin's chapter in this book.

## REFERENCES

Ahmadiani, S., & Nikfar, S. (2016). Challenges of access to medicine and the responsibility of pharmaceutical companies: A legal perspective. *DARU Journal of Pharmaceutical Sciences, 24,* 13. doi:10.1186/s40199-016-0151-z

Anand, S., Peter, F., & Sen, A. (Eds.). (2004). *Public health, ethics, and equity.* Oxford: Oxford University Press.

Benzeval, M., Judge, K., & Whitehead, M. (Eds.). (1995). *Tackling inequalities in health: An agenda for action.* London: King's Fund.

Beyrer, C., Villar, J. C., Suwanvanichkij, V., Singh, S.,. Baral, S. D., & Mills, E. J. (2007). Neglected diseases, civil conflicts, and the right to health. *The Lancet, 370,* 619–627. doi:10.1016/S0140-6736(07)61301-4

Brady O. J., Gething, P. W., Bhatt, S., Messina, J. P., Brownstein, J. S., Hoen, A. G., … Hay, S. I. (2012). Refining the global spatial limits of dengue virus transmission by evidence-based consensus. *PLoS Neglected Tropical Diseases, 6*(8), e1760. doi:10.1371/journal.pntd.0001760

Coates, T., Richter, T., & Caceres, C. (2008). Behavioural strategies to reduce HIV transmission: How to make them work better. Geneva: World Health Organization. Retrieved from https://www.who.int/hiv/events/artprevention/coates.pdf

Cohen, J. C. (2002). Developing states' response to the pharmaceutical imperatives of the TRIPS agreement. In B. Granville (Ed.), *The economics of essential medicines* (pp. 115–136). London: Chatham House (Royal Institute of International Affairs).

Cook, R. J., & Dickens, B. M. (2003). Access to emergency contraception. *Journal of Obstetrics and Gynecology Canada, 25*(11), 914–916. doi:10.1016/S1701-2163(16)30238-9

Cook, R. J., Dickens, B. M., & Fathalla, M. F. (2003). *Reproductive health and human rights: Integrating medicine, ethics, and law.* Oxford and New York: Clarendon Press.

Cook, R. J., Dickens, B. M., Ngwena, C., & Plata, M. I. (2001). The legal status of emergency contraception. *International Journal of Gynecology and Obstetrics, 75*(2), 185–191. doi:10.1016/S0020-7292(01)00481-7

Deber, R. (1999). The use and misuse of economics. In M. A. Somerville & J. R. Saul (Eds.), *Do we care? Renewing Canada's commitment to health: Proceedings of the first directions for Canadian health care conference* (pp. 53–68). Montreal: McGill-Queen's University Press.

Degener, T. (1995). Disabled persons and human rights: The legal framework. In T. Degener & Y. Koster-Dreese (Eds.), *Human rights and disabled persons: Essays and relevant human rights instruments* (vol. 40, pp. 9–39). Dordrecht, Netherlands: Martinus Nijhoff.

*Eldridge v. British Columbia (Ministry of Health)*, 1997 3 SCR 624 (CanLII). Retrieved from https://www.canlii.org/en/ca/scc/doc/1997/1997canlii327/1997canlii327.html

Fidler, D. P. (2000). The globalization of public health. In D.P. Fidler (Ed.), *International law and public health: Materials on and analysis of global health jurisprudence* (pp. 16–23). Ardsley, NY: Transnational Publishers.

Foucault, M. (1980). *Power/knowledge: Selected interviews and other writings, 1972–1977.* C. Gordon (Ed.). New York: Pantheon Books.

Gostin, L. O., & Taylor, A. L. (2008). Global health law: A definition and grand challenges. *Public Health Ethics, 1*(1), 53–63. doi:10.1093/phe/phn005

Hunt, P. (2003a). *Economic, social, and cultural rights: The right of everyone to the enjoyment of the highest attainable standard of physical and mental health.* Geneva: United Nations.

Hunt, P. (2003b). The UN Special Rapporteur on the right to health: Key objectives, themes and interventions. *Health and Human Rights, 7*(1). doi:10.2307/4065415

Kindhauser, M. K. (Ed.). (2003). *Communicable diseases cluster, communicable diseases 2002: Global defence against the infectious disease threat.* Geneva: World Health Organization. Retrieved from https://apps.who.int/iris/bitstream/handle/10665/42572/9241590297.pdf?sequence=1&isAllowed=y

Kinney, E. D. (2000). The international human right to health: What does this mean for our nation and world. *Indiana Law Review, 34,* 1457–75.

Lexchin, J. (2013). Canada and access to medicines in developing countries: Intellectual property rights first. *Globalization and Health, 9*(1), 42. doi:10.1186/1744-8603-9-42

Lock, M. (1995). Transcending mortality: Organ transplants and the practice of contradictions. *Medical Anthropology Quarterly, 9*(3), 390–393. doi:10.1525/maq.1995.9.3.02a00060

Mann, J. M. (1999a). Health and human rights. In J. M. Mann, S. Gruskin, M. A. Grodin, & G. J. Annas (Eds.), *Health and human rights: A reader* (pp. 7–20). New York: Routledge.

Mann, J. M. (1999b). Human rights and AIDS: The future of the pandemic. In J. M. Mann, S. Gruskin, M. A. Grodin, & G. J. Annas (Eds.), *Health and human rights: A reader* (pp. 216–226). New York: Routledge.

The Mental Health Commission of Canada. (2018). *Building for the future.* Ottawa: Mental Health Commission of Canada.

*Moore v. British Columbia (Education)*, 2012 SCC 61, [2012] 3 SCR 360. Retrieved from https://scc-csc.lexum.com/scc-csc/scc-csc/en/item/12680/index.do

Mosoff, J., & Grant, I. (1999). *Intellectual disability and the Supreme Court: The implications of the Charter for people who have a disability.* Toronto: Canadian Association for Community Living.

Rioux, M. H. (2003). On second thought: Constructing knowledge, law, disability, and inequality. In S. S. Herr, L. O. Gostin, & H. H. Koh (Eds.), *The human rights of persons with intellectual disabilities: Different but equal* (pp. 287–317). Oxford: Oxford University Press.

Rioux, M. H., Pinto, P. C., & Parekh, G. (Eds.). (2015). *Disability, rights monitoring, and social change: Building power out of evidence.* Toronto: Canadian Scholars' Press.

UN Committee on Economic, Social, and Cultural Rights (CESCR). (1994). *Eleventh session, general comment no. 5; Persons with disabilities.* UN Doc. E/1995/22.

UN Committee on Economic, Social, and Cultural Rights (CESCR). (2000). *Twenty-second session, Geneva, 25 April–12 May, general comment no. 14: The right to the highest attainable standard of health. (Art. 12 of the Covenant).* UN Doc. E/C.12/2000/4.

UN Committee on the Rights of the Child (CRC). (2003). *Thirty-third session, 19 May–6 June, general comment No. 4: Adolescent health and development in the context of the Convention on the Rights of the Child.* UN Doc. CRC/GC/2003/4.

UN Department of Economic, Social Information, and Policy Analysis. (1995). *Population and development: Programme of action adopted at the International Conference on Population and Development, Cairo, 5–13 September 1994.* New York: United Nations, Department for Economic, Social Information, and Policy Analysis.

UN Department of Public Information. (1996). *The Beijing Declaration and the platform for action: Fourth World Conference on Women, Beijing, China, 4–15 September 1995.* New York: United Nations, Department of Public Information.

UN Development Programme. (2000). *Human development report 2000: Human development and human rights.* New York and Oxford: Oxford University Press.

UN Economic and Social Council (ECOSOC), Commission on Human Rights. (2003). *Report of the Special Rapporteur, 59th Session, 13 February. The right of everyone to the enjoyment of the highest attainable standard of physical and mental health.* UN Doc. E/CN.4/2003/58.

UN General Assembly. (1966). *International Covenant on Economic, Social, and Cultural Rights (ICESCR), Twenty-first session,* Resolution 2200A/21. UN Doc. A/6316.

UN General Assembly. (1979). *Convention on the Elimination of All Forms of Discrimination against Women (CEDAW), 18 December,* Resolution 34/180.

UN General Assembly. (1991). *Principles for the protection of persons with mental illness and the improvement of mental health care,* 75th Plenary Meeting, 17 December, Resolution 46/119. UN Doc. A/RES/46/119. Retrieved from www.un.org/documents/ga/res/46/a46r119.htm

UN General Assembly. (1993). *Declaration on the Elimination of Violence against Women (UNDEVW),* 85th Plenary Meeting, Preamble, 20 December, Resolution 48/104. UN Doc. A/RES/48/104. Retrieved from https://www.un.org/documents/ga/res/48/a48r104.htm

UN General Assembly. (2003). *Human rights situations: Human rights situations and reports of Special Rapporteurs and Representatives, Fifty-eighth session, 10 October.* UN Doc. A/58/427.

UN Office of the High Commissioner for Human Rights. (1998). *HIV/AIDS and human rights, international guidelines: Second international consultation on HIV/AIDS and human rights, Geneva, 23–25 September 1996.* UN Doc. HR/PUB/98/1. New York: United Nations.

UN Office of the High Commissioner for Human Rights. (2009). *2009 report: Activities and results.* New York: Author. Retrieved from https://www.ohchr.org/Documents/Publications/I_OHCHR_Rep_2009_complete_final.pdf

UN Office of the High Commissioner for Human Rights. (2018). *Fact sheet no. 31: The right to health*. New York: Author. Retrieved from https://www.ohchr.org/Documents/Publications/Factsheet31.pdf

World Health Organization. (1946). *Constitution of the World Health Organization*. Retrieved March 5, 2019, from http://apps.who.int/gb/bd/PDF/bd47/EN/constitution-en.pdf?ua=1

World Health Organization. (1948). *Preamble to the Constitution of the WHO, as adopted by the International Health Conference, New York, 19–22 June, 1946; signed on 22 July 1946 by the representatives of 61 states (Official records of the World Health Organization, no. 2, p. 100) and entered into force on 7 April 1948.* Geneva: Author.

World Health Organization. (1978). *Declaration of Alma-Ata, International Conference on Primary Health Care, Alma-Ata, USSR, 6–12 September.*

World Health Organization. (2002). *Health and human rights.* Health and Human Rights Publication Series 1. Geneva: Author.

World Health Organization. (2011). *World report on disability.* Geneva: World Health Organization and World Bank. Retrieved from https://www.who.int/disabilities/world_report/2011/report.pdf?ua=1.

World Health Organization. (2017). Global Health Observatory (GHO) data: HIV/AIDS. Geneva: Author. Retrieved from https://www.who.int/gho/hiv/en/

World Health Organization. (2018). Dengue and severe dengue (February). WHO Fact Sheet. Retrieved from http://www.who.int/en/news-room/fact-sheets/detail/dengue-and-severe-dengue

# CHAPTER 5

## Researching Health: Knowledge Perspectives, Methodologies, and Methods

*Toba Bryant, Dennis Raphael, and Marcia Rioux*

## INTRODUCTION

In the previous chapters, four broad approaches to understanding health, illness, and health care were presented. Each of these represents a way of making sense of these issues and identifying means of improving health. But what is the nature of knowledge about these health, illness, and healthcare issues, and how is such knowledge created? How do we identify sources of health and illness, decide which healthcare delivery gets the best results, and understand the way in which health-related policy is created? Despite the common belief that there are objective "facts" about the world that can be observed and acted upon, this is not really the case. In reality, facts are very much a result of how we understand the nature of the world. There are different ways of thinking about the nature of the world and how we come to know about it, and this is especially the case when it comes to the issues discussed in this volume.

Ways of thinking about what constitutes knowledge about the world and how we come to acquire it are known as knowledge perspectives (Bryant, 2016). A knowledge perspective can be defined as a set of basic beliefs or assumptions about knowledge and how it is created. Each health approach—epidemiology, sociology, political economy, and human rights—aligns with one or more of these particular knowledge perspectives.

## KNOWLEDGE PERSPECTIVES IN HEALTH STUDIES

There are three primary approaches to research and inquiry that are useful for understanding how health, illness, and healthcare issues can be studied. These approaches are positivism, idealism, and realism (Wilson, 1983d). A summary of their features is provided in Box 5.1.

## Box 5.1: Knowledge Perspectives in Health Studies

**Key Questions**

- *Ontological*: What is the nature of the knowable? Or what is the nature of reality?
- *Epistemological*: What is the nature of the relationship between the knower (the inquirer) and the known (or knowledge)?
- *Methodological*: How should the inquirer go about finding out this knowledge?

**Positivism**

- Research methods developed for the natural sciences are also appropriate for health studies.
- Research should aim to develop general principles and laws that identify straightforward causes and effects.
- Research should focus on the readily observable and measurable.
- There is a distinction between values and facts such that inquiry is value-free.
- Focus on individual characteristics rather than broader community and societal features.
- Emphasis on experimental methods, surveys, and observations that produce numbers subjected to statistical analysis.
- Examples of research questions:
  - What behaviours are associated with morbidity and mortality?
  - Which drugs are most effective at treating disease?
  - Which aspects of primary care best promote health and prevent disease?

**Idealism**

- Research should explore the meanings that individuals place on events.
- Research should identify the multiple realities held by individuals.
- Individuals, communities, and even whole societies subscribe to the realities created by their understandings.
- Research should examine how individuals' understandings are shaped by their environments.
- These understandings are real in that they shape behaviours.
- The emphasis is on ethnographic methods whereby individuals' understandings of the world are made explicit through open-ended interviews, diaries, focus groups, and detailed observations.
- The focus is on the lived experiences of health and health care and how these shape individuals' place and actions in the world.
- Examples of questions:
  - How do people understand the causes of their illness and the best means of managing it?

- Why do some people continue their treatment while others do not?
- How do health workers and policy-makers conceive the role of the healthcare system?

**Realism**

- Research should identify the background structures and processes of society that distribute resources among different groups.
- The interpretations individuals have are shaped by these societal structures and processes.
- Research can investigate how individuals can transcend these factors, acting to change their world.
- Research can identify how people come to have faulty understandings of their world, exhibiting what is called "false consciousness."
- Research can employ a variety of methods to identify the social structures and processes that shape both phenomena and individuals' understandings of these phenomena.
- Research can examine how identifying these social structures and processes can lead to social change.
- Examples of questions:
  - What are the public policies that lead to some groups living longer with less illness than others?
  - How does the drug industry shape the marketing and prescribing of drugs in different forms of the welfare state?
  - How do different health workers come to have differing roles in the organization and delivery of primary health care?

*Sources:* Adapted from Wilson, J. (1983d). *Social theory.* Englewood Cliffs, NJ: Prentice Hall; and Lincoln, Y., & Guba, E. (1985). *Naturalistic inquiry.* Newbury Park, CA: Sage Publications.

## Positivism

In the field of health studies, there are many ways to understand how health and illness come about and to examine the organization and delivery of health care. For many health researchers, a primary approach is to focus upon clearly observable aspects of the world in order to identify patterns between "causes" and "effects." Positivism is an approach that formed the basis for many of the great discoveries in the physical sciences in the 18th century (Wilson, 1983b). The scientific methods applied, such as experimentation, observation, and statistical analysis of numerical data, usually include *quantitative research methods.*

Traditional epidemiology (see Chapter 1) shares many features with positivist science. When considering issues such as the causes of illness, epidemiology's tendency is toward a reductionism that leads to observation, measurement, and analysis of individual characteristics (e.g., biomedical indicators, risk behaviours, etc.). Clinical epidemiology focuses on the effects of specific treatment regimens such as surgeries, pharmaceuticals, and other healthcare interventions. Social epidemiology, however (see Box 5.2), moves beyond these narrow preoccupations to consider broader societal issues (Berkman, Kawachi, & Glymour, 2014) but is still limited in its dependence on identifying "cause" and "effect relations" through statistical analysis of quantitative data (Bambra, 2009).

Positivist science is associated with the application of experimental designs and other quantitative methodologies and avoiding *normative* judgments—that is, avoiding saying how the world *should* be instead of simply describing how it is. It has proven useful for describing the distribution and precursors of health and illness, evaluating the effects of healthcare innovations and treatments, identifying some causes of health and illness, and specifying the form healthcare systems take. Against this, positivist science takes little account of humans' abilities to interpret their world in various ways and how these understandings shape the organization of healthcare systems, the experience of illness, and adoption of health-related behaviours (Popay & Williams, 1994). Positivist science can also be argued to avoid analysis of the less-than-obvious underlying structures and processes of society—the main preoccupations of sociological and political economy

**Box 5.2**: Social Epidemiology

Social epidemiology is the systematic and comprehensive study of health, well-being, social conditions or problems, and diseases and their determinants, using epidemiology and social science methods to develop interventions, programs, policies, and institutions that may reduce the extent, adverse impact, or incidence of a health or social problem and promote health. This definition provides evidence-based methods for public health activism. Social problems are specifically included in this definition because many of today's challenges in public health, including obesity, infectious diseases, violence, child abuse, and drug use, are associated with both personal behavior and macro trends in the social structure such as the distribution of wealth, social resources, and exposure to media and market forces. Furthermore, those who specifically study social problems can enrich their research and practice through the methods of social epidemiology, revealing how social problems are intrinsically linked to the health status of populations. Social epidemiology is the combination of epidemiology (the study of the distribution and determinants of disease and injury in human populations) with the social and behavioral sciences.

*Source*: Cwikel, J. (2006). *Social epidemiology: Strategies for public health activism* (p. 4). New York: Columbia University Press.

approaches (Chapters 2 and 3)—finding these to be beyond its scope. It does not usually consider issues of power and influence and how certain sectors of society may come to violate the human rights of others (Chapter 4).

## Idealism

Two schools of thought challenge a positivist approach. One school of thought is concerned with humans' interpretations and understandings of the world and goes by the names of idealism, constructivism, and interpretivism (Wilson, 1983a). This approach originated in sociology, but has been applied across many fields of study, including health studies. It has proven helpful in understanding patients' experience of illness, explaining how organizations such as governments and hospitals, as well as healthcare providers, make decisions about service delivery. It has also been useful for identifying the way in which ideas about health, illness, and health care shape the health of different groups in society as well as the organization and form of the healthcare system.

The data in idealism are people's ideas and understandings as collected through observations, interviews, diaries, and document analysis. A key concept is that ideas and understandings differ among individuals, groups, and even entire societies, and that these ideas and understandings have real consequences, which is a challenge to the positivist idea that a single objective reality of objective facts exists. Analyzing people's ideas and understandings, it is argued, may be more useful for understanding some health issues than objective data collected through the positivist approach. The methods applied for this type of research are usually called *qualitative research methods*.

## Realism

A third knowledge perspective is concerned with the identification and analysis of underlying—that is, not immediately observable—societal structures and processes and how these determine the distribution of economic, social, and political resources. It is also concerned with the understandings people have about these societal structures and processes and the resource distributions that result from these structures and processes. This third approach is variously known as realism, structuralism, or materialism (Wilson, 1983c). Researchers in this tradition employ a range of research methods, but its key aspect is the application of *critical theory*, an approach that aims to critique society, social structures, and systems of power as a way to understand and to move toward the realization of egalitarianism.

Realism's primary thesis is that the analysis of health, illness, and healthcare issues cannot be limited to the concrete and observable, nor can they be focused solely upon people's understandings of these issues. Instead, realism strives to identify how economic and political structures and processes such as the operation of the economic system and the laws and regulations made by governments result in the existence of different entitlements between different groups with subsequent differences in health outcomes. These differences exist among workers, managers, and owners, men and women, visible minorities and white members of society, urban and rural dwellers, and others with marginalized statuses. Realism is also interested in how different kinds of healthcare systems emerge. The political economy and human rights approaches to understanding health, illness, and health care are most closely aligned with this paradigm. But much sociological analysis and even some epidemiological approaches draw upon *critical theory* to illuminate health, illness, and healthcare issues.

## COMPONENTS OF A KNOWLEDGE PERSPECTIVE

Positivism, idealism, and realism consist of three somewhat overlapping components: ontology, epistemology, and methodology (Lincoln & Guba, 1985). These components illuminate how knowledge can be generated in health studies. Table 5.1 shows linkages between the four health studies approaches of epidemiology, sociology, political economy, and human rights and these knowledge paradigm components.

### Ontology

Ontology refers to a paradigm's core belief system about the nature of the world and its components (Guba, 1990). *What exactly are the aspects of the world that we can come to know?* Related to this is the values position of: *What are the specific aspects of this world that are worth knowing?* In every discipline, there are different views of what is worth knowing about the world, and this is particularly the case when issues such as health, illness, and health care are considered. In regards to health care and the delivery of services, one of the key issues is how to monitor this process. Should we be looking at the number of services provided or the impact of those services on health status? Should we be looking at the number of people who survive cancer or the quality of life in the process?

The ontology of traditional epidemiology is closely aligned with the *positivist* approach in that what is worth knowing consists of measurable biomedical and physiological indicators of cell, organ, and body systems whose impairment leads to disease. In the

**Table 5.1:** Linkages between the Health Studies Approaches of Epidemiology, Sociology, Political Economy, and Human Rights and the Knowledge Perspectives of Positivism, Idealism, and Realism

| Health Studies Approach | Knowledge Perspective |
|---|---|
| Epidemiology | Primarily positivist |
| Sociology | Various schools use differing paradigms |
| Political economy | Primarily realist |
| Human rights | Primarily realist |

health sciences, this view is clearly dominant and reflects the understandings held by most healthcare professionals.

Understandings of the nature of reality (what is worth knowing about health, illness, and health care and how to promote it) held by the other health paradigms—sociological (i.e., what is important is the organization and operation of society and individuals' beliefs), political economy (i.e., what is important is the distribution of influence and power), and human rights (i.e., what is important is adherence to the most equitable standard of health)—clearly overlap. The political economy approach is most aligned with *realism* and sociology with both *realism* and *interpretivism*, while human rights arguably is aligned with *realism*.

## Epistemology

Epistemology refers to how the inquirer—that is, the epidemiologist, sociologist, political economist, or human rights scholar—who wishes to understand health, illness, and health care creates knowledge about these matters through research and other inquiries. What research approaches can usefully be applied to learn about the world? Is important knowledge best gained through the methodology of objective observation and experimentation as developed and applied in the natural sciences of biology, chemistry, and physics or through other methodologies? *Positivism* and the epidemiological approach are closely aligned with the methodology of objective observation and experimentation.

For some sociological approaches, important knowledge is to be gained through understanding the personal experiences of individuals who are affected by health, illness, and healthcare issues. This focus—indicative of *interpretivism*—is directed toward understanding how patients, healthcare providers, and policy-makers see the world and how these understandings shape their outlook and behaviours. The methodology applied here is that of understanding people's lives through shared observations, extensive interviews, and discussion.

*Realism*—the view that the most important knowledge can be gained by identifying the societal structures or institutions that shape the distribution of economic, political, and social resources among the population—is closely aligned with the political economy perspective. What is it about different economic and political systems that leads to certain segments of the population achieving health and receiving good health care while other segments fare rather less well? Finally, should analysis—the human rights perspective—be guided by consideration of the ethical principles that guide policy-makers' decisions within these economic and political systems? Can these ethical principles allow for the making of judgments about the best means of promoting health and delivering healthcare services? Are the services delivered in a framework based on autonomy, dignity, equality, and respect for difference?

Epistemology therefore represents a key aspect of the knowledge creation process shaping how knowledge is acquired and understood. Epistemology leads to the application of different means of learning about health, illness, and health care. The epidemiological, sociological, political economy, and human rights approaches may represent differing epistemologies, therefore leading to differing research approaches—or methodologies—for gaining knowledge about health, illness, and health care.

## Methodology

Methodology is about the kinds of research tools that can be employed to acquire knowledge about the world. The *positivist* tool kit consists of experimental methods that focus on observation and manipulation of specific aspects of the world specified in the form of concrete indicators, measures, and variables. These data are then placed into statistical models that strive to identify cause-and-effect relationships. These methods are the mainstay of the epidemiological approach.

The *idealist* tool kit consists of methods that have the researchers interact with the subjects of study to examine their lived experiences. The emphasis here is on ascertaining the meanings people have of events in their world and discovering how these shape their behaviour. Data are in the form of words and observations, themes, and ideas. These methods are the tools employed by some schools of sociological thought. The *realist* tool kit is concerned with critical analyses of the organization of society and how this organization shapes the healthcare system and the determinants of health. The emphasis here is on critical reasoning and analysis of societal structures and institutions and whether these analyses make sense. The realist tool kit is the mainstay of the political economy and the human rights approaches to knowledge generation.

As well as the above, legal and ethical analysis and monitoring of outcomes can ascertain whether a society and its institutions are meeting the goals of providing basic healthcare rights rights to its citizens through the provision of health care and other health-related public policies—the human rights approach. All these different ways of understanding the world—through the aspects of ontology, epistemology, and methodology—shape how we come to study health, illness, and healthcare issues.

## DETERMINING THE VALUE OF THESE APPROACHES AND PERSPECTIVES

How is it determined which of the epidemiological, sociological, political economy, or human rights approaches and the associated knowledge perspectives of positivism, idealism, or realism are correct? Rather than asking whether an approach or knowledge perspective is *correct*, perhaps the better question to ask is whether an approach or knowledge perspective is *useful*. And any approach or perspective's usefulness will be determined in large part from: (1) the frame of reference held by the individual doing the inquiry, and (2) the specific question about health, illness, and health care that is being asked.

Knowledge perspectives themselves shape the form of inquiry. These disciplinary traditions, as well as societal values, also shape what is considered to be an appropriate area and method of inquiry. Positivist approaches focus on objective qualities of immediate environments. Interpretivist approaches focus on people's understandings. Realism is concerned with societal structures and their effects. Additionally, one's training as an epidemiologist, sociologist, political economist, or human rights analyst shapes how one defines and carries out an area of inquiry. Consider how much emphasis is given—with resultant research activity, public policy action, and media coverage—to lifestyle approaches to combat obesity as opposed to understanding how deteriorating living conditions shape Canadians' health.

In essence, an approach or paradigm can be assessed as being useful in terms of how its analytical lens, its methods, and findings answer the following questions:

- Does the approach or perspective and its methods explain the phenomena chosen to be of interest?
- Does the approach or perspective allow the making of predictions concerning the phenomena?
- Does the approach or perspective point the way to further areas of fruitful inquiry?
- Does the approach or perspective point the way to means of improving the situation?
- Does the approach recognize diverse knowledge, acknowledging understanding from countries and scholars of both the global North and South, and does it recognize the importance of diversity and intersectionality?

These are not easy questions to answer. Indeed, many researchers in health studies do not even consider these questions and simply carry out research and inquiry within one selected approach or perspective without acknowledging the limitations of the approach and perspective. Box 5.3 contains some thoughts from one eminent sociologist of what a mature study of society should entail. What are the implications of these ideas for the study of health, illness, and healthcare issues?

In the remainder of this chapter, an overview of the tools available for research and inquiry in health studies is provided. The tools are placed within the context of both the approaches provided in Chapters 1–4 and the three knowledge paradigms of positivism, idealism, and realism. Like the construction activity of building a house, some tools will be more appropriate for certain tasks and questions, and less appropriate for others.

# QUANTITATIVE METHODS IN HEALTH STUDIES

Aligned with the positivist approach, the primary aspect of quantitative approaches is the identification, measurement, and statistical analysis of aspects of the world, normally

**Box 5.3:** C. Wright Mills on the Key Questions Facing Social Scientists

No social study that does not come back to the problems of biography, of history and of their intersections within a society has completed its intellectual journey. Whatever the specific problems of the classic social analysts, however limited or however broad the features of social reality they have examined, those who have been imaginatively aware of the promise of their work have consistently asked three sorts of questions:

1. What is the structure of this particular society as a whole? What are its essential components, and how are they related to one another? How does it differ from other varieties of social order? Within it, what is the meaning of any particular feature for its continuance and for its change?

2. Where does this society stand in human history? What are the mechanics by which it is changing? What is its place within and its meaning for the development of humanity as a whole? How does any particular feature we are examining affect, and how is it affected by, the historical period in which it moves? And this period—what are its essential features? How does it differ from other periods? What are its characteristic ways of history-making?

3. What varieties of men and women now prevail in this society and in this period? And what varieties are coming to prevail? In what ways are they selected and formed, liberated and repressed, made sensitive and blunted? What kinds of "human nature" are revealed in the conduct and character we observe in this society in this period? And what is the meaning for "human nature" of each and every feature of the society we are examining?

*Source:* Mills, C. W. (1990). *The sociological imagination* (pp. 6–7). New York: Oxford University Press. Originally published 1959.

designated with the term "indicator," "measurement," or "variable." Quantitative approaches are used to generate knowledge in the epidemiological, sociological, political economy, and human rights approaches, but the emphasis, and the form these methods and analyses of findings take, systematically differs among the approaches.

## Epidemiological Methods

Epidemiologists are primarily concerned with the distribution and causes of disease. One of their primary efforts is focused on isolating the causes of illness. Clinical epidemiologists are concerned with ascertaining the effects of treatments. In their interests to isolate specific causes and effects, their methods consist of two key aspects: experimental design and statistical analyses. There is a prevailing tendency in epidemiological research to focus on the concrete and observable as compared to the abstract and conceptual.

### Basic Epidemiological Terms

There are some unique terms that are common to epidemiological research. *Mortality* refers to the number—reported as a rate or proportion of a given population—of individuals who die from a disease or injury. *Morbidity* refers to the number of individuals who suffer from an affliction, such as the number of people with a specific illness or who suffer an injury.

*Incidence* refers to the number of new cases as a proportion of the population within a designated time period. *Prevalence* refers to the total number of cases within a designated population at a designated time. One example would be that the incidence (or new cases) of type 2 diabetes among men over 20 years is 8.5/1,000 and the prevalence (or existing cases) of type 2 diabetes among men over 20 years is 76/1,000.

### Epidemiological Research Design

Experimental design is about arranging data collection such that a specific cause or treatment can be determined to have a specific effect or outcome. Some of the primary methods applied in the search for the causes of illness are: case-control, cross-sectional, and prospective or longitudinal studies. Box 5.4 outlines the key features of these data collection designs.

In each method, the emphasis is on specifying actual causes of outcome. And consistent with assumptions of the positivist approach, variables of interest are usually concrete and observable rather than abstract and conceptual. Critiques of the approach are available (Davey Smith & Ebrahim, 2001).

### Epidemiological Statistical Analysis

Analyses attempt to calculate the risk that a particular outcome will occur as a function of a predictor variable. Examples of analysis outcomes are risk ratios, odds ratios, relative and absolute risk, and attributable risk. Univariate analyses look at one association at a time. Multivariate analyses look at a combination of associations at a single time and identify which are the most important associations. Logistic regression is a widely used technique to achieve these objectives, in which the outcome variable is the presence or absence of a disease.

### Examples of Epidemiological Approaches

Three examples of the traditional epidemiological approach are provided. As noted, social epidemiologists move beyond these narrow preoccupations, but these investigations represent a minority of epidemiological investigations.

*Tobacco use and lung cancer*: An enormous literature has accumulated that documents the relationship between tobacco use and the incidence of and mortality from tobacco use. These investigations range from animal studies of the effects of tobacco upon rats and other animals right through to prospective studies that show that over time, tobacco users are more likely to develop and succumb to lung cancer.

## Box 5.4: Research Designs in Epidemiology

*Case control*: A study that compares two groups of people, those with the disease or condition under study (cases) and a very similar group of people who do not have the disease or condition (controls). Researchers study the medical and lifestyle histories of the people in each group to learn what factors may be associated with the disease or condition. For example, one group may have been exposed to a particular substance that the other was not. Also called retrospective study.

*Cross-sectional study*: A cross-sectional study aims to describe the relationship between diseases (or other health-related states) and other factors of interest as they exist in a specified population at a particular time without regard for what may have preceded or precipitated the health status found at the time of the study.

*Experimental design*: A blueprint of the procedure that enables the researcher to test their hypothesis by reaching valid conclusions about relationships between independent and dependent variables. It refers to the conceptual framework within which the experiment is conducted.

*Experimental research*: A researcher's attempt to maintain control over all factors that may affect the result of an experiment. In doing this, the researcher attempts to determine or predict what may occur.

*Prospective or longitudinal study*: A research study that follows over time groups of individuals who are alike in many ways, but differ by a certain characteristic (for example, female nurses who smoke and those who do not smoke) and compares them for a particular outcome (such as lung cancer).

*Sources:* National Cancer Institute. (2009). *Dictionary of cancer terms.* Retrieved from http://www. cancer.gov/Templates/db_alpha.aspx?CdrID=348989; *Encyclopedia of public health.* (2009). Retrieved from http://www.answers.com/topic/synchronic-study; and Module 13 Experimental Research and Design, Oklahoma State University. Retrieved from http://www.okstate.edu/ag/agedcm4h/academic/aged5980a/5980/newpage2.htm

*Race and cancer survival*: In Canada and the U.S., a literature has accumulated that indicates that people of different races (e.g., Black, White, Asian, etc.) differ in their likelihood of succumbing to various forms of cancers. Focus has been on detailing whether these differences are due to delays in diagnosis, differences in treatments, or differing attitudes of healthcare providers to members of racial groups (see Chapter 7).

*Effectiveness of treatments for prostate cancer*: A lively area of activity is concerned with relative effectiveness of various forms of treatment (e.g., surgery, radiation, drugs, no treatment) for diagnosed prostate cancer. Amazingly, there is controversy as to whether any treatment is more effective than simply monitoring the patient.

## Social Science Quantitative Methods

Many social scientists have adapted the basic provisions of positivist science in their application of social science concepts to the study of health, illness, and health care. What distinguishes these approaches from epidemiological methods is a greater willingness to recognize sociological and psychological concepts as relevant to health studies, and a willingness to consider social and structural aspects of society such as the distribution of income and wealth as precursors to illness and the organization and delivery of healthcare services. Social scientists also utilize a somewhat different tool kit of research designs and statistical analyses than those seen in the epidemiological approach.

### Social Science Research Design

The primary aspect of social science research design is a use of designs that focus on broader indicators such as individuals' personality and behavioural characteristics, measures of organizational functioning, and indicators of societal functioning. Additionally, there is much greater use of what are termed parametric statistics (i.e., using measures that are continuous in their distribution [e.g., the degree of leadership in a hospital] rather than dichotomous indicators [e.g., the presence or absence of disease or effectiveness or ineffectiveness of a treatment]).

*Experimental design*: The focus here is on experiments where individuals are assigned to differing experimental conditions or treatments. The emphasis is on random assignment of individuals to conditions.

*Quasi-experimental design*: In this approach, researchers try to make sense of real-life experiments in which individuals already exist under differing conditions such as good or poor housing or enlightened or regressive management approaches, or are members of different groups (e.g., class, racial, or gender). Individuals cannot be ethically assigned to these differing groups, yet quasi-experimental forms of analyses are available to identify potential treatment effects.

*Cross-sectional and longitudinal designs*: These designs refer to the temporal dimension. In cross-sectional studies, the association of two measures or indicators is looked at for one point in time. Then arguments are made of how one factor can be hypothesized to cause or influence the other. In longitudinal studies, individuals are followed over time on a series of measures. Introduction of the temporal dimension allows greater confidence in assuming that one factor is causing the other. But even in this approach, other unobserved factors may be causing the apparent association of one measure with another.

### Statistics and Statistical Analysis

Social science statistical analyses are specified by their focus on identifying relationships among continuous rather than dichotomous measures.

*Univariate measures of similarity and difference*: Some examples of these techniques are correlation coefficients for examination of similarity and t-tests and analyses of variance for examining differences between groups on some measure. These approaches look at one predictor and outcome at a time.

*Multivariate measures of similarity and difference*: Multiple correlation coefficients and multivariate analyses of variance allow for the ascertaining of the effects of a series of predictors upon an outcome. Multiple regression is a very common approach that looks at the amount of variation in an outcome measure explained by a series of predictor measures. More advanced methods are factor analysis, discriminant analysis, and cluster analysis.

### Examples of Social Science Quantitative Approaches

Social science analyses are usually broader in their scope than epidemiological analyses.

*Social isolation and mortality among older people*: A number of studies have shown that older people with fewer social contacts are more likely to die sooner than those with more contacts. These effects are important even after controlling for a large number of other measures, such as social class, education, and lifestyle behaviours.

*Community cohesion and community health*: Studies have shown that communities in which people have greater contact with each other show better health and social outcomes than communities in which people have fewer contacts. These findings may be influenced by the level of government supports provided to communities.

*Welfare states and population health*: Studies show that nations where governments provide more supports in services and benefits show better indicators of health. These indicators include life expectancy, levels of infant mortality, and crime rates.

## Social Science Qualitative Approaches

Social scientists also apply non-quantitative approaches to understanding health issues. These approaches are aligned with the approach of idealism and aim to understand individuals' perceptions of reality.

### Ethnographies

In ethnography there is an extensive attempt to understand the culture within which individuals live. These cultures can be concerned with neighbourhoods, offices, schools, or any other place in which individuals interact. These understandings can come about through open-ended interviews, examination of documents and surroundings, arts-based investigations, and observations of individuals in their environments. The raw data are people's words or illustrations and the observations of the researcher.

### Participant Observation

This approach is about the researcher actually participating in the everyday kinds of activities in which the people of interest participate. Researchers, usually cultural anthropologists, may not identify themselves as researchers. One famous study had researchers joining a Doomsday cult to understand why people join these kinds of groups (Festinger, Riecken, & Schacter, 1956). The experiences the researcher has provide the raw data for these kinds of research inquiries.

### Open-Ended Interviews and Focus Groups

These are more specific methods that allow for specification of the perceptions individuals have about an area of interest. The primary data are the words spoken by individuals in one-on-one interviews or in groups of similar people. For example, people can explain how they cope with an illness or disease, sometimes in an interview and other times during a focus group discussion with others with the same health status. Interviews can be had with elected officials about what they see as the government's role in making sure citizens have their basic needs met through public policy action.

### Discourse Analysis

This methodology is a detailed examination of the contents of printed documents. These documents can be books, media stories, agency mission statements, or government laws and regulations. The task is to identify key concepts or ideas embedded in these documents. For example, many government and disease association documents talk about the importance of providing people with the resources necessary to be healthy, but then go on to ignore these larger issues and argue that if people adopted healthy lifestyles they could avoid disease and illness.

## Qualitative Data Analysis

The primary approach is to identify themes or ideas that are present in the data collected through these methods. It is here that the researcher acts as an analyst in trying to make sense of what they have heard, read, or observed. The researcher approaches a study with some expectations of what might be present but remains open to the presence of novel themes or concepts that might emerge from the analysis of data.

## Examples of Social Sciences Qualitative Approaches

*Why teenagers use tobacco*: In a series of studies, teenagers were asked about the factors associated with their smoking. These study results showed that there are many reasons why teenagers smoke. These include issues of identify formation, building relationships and friendships, and resisting what they perceive as illegitimate authority on the part of teachers and school officials.

*Community quality of life study*: In a series of studies as to what makes a neighbourhood good for your health, individuals identified friendly and helpful neighbourhoods; the presence of community agencies and organizations; and governmental responsiveness and support of employment and income security.

*Newspaper coverage of health issues:* Recent studies have documented how Canadian newspapers ignore the social determinants of health and focus on healthcare service issues and lifestyle factors. Numerous barriers to having a broader approach to health reported in the media were identified.

# CRITICAL ANALYSIS IN HEALTH STUDIES

Critical analysis is more of a conceptual approach than an actual research methodology (Fay, 1987). Aligned with realism, it is concerned with identifying societal structures and institutions that distribute power and influence unequally. Critical analysis is broader than a political economy approach, which focuses on the political and economic institutions of society. Critical analysis includes issues such as the perception and meanings of disability, how the healthcare system privileges some kinds of professionals over others, and how scientific discourse itself is shaped (Rioux & Bach, 1994). Critical analysis employs all of the methods described above, but its distinguishing characteristic is its concern with uncovering structures of domination and oppression. Its gaze is firmly focused on the abstract and the conceptual rather than the concrete and observable. A key characteristic of this critical social research, which is also found in some of the other approaches to health research, is that it "positively allie[s] itself with oppressed groups" (Barnes, 2003, p. 6). It recognizes underlying issues of social justice as inherent conditions of the design and the implementation of research and "has a transformative aim" (Barnes, 2003, p. 6).

## Political Economy Approach

Commonly included in the critical analysis approach is a particular focus on how political and economic systems lead to unequal distributions of influence, power, and health. Political economists focus on the *control of material resources and production* through analysis of economic structures concerned with finance and commerce and *control of human resources and people* through analysis of political structures of the state (executive, judiciary, civil service, police, military, etc.). These structures are supported by the *control of ideas and knowledge*, which occurs through the dominant ideas of a society (e.g., its religion, mass media, education and science, etc.).

## Class, Gender, and Race Analyses

Within these analyses, special attention is given to how social class, gender, and race affect the allocation of influence, power, and health. There are systematic differences in influence, power, and health among upper-class, middle-class, and working-class Canadians, between men and women, and between Canadians of colour and Canadians of European descent or African descent. What are these differences? How do they come about? What can be done to reduce them? These questions are the central foci of these analyses.

## Historical Analysis

Historical analysis is concerned with identifying the specific characteristics of historical times that interact with societal structures to lead to various health outcomes and healthcare system characteristics. Much of this has to do with the forces driving economic and political change. By understanding where we have come from, we can help to identify where we might be going on a variety of health and healthcare issues. This is the kind of analysis outlined in Box 5.3.

## Examples of Critical Analysis

*Growing social and health inequalities in Canada*: Income and wealth inequality has been growing in Canada. Such differences are important as they usually translate into differences in health status among the population. Research has suggested that much of this has to do with an increasing imbalance among the business, labour, and civil society sectors in influence and power. Why this has occurred and what can be done to reverse it has been the subject of much health-related research (Raphael, 2015).

*Male and female differences in income and wealth*: Women consistently have lower income and less wealth than men. Why this is the case is the focus of inquiries in the labour and employment structure and the importance and value ascribed to male and female occupations. While women live longer than men, they are more likely to experience a number of diseases and illnesses that can be traced back to these income and wealth inequalities.

*Increasing poverty rates among immigrants of colour to Canada*: Immigrants of colour are much more likely to experience poverty than immigrants of European descent. This is the case despite these immigrants having excellent education credentials and fluency in one or the other official languages. These trends have intensified over the past 20 years such that immigrants of colour are the most likely to experience deteriorating health status after their arrival in Canada.

# HUMAN RIGHTS ANALYSIS

Human rights analysis uses, to some extent, all of the particular approaches discussed above. Within these analyses, special attention is given to the determination of how the health status at the international level, the national level, and the individual level, as well as by identifiable groups and in various societies, is measured to understand whether it is equitably achievable. At a minimum it looks at whether the norm of non-discrimination in the provision of healthcare services is met based on such factors as social class, gender, and race. Hunt (2003) maintains that there are a number of categories of right to health indicators, including structural indicators, process indicators, and outcome indicators (see Chapter 4, this volume).

In each of these areas, there has to be "an accountability for the State to explain what it is doing and how it is moving as expeditiously and effectively as possible toward the realization of the right to health for all" (United Nations High Commissioner for Human Rights and the World Health Organization, 2008). A framework on the right to health requires the capacity to measure compliance with a human rights approach to health nationally and under international norms and standards.

## Examples of Human Rights Analysis

Two examples that illustrate the link between these concepts and how research questions are identified can be seen in the following two issues.

*Equitable access to pharmaceuticals to treat HIV/AIDS in Africa and Asia*: HIV/AIDS drugs are differentially available between the rich and poor nations and within countries. Fundamental to the right to health is making medicines available where they are needed and making sure that the medicines are being adequately and equitably distributed so that those who are most vulnerable—including sex trade workers and HIV/AIDS mothers, those who are living in rural areas, and those who cannot afford private health care—are provided with needed drugs. Research would focus on identifying whether these gaps exist, why they exist, and what can be done to reduce gaps.

*Access to health services*: At the level of service delivery, there has to be a fair process for triaging and delivering health services and health benefits. People with disabilities, people who are poor, and women do not have the same access to health services, to organ transplants, and even to life as do others in many societies. Again, research would focus on identifying whether these differences exist, why they exist, and what can be done to reduce them. Research would also focus on whether people have choice in receiving health care and are treated with dignity as this impacts their health outcomes.

# CONCLUSIONS

Research and inquiry in health studies can be carried out within a variety of knowledge paradigms. These knowledge paradigms fundamentally shape which issues will be identified for inquiry, how such inquiry will be carried out, and the actual methods that will be applied in the course of inquiry. Positivist approaches have traditionally dominated health studies. Applying *quantitative* methods from the natural sciences, these approaches rely on experimental designs and statistical methods to identify relationships between causes and outcomes.

Approaches associated with *positivism* have been criticized as overly narrow and neglecting the importance of human understandings and societal structures. *Idealism* identifies the importance of these understandings and provides a rationale for applying qualitative methods for attaining and analyzing these understandings. The methods include open-ended interviews, detailed observations, and analyses of documents and other texts.

*Realism* directs attention to societal structures and institutions and how these shape the distribution of economic and political resources and the understandings that people have of the world. Critical analysis is the general manner in which these structures can be exposed and acted upon. Realist approaches can employ a whole range of methods, including quantitative and qualitative methods.

The *human rights* approach is a specific form of critical analysis. Its focus is upon human rights and their realizations. Ethical principles and human rights concepts direct attention to important issues and suggest means of carrying out inquiry. The goal is to provide all people with the opportunities for health and fulfillment identified in various human rights declarations and documents and delivered in ethical ways.

## CRITICAL THINKING QUESTIONS

1. What would be the implications for health studies of limiting analysis to a positivist approach?
2. What would be the implications for health studies of limiting analysis to an idealist approach?
3. What would be the implications for health studies of limiting analysis to a realist approach?
4. Why do you think that positivist approaches dominate in health studies?
5. Which approach seems the most relevant to you in terms of understanding health outcomes?

## FURTHER READINGS

Bryman, A., & Teevan, J. (2005). *Social research methods* (Canadian ed.). Toronto: Oxford University Press.
This book provides students with the conceptual building blocks and essential tools for conducting quantitative and qualitative research. Tackling complex, subtle, and methodological issues in ways that require reflection rather than regurgitation, this text challenges students to think freely, critically, and creatively.

Lincoln, Y., & Guba, E. (1985). *Naturalistic inquiry*. Newbury Park, CA: Sage.
*Naturalistic Inquiry* provides social scientists with a basic but comprehensive rationale for non-positivistic approaches to research. It confronts the basic premise underlying the scientific tradition that all questions can be answered by employing empirical, testable, replicable research techniques associated with traditional positivistic inquiry. They suggest an alternative approach supporting the use of the "naturalistic" paradigm.

Norman, G., & Steiner, D. (2008). *Biostatistics: The bare essentials*. Toronto: McGraw-Hill Ryerson.

This book translates biostatistics in the health sciences literature with clarity and irreverence. It is a practical guide that describes every statistical test you may encounter, with careful conceptual explanations.

Rioux, M., Basser, L., & Jones, M. (Eds.). (2018). *Critical perspectives on human rights and disability law.* The Hague, Netherlands: Martinus Nijhoff.
A collection of original articles from researchers around the world examining emerging frameworks for theorizing and researching disability. Topics include a critical analysis of disability within a broader policy framework and linkages among disability, gender, race, and class.

Wilson, J. (1983). *Social theory.* Englewood Cliffs, NJ: Prentice Hall.
An excellent book that provides an overview of no less than 16 approaches to understanding and carrying out research. Its particular strength is the focus on positivism, idealism, and realism. It is no longer in print, but can be bought used online.

## RELEVANT WEBSITES

**Colorado State University Writing Guides: Overview: Ethnography, Observational Research, and Narrative Inquiry**
http://writing.colostate.edu/guides/research/observe/index.cfm
This site provides an overview of methodologies that employ a range of qualitative techniques to explore the behaviours of groups.

**Colorado State University Writing Guides: Overview: Experimental and Quasi-Experimental Research**
http://writing.colostate.edu/guides/research/experiment/
An overview of methodologies that employ a range of experimental and quasi-experimental methods techniques.

**Resource Collection on Human Rights Education and Training**
https://www.ohchr.org/EN/Issues/Education/Training/Pages/Collection.aspx
The Office of the High Commissioner for Human Rights (OHCHR) has developed a specialized public-access Resource Collection on Human Rights Education and Training, which is part of the OHCHR Library.

**International Institute for Qualitative Methodology (IIQM)**
https://www.ualberta.ca/international-institute-for-qualitative-methodology
The International Institute for Qualitative Methodology (IIQM) is an interdisciplinary institute based at the University of Alberta, in Edmonton, Alberta, Canada, but serves qualitative researchers around the world. IIQM was founded in 1998, with the primary

goal of facilitating the development of qualitative research methods across a wide variety of academic disciplines.

**SAGE Publications Research Methods**

https://us.sagepub.com/en-us/nam/sage-research-methods

SAGE Research Methods is the essential online resource for anyone doing research or learning how to do research. SAGE Research Methods provides information on writing a research question, conducting a literature review, choosing a research method, collecting and analyzing data, and writing up the findings. Coverage spans the full range of research methods used in the social and behavioural sciences, plus a wide range of methods commonly used in science, technology, medicine, and the humanities.

## GLOSSARY

**Critical theory:** "The central principles of critical theory can perhaps be defined most clearly in contrast to some of the principles of twentieth-century positivism—indeed its proponents sometimes referred to it as negative philosophy. As opposed to the idea that knowledge comes from our sense-experience, critical theory is a form of rationalism; that is, critical theorists maintain that the source of our knowledge and the source of our common humanity is the fact that we are all rational beings" (Marshall, 1998).

**Epidemiology:** "… the study of the distribution of disease as well as its determinants and consequences in human populations. It uses statistical methods to answer questions on how much disease there is, what specific factors put individuals at risk, and how severe disease outcomes are in patient populations, in order to inform public health policy-making. The term 'disease' encompasses not only physical or mental illnesses but also behavioural patterns with negative health consequences, such as substance abuse or violence" (Ritzer & Ryan, 2011, p. 192).

**Human rights approach:** The goal of a human rights approach is to ensure the equal dignity and equal effective enjoyment of all human rights by all people, including the right to health. All people have the right to participate and to exercise self-determination as equals in society.

**Naturalistic inquiry:** Naturalistic inquiry refers to various forms of qualitative research that assume human constructions of reality are more meaningful to study than physical realities when dealing with human issues.

**Positivism:** "Positivism is, above all, a philosophy of science. As such, it stands squarely within the empiricist tradition. Metaphysical speculation is rejected in favour of 'positive' knowledge based on systematic observation and experiment. The methods of science can give us knowledge of the laws of coexistence and succession of phenomena but can never penetrate to the inner 'essences' or 'natures' of things" (Marshall, 1998).

## REFERENCES

Bambra, C. (2009). Changing the world? Reflections on the interface between social science, epidemiology and public health. *Journal of Epidemiology and Community Health, 63*(11), 867–868. doi:10.1136/jech.2009.087221

Barnes, C. (2003). What a difference a decade makes: Reflections on doing emancipatory disability research. *Disability and Society, 18*(1), 3–17. doi:10.1080/713662197

Berkman, L. F., Kawachi, I., & Glymour, M. M. (Eds.). (2014). *Social epidemiology* (2nd ed.). Oxford: Oxford University Press.

Bryant, T. (2016). *Health policy in Canada* (2nd ed.). Toronto: Canadian Scholars' Press.

Davey Smith, G., & Ebrahim, S. (2001). Epidemiology—Is it time to call it a day? *International Journal of Epidemiology, 30*(1), 1–11. doi:10.1093/ije/30.1.1

Fay, B. (1987). *Critical social science: Liberation and its limits.* Ithaca, NY: Cornell University Press.

Festinger, L., Riecken, H. W., & Schacter, S. (1956). *When prophecy fails: A social and psychological study of a modern group that predicted the destruction of the world.* New York: Harper-Torchbooks.

Guba, E. (Ed.). (1990). *The paradigm dialog.* Newbury Park, CA: Sage.

Hunt, P. (2003). *Economic, social and cultural rights: The right of everyone to the enjoyment of the highest attainable standard of physical and mental health.* Geneva: United Nations.

Lincoln, Y., & Guba, E. (1985). *Naturalist inquiry.* Newbury Park CA: Sage.

Marshall, G. (1998). Critical theory. In *A Dictionary of sociology.* New York: Oxford University Press.

Popay, J., & Williams, G. H. (Eds.). (1994). *Researching the people's health: Social research and health care.* London, U.K.: Routledge.

Raphael, D. (2015). The political economy of health: A research agenda for addressing health inequalities in Canada. *Canadian Public Policy, 41*(Suppl. 2), S17–S25.

Rioux, M., & Bach, M. (Eds.). (1994). *Disability is not measles: New research paradigms in disability.* Toronto: Roeher Institute.

Ritzer, G., & Ryan, J. (2011). *The concise encyclopedia of sociology.* Malden, MA: Blackwell Publishing.

Sung, H. (2007). Epidemiology. In G. Ritzer (Ed.), *The Blackwell encyclopedia of sociology.* doi:10.1002/9781405165518.wbeose055.

United Nations High Commissioner for Human Rights and the World Health Organization. (2008). *Fact Book No. 31.* Geneva: United Nations.

Wilson, J. (1983a). Idealism. In J. Wilson (Ed.), *Social theory* (pp. 106–121). Englewood Cliffs, NJ: Prentice Hall.

Wilson, J. (1983b). Positivism. In J. Wilson (Ed.), *Social theory* (pp. 11–18). Englewood Cliffs NJ: Prentice Hall.

Wilson, J. (1983c). Realism. In J. Wilson (Ed.), *Social theory* (pp. 166–175). Englewood Cliffs NJ: Prentice Hall.

Wilson, J. (1983d). *Social theory.* Englewood Cliffs, NJ: Prentice Hall.

# PART II

## SOCIAL DETERMINANTS OF HEALTH

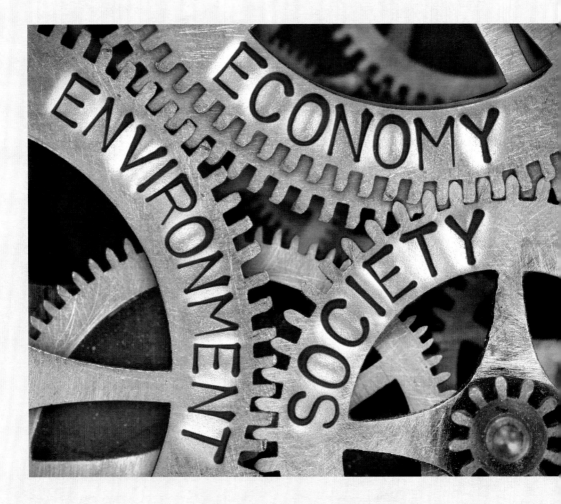

There is increasing recognition that the mainsprings of health are to be found in the manner in which societies are organized and resources distributed among the population. The concept of the social determinants of health is an illustration of how the various paradigms by which health, illness, and health care can be examined contribute to furthering our understanding of these issues.

A focus upon society and its characteristics as a source of health is clearly a subordinate approach to these issues. Governmental, public, and the media's concerns are firmly entrenched within a medical model of health, whereby the body is a machine that is either running well or in need of repair. If the body is free of illness, the person is healthy. If it is either infected with pathogens or afflicted with system or organ-malfunctioning disease, illness occurs. The remedy for such disease and illness is found in medical or curative care, which is located in the healthcare system and administered by doctors and nurses.

The allocation of government spending to the healthcare system, research activities, and disease foundations reflects this commitment to the medical model. The preoccupation of all key players—the public, the media, and governments—with the medical model ensures that issues related to health and health care will receive primary attention. These strong tendencies are reinforced by increasing governmental adherence to public policy approaches associated with neo-liberalism, the belief that the marketplace is the best arbiter of societal resources, and that citizens are best viewed as individual consumers rather than members of a communal whole. Individualism focuses attention on people and their bodies rather than the societal structures and the political, economic, and social forces that create either health or disease.

In Chapter 6, Dennis Raphael defines and identifies the social determinants of health. He provides evidence that factors such as the distribution of income, the provision of housing and food security, and the security of employment and the quality of working conditions are the primary determinants of health. These social determinants of health help explain increases in health in countries such as Canada over the past century, differences among Canadians, and why Canadians are healthier than Americans but less healthy than citizens of nations of Northern Europe. Despite this evidence, governments and the media pay little attention to these determinants. Raphael shows how each of the perspectives identified in Part I of this volume contributes to understanding these issues and identifies key questions that need to be considered.

In Chapter 7, Ambreen Sayani explores social class and how it shapes health and produces inequalities in health. She provides definitions of social class and notes that social class is rarely explicitly considered in the health literature. Rather, socio-economic status (SES), as measured by income, education, and occupation, is most often considered in relation to various health outcomes. She provides explanations for the SES and health relationship. Specific analysis is then made about how SES comes to be related to all aspects of cancer incidence and care, with special focus on breast cancer. While the focus of her chapter draws out the links between social class and health inequalities using cancer as an example, the theoretical underpinnings and concepts presented can be applied to almost any illness.

In Chapter 8, Ann Pederson and Stefanie Machado explore the interactions of gender and ethnicity/race with health. They examine how gender and ethnicity/race shape the health of im/migrant and Indigenous women and girls and thereby identify the commonalities as well as differences in how their respective social locations and positioning contribute to health and access to health care. They provide details as to the health of those occupying these social locations and then suggest means of responding to these situations through various health promotion approaches. Key to this is understanding the lived experiences of women, Indigenous peoples, and im/migrants in Canada. The authors suggest greater focus upon aspects of resiliency as opposed to vulnerabilities will facilitate such health promotion activities.

Finally, in Chapter 9, Toba Bryant shows how the quality of various social determinants of health is influenced by governments' public policies. She compares the public policies of Canada, the U.S., the United Kingdom, Sweden, and Norway, and their differential impact on health determinants. She traces the political, economic, and social influences that lead governments to take one public policy position rather than another. Political ideology and political and social organization are strong influences upon public policy. Policies developed and implemented in nations oriented toward neo-liberal nations, such as Canada, the U.S., and the U.K., are not as supportive of health as those of social democratic nations. The public policies taken in the U.S. in particular lead to greater incidence of poverty, larger income and wealth gaps between rich and poor, and poorer population health than what is seen in Canada.

# CHAPTER 6

## Social Determinants of Health

*Dennis Raphael*

## INTRODUCTION

A main theme of this volume is that the health of individuals and societies and the delivery of health care are strongly determined by the organization of societies and how these societies distribute material resources among their members. In this chapter, the focus is on how the social determinants of health—that is, the living and working conditions individuals experience—are the primary factors shaping their health. This idea is accepted by each of the epidemiological, sociological, political economy, and human rights approaches to understanding health. The social determinants of health concept and the research that documents its importance illustrate how analysis of health issues requires an interdisciplinary approach to understanding health, illness, and health care.

The idea that societal factors—of which one of the most important is how income and wealth are distributed within a society—are important determinants of health is not new. As early as the 4th century BC, the Greek philosopher Plato stated:

> The form of law which I should propose as the natural sequel would be as follows: In a state which is desirous of being saved from the greatest of all plagues—not faction, but rather distraction—there should exist among the citizens neither extreme poverty, nor, again, excess of wealth, for both are productive of both these evils. Now the legislator should determine what is to be the limit of poverty or wealth. Let the limit of poverty be the value of the lot; this ought to be preserved, and no ruler, nor any one else who aspires after a reputation for virtue, will allow the lot to be impaired in any case. This the legislator gives as a measure, and he will permit a man to acquire double or triple, or as much as four times the amount of this. (Plato, 360 BC/2010)

The modern study of the social determinants of health began with the writings of Rudolph Virchow and Friedrich Engels during the mid-19th century. Virchow's *Report on the Typhus Epidemic in Upper Silesia* (1848/1985) and Engels's *The Condition of the Working Class in England* (1845/1987) not only made explicit the link between living and working conditions and health but also explored the political and economic structures in society that create differences in these conditions that lead to health inequalities. Over 150 years ago, Virchow (1848/1985) stated, "Do we not always find the diseases of the populace traceable to defects in society?" (p. 117), while Engels (1845/1987) noted, "That a class which lives under the conditions already sketched and is so ill-provided with the most necessary means of subsistence, cannot be healthy and can reach no advanced age is self-evident" (p. 128).

International interest in the social determinants of health led the World Health Organization (WHO) to create a Commission on Social Determinants of Health (WHO, 2008). Its final report, *Closing the Gap in a Generation: Health Equity through Action on the Social Determinants of Health*, succinctly summarizes the importance of these determinants of health and how these come about (Commission on Social Determinants of Health, 2008; see Box 6.1).

## Box 6.1: The Commission Calls for Closing the Health Gap in a Generation

Social justice is a matter of life and death. It affects the way people live, their consequent chance of illness, and their risk of premature death. We watch in wonder as life expectancy and good health continue to increase in parts of the world and in alarm as they fail to improve in others. A girl born today can expect to live for more than 80 years if she is born in some countries, but less than 45 years if she is born in others. Within countries there are dramatic differences in health that are closely linked with degrees of social disadvantage. Differences of this magnitude, within and between countries, simply should never happen.

These avoidable inequities in health arise because of the circumstances in which people grow, live, work, and age, and the systems put in place to deal with illness. The conditions in which people live and die are, in turn, shaped by political, social, and economic forces.

Social and economic policies have a determining impact on whether a child can grow and develop to its full potential and live a flourishing life, or whether his or her life will be blighted. Increasingly the nature of the health problems that rich and poor countries have to solve is converging. The development of a society, rich or poor, can be judged by the quality of its population's health, how fairly health is distributed across the social spectrum, and the degree of protection provided from disadvantage as a result of ill health.

In the spirit of social justice, the Commission on Social Determinants of Health was set up by the World Health Organization (WHO) in 2005 to marshal the evidence on what can be done to promote health equity, and to foster a global movement to achieve it.

As the commission has done its work, several countries and agencies have become partners seeking to frame policies and programs across the whole of society that influence the social determinants of health and improve health equity. These countries and partners are in the forefront of a global movement.

The commission calls on the WHO and all governments to lead global action on the social determinants of health with the aim of achieving health equity. It is essential that governments, civil society, the WHO, and other global organizations now come together in taking action to improve the lives of the world's citizens. Achieving health equity within a generation is achievable, it is the right thing to do, and now is the right time to do it.

*Source:* Commission on the Social Determinants of Health. (2008). Preface. *Closing the gap in a generation: Health equity through action on the social determinants of health.* Geneva: WHO.

Canada had been a leader in developing social determinants of health concepts, at least until the beginning of the 21st century (Restrepo, 2000). But Canada has been rather less successful than other wealthy nations in putting these concepts into action (Bryant, Raphael, Schrecker, & Labonte, 2011). Instead, the application of these concepts in the service of health has taken place in many European nations by being integrated into their public policies. In Canada, however, the approach remains subordinate to traditional medical and behavioural paradigms of health, illness, and health care (see Chapter 16, this volume).

**Box 6.2:** Rudolph Virchow and the Social Determinants of Health

German physician Rudolph Virchow's (1821–1902) medical discoveries were so extensive that he is known as the "father of modern pathology." But he was also a trailblazer in identifying how societal policies determine health. In 1848, Berlin authorities sent Virchow to investigate the epidemic of typhus in Upper Silesia. His *Report on the Typhus Epidemic Prevailing in Upper Silesia* argued that lack of democracy, feudalism, and unfair tax policies in the province were the primary determinants of the inhabitants' poor living conditions, inadequate diet, and poor hygiene that fuelled the epidemic.

Virchow stated, "Disease is not something personal and special, but only a manifestation of life under modified (pathological) conditions." Arguing that "medicine is a social science and politics is nothing else but medicine on a large scale," Virchow drew the direct links between social conditions and health. He argued that improved health required recognition that "if medicine is to fulfil her great task, then she must enter the political and social life. Do we not always find the diseases of the populace traceable to defects in society?" (Virchow, 1848/1985).

The authorities were not happy with the report, and Virchow was relieved of his government position. But he continued his pathology research within university settings and went on to a parallel career as a member of Berlin City Council and the Prussian Diet, where he focused on public health issues consistent with his Upper Silesia report. Virchow also bitterly opposed Otto Von Bismarck's plans for national rearmament and was challenged to a duel by the said gentleman. Virchow declined participation.

## WHAT ARE SOCIAL DETERMINANTS OF HEALTH?

The term *social determinants of health* grew out of researchers' search for the specific mechanisms by which members of different socio-economic groups come to experience varying degrees of health and illness (Doyal & Pennell, 1979; Graham, 2004; Tarlov, 1996). Everywhere, individuals of different socio-economic status show profoundly different levels of health and incidence of disease.

Another stimulus to investigating social determinants of health was the finding of national differences in overall health. For example, the health status of Americans—using indicators such as life expectancy, infant mortality, and death by childhood injury rates—compares unfavourably to citizens in most wealthy nations (see Chapter 1, this volume). In contrast, the health status of Norwegians is generally superior to that seen in most nations (Raphael, 2012). It was hypothesized that perhaps the same factors that explain health differences among groups within nations could also explain health differences among national populations.

A variety of approaches to the social determinants of health exist, and all are concerned with the organization and distribution of economic and social resources among the population. See Figure 6.1 for one influential example that places the social determinants of health in broader context. The *Ottawa Charter for Health Promotion* identifies the *prerequisites for health* as peace, shelter, education, food, income, a stable ecosystem, sustainable resources, social justice, and equity (WHO, 1986). A British working group charged with the specific task of identifying *social determinants of health* named the social (class health) gradient, stress, early life, social exclusion, work, unemployment, social support, addiction, food, and transport (Wilkinson & Marmot, 2003). And the U.S. Centers for Disease Control and Prevention (CDC) highlight *social determinants of health* of economic stability, education, social and community context, health and health care, and neighbourhood and built environments (CDC, 2018).

Canadian workers synthesized these formulations to identify 16 *social determinants of health*: early life, education, disability, employment and working conditions, food security, gender, geography, healthcare services, housing, immigrant status, income and its distribution, Indigenous descent, race, social safety net, social exclusion, and unemployment

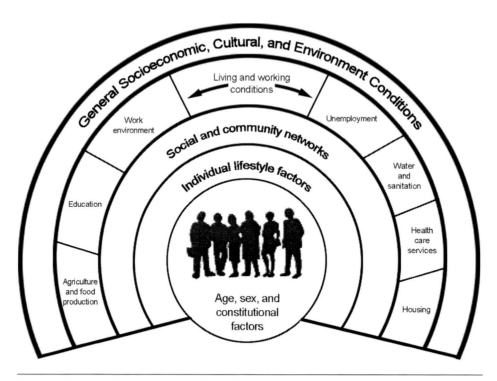

**Figure 6.1:** Social Determinants of Health in Broader Perspective

*Source:* Dahlgren, G., & Whitehead, M. (1991). *Policies and strategies to promote social equity in health.* Stockholm, Sweden: Institute for Futures Studies.

and employment security (Raphael, 2016c). These determinants are especially relevant to understanding and improving the health of Canadians. Evidence indicates that the health-related effects of each and every one of these factors equals or exceeds the influence of the so-called lifestyle or behavioural risk factors such as tobacco and alcohol use, diet, weight, and physical activity, a conclusion stated as early as the mid-1970s (Marmot, Rose, Shipley, & Hamilton, 1978).

## WHAT IS THE EVIDENCE CONCERNING THE SOCIAL DETERMINANTS OF HEALTH?

Research that examines the importance of the social determinants of health provides insights into: (1) the general improvement in health among citizens in developed nations over the past 100 years; (2) the health inequalities observed among populations within nations; and (3) the differences in overall national health among both developed (e.g., Norway vs. Canada vs. the U.S.) and developing nations (e.g., Cuba vs. Argentina vs. Brazil).

## The Social Determinants of Improved Health among Canadians Since 1900

Profound improvements in health status have occurred in industrialized nations such as Canada since 1900. Many believe that access to improved medical care is responsible for these differences, but best estimates are that only 10%–15% of increased longevity since 1900 in wealthy nations is due to improved health care (McKinlay & McKinlay, 1987). As one illustration, the advent of vaccines and medical treatments is usually held responsible for the profound declines in mortality from infectious diseases in Canada since 1900. But by the time vaccines for diseases such as measles, influenza, and polio and treatments for scarlet fever, typhoid, and diphtheria appeared, dramatic declines in mortality had already occurred (McKinlay & McKinlay, 1987).

Improvements in behaviour (e.g., reductions in tobacco use, changes in diet, increased exercise, etc.) have also been hypothesized as responsible for improved longevity, but most analysts conclude that improvements in health are due to the improving material conditions of everyday life experienced by Canadians since 1900 (McKeown, 1976; McKeown, Record, & Turner, 1975). These improvements have occurred in the areas of early childhood, education, food processing and availability, health and social services, housing, and employment security and working conditions, all clearly being the social determinants of health.

## The Social Determinants of Health Inequalities among Canadians

Despite dramatic improvements in health in general, significant inequalities in health among Canadians persist (Tjepkema, Wilkins, & Long, 2013). Access to essential medical procedures is guaranteed by medicare in Canada. Nevertheless, access to care issues are common, and this is particularly the case with regard to required prescription medicines where income is a strong determinant of such access (McGibbon, 2016; Raphael, 2011b). It is believed, however, that healthcare issues account for a relatively small proportion of health status differences among Canadians (Siddiqi & Hertzman, 2007). As for differences in health behaviours (e.g., tobacco and alcohol use, diet, physical activity, etc.), studies from as early as the mid-1970s—reinforced by many more studies since then—find their impact upon health to be less important than social determinants of health such as income and other aspects of living conditions (Marmot et al., 1978; Marmot, Shipley, Brunner, & Hemingway, 2001; Nettleton, 1997; Raphael, 2007).

Indeed, evidence indicates that health differences among Canadians result primarily from experiences of qualitatively different living and working conditions associated with the social determinants of health. As just one example, consider the magnitude of differences in health that are related to the social determinant of health of income. Income is especially important as it serves as a marker of different experiences with many social determinants of health (Raphael, 2016a). Income is a determinant of health in itself, but it is also a determinant of the quality of early life, education, employment and working conditions, and food security. Income also is a determinant of the quality of housing, the need for a social safety net, the experience of social exclusion, and the experience of unemployment and employment insecurity across the lifespan. Also, a key aspect of Indigenous life and the experience of women in Canada is their greater likelihood of living under conditions of low income (Raphael, 2011e; Smylie & Firestone, 2016).

Income is a prime determinant of Canadians' premature years of life lost and premature mortality from a range of diseases (Auger & Alix, 2016; Tjepkema et al., 2013). Numerous studies indicate that income levels during early childhood, adolescence, and adulthood are all independent predictors of who develops and eventually succumbs to disease (Benzeval, Dilnot, Judge, & Taylor, 2001; Benzeval & Judge, 2001; Davey Smith, 2003; Judge & Paterson, 2001).

A 2013 report by Statistics Canada further highlights how important income is as a social determinant of health. The study shows that income differences are associated with the excess deaths of 40,000 Canadians a year (Tjepkema et al., 2013). That's equal to 110 Canadians dying prematurely each day. How does this report arrive at this conclusion? Researchers followed 2.7 million Canadians over a 16-year period and calculated death rates from a wide range of diseases and injuries as a function of the person's income. Canadians in the study were divided into five quintiles of approximately equal numbers from poorest to wealthiest.

It then compared the number of deaths of the wealthiest 20% of Canadians to the other 80% of Canadians. It concluded that if all Canadians were as healthy as the top 20% of Canadian income earners, there would be approximately 40,000 fewer deaths each year. Of these, 25,000 fewer deaths would be among Canadian men and 15,000 among Canadian women. These numbers are comparable to eliminating all deaths from a major killer of Canadians, coronary artery disease. The report also calculates the relative rate of mortality, comparing the likelihood of death between someone in the poorest 20% of Canadians and one of the wealthiest 20% of Canadians. Overall, this figure is 1.67 for men and 1.52 for women, indicating that a poor male has a 67% greater chance of dying each year and a poor woman has a 52% greater chance of dying each year than their wealthy counterparts. That's an overall excess death rate of 19.4% for men and 16.6% for women.

The study goes into further detail, outlining income-related statistics for specific diseases. Table 6.1 shows the greater risk associated with being poor as compared to wealthy and excess mortality associated with income differences between the wealthy and all other Canadians for various diseases and injuries. Poor Canadian males have a 67% greater chance of dying each year from heart disease than their wealthy counterparts. For women, it's a difference of 53%. The excess cardiovascular deaths each year associated with not being as healthy as the wealthy are 19% for men and 18% for women.

In relation to mortality from diabetes, the figures are even more striking. Poor Canadian men have a 150% greater chance and poor women a 160% greater chance of dying from diabetes each year than wealthy Canadians. This means that if all Canadians were as healthy as wealthy Canadians, there would be nearly 40% fewer deaths from diabetes

**Table 6.1:** Greater Risk of Dying Associated with Being Poor as Compared to Wealthy (RR) and Excess Deaths Associated with Income Inequality for Various Diseases and Injuries among Canadians

| Disease | RR[1] | | Excess Deaths[2] (%) | |
|---|---|---|---|---|
| | **Men** | **Women** | **Men** | **Women** |
| Cardiovascular disease | 1.67 | 1.53 | 19 | 18 |
| Cancers | 1.46 | 1.30 | 16 | 11 |
| Diabetes | 2.49 | 2.64 | 36 | 38 |
| Respiratory disease | 2.31 | 2.11 | 37 | 30 |
| HIV/AIDS | 3.57 | 11.10 | 39 | 69 |
| Injuries | 1.88 | 1.83 | 18 | 17 |

*Notes:* 1. Inter-quintile rate ratio between poorest and wealthiest = (Q1—Poorest)/Q5—Wealthiest);
2. % excess deaths due to differences between wealthy and all other Canadians = [100*(Total-Q5)/Total]

*Source:* Adapted from Tjepkema, M., Wilkins, R., & Long, A. (2013). Cause-specific mortality by income adequacy in Canada: A 16-year follow-up study. *Health Reports, 24*(7), 14–22, Tables 2 and 3, pp. 17–18.

and nearly 20% fewer deaths from cardiovascular disease every year. Similar numbers showing a profound difference between wealthy and poor Canadians and between wealthy and all other Canadians appear for virtually every known disease that can kill Canadians, including cancer, respiratory disease, injuries, HIV/AIDS, and many more.

The Statistics Canada report also makes clear that these differences in health outcomes are primarily due to the material living circumstances and the psychosocial stresses associated with not being as well-off as the wealthiest 20% of Canadians, not differences in health-related behaviours: "Income influences health most directly through access to material resources such as better quality food and shelter" (Tjepkema et al., 2013, p. 14).

While governments, medical researchers, and healthcare workers emphasize the importance of traditional adult risk factors (e.g., cholesterol levels, diet, physical activity, and tobacco and alcohol use), it is well established that these are relatively poor predictors of heart disease, stroke, and type 2 diabetes rates among populations (Chaufan, 2008; Davey Smith, Ben-Shlomo, & Lynch, 2002; Lawlor, Ebrahim, & Smith, 2002). The factors making a difference are living under conditions of material deprivation as children and adults, stress associated with such conditions, and the adoption of health-threatening behaviours as means of coping with these difficult circumstances (Benzeval, Judge, & Whitehead, 1995). In fact, difficult living circumstances during childhood are especially good predictors of these diseases (Barker, Osmond, Winter, Margetts, & Simmonds, 1989; Davey Smith & Hart, 2002; Eriksson, Forsén, Tuomilehto, Osmond, & Barker, 2001; Eriksson et al., 1999).

In addition to predicting adult incidence and death from disease, income differences—and the other social determinants of health related to income—are also related to the health of Canadian children and youth. Canadian children living in low-income families are more likely to experience greater incidence of a variety of illnesses, hospital stays, accidental injuries, mental health problems, lower school achievement and dropping out of school early, and family violence and child abuse, among other problems (Raphael, 2010a, 2010b, 2010c, 2010d). In fact, low-income children show higher incidences of just about any health-, social-, or education-related problem, however defined. These differences in problem incidence occur across the income range, but are most concentrated among low-income children (Raphael, 2016b).

One way to think about the different approaches to the determinants of health is presented in Box 6.3. In one approach, the focus is on so-called lifestyle choices. In the other, there is a concern with the social determinants of health.

## The Social Determinants of Health Differences between Nations

Profound differences in overall health status exist between developed and developing nations. Much of this has to do with the lack of the basic necessities of life (food, water, sanitation, primary health care, etc.) common to developing nations (Gordon, 2010). Yet among developed nations such as Canada, there are significant differences in health status indicators such as life expectancy, infant mortality, incidence of disease, and death from injuries (Raphael, 2011d). An excellent example is comparison of health status differences and the social determinants of these health status differences among Canada, the United States, and Norway.

Table 6.2 shows how Canada, the U.S., and Norway fare on several social determinants of health and indicators of overall population health. Scholarship has noted that the U.S. takes an especially laissez-faire approach to providing various forms of security (employment, food, income, and housing) and health and social services, while Norway's welfare state makes extraordinary efforts to provide security and services. The sources of these differences in public policy appear to be in differing commitments to citizen support informed by the political ideologies of governing parties within each nation.

Emerging scholarship is specifically focused on how national approaches to security provision to citizens influence health by shaping the quality of numerous social determinants of health. Nations such as Norway, whose policies reduce unemployment, minimize income and wealth inequality, and address numerous social determinants of health, show evidence of improved population health using indicators such as infant mortality and life expectancy. At the other end, nations with minimal commitments to such efforts, such as the United States, show rather worse indicators of population health.

Finally, poverty is an especially important indicator of how various social determinants of health combine to influence health. Using child—that is, family—poverty rates

**Box 6.3:** Which Tips for Better Health Are Consistent with Research Evidence?

The messages given to the public by governments and health workers are influenced by the ways in which health issues are understood. Contrast the two sets of messages provided below. The first set assumes individuals can control the factors that determine their health. The second set assumes the most important determinants of health are beyond the control of most individuals. Which set of tips is most consistent with the evidence provided in this book?

The Traditional 10 Tips for Better Health (Donaldson):
1. Don't smoke. If you can, stop. If you can't, cut down.
2. Follow a balanced diet with plenty of fruit and vegetables.
3. Keep physically active.
4. Manage stress by, for example, talking things through and making time to relax.
5. If you drink alcohol, do so in moderation.
6. Cover up in the sun, and protect children from sunburn.
7. Practice safer sex.
8. Take up cancer-screening opportunities.
9. Be safe on the roads: follow the Highway Code.
10. Learn the First Aid ABCs: airways, breathing, circulation.

The Social Determinants 10 Tips for Better Health (Gordon):
1. Don't be poor. If you can, stop. If you can't, try not to be poor for long.
2. Don't have poor parents.
3. Own a car.
4. Don't work in a stressful, low-paid manual job.
5. Don't live in damp, low-quality housing.
6. Be able to afford to go on a foreign holiday and sunbathe.
7. Practice not losing your job, and don't become unemployed.
8. Take up all benefits you are entitled to, if you are unemployed, retired or sick or disabled.
9. Don't live next to a busy major road or near a polluting factory.
10. Learn how to fill in the complex housing benefit/asylum application forms before you become homeless and destitute.

*Sources:* Donaldson, L. (1999). *Ten tips for better health* (London: Stationary Office); Gordon, D. (1999). *Ten tips for better health.* Message posted on the Spirit of 1848 Listserv.

**Table 6.2:** Norway, Canada, and U.S. Rankings on Selected Social Determinants of Health and Indicators of Population Health in Comparison to Other OECD Nations (c. 2015–2017) (n=34)

| | Measure Ranking (1 is best) | | |
| --- | --- | --- | --- |
| | **Norway** | **Canada** | **USA** |
| *Social Determinants of Health* | | | |
| % living in poverty[1] | 7 | 23 | 33 |
| Income inequality[1] | 6 | 20 | 33 |
| Public social expenditure[2] | 10 | 27 | 23 |
| Minimum-income benefit (single person)[3] | 15 | 28 | 30 |
| Minimum-income benefit (couple)[3] | 12 | 27 | 30 |
| *Health* | | | |
| Life expectancy[4] | 4 | 14 | 27 |
| Infant mortality[4] | 5 | 30 | 33 |
| Low birthweight[4] | 5 | 14 | 31 |
| Child well-being[5] | 1 | 25 | 37 |

*Notes:* (1) 2016/2017 data from OECD. (2019). Income inequality. Retrieved from https://data.oecd.org/inequality/income-inequality.htm; (2) 2016/2017 data from OECD. (2019). Public social expenditure. Retrieved from http://www.oecd.org/social/expenditure.htm; (3) 2015 data from OECD. (2019). Benefits and wages. Retrieved from http://www.oecd.org/els/benefits-and-wages-statistics.htm; (4) 2016 data from OECD. (2019). Health status. Retrieved from https://stats.oecd.org/Index.aspx?DataSet Code=HEALTH_STAT&_ga=2.69825936.1093734741.1547505112-339343583.1547505112; (5) 2016 data from UNICEF Canada. (2017). *UNICEF report card 14: Canadian Companion, Oh Canada! Our kids deserve better.* Toronto: UNICEF Canada. Retrieved from https://www.unicef.ca/sites/default/files/2017-06/RC14%20Canadian%20Companion_0.pdf

as an important social determinant of both child and eventual adult health, Canada does not fare well in relation to European nations (see Figure 6.2).

## MECHANISMS AND PATHWAYS BY WHICH SOCIAL DETERMINANTS OF HEALTH INFLUENCE HEALTH

To secure attention to the social determinants of health and build support for improving their quality and equitable distribution, it is important to understand how social determinants of health come to influence health and cause disease. How do social determinants of health "get under the skin" to influence health? The very influential U.K. *Black* and *Health Divide* reports considered two primary mechanisms for understanding this process: *cultural/behavioural* and *materialist/structuralist* (Townsend, Davidson, & Whitehead, 1992).

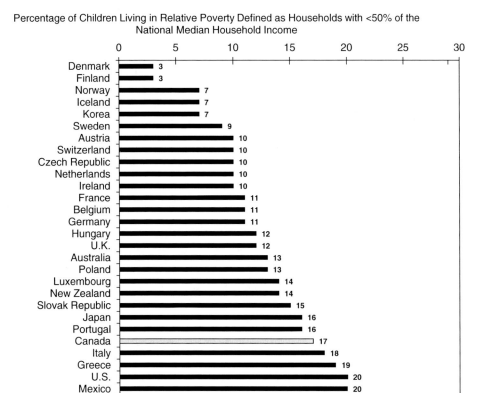

**Figure 6.2:** Child Poverty in Wealthy Nations, 2017 or Latest Year

*Source:* Adapted from Organisation for Economic Co-operation and Development. (2019). *Poverty rate.* Retrieved May 1, 2019, from https://data.oecd.org/inequality/poverty-rate.htm

The *cultural/behavioural explanation* was that individuals' behavioural choices (e.g., tobacco and alcohol use, diet, physical activity, etc.) were responsible for their developing and dying from a variety of diseases. Both the *Black* and *Health Divide* reports, however, showed that behavioural choices are heavily structured by one's material conditions of life. And—consistent with mounting evidence—these behavioural risk factors account for a relatively small proportion of variation in the incidence and death from various diseases. The *materialist/structuralist* explanation emphasizes the material conditions under which people live their lives. These conditions include availability of resources to access the amenities of life, working conditions, and quality of available food and housing, among others.

The author of the *Health Divide* concluded that: "The weight of evidence continues to point to explanations which suggest that socio-economic circumstances play the major part in subsequent health *differences* (Whitehead, 1992, p. 336). Despite this conclusion and increasing evidence in favour of this view, much of the Canadian public discourse on health and disease remains focused on "lifestyle" approaches to disease prevention (Raphael et al., 2018).

These *materialist/structuralist* conceptualizations have been refined such that analysis is now focused upon three frameworks by which social determinants of health come to influence health (Bartley, 2016). These frameworks are: (1) materialist, (2) neo-materialist, and (3) psychosocial comparison. The materialist explanation is about how living conditions—and the social determinants of health that constitute these living conditions—shape health. The neo-materialist explanation extends the materialist analysis by asking how these living conditions come about. The psychosocial comparison explanation considers whether people compare themselves to others and how these comparisons affect health and well-being.

## Materialist Approach: Conditions of Living as Determinants of Health

In this argument, individuals experience varying degrees of positive and negative exposures over their lives that accumulate to produce adult health outcomes (Shaw, Dorling, Gordon, & Davey Smith, 1999). Overall wealth of nations is a strong indicator of population health, but within nations, socio-economic position is a powerful predictor of health as it is an indicator of material advantage or disadvantage over the lifespan (Graham, 2007). Material conditions of life determine health by influencing the quality of individual development, family life and interaction, and community environments. Material conditions of life lead to differing likelihood of physical (infections, malnutrition, chronic disease, and injuries), developmental (delayed or impaired cognitive, personality, and social development), educational (learning disabilities, poor learning, early school leaving), and social (socialization, preparation for work, and family life) problems (Raphael, 2016b).

Material conditions of life also lead to differences in psychosocial stress (Brunner & Marmot, 2006). The fight-or-flight reaction—chronically elicited in response to threats such as income, housing, and food insecurity, among others—weakens the immune system, leads to increased insulin resistance, greater incidence of lipid and clotting disorders, and other biomedical problems that are precursors to adult disease.

Adoption of health-threatening behaviours is a response to material deprivation and stress (Jarvis & Wardle, 2003). Environments determine whether individuals take up tobacco, use alcohol, experience poor diets, and have low levels of physical activity. Tobacco and excessive alcohol use, and carbohydrate-dense diets are also means of coping with difficult circumstances (Wilkinson, 1996). Materialist arguments help us understand the sources of health inequalities among individuals and nations and the role played by the social determinants of health.

## Neo-materialist Approach: Conditions of Living and Social Infrastructure as Determinants of Health

Exposures to the material conditions of life are important for health, but why are these material conditions so unequally distributed among the Canadian population, but less so elsewhere (Graham, 2004)? The neo-materialist approach is concerned with how nations, regions, and cities differ on how economic and other resources are distributed among the population (Lynch, Davey Smith, Kaplan, & House, 2000). Some jurisdictions have more egalitarian distribution of resources so that there are fewer poor people, and the gaps among the population in their exposures to the social determinants of health are narrower than places where there are more poor people and the gaps among the population are greater.

In the U.S., states and cities with more unequal distributions of income have more low-income people and greater income gaps between rich and poor. They invest less in public infrastructure such as education, health and social services, health insurance, and supports for the unemployed and those with disabilities, and spend less on education and libraries. All of these issues contribute to the quality of the social determinants of health to which people are exposed. Such unequal jurisdictions have much poorer health profiles than more egalitarian places (Kaplan, Pamuk, Lynch, Cohen, & Balfour, 1996; Lynch et al., 1998).

Canada has a smaller proportion of lower-income people, a smaller gap between rich and poor, and spends relatively more on public infrastructure than the U.S. (Raphael, 2011a). Not surprisingly, Canadians enjoy better health than Americans as measured by infant mortality rates, life expectancy, and death rates from childhood injuries. Neither nation does as well as Norway, where distribution of resources is much more egalitarian, low-income rates are very low, and health indicators are among the best in the world (Raphael, 2012).

The neo-materialist view, therefore, directs attention to both the effects of living conditions—the social determinants of health—on individuals' health and the societal factors that determine the quality of the distribution of these social determinants of health. How a society decides to distribute resources among citizens is especially important.

## Social Comparison Approach: Hierarchy and Social Distance as Determinants of Health

The argument here is that the social determinants of health play their role through citizens' interpretations of their standings in the social hierarchy (Kawachi & Kennedy, 2002; Tarlov, 1996). There are two mechanisms by which this occurs.

At the individual level, the perception and experience of one's status in unequal societies lead to stress and poor health. Comparing their status, possessions, and other life circumstances to those who are better off than themselves, individuals experience feelings of shame, worthlessness, and envy that have psychobiological effects upon health. These processes involve direct disease-producing effects upon neuro-endocrine, autonomic and metabolic, and immune systems (Brunner & Marmot, 2006). These comparisons can also lead to attempts to alleviate such feelings by overspending, taking on additional employment that threatens health, and adopting health-threatening coping behaviours such as overeating and using alcohol and tobacco (Kawachi & Kennedy, 2002).

At the communal level, widening and strengthening of hierarchy weakens social cohesion, a determinant of health (Kawachi & Kennedy, 1997). Individuals become more distrusting and suspicious of others, with direct stress-related effects on the body. Such attitudes can also weaken support for communal structures such as public education, health, and social programs. An exaggerated desire for tax reductions on the part of the public can weaken public infrastructure.

This approach directs attention to the psychosocial effects of public policies that weaken the social determinants of health. But these effects may be secondary to how societies distribute material resources and provide security to their citizens, processes described in the materialist and neo-materialist approaches. Material aspects may be paramount, and the stresses associated with deprivation simply add to the toll on individuals' bodies.

## THE IMPORTANCE OF A LIFE-COURSE PERSPECTIVE

Traditional approaches to health and disease prevention have a distinctly non-historical here-and-now emphasis. Usually adults, and increasingly adolescents and youth, are urged to adopt "healthy lifestyles" as a means of preventing the development of chronic diseases such as heart disease and diabetes, among others (Chronic Disease Prevention Alliance of Canada, 2003; Health Canada, 2003). In contrast to these approaches, life-course approaches emphasize the accumulated effects of experience across the lifespan in understanding the maintenance of health and the onset of disease. It has been argued from as early as 1997 that:

> The prevailing aetiological model for adult disease which emphasizes adult risk factors, particularly aspects of adult life style, has been challenged in recent years by research that has shown that poor growth and development and adverse early environmental conditions are associated with an increased risk of adult chronic disease. (Kuh & Ben-Shlomo, 1997, p. 3)

More specifically, it is apparent that the economic and social conditions—the social determinants of health—under which individuals live their lives have a cumulative effect upon the probability of developing any number of diseases. This has been repeatedly demonstrated in longitudinal studies—the U.S. National Longitudinal Survey, the West of Scotland Collaborative Study, Norwegian and Finnish linked data—which follow individuals across their lives (Blane, 2005). This has been most clearly demonstrated in the case of heart disease and stroke and type 2 diabetes (Raphael et al., 2003; Raphael & Farrell, 2002).

One volume brings together some of the important work concerning the importance of a life-course perspective for understanding the importance of social determinants (Davey Smith, 2003). Adopting a life-course perspective directs attention to how social determinants of health operate at every level of development—early childhood,

childhood, adolescence, and adulthood—to immediately influence health as well as provide the basis for health or illness during later stages of the life course.

Hertzman outlines three health effects that have relevance for a life-course perspective (Hertzman & Boyce, 2010). *Latent effects* are biological or developmental early life experiences that influence health later in life. Low birth weight, for instance, is a reliable predictor of incidence of cardiovascular disease and adult-onset diabetes in later life. Experience of nutritional deprivation during childhood has lasting health effects.

*Pathway effects* are experiences that set individuals onto trajectories that influence health, well-being, and competence over the life course. As one example, children who enter school with delayed vocabulary are set upon a path that leads to lower educational expectations, poor employment prospects, and greater likelihood of illness and disease across the lifespan. Deprivation associated with poor-quality neighbourhoods, schools, and housing sets children off on paths that are not conducive to health and well-being.

*Cumulative effects* are the accumulation of advantage or disadvantage over time that manifests itself in poor health. These involve the combination of latent and pathways effects. Adopting a life-course perspective directs attention to how social determinants of health operate at every level of development—early childhood, childhood, adolescence, and adulthood—to both immediately influence health and provide the basis for health or illness later in life.

## THE IMPORTANCE OF PUBLIC POLICY AND POLICY ENVIRONMENTS

Much social determinants of health research simply focuses on determining the relationship between a social determinant of health and health status, so a researcher may document that lower income is associated with adverse health outcomes among parents and their children. Or a researcher may demonstrate that food insecurity and living in crowded housing are related to poor health status among parents and children, and so on. This is what is termed a depoliticized approach in that it says little about how these poor-quality social determinants of health come about (Raphael, 2015).

The quality and distribution of the social determinants of health do not exist in a vacuum. They are usually a result of public policy decisions made by governing authorities. As one example, consider the social determinant of health of early life. Early life is shaped by the availability of sufficient material resources that assure adequate educational opportunities, food, and housing, among other needs. Much of this has to do with the employment security and the quality of working conditions and wages. The availability of quality, regulated child care is an especially important policy option in support of early life (Esping-Andersen, 2002). These are not issues that usually come under individual control. A policy-oriented approach places such findings within a broader societal context.

Yet it is not uncommon to see governmental and other authorities individualize these issues. Governments may choose to understand early life as being primarily about parenting behaviours. They then focus upon promoting more sensitive parenting and encourage parents to read to their children. They can see early life solely in terms of physical activity, urging parents and schools to foster exercise among children rather than providing the financial resources necessary for health (Raphael et al., 2018). Indeed, for every social determinant of health, individualized manifestations are common. There is little evidence to suggest the efficacy of such approaches for improving the health of those most vulnerable to illness in the absence of efforts to modify their adverse living and working conditions.

## POLITICS, POLITICAL IDEOLOGY, AND THE SOCIAL DETERMINANTS OF HEALTH

Considering the evidence of the importance of the social determinants of health, how can we explain why certain nations take up this information and apply it in the formulation of public policy while others do not? Another way of considering this issue is to ask why there is such a gap between knowledge and action on the social determinants of health in Canada.

One way to think about this is to consider the idea of the welfare state and the political ideologies that shape its form in Canada and elsewhere. The concept of the welfare state is about the extent to which governments or the state use their power to provide citizens with the means to live secure and satisfying lives (see Chapter 3, this volume). Every developed nation has some form of the welfare state. Two important questions are: (1) How developed is this welfare state? and (2) What are the implications of the welfare state for the social determinants of health?

Two literatures inform this analysis. The first concerns the three forms of the modern welfare state. Esping-Andersen (1990, 1999) identifies three distinct clusters of welfare regimes among wealthy developed nations: social democratic (e.g., Sweden, Norway, Denmark, and Finland); liberal (Australia, Canada, Ireland, New Zealand, U.S., and U.K.); and conservative (France, Germany, Netherlands, and Belgium, among others). There is high government intervention, and strong welfare systems, in the social democratic countries and rather less in the liberal. Conservative nations fall midway between these others in service provision and citizen supports.

Social democratic nations have very well-developed welfare states that provide a wide range of universal and generous benefits (Olsen, 2010). They expend more of national wealth in supports and services. They are proactive in supporting labour, are family-friendly, and have gender equity-supporting policies. Liberal nations spend rather less on supports and services. They offer modest universal transfers and modest social-insurance plans. Benefits are provided primarily through means-tested assistance whereby these benefits are provided only to the least well-off. How do these forms of the welfare state come about? How do they shape the social determinants of health?

There is empirical support for the hypotheses that the social determinants of health and health status outcomes are of higher quality in the social democratic rather than the liberal nations (Raphael, 2011d). Some of these indicators are spending on supports and services, equitable distribution of income, and wealth and availability of services in support of families and individuals. Health indicators include life expectancy and infant mortality.

Could this general approach to welfare provision shape Canadian receptivity to the concepts developed in this volume? And, if so, what can be done to improve receptivity to and implementation of these concepts? The final chapter of this volume revisits these issues.

## WHAT KEY ISSUES ARE SUGGESTED BY EACH HEALTH PERSPECTIVE?

### Epidemiological Perspectives: Providing the "Hard" Evidence

Epidemiologists are concerned with identifying the determinants of individual and population health. Much of this is concerned with identifying individual biomedical and behavioural risk factors associated with disease such as cholesterol and glucose levels, weight, tobacco and alcohol use, diet, and sedentary behaviour (see Chapter 1, this volume). Individual-oriented approaches can also focus upon characteristics of individuals such as income, educational levels, occupational classification, individual control and empowerment, or attitudes and values and how these come to be related to health.

Social epidemiologists have expanded their analysis to broader concerns with environments, social conditions, and even the political context within which environments are created and sustained (Berkman, Kawachi, & Glymour, 2014). Within these frameworks, the key issues are the nature of environmental structures that influence health and the pathways by which these environmental structures come to influence health. These structural approaches are concerned with how societal structures mediate the social determinants and health relationship.

### *Horizontal Structures That Influence Health*

Horizontal structures are the more immediate factors that shape health and well-being (Mikkonen & Raphael, 2010). Some horizontal structures, for example, are the quality of childhood and family environments; the nature of work and workplace conditions; the quality and availability of housing; and the availability of resources for food, recreation, and educational resources. Similarly, a neighbourhood with few economic resources may have low levels of social organization or community cohesion.

### *Vertical Structures That Influence Health*

Vertical structures are the more distant macro-level issues that influence health and well-being. Vertical structures are the political, economic, and social forces that determine in large part the quality of the horizontal structures described above (Raphael, 2015). These forces are manifested in a jurisdiction's approaches to employment, training, income, social welfare, and tax policies. There are clear national, regional, and municipal differences in how these policy issues are addressed.

*Pathways and Mechanisms*

How do social determinants of health get "under the skin" to influence health? How do differences in conditions of living come about in the first place? These are questions about the pathways between environmental conditions and health. A study of how Canadian researchers conceptualize a prime social determinant of health—income and its distribution—and its relationship to health found that much of the research failed to take account of perspectives concerned with horizontal and vertical social structures (Raphael et al., 2005). Among 241 studies about income and health, only 16% focused on horizontal structures and 10% on vertical structures. An additional 14% focused on both kinds of structures, leaving 60% of studies neglecting these issues.

Concerning pathways linking income to health, 29% of studies simply noted that social class or education-related group memberships were related to income and health, and 28% were focused on behavioural risk factors. Only 33% were concerned with materialist or neo-materialist interpretations of the relationship between income and health, and only 22% were concerned with political-economic pathways. What are the reasons that epidemiologists limit themselves to these narrow analyses?

## Sociological Perspectives: Understanding the Gap between Knowledge and Action

Considering what we know about the social determinants of health, why is there so little action on these issues in Canada? Sociological perspectives offer us some insights into these issues.

*Psychological Constructs and Issues*

Sociologists have explored how we come to understand our world (see Chapter 2, this volume). The view that reality is socially constructed—that is, our understandings of the world are not given by nature but are chosen—is important for understanding how health and the determinants of health are conceptualized and, once so conceptualized, acted upon. Why is it that the social determinants of health are not the primary understandings held by the public, health workers, and government policy-makers? What are the political, economic, and social forces that shape our understandings of the world? Who benefits from our holding certain world views of the causes of illness?

*Disciplinary Approaches: Professions*

Professions differ profoundly on how they address issues of health, illness, and health care. Labonté (1993) suggests that health and health care can be viewed within three general frameworks: the biomedical, lifestyle, and socio-environmental. In the biomedical approach, emphasis is on high-risk groups, screening of one sort or another, and health-care delivery. The behavioural approach focuses on high-risk attitudes and behaviours and developing programs that educate and support individuals to change behaviours.

The socio-environmental approach focuses on risk conditions and considers how individuals adjust to these conditions or move to change them.

Clearly, the dominant paradigm among healthcare workers and researchers has been the biomedical. Public health has been focused on the behavioural, but this may be changing (Raphael & Sayani, 2017). Increasingly, public health units are addressing broader social determinants of health and the public policies that shape their quality and equitable distribution (Brassolotto, Raphael, & Baldeo, 2014; Raphael & Brassolotto, 2015; Raphael, Brassolotto, & Baldeo, 2015). How can these efforts be supported and converted into more health-promoting public policy?

### Institutional Mandates and Political Issues

Why do healthcare and public health organizations that emphasize the medical and behavioural approaches receive the greatest share of funding and public support (Kirkland & Raphael, 2018; Raphael et al., 2018)? Is it because governments welcome an approach that downplays their responsibility in addressing the social determinants of health? Given this reality, how can health care and public health be further supported in addressing the social determinants of health?

## Political Economy Perspectives: Identifying the Political and Economic Context

While sociological approaches direct attention to broader political and economic structures that influence health, it is the field of political economy that is devoted to exploring these issues and their influence upon health. It is an undeveloped area with few active health researchers. Particularly important issues are power relationships, government ideology and public policy, and welfare state typologies (Raphael, 2015). Also of increasing interest is the role played by economic globalization and trade agreements.

### Power Relationships

Hofrichter's (2003) volume provides an excellent overview of how issues of class, gender, and race come to influence health in developed nations. Chapters 7 and 8 in this volume consider how class, gender, and race come to influence health in Canada. In these analyses, class, gender, and race are not simply indicators of individuals' characteristics as much as markers of the power individuals within particular groups have within society.

It has also been pointed out that power relationships within a society are more equalized when labour unions and the "left" within a nation have more influence. Nations where a greater proportion of citizens are members of unions and are covered by collective agreements have lower overall poverty rates (see Figure 6.3).

Within nations, union membership also affects the quality of the social determinants of health. In Canada, for example, Canadians who are members of unions have higher incomes, as well as other benefits, that are social determinants of health

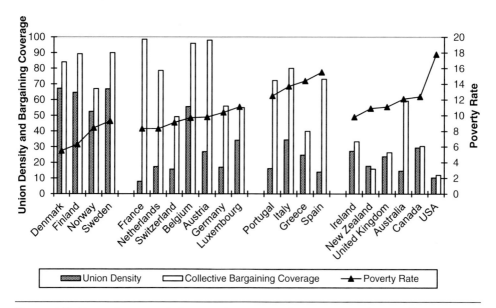

**Figure 6.3:** Union Density, Collective Agreement Coverage, and Overall Poverty Rates, Selected OECD Nations, 2017

*Source:* Adapted from OECD. (2019). Trade union members and union density. Retrieved from https://stats.oecd.org/Index.aspx?DataSetCode=TUD; and OECD. (2019). Poverty rate. Retrieved from https://data.oecd.org/inequality/poverty-rate.htm

(Jackson & Thomas, 2017). Another way in which power is more equally distributed is through adoption of proportional representation in elections. Nations in which this is established show greater commitment to income distribution and provision of public services to their citizens (see Chapter 9, this volume).

### Governmental Ideology and Public Policy

Raphael and Bryant, in Chapter 3, point out how social determinants of health such as income and income inequality, as well as housing, food security, and health and social services, are heavily influenced by the ideology of the government of the day. They consider how neo-liberalism—through its emphasis on the market as the arbiter of societal values and resource allocations—supports regressive political and economic forces. Implementing neo-liberal economic policies fosters income and wealth inequalities, weakens social infrastructure, dissipates social cohesion, and threatens civil society.

### Welfare States and Their Variants

Esping-Andersen (1990, 1999) has identified what he calls the three worlds of welfare capitalism: social democratic, conservative, and liberal. The social democratic welfare states (Finland, Sweden, Denmark, and Norway) emphasize universal welfare rights and provide generous benefit entitlements. The conservative welfare states (France, Germany, Spain, and Italy) also offer generous benefits, but provide these based on employment status with emphasis on male primary breadwinners. The liberal Anglo-Saxon economies (Australia, New Zealand, the U.K., the U.S., Canada, and Ireland) provide only modest benefits and step in only when the market fails to provide adequate supports. These liberal states depend on means-tested benefits targeted to only the least well-off. There are many differences in public policy among these types (see Table 6.1 earlier in this chapter and Chapter 9, this volume).

### *Health Impacts of Globalization and Trade Agreements*

Teeple (2000) sees increasing income and wealth inequalities and the weakening of infrastructure within Canada and elsewhere as resulting from the ascendance of concentrated monopoly capitalism and corporate globalization. Transnational corporations apply their increasing power to oppose aspects of the welfare state to reduce labour costs. With such a power shift, business has less need to develop political compromises with labour and governments. Important questions raised by this perspective include: To what extent is the weakening of the welfare state inevitable? What is the role that trade agreements play in the weakening of the welfare state?

## Human Rights Perspectives: Providing the Legal and Moral Justifications for Action

Canada is signatory to many international covenants that guarantee the provision of citizen supports that show commonalities with the social determinants of health. The *Universal Declaration on Human Rights* states:

> Everyone has the right to a standard of living adequate for the health and well-being of himself and of his family, including food, clothing, housing and medical care and necessary social services, and the right to security in the event of unemployment, sickness, disability, widowhood, old age or other lack of livelihood in circumstances beyond his control. (United Nations, 1948, p. 7)

Similarly, the 1995 *Declaration of the International Summit for Social Development* identified the following commitments:

> Achieving specified target dates which have been agreed previously at the international level for meeting basic human needs such as food, shelter, water, sanitation, health care, and education, and in relation to areas such as South Asia which have substantial concentrations of people in poverty.
>
> Ensuring adequate economic and social protection during periods of vulnerability such as unemployment, ill health, maternity, child-rearing and old age. (United Nations, 1995)

Non-governmental organizations consistently report that Canada does not live up to its commitments to these international agreements. Indeed, conditions either continue to deteriorate or stagnate, yet governments do little in response to these negative reports. How can Canadian governmental authorities be called to account (Raphael, Komakech, Bryant, & Torrence, 2018)?

### Social Justice and Health Equity

Issues of health equity and the role played by social determinants of health that lead to such inequity are rooted in concepts of social justice (Braveman & Gruskin, 2003). There are two reasons why a concept of social justice is important in considering the roots of differences in health:

> First, social justice demands an equitable distribution of collective goods, institutional resources (such as social wealth), and life opportunities. ... Second, social justice calls for democracy—the empowerment of all social members, along with democratic and transparent structures to promote social goals. This is another way of describing political equality. (Hofrichter, 2003, p. 13)

The focus on justice and fairness in discussions of health, illness, and health care is an important contribution of the human rights approach. What role can moral, legal, and human rights arguments play in promoting the quality of the social determinants of health? How useful can these arguments be in provoking the public to advocate for more public policies that support health?

## WHAT ARE AREAS OF NEEDED INQUIRY?

In addition to the questions raised in the sections above, there are some key areas that could benefit from inquiry applying a social determinants of health framework.

- *Recovery from illness and rehabilitation*: While it is well-established that social determinants of health are excellent predictors of illness and diseases, we know little about how these same health determinants lead to recovery from illness.
- *Organization and activities of public health units*: Many public health units in Canada are taking the social determinants of health into their work (Raphael et al., 2015; Raphael & Sayani, 2017). What can they do to influence the making of public policy to improve the quality and equitable distribution of the social determinants of health?
- *Concept representation and the media*: There has been little penetration of the social determinants of health into the media (Raphael, 2011c). The overwhelming proportion of coverage in the written press, radio, or television is on biomedical

research and behavioural risk factors. We need to understand why the press is so limited in its health-related coverage. What are the barriers to fostering reporters' understanding of the social determinants of health?

- *Public understanding and action*: Considering media coverage of health, we should not be surprised to find the public has little understanding of the social determinants of health (Conference Board of Canada, 2012; Shankardass, Lofters, Kirst, & Quiñonez, 2012). One study asked 601 residents of Hamilton, Ontario, to identify up to seven causes of heart disease (Paisley, Midgett, Brunetti, & Tomasik, 2001). In response to this open-ended question, only one respondent out of 601—and only one of 4,200 potential responses—identified poverty as a cause of heart disease. How can we go about educating Canadians about the social determinants of health?

- *Links between evidence and policy (in)action*: Raphael (2015) argues that social determinants of health continue to be a marginalized approach to developing public policy. While policy-makers are aware of the importance of these concepts, governments do not institute health-promoting social policies. Is the creation of healthy public policy primarily about health? Or is healthy public policy primarily about politics?

## CONCLUSIONS

The social determinants of health concept offers a window into both the micro-level processes by which social structures lead to individual health or illness and the macro-level processes by which power relationships and political ideology shape the quality of these social structures. The epidemiological approach directs attention to the pathways that link these social structures to health and illness.

The sociological approach directs attention to how we develop explanations and actions to address the causes and treatment of disease and illness. The political economy perspective forces us to ask questions about power and politics, and how economics shapes the organization of society and the distribution of wealth and other resources. Finally, the human rights approach asks about the values that determine the type of society we live in and our commitments to providing every citizen with the resources necessary to realize health and well-being, and achieve our full human potential. The social determinants of health is a rich area for both sociological inquiry and political and social action to improve health, healthcare services, and society in general.

### CRITICAL THINKING QUESTIONS

1. Review the health-related stories of your local newspaper over the next five days. If you based your understanding of the determinants of health on these stories, what would be your views of what makes some people healthy and others ill?

2.  What evidence is available concerning the extent of housing, food, employment, and income insecurity in your area? Have conditions been improving or declining?
3.  To what extent is the discipline in which you are studying addressing issues related to the social determinants of health? What could be done to increase your discipline's emphasis in this area?
4.  What could be done to improve the public's understanding of the importance of the social determinants of health? What should be the role of your local public health unit or healthcare professionals?
5.  To what extent is public policy in your nation, region, or city concerned with improving the quality of various social determinants of health? Why are other nations more concerned with integrating the social determinants of health into public policy?

## FURTHER READINGS

Bartley, M. (2016). *Health inequality: An introduction to theories, concepts, and methods* (2nd ed.). Cambridge, U.K.: Polity Press.
Large differences in life expectancy exist between the most privileged and the most disadvantaged social groups in industrial societies. This book assists in understanding the four most widely accepted theories of what lies behind inequalities in health: behavioural, psychosocial, material, and life-course approaches.

Davey Smith, G. (2003). *Health inequalities: Life-course approaches.* Bristol, U.K.: Policy Press.
The life-course perspective on adult health and health inequalities is an important development in epidemiology and public health. This volume presents innovative, empirical research that shows how social disadvantage throughout the life course leads to inequalities in life expectancy, death rates, and health status in adulthood.

Hofrichter, R. (2003). *Health and social justice: Politics, ideology, and inequity in the distribution of disease.* San Francisco: Jossey-Bass.
This volume offers a collection of articles written by contributors from the fields of sociology, epidemiology, public health, ecology, politics, and advocacy. Each article explores a particular aspect of health inequalities and demonstrates how these are rooted in injustices of racism, sex discrimination, and social class.

Raphael, D. (2016). *Social determinants of health: Canadian perspectives* (3rd ed.). Toronto: Canadian Scholars' Press.
This book summarizes how socio-economic factors affect the health of Canadians, surveys the current state of 16 social determinants of health across Canada, and provides an analysis of how these determinants affect Canadians' health.

## RELEVANT WEBSITES

### The Broadbent Institute
http://www.broadbentinstitute.ca/
The Broadbent Institute is Canada's leading progressive, independent organization championing change through the promotion of democracy, equality, and sustainability, and the training of a new generation of leaders.

### Canadian Centre for Policy Alternatives
www.policyalternatives.ca
The centre monitors developments and promotes research on economic and social issues facing Canada. It provides alternatives to the views of business research institutes and many government agencies by publishing research reports, sponsoring conferences, organizing briefings, and providing informed comment on the issues of the day from a non-partisan perspective.

### Commission on Social Determinants of Health
www.who.int/social_determinants/en/
The Commission on Social Determinants of Health supports countries and global health partners to address the social factors leading to ill health and inequities. It draws the attention of society to the social determinants of health that are known to be among the worst causes of poor health and inequalities among and within countries. The determinants include unemployment, unsafe workplaces, urban slums, globalization, and lack of access to health systems.

### Public Health Agency of Canada: Social Determinants of Health and Health Inequalities
http://www.phac-aspc.gc.ca/ph-sp/determinants/index-eng.php
This site provides details about how population health aims to improve the health of the entire population by acting upon the broad range of factors and conditions that influence health.

### National Collaborating Centre on the Determinants of Health
http://www.nccdh.ca/
The centre provides the Canadian public health community with knowledge and resources to take action on the social determinants of health, to close the gap between those who are most and least healthy. They work with the public health field to move knowledge into action—in practice, in policy, and in decision-making—to achieve societal improvements that result in health for all.

## GLOSSARY

**Equity in health:** An ethical value grounded in the ethical principle of distributive justice and consonant with human rights principles. Equity in health can be defined as the absence of disparities in health (and in its key social determinants) that are systematically associated with social advantage or disadvantage. Health inequities systematically put populations who are already socially disadvantaged by virtue of being poor, female, or members of a disenfranchised racial, ethnic, or religious group at further disadvantage with respect to their health (Braveman & Gruskin, 2003).

**Poverty:** The condition whereby individuals, families, and groups in the population lack the resources to obtain the type of diet, participate in the activities, and have the living conditions and amenities that are customary, or at least widely encouraged or approved, in the societies to which they belong (Townsend, 1993). Poverty can be considered in terms of absolute poverty, whereby individual and families do not have enough resources to keep "body and soul together," or relative poverty, whereby they do not have the ability to participate in common activities of daily living (Gordon & Townsend, 2000).

**Public policy:** A course of action or inaction chosen by public authorities to address a given problem or interrelated set of problems. Policy is a course of action that is anchored in a set of values regarding appropriate public goals and a set of beliefs about the best way of achieving those goals. The idea of public policy assumes that an issue is no longer a private affair (Wolf, 2005).

**Social determinants of health:** The economic and social conditions that influence the health of individuals, communities, and jurisdictions. Social determinants of health determine whether individuals stay healthy or become ill and the extent to which a person or community possesses the physical, social, and personal resources to identify and achieve personal aspirations, satisfy needs, and cope with the environment. Social determinants of health include conditions of childhood, availability and quality of income, food, housing, employment, and health and social services (Raphael, 2007).

**Welfare state:** A state in which organized power is deliberately used to modify the play of market forces in at least three directions: (1) by guaranteeing individuals and families a minimum income irrespective of the market value of their work or property; (2) by narrowing the extent of security by enabling individuals and families to meet certain social contingencies (for example, sickness, old age, and unemployment) that lead otherwise to individual and family crises; (3) by ensuring that all citizens without distinction of status or class are offered the best standards available in relation to a certain agreed range of social services (Briggs, 1961).

## REFERENCES

Auger, N., & Alix, C. (2016). Income, income distribution, and health in Canada. In D. Raphael (Ed.), *Social determinants of health: Canadian perspectives* (3rd ed., pp. 90–109). Toronto: Canadian Scholars' Press.

Barker, D. J. P., Osmond, C., Winter, P. D., Margetts, B., & Simmonds, S. J. (1989). Weight in infancy and death from ischemic heart disease. *The Lancet, 334*(8663), 577–580. doi:10.1016/S0140-6736(89)90710-1

Bartley, M. (2016). *Health inequality: An introduction to concepts, theories, and methods* (2nd ed.). Cambridge, U.K.: Polity Press.

Benzeval, M., Dilnot, A., Judge, K., & Taylor, J. (2001). Income and health over the lifecourse: Evidence and policy implications. In H. Graham (Ed.), *Understanding health inequalities* (pp. 96–112). Buckingham, U.K.: Open University Press.

Benzeval, M., & Judge, K. (2001). Income and health: The time dimension. *Social Science and Medicine, 52*(9), 1371–1390. doi:10.1016/S0277-9536(00)00244-6

Benzeval, M., Judge, K., & Whitehead, M. (Eds.). (1995). *Tackling inequalities in health: An agenda for action*. London: Kings Fund.

Berkman, L. F., Kawachi, I., & Glymour, M. M. (Eds.). (2014). *Social epidemiology* (2nd ed.) Oxford: Oxford University Press.

Blane, D. (2005). The life course, the social gradient and health. In M. G. Marmot & R. G. Wilkinson (Eds.), *Social determinants of health* (2nd ed., pp. 54–77). Oxford: Oxford University Press.

Brassolotto, J., Raphael, D., & Baldeo, N. (2014). Epistemological barriers to addressing the social determinants of health among public health professionals in Ontario, Canada: A qualitative inquiry. *Critical Public Health, 24*(3), 321–336. doi:10.1080/09581596.2013.820256

Braveman, P., & Gruskin, S. (2003). Defining equity in health. *Journal of Epidemiology and Community Health, 57*(4), 254–258. doi:10.1136/jech.57.4.254

Briggs, A. (1961). The welfare state in historical perspective. *European Journal of Sociology, 2*(2), 221–258. doi:10.1017/S0003975600000412

Brunner, E., & Marmot, M. G. (2006). Social organization, stress, and health. In M. Marmot & R. Wilkinson (Eds.), *Social determinants of health* (2nd ed., pp. 6–30). Oxford: Oxford University Press.

Bryant, T., Raphael, D., Schrecker, T., & Labonte, R. (2011). Canada: A land of missed opportunity for addressing the social determinants of health. *Health Policy, 101*(1), 44–58. doi:10.1016/j.healthpol.2010.08.022

Centers for Disease Control and Prevention. (2018). *Social determinants of health: Know what affects health*. Retrieved September 1, 2018, from https://www.cdc.gov/socialdeterminants/

Chaufan, C. (2008). What does justice have to do with it? A bioethical and sociological perspective on the diabetes epidemic. *Bioethical Issues, Sociological Perspectives, 9*, 269–300.

Chronic Disease Prevention Alliance of Canada. (2003). *Who we are*. Retrieved April 16, 2003, from http://www.chronicdiseaseprevention.ca/content/about_cdpac/mission.asp

Commission on Social Determinants of Health. (2008). *Closing the gap in a generation: Health equity through action on the social determinants of health*. Geneva: World Health Organization.

Conference Board of Canada. (2012). *Canadians see their own behaviour and lifestyle as the key to their health, not socio-economic factors*. Retrieved December 1, 2012, from http://www.conferenceboard.ca/press/newsrelease/12-10-16/

Canadians_see_their_own_Behaviour_and_Lifestyle_as_the_Key_to_their_Health_not_
Socio-Economic_Factors.aspx

Davey Smith, G. (Ed.). (2003). *Health inequalities: Lifecourse approaches.* Bristol, U.K.: Policy
Press.

Davey Smith, G., Ben-Shlomo, Y., & Lynch, J. (2002). Life course approaches to inequalities
in coronary heart disease risk. In S. A. Stansfeld & M. Marmot (Eds.), *Stress and the heart:
Psychosocial pathways to coronary heart disease* (pp. 20–49). London: BMJ Books.

Davey Smith, G., & Hart, C. (2002). Life-course approaches to socio-economic and behavioural
influences on cardiovascular disease mortality: The collaborative study. *American Journal of
Public Health, 92*(8), 1295–1298.

Doyal, L., & Pennell, I. (1979). *The political economy of health.* London: Pluto Press.

Engels, F. (1987). *The condition of the working class in England.* New York: Penguin Classics.
Originally published 1845.

Eriksson, J., Forsén, T., Tuomilehto, J., Osmond, C., & Barker, B. (2001). Early growth and
coronary heart disease in later life: Longitudinal study. *British Medical Journal, 322*(7292),
949–953. doi:10.1136/bmj.322.7292.949

Eriksson, J. G., Forsén, T., Tuomilehto, J., Winter, P., Osmond, C., & Barker, D. J. P. (1999).
Catch-up growth in childhood and death from coronary heart disease: Longitudinal study.
*British Medical Journal Clinical Research, 318*(7181), 427–431. doi:10.1136/bmj.318.7181.427

Esping-Andersen, G. (1990). *The three worlds of welfare capitalism.* Princeton, NJ: Princeton
University Press.

Esping-Andersen, G. (1999). *Social foundations of postindustrial economies.* New York: Oxford
University Press.

Esping-Andersen, G. (2002). A child-centred social investment strategy. In G. Esping-Andersen
(Ed.), *Why we need a new welfare state* (pp. 26–67). Oxford U.K.: Oxford University Press.

Gordon, D. (2010). Determinants of health equity in developing nations. *Social Alternatives,
29*(2), 28–33.

Gordon, D., & Townsend, P. (Eds.). (2000). *Breadline Europe: The measurement of poverty.* Bristol,
U.K.: Policy Press.

Graham, H. (2004). Social determinants and their unequal distribution: Clarifying policy
understandings. *Milbank Quarterly, 82*(1), 101–124.

Graham, H. (2007). *Unequal lives: Health and socioeconomic inequalities.* New York: Open
University Press.

Health Canada. (2003). *Healthy living strategy.* Retrieved April 16, 2003, from http://www.hc-sc.
gc.ca/english/media/releases/2003/2003_14.htm

Hertzman, C., & Boyce, T. (2010). How experience gets under the skin to create gradients in
developmental health. *Annual Review of Public Health, 31,* 329–347.

Hofrichter, R. (2003). The politics of health inequities: Contested terrain. In *Health and social justice: A
reader on ideology, and inequity in the distribution of disease* (pp. 1–56). San Francisco: Jossey-Bass.

Jackson, A., & Thomas, M. P. (2017). *Work and labour in Canada: Critical ossues* (3rd ed.). Toronto:
Canadian Scholars' Press.

Jarvis, M. J., & Wardle, J. (2003). Social patterning of individual health behaviours: the case of cigarette smoking. In M. G. Marmot & R. G. Wilkinson (Eds.), *Social determinants of health* (2nd ed., pp. 224–237). Oxford: Oxford University Press.

Judge, K., & Paterson, I. (2001). *Treasury Working Paper: Poverty, income inequality and health.* Wellington, NZ: Government of New Zealand.

Kaplan, G. A., Pamuk, E. R., Lynch, J. W., Cohen, R. D., & Balfour, J. L. (1996). Income inequality and mortality in the United States: Analysis of mortality and potential pathways. *Britich Medical Journal, 312*(7037), 999–1003. doi:10.1136/bmj.312.7037.999

Kawachi, I., & Kennedy, B. (2002). *The health of nations: Why inequality is harmful to your health.* New York: New Press.

Kawachi, I., & Kennedy, B. P. (1997). Socioeconomic determinants of health: Health and social cohesion: Why care about income inequality? *British Medical Journal, 314*(7086), 1037–1040. doi:10.1136/bmj.314.7086.1037

Kirkland, R., & Raphael, D. (2018). Perpetuating the utopia of health behaviourism: A case study of the Canadian Men's Health Foundation's Don't Change Much initiative. *Social Theory & Health, 16*(1), 1–19. doi:10.1057/s41285-017-0040-7

Kuh, D., & Ben-Shlomo, Y. (Eds.). (2004). *A life course approach to chronic disease epidemiology* (2nd ed.). Oxford: Oxford University Press.

Labonte, R. (1993). *Health promotion and empowerment: Practice frameworks.* Toronto: Centre for Health Promotion and ParticipAction.

Lawlor, D., Ebrahim, S., & Smith, G. D. (2002). Socioeconomic position in childhood and adulthood and insulin resistance: Cross sectional survey using data from British women's heart and health study. *British Medical Journal, 325*(7368), 805–807. doi:10.1136/bmj.325.7368.805

Lynch, J. W., Kaplan, G. A., Pamuk, E. R., Cohen, R. D., Heck, K. E., Balfour, J. L., & Yen, I. H. (1998). Income inequality and mortality in metropolitan areas of the United States. *American Journal of Public Health, 88*(7), 1074–1080. doi:10.2105/AJPH.88.7.1074

Lynch, J. W., Davey Smith, G., Kaplan, G. A., & House, J. S. (2000). Income inequality and mortality: Importance to health of individual income, psychosocial environment, or material conditions. *British Medical Journal, 320*(7243), 1200–1204. doi:10.1136/bmj.320.7243.1200

Marmot, M., Rose, G., Shipley, M., & Hamilton, P. J. S. (1978). Employment grade and coronary heart disease in British civil servants. *Journal of Epidemiology and Community Health, 32*(4), 244–249. doi:10.1136/jech.32.4.244

Marmot, M., Shipley, M., Brunner, E., & Hemingway, H. (2001). Relative contribution of early life and adult socioeconomic factors to adult morbidity in the Whitehall II Study. *Journal of Epidemiology and Community Health, 55*(5), 301–307. doi:10.1136/jech.55.5.301

McGibbon, E. (2016). Oppressions and access to health care: Deepening the conversation. In D. Raphael (Ed.), *Social determinants of health: Canadian perspectives* (3rd ed., pp. 491–520). Toronto: Canadian Scholars' Press.

McKeown, T. (1976). *The role of medicine: Dream, mirage, or nemesis.* London: Nuffield Provincial Hospitals Trust.

McKeown, T., Record, R. G., & Turner, R. D. (1975). An interpretation of the decline in mortality in England and Wales during the twentieth century. *Population Studies, 29*(3), 391–422. doi:10.1080/00324728.1975.10412707

McKinlay, J., & McKinlay, S. M. (1987). Medical measures and the decline of mortality. In H. D. Schwartz (Ed.), *Dominant issues in medical sociology* (2nd ed., pp. 7–19). New York: Random House.

Mikkonen, J., & Raphael, D. (2010). *Social determinants of health: The Canadian facts.* Retrieved November 1, 2010, from http://thecanadianfacts.org

Nettleton, S. (1997). Surveillance, health promotion and the formation of a risk identity. In M. Sidell, L. Jones, J. Katz, & A. Peberdy (Eds.), *Debates and dilemmas in promoting health* (pp. 314–324). London: Open University Press.

Olsen, G. M. (2010). *Power and inequality: A comparative introduction.* Toronto: Oxford University Press.

Paisley, J. A., Midgett, C., Brunetti, G., & Tomasik, H. H. (2001). Heart health Hamilton-Wentworth survey: Programming implications. *Canadian Journal of Public Health, 92*(6), 443–447.

Plato. (2010). *The Laws: Books 1–6.* Retrieved November 30, 2009, from http://www.greektexts. com/library/Plato/laws_(books_1_-_6)/eng/317.html. Originally published 360 BC.

Raphael, D. (2007). Poverty and health: Mechanisms and pathways. In D. Raphael (Ed.), *Poverty and policy in Canada: Implications for health and quality of life* (pp. 239–268). Toronto: Canadian Scholars' Press.

Raphael, D. (2010a). The health of Canada's children. Part 1: Canadian children's health in comparative perspective. *Paeditrics and Children's Health, 15*(1), 23–29.

Raphael, D. (2010b). The health of Canada's children. Part II. Health mechanisms and pathways. *Paediatrics and Child Health, 15*(2), 71–76. doi:10.1093/pch/15.1.23

Raphael, D. (2010c). The health of Canada's children. Part III. Public policy and the social determinants of children's health. *Paediatrics and Child Health, 15*(3), 143–149. doi:10.1093/pch/15.3.143

Raphael, D. (2010d). The health of Canada's children. Part IV. Towards the future. *Paediatrics and Child Health, 15*(4), 199–204. doi:10.1093/pch/15.4.199

Raphael, D. (2011a). Canadian public policy and poverty in international perspective. In D. Raphael (Ed.), *Poverty in Canada: Implications for health and quality of life* (2nd ed., pp. 374–405). Toronto: Canadian Scholars' Press.

Raphael, D. (2011b). Interactions with the social assistance and health care systems. In D. Raphael (Ed.), *Poverty in Canada: Implications for health and quality of life.* (2nd ed., pp. 186–219). Toronto: Canadian Scholars' Press.

Raphael, D. (2011c). Mainstream media and the social determinants of health in Canada: Is it time to call it a day? *Health Promotion International, 26*(2), 220–229. doi:10.1093/heapro/dar008

Raphael, D. (2011d). The political economy of health promotion: part 2, national provision of the prerequisites of health. *Health Promotion International, 28*(1), 112–132. doi:10.1093/heapro/dar058 vRaphael, D. (2011e). Who is poor in Canada? In D. Raphael (Ed.), *Poverty in Canada: Implications for health and quality of life* (2nd ed., pp. 62–89). Toronto: Canadian Scholars' Press.

Raphael, D. (2015). Beyond policy analysis: The raw politics behind opposition to healthy public policy. *Health Promotion International, 30*(2), 380–396. doi:10.1093/heapro/dau044

Raphael, D. (2016a). *About Canada: Health and illness* (2nd ed.). Winnipeg: Fernwood Publishing.

Raphael, D. (2016b). Early child development and health. In D. Raphael (Ed.), *Social determinants of health: Canadian perspectives* (3rd ed., pp. 218–239). Toronto: Candian Scholars' Press.

Raphael, D. (Ed.). (2009). *Social determinants of health: Canadian perspectives* (2nd ed.). Toronto: Canadian Scholars' Press.

Raphael, D. (Ed.). (2012). *Tackling health inequalities: Lessons from international experiences.* Toronto: Canadian Scholars' Press.

Raphael, D. (Ed.). (2016c). *Social determinants of health: Canadian perspectives* (3rd ed.). Toronto: Canadian Scholars' Press.

Raphael, D., Anstice, S., Raine, K., McGannon, K. R., Rizvi, S. K., & Yu, V. (2003). The social determinants of the incidence and management of type 2 diabetes mellitus: Are we prepared to rethink our questions and redirect our research activities? *Leadership in Health Services, 16*(3), 10–20. doi:10.1108/13660750310486730

Raphael, D., & Brassolotto, J. (2015). Understanding action on the social determinants of health: A critical realist analysis of in-depth interviews with staff of nine Ontario public health units. *BMC Research Notes, 28*(8), 105. doi:10.1186/s13104-015-1064-5

Raphael, D., Brassolotto, J., & Baldeo, N. (2015). Ideological and organizational components of differing public health strategies for addressing the social determinants of health. *Health Promotion International, 30*(4), 855–867. doi:10.1093/heapro/dau022

Raphael, D., Chaufan, C., Bryant, T., Bakhsh, M., Bindra, J., Puran, A., & Saliba, D. (2018). The cultural hegemony of chronic disease association discourse in Canada. *Social Theory & Health, 17,* 172–191. doi:10.1057/s41285-018-0072-7

Raphael, D., & Farrell, E. S. (2002). Beyond medicine and lifestyle: Addressing the societal determinants of cardiovascular disease in North America. *Leadership in Health Services, 15*(4), 1–5. doi:10.1108/133660750210452143

Raphael, D., Komakech, M., Bryant, T., & Torrence, R. (2018). Governmental illegitimacy and incompetency in Canada and other liberal nations: Implications for health. *International Journal of Health Services, 49*(1), 17–36. doi:10.1177/0020731418795136

Raphael, D., Macdonald, J., Labonte, R., Colman, R., Hayward, K., & Torgerson, R. (2005). Researching income and income distribution as a determinant of health in Canada: Gaps between theoretical knowledge, research practice, and policy implementation. *Health Policy, 72*(2), 217–232. doi:10.1016/j.healthpol.2004.08.001

Raphael, D., & Sayani, A. (2017). Assuming policy responsibility for health equity: Local public health action in Ontario, Canada. *Health Promotion International, 34*(2), 215–226. doi:10.1093/heapro/dax073

Restrepo, H. E. (2000). Introduction. In H. E. Restrepo (Ed.), *Health promotion: An anthology* (pp. ix–xi). Washington, DC: Pan American Health Organization.

Shankardass, K., Lofters, A., Kirst, M., & Quiñonez, C. (2012). Public awareness of income-related health inequalities in Ontario, Canada. *International Journal for Equity in Health, 11*(1), 26. doi:10.1186/1475-9276-11-26

Shaw, M., Dorling, D., Gordon, D., & Davey Smith, G. (1999). *The widening gap: Health inequalities and policy in Britain*. Bristol, U.K.: Policy Press.

Siddiqi, A., & Hertzman, C. (2007). Towards an epidemiological understanding of the effects of long-term institutional changes on population health: A case study of Canada versus the USA. *Social Science & Medicine, 64*(3), 589–603. doi:10.1016/j.socscimed.2006.09.034

Smylie, J., & Firestone, M. (2016). The health of Indigenous Peoples. In D. Raphael (Ed.), *Social determinants of health: Canadian perspectives* (3rd ed., pp. 434–466). Toronto: Canadian Scholars' Press.

Tarlov, A. (1996). Social determinants of health: The sociobiological translation. In D. Blane, E. Brunner & R. Wilkinson (Eds.), *Health and social organization: Towards a health policy for the twenty-first century* (pp. 71–93). London: Routledge.

Teeple, G. (2000). *Globalization and the decline of social reform: Into the twenty-first century*. Aurora, ON: Garamond Press.

Tjepkema, M., Wilkins, R., & Long, A. (2013). Cause-specific mortality by income adequacy in Canada: A 16-year follow-up study. *Health Reports, 24*(7), 14–22.

Townsend, P. (1993). *The international analysis of poverty*. New York: Harvester Wheatsheaf.

Townsend, P., Davidson, N., & Whitehead, M. (Eds.). (1992). *Inequalities in health: The Black Report and the Health Divide* (3rd ed.). New York: Penguin Books.

United Nations. (1948). *Universal Declaration of Human Rights*. New York: Author.

United Nations. (1995). *Commitments of the U.N. World Summit on Social Development*. Copenhagen: Author.

Virchow, R. (1985). Report on the typhus epidemic in Upper Silesia. In L. J. Rather (Ed.), *Collected essays by Rudolph Virchow on public health and epidemiology, Volume 1* (pp. 205–319). Canton, MA: Science History Publications. Originally published 1848.

Whitehead, M. (1992). The health divide. In P. Townsend, N. Davidson, & M. Whitehead (Eds.), *Inequalities in health: The Black Report and the Health Divide* (pp. 215–281). New York: Penguin Books.

Wilkinson, R. (1996). *Unhealthy societies: The afflictions of inequality*. New York: Routledge.

Wilkinson, R., & Marmot, M. (2003). *Social determinants of health: The solid facts*. Retrieved from http://www.euro.who.int/document/e81384.pdf

Wolf, R. (2005). *What is public policy?* Queen's University. Retrieved April 15, 2012, from http://ginsler.com/toolbox/

World Health Organization. (1986). *Ottawa Charter for Health Promotion*. Retrieved June 14, 2011, from http://www.who.int/hpr/NPH/docs/ottawa_charter_hp.pdf

World Health Organization. (2008). *Commission on the Social Determinants of Health*. Retrieved March 15, 2008, from http://www.who.int/social_determinants/en/

# CHAPTER 7

## Social Class and Health Inequalities

*Ambreen Sayani*

## INTRODUCTION

The purpose of this chapter is to describe how social class is defined and conceptualized in relation to inequalities in health. In its simplest form, social class refers to the hierarchical ranking of groups of people. In terms of health, the availability of resources, or opportunity of choice, that is implied in relation to social ranking results in varying health outcomes between the social classes. Indeed, social observations spanning over a century and, more recently, research conducted over the past four decades demonstrate that lower social classes experience a wider array of health problems and higher rates of mortality and morbidity than more privileged social classes.

This chapter will begin by unpacking the meaning of social class and providing a brief description of the ways in which social class is measured and used for analysis in social science and health research. This discussion is continued in the context of health inequalities with an introduction to the theories that underpin our understanding of the link between social class and health inequalities. Since you will be using these foundational concepts to both understand and design your own work, this background will allow you to compare different approaches to solving social class–based health inequalities and identify alternatives to current interventions.

Social inequalities in health are evident for many health problems and illnesses, such as cardiovascular disease (Lemstra, Rogers, & Moraros, 2015), diabetes (Dinca-Panaitescu et al., 2012), mental health (Muntaner, Eaton, & Diala, 2000), and oral health (Gomaa et al., 2017; Raphael, 2018). The focus of this chapter is to illuminate how the living and working conditions associated with social class impact cancer-related health outcomes. This is important, given that recent statistics point out that one in every two Canadians will face a diagnosis of cancer over their lifetime, and eventually one in four will die of the disease (Canadian Cancer Society's Advisory Committee on Cancer Statistics, 2017). As you will see, social class plays a profound role in susceptibility to cancer by influencing exposure to a variety of risk factors and risk conditions. Furthermore, social class influences the ability to engage with and reap benefits of universally available health care (Sayani, 2017). For some cancers more than others, mortality and survival after diagnosis are correlated with social class.

Social processes group people in ways that shape their life chances. Since social stratification occurs as a result of deliberate political and economic decisions, it can therefore be undone to the extent that class differences are minimal (Raphael, 2009). The ability to do so rests on the political will of future stakeholders. It is my hope that this chapter will give you both answers, as well as the tools with which to ask meaningful questions.

## UNDERSTANDING SOCIAL CLASS

Simply speaking, a social class is a group of people that occupy a similar rank in terms of economic (wealth), social (personal networks), or cultural (knowledge) capital (Crompton, 2008; McCartney, Collins, & Mackenzie, 2013; Savage, 2015). From a sociological perspective, these ranks are understood to be based on the stratification of society in relation to the economic mode of production. This means that the power or privilege to control income-generating resources inherently places certain individuals at a higher rank, or social class, than those who do not have access to these possibilities.

Karl Marx (1818–1883) was the first to categorize society within this context. For Marx, society is made up of two groups: those that own and control the means of economic production, called the bourgeoisie; and workers that must sell their labour power to the bourgeoisie to survive, called the proletariat (Marx & Engels, 1846/2011). Since these groups are locked in a struggle for material resources such that one group can only materially benefit at the expense of the other, class conflict leads to the bourgeoisie dominating and subordinating the proletariat. Subsequently, there is exploitation of the lower social class, the proletariat, by the bourgeoisie, via their control of workers' labour efforts.

Max Weber (1864–1920), like Marx, believed in the economic stratification of society. However, for Weber (1978/2013) social classes were also created by the differential distribution of prestige and political power, in addition to economic power. Through this perspective, then, social stratification occurs through the ownership of property or assets; privilege of education and skills; and/or the power to influence and control decision-making. Therefore, the life chances, or realm of choices and opportunities available, between the social classes vary immensely, such that higher social classes have a greater likelihood of securing not only higher income and wealth but also the political power and influence to assure themselves a better quality of life and better overall health.

Twenty-first-century critiques of Marx and Weber's perspectives on social class structure claim that their focus on economic means and assets as a pivotal driver of social stratification ignores other competing elements of social identity such as ethnicity, gender, and race (Crompton, 2008). Indeed, contemporary sociologists such as Erik Olin Wright have pointed out that classifying society into the bourgeoisie, proletariat, and petty bourgeoisie (those that control their own means of production but do not control the labour power of others) is overly simplistic. Wright (2005) has added further categories of social class to include: (1) managers that oversee the process of production, though they do not own the mode of production; and (2) the self-employed who may not own the means of production per se but can control their own labour-power. Others, such as Pierre Bourdieu, shift the categorization of social class from that driven by economic production to one that is based in broader social relations. According to Bourdieu (1973), life chances depend as much on social and cultural capital as on economic means. Therefore, emphasis is simultaneously placed on connections and networks (social capital), as well as cultural knowledge and credentials (cultural capital; Crompton, 2008).

At this point it is important to ask two questions: Why does social class matter? And why does it increasingly matter? For starters, not only does social class determine life chances and ultimately health outcomes (as we will discuss throughout the rest of this chapter), but social class also matters because societies that have higher levels of social stratification (Muntaner et al., 2010) are more likely to have poorer levels of social cohesion, greater societal distrust, and higher incidences of crime (Wilkinson & Pickett, 2010).

And why is this increasingly important? The past two decades have seen a sharp polarization of economic assets such that the wealthiest 87 families in Canada now collectively own 4,448 times more wealth than the average Canadian family (Macdonald, 2018). In addition, the value of this wealth is equivalent to that of 12 million of the lowest-income Canadian families combined (Macdonald, 2018). The rich have the resources (economic, social, and cultural capital) to get richer. But this is at the expense of other social classes. Approximately 14 million of the Canadian population are currently classed as living with low income (or in poverty, using international definitions; Statistics Canada, 2017b). Would it surprise you that recent immigrants, Indigenous peoples, the disabled, and the elderly are more likely to fall into this group of low-income people? And would you be shocked to learn that, at present, close to one in five children in Canada are living in poverty (Statistics Canada, 2017a)?

Rising stratification, closely related to growing income inequality, has many consequences. The focus of the rest of this chapter is to draw out the links between social stratification and health, but the aim is also to encourage you to think critically about the impact on the overall well-being of Canadians as rising income inequality creates greater stratification between the social classes.

## MEASURING SOCIAL CLASS

To track developments, test theory, conduct research, and design policy interventions, it is important to have a means of measuring important variables such as social class and relevant outcomes such as health status. This way, any changes over time, possible explanations and solutions, or even the success/failure of programs can be brought to the limelight and relevant authorities can be held accountable for their policies and programs.

However, measuring social class is easier said than done. As you have now learned, social class can be linked to the economic mode of production and the subsequent conflict between the proletariat and bourgeoisie. Given that employment rank can reflect a similar phenomenon, many research studies, particularly those originating from the U.K. (McCartney et al., 2018), use "occupation" as an individual indicator of social class. Occupations can be categorized based on level of individual skill, such as unskilled (social class V), partly skilled (social class IV), skilled manual and non-manual (social class III), intermediate (social class II), and professional (social class I; Townsend, Davidson, & Whitehead, 1999). Classifications based on skill and rank have an added advantage of inculcating the concept of social prestige and power hierarchy into the analysis. As such, contemporary occupation-based class typologies include survey questions that assess the decision-making authority and supervisory control of employees (Wright, 2005).

Another way to operationalize social class is to measure "education." Measuring education is attractive because it is easy to record, stable over time, and has shown to correlate well with health outcomes (Krieger, Williams, & Moss, 1997). Education can be used as a continuous measure (where it is recorded as number of years of education), or it can be used as a categorical measure, such that people can be classed at meaningful timepoints such as the completion of high school or university. Focusing on education, however, can deflect attention from important aspects of income distribution that involve issues of power and influence available to those of differing education levels and why such differences exist (Raphael, 2007).

In practice, you will find that many Canadian studies measure social class by estimating individual income. The analysis of income against health indicators also shows a strong correlation, such that individuals with lower income consistently demonstrate poorer health-related outcomes (Krieger et al., 1997). Since individual-level income data obtained through survey data are usually incomplete, additional strategies are used to circumvent this problem, including estimations of income at the neighbourhood or regional level (Krieger et al., 1997). Some measurement techniques gauge personal wealth and prestige through survey questions that weigh ownership of assets such as a car, garden, or home (Townsend et al., 1999).

In essence, you will find that there is a myriad of ways in which to operationalize social class into a measurement. As you read through research studies, try to identify which technique is being used and what underlying assumptions have been made about the conceptualization of social class as a phenomenon. Also try to think of ways in which the conceptualization may fall short. For example, how valid are occupational class stratifications in current neo-liberal market-driven workplaces? This is significant given that de-industrialization and outsourcing of service sector jobs have led to a change in the demographic profile of the traditional employee (Crompton, 2010). In addition, women now constitute nearly half of the employed workforce (Crompton, 2010). Would a simple categorization by occupation suffice, when other elements of race, age, and gender may be more important variables in constructing social class? Consider education.

While education has been shown to correlate well with health outcomes so far (Krieger et al., 1997), will it continue to hold the same statistical power in the current era of corporate down-sizing with the precarious nature of available jobs? How about income? What aspects of social class are tapped into when income is measured at the personal level versus household and regional level? This is also important, as studies have shown that individuals with relatively higher incomes living in deprived neighbourhoods have health outcomes similar to those who are impoverished (Diez Roux et al., 2001).

It is important to consider how social forces interact to shape access to resources by creating conditions of relative advantage and disadvantage. Contemplate which elements of social class are captured in research studies and reflect on which aspects have been left out. I also encourage you to deliberate over research findings, answers, and interpretations that are offered by researchers via their study and analysis. Consider how often studies move from the passive description of social inequalities in health to a critical exploration of why the inequalities are happening.

Let's take the example of social inequalities in lung cancer risk and mortality. Studies have demonstrated the link between smoking and lung cancer mortality (Peto et al., 2000) and subsequently concluded that to reduce the incidence of lung cancer, it is important to focus on smoking cessation. Indeed, this is correct. However, another way to problematize this situation is to ask: Which population group smokes the most and is therefore at highest risk for lung cancer? Studies have illuminated that lower social classes are more likely to be smoking than their socially advantaged counterparts (Hart et al., 2001). We can delve into this further and consider which resources would best help individuals from lower social classes to quit smoking: a free supply of nicotine patches or long-term employment in a stable job? We get answers to the questions that we ask; it is therefore of utmost importance that we consider the limitations of our questions and the implications of our answers on people's lives.

## SOCIAL CLASS AND HEALTH

Social observations spanning over a century have illuminated the plight of the working classes, and particularly the poor in terms of their limited access to resources and higher rates of morbidity and mortality (Engels, 1845/1987; Virchow, 1848/1985). What is it about their conditions of relative and absolute deprivation that lead to these health outcomes? Models proposed by Bartley (2004, 2016) categorize the links between social inequality and health inequality into cultural-behavioural, psychosocial, material, and life-course explanatory theories. These are described in further detail below and summarized in Box 7.1.

### Cultural-Behavioural

This model posits that differences in health outcomes between social classes are a result of differences in health-related behaviours. The "hard" version of this theory causally links these two patterns together, such that poor health habits of lower social classes lead to worse health (Macintyre, 1997). The "soft" version of this theory acknowledges that behaviour patterns and health outcomes are linked, but not via simple causation (Macintyre, 1997). From this perspective, lifestyle choices (diet, exercise, smoking, and alcohol consumption) and other health-promoting activities, such as the use of preventative health services (vaccinations and screening), are class-based. As a result, conditions of social disadvantage are more likely to be associated with a higher risk of behaviours that are damaging to health (Scambler, 2012; Scott-Samuel & Smith, 2015). Since economic, cultural, and social stratification produces class differences, it follows that these processes themselves drive the adverse health behaviours of lower social classes, yet this reality is usually downplayed. The cultural-behavioural model of health inequities has been described as individual-level or agency-based (Øversveen, Rydland, Bambra, & Eikemo, 2017).

## Psychosocial

Psychosocial explanations of health inequities posit that differences in health outcomes are based on micro-level responses to social forces, such as social position, and/or macro-level societal structures, such as social cohesion (World Health Organization, 2010). Therefore, depending on one's hierarchical situation on a social ladder of prestige, power, and privilege, chronic feelings of subordination, marginalization, and oppression can lead to activation of the stress response, resulting in a higher predisposition to disease (Cassel, 1976; Marmot & Wilkinson, 2001; Wilkinson, 1997). Furthermore, higher levels of income inequality are associated with greater levels of distrust, poor community resources, higher levels of crime, and an overall lack of social cohesion, resulting in unhealthy living conditions (Wilkinson, 1999a, 1999b; Wilkinson & Pickett, 2006). The psychological explanations of health inequities are strongly anchored to the belief that social inequalities create alterations in the body's susceptibility to disease (Cassel, 1976), and that this predisposition drives poorer health outcomes for the socially disadvantaged.

## Materialist

Materialist explanations of health inequities are rooted in the political economy of health framework, and place emphasis on the "ability to choose" within the limitations of one's choices. As a result, materialists are less concerned with agency and focus more on the structural forces that influence agency (Øversveen et al., 2017). From this perspective, micro-level structures, such as individual income, directly impact the ability to avoid risk, prevent injury/illness, and access health resources (World Health Organization, 2010). And at the macro-level, disinvestment of the government from social spending affects the quality and distribution of the social determinants of health, which indirectly affects health outcomes (World Health Organization, 2010).

The social production of diseases has been well recognized for several centuries, through the works of Friedrich Engels (1820–1895) and Rudolph Virchow (1821–1902), and contemporary debates around social hierarchy and health inequities are geared around the typology of the welfare state (Esping-Andersen, 1990). From this theoretical perspective, liberal states, which support a market-driven economy and commodification of public assets, and promote individual responsibility with minimal state intervention, classically have higher degrees of socio-economic inequality, through a lack of public policies that can enhance the social determinants of health (Coburn, 2000; Coburn, 2004; Muntaner et al., 2011; Navarro, 2007, 2009; Raphael & Bryant, 2006). The resurgence of neo-liberal ideology has only heightened these problematic aspects of society (see Coburn, this volume).

## Life Course

The life-course model illuminates how embodiment, or internalization of social phenomenon into the body, is a continuous and dynamic process. As such, past historical events profoundly influence exposure to risk, vulnerability to disease, and opportunity to access timely care (World Health Organization, 2010). The life-course model has been further categorized into (1) the "critical periods" model, in which exposure during certain sensitive periods of development leave a permanent biological mark on the body; and (2) the "accumulation of risk" model, in which the intensity and frequency of exposures to risk are injurious to health through their cumulative effect rather than a single event (Ben-Shlomo & Kuh, 2002). Other authors (e.g., Blane, 2005) have considered the life-course perspective from a critical sociological lens. These analyses highlight how critical social transitions (such as moving from education to attaining a job) represent pivotal moments in upward social mobility, and how a failure to transition leads to clustering and accumulation of social disadvantage (such as lack of education leading to fewer work prospects, resulting in lower income that results in poor housing conditions, etc.).

# SOCIAL CLASS AND CANCER

Over the years, advances in cancer diagnosis and treatment modalities have meant that more and more people are surviving cancer. Key to the successful treatment of cancer and long-term disease-free survival is the timely diagnosis and treatment of early stage tumours (Canadian Cancer Statistics Advisory Committee, 2018). Tumours that are found at a later stage, or after metastasis to other body sites, have distinctly poorer prognosis. For cancer, adequate and timely access to health care plays a crucial role in the ability to survive cancer and maintain a good quality of life (Canadian Cancer Statistics Advisory Committee, 2018).

Canadians boast a publicly funded healthcare system, where 70% of healthcare costs are picked up by the state through revenue generated by citizen taxation (Marchildon, 2013). The remaining 30% of healthcare costs are funded through employer-based health insurance plans or are incurred as out-of-pocket expenses (Marchildon, 2013). In Canada,

**Box 7.1:** Explanations for the Social Class and Health Inequalities Relationship

**Cultural-behavioural**

1. Differences in health outcomes between social classes are a result of differences in health-related behaviours.
2. Lifestyle choices and participation in health-promoting practices are different among different social classes.
3. Conditions of social disadvantage are more likely to be associated with a higher risk of health-damaging behaviours.
4. Socio-political forces typically shape social stratification and hence shape health behaviour patterns.

**Psychosocial**

1. Social inequalities create alterations in the body's susceptibility to disease.
2. Chronic feelings of subordination and oppression can lead to an activation of the stress response and a higher predisposition to disease.
3. The position one occupies on a ladder of social privilege will determine the extent of deprivation endured.
4. Socio-political forces shape the distribution of power, privilege, and prestige, and hence drive social hierarchy.

**Materialist**

1. Access to material resources influences ability to choose and benefit from health resources.
2. Material resources enable individuals to avoid risk, prevent injury/illness, and seek health care.
3. The social determinants of health, such as income and education, are examples of material resources.
4. Jurisdictional policies determine the quality and distribution of the social determinants of health and hence shape health outcomes through mediating resource allocation.

**Life Course**

1. Historical events over an individual's lifespan determines vulnerability to disease and health outcomes.
2. Risks can accumulate over time, such that the cumulative effect of multiple exposures reflects in poor health.
3. Risk exposure during critical periods of development can lead to permanent biological injury.
4. Socio-political forces influence risk throughout the life course, and hence leave their imprint on the body through the embodiment of risk to influence health outcomes.

organized screening programs for cervical, breast, and colorectal cancer exist in all provinces (Canadian Partnership Against Cancer, 2015). Canadians are also spending an increasing amount of their healthcare dollars on hospital-based cancer treatment. It has been estimated that hospital-associated healthcare costs, primarily for chemotherapy and radiotherapy, increased from $2.9 billion in 2005 to approximately $7.5 billion in 2012 (de Oliveira et al., 2018). Annually, Canadians spend an average of $500 million funding innovative cancer research-based studies (Canadian Cancer Research Alliance, 2017).

According to recent statistics, approximately 200,000 new cases of cancer are diagnosed every year in Canada (Canadian Cancer Society's Advisory Committee on Cancer Statistics, 2017). The average five-year survival for all cancers combined is 60%, and approximately 80,000 cancer-related deaths occur annually. While these numbers paint an important picture, they tell us little about who is more likely to get cancer, and indeed, even who is more likely to die of cancer and under what circumstances.

In Canada, evidence spanning several decades demonstrates that cancer-related health outcomes are dependent on social class. Those who have higher levels of social advantage, such as those who have higher levels of income, are more likely to survive cancer (Booth, Li, Zhang-Salomons, & Mackillop, 2010; Mackillop, Zhang-Salomons, Groome, Paszat, & Holowaty, 1997). This finding persists even if tumours are diagnosed at a similar stage.

What does this mean? It means that someone with a stage-two tumour from a lower social class is more likely to die of their cancer than someone with a stage-two tumour from a higher social class.

Despite all our advances in health care, individuals who are socially disadvantaged are more likely to die of cancer than those who are socially advantaged. And this is a finding that has persisted over time (Booth et al., 2010; Mackillop et al., 1997). From this observation, one can assume that access to health care is important, but that a focus on health care alone will not be enough to solve inequalities in cancer risk, mortality, and survival. Solving inequalities in cancer-related health outcomes that are driven primarily by differences in social circumstance requires a political commitment to change the living and working conditions of people susceptible to and suffering from cancer.

## CONNECTING THEORY WITH PRACTICE: A CLOSER LOOK AT BREAST CANCER IN CANADA

Breast cancer is the most commonly occurring cancer in Canadian women, and approximately 70 women across the country face the diagnosis each day (Canadian Cancer Society's Advisory Committee on Cancer Statistics, 2017). While women are more likely to die of lung cancer, breast cancer comes in as the second leading cause of cancer-related deaths in females (Canadian Cancer Society's Advisory Committee on Cancer Statistics, 2017). Overall, mortality rates due to breast cancer have declined over time, and this has been primarily due to advances in diagnostic procedures and treatment regimes (Edwards et al., 2005; Holford, Cronin, Mariotto, & Feuer, 2006).

Women from higher social classes (as measured by income levels), are more likely to be diagnosed with breast cancer (Canadian Partnership Against Cancer, 2012). This has been attributed primarily to the higher levels of disease awareness and increased use of screening mammography services by the socially advantaged (Canadian Partnership Against Cancer, 2012). Interestingly, despite a higher incidence rate of breast cancer amongst higher social classes, women who are socially advantaged have a 5% higher relative survival rate compared to their socially disadvantaged counterparts (Canadian Partnership Against Cancer, 2012).

What does this tell us? It tells us that even though universally available provincial screening programs allow us to detect breast cancers early, this is not enough to equalize the difference in health outcomes experienced by women of different social classes.

This section will now focus on drawing the links between the theoretical models that we discussed earlier (Bartley, 2004) and actual practice implications using breast cancer as an example.

## Cultural-Behavioural

The cultural-behavioural model posits that the distinct health behaviours of different social groups are a result of their class location. As a result, lower social classes are more likely to have poorer health habits, and therefore endure worse health outcomes. Habits most often include reference to lifestyle-based choices, such as diet, exercise, smoking, and alcohol consumption; and can also include participation in health promotion activities, such as vaccination and screening for cancer.

For breast cancer, smoking for long periods, as well as exposure to second-hand smoke, has been associated with a higher risk of breast cancer (Terry & Rohan, 2002). In addition, alcohol consumption has been directly linked with cancer such that the amount of alcohol consumed is directly proportional to the risk of developing breast cancer (Berkey et al., 2010). Obesity is associated with worse breast cancer–related health outcomes, such that obese women are at a higher risk of breast cancer, have more advanced stage tumours at diagnosis, and a greater likelihood of metastasis and early death (Neuhouser et al., 2015).

A nutritious diet that is rich in fresh fruits and fibre has been shown to reduce the incidence of breast cancer (Su et al., 2010), while increased levels of physical activity are protective against both premenopausal (Maruti, Willett, Feskanich, Rosner, & Colditz, 2008) and postmenopausal breast cancer (Fournier et al., 2014).

Cancer care experts, including public health promotion experts, place emphasis on the role of "risk," and the importance of identifying personal risk factors and making changes to personal lifestyles (Cancer Care Ontario, n.d.) to reduce the likelihood of developing cancer. While it is important to quit smoking, drink less alcohol, eat well, and get plenty of exercise, these recommendations are unlikely to have any significant effect on influencing individual behaviour change (Scott-Samuel & Smith, 2015). This is particularly so for social groups where these behaviour choices are patterned by aspects of social structure such as distribution of income and wealth and the extent to which society provides people with the resources necessary for health through provision of adequate wages and child care, and access to food and housing (Daykin & Naidoo, 1995). Smoking, for example, is heavily class-based. Low income, a lack of social supports, and the physical and emotional toil of care-giving are prevalent among women from lower social classes. Smoking for this group of women is a coping mechanism to deal with the stressors of daily life (Daykin & Naidoo, 1995).

In Canada, women living in low-income neighbourhoods are more likely to smoke and are also more likely to be obese (Canadian Partnership Against Cancer, 2014). In addition, women from lower-income groups are less aware of cancer screening programs (Canadian Partnership Against Cancer, 2012) and are less likely to undergo mammography screening for breast cancer (Canadian Partnership Against Cancer, 2012).

At this point, it is important to consider the different ways of intervening to improve population health: on the one hand, we can try to reach all individuals and coach them to change their lifestyles and health choices; on the other hand, we can work to change societal structures so that fewer people live in the dire social circumstances that shape their poor health habits. These approaches are inherently different. For one, the focus is on individuals (what we will call the midstream of disease management), and for the other, the focus is on society, politics, and the global forces that shape the economic distribution of wealth (the upstream of health determinants; Turrell, Oldenburg, McGuffog, & Dent, 1999).

## Psychosocial

The psychosocial explanation of health inequities posits that differences in health outcomes between social groups are due to changes in the body's susceptibility to disease (Cassel, 1976; McEwen, 1998). For cancer, a chronic activation of the body's stress response can lead to a down regulation of the immune system, enabling tumour growth (Woods, Rachet, & Coleman, 2006). Put simply, the immune system is less responsive and allows the tumour to grow. Indeed, studies have demonstrated that socially disadvantaged cancer patients have compromised immune systems (Groome, Schulze, Keller, & Mackillop, 2008) and more aggressive tumours that are difficult to treat (Booth et al., 2010).

Recent reports in Canada highlight how currently approximately 12% of the population lives with low income (Statistics Canada, 2017b). This population group is more likely to contain members of ethnic minority groups, Indigenous people, the elderly, and the disabled (Statistics Canada, 2017b). Women are particularly vulnerable to economic hardship, and as a result women are more likely than men to experience poverty and homelessness (Bezanson, 2006). When women are employed, they are more likely to be working in precarious jobs (Bezanson, 2006) and are subject to discrimination and unequal pay for equal work (Pay Equity Commission, 2011).

Social polarization of ethnic minority groups into racial ghettos and economically deprived enclaves (Smith & Ley, 2008) influences the ability of residents to access recreation and health care (Prince et al., 2012). In addition, discrimination against groups based on their social identity can lead to higher levels of stress (Harwood & Sparks, 2003). This is often compounded with feelings of marginalization and deprivation, as well as cultural misgivings about the health system (Gerend & Pai, 2008). Furthermore, there is evidence of differential and inappropriate healthcare management of patients based on social class (Woods et al., 2006).

How are these findings associated with breast cancer? Women with access to social supports, such as those women in a marital relationship (Meng, Maskarinec, & Wilkens, 1997), tend to have better overall survival. It is hypothesized that this is because of timely diagnosis and compliance with treatment (Woods et al., 2006). In addition, even though most women with breast cancer are likely to report psychosocial stress and anxiety, women who are socially disadvantaged are more likely to continue to report mental distress years after receiving their diagnosis (Macleod, Ross, Fallowfield, & Watt, 2004). Low-income women with breast cancer are also more likely be diagnosed with clinical depression (Ramírez et al., 1993). Not surprisingly, women from lower social classes report higher levels of anxiety in relation to financial, health, and family problems (Macleod et al., 2004). But perhaps most significantly, it has been reported that women who report higher levels of depression are more likely to have a tumour recurrence, as well as poorer survival (Watson, Haviland, Greer, Davidson, & Bliss, 1999).

What can be done to resolve psychosocially mediated health differences? Many interventions have focused on correctly identifying women who report mental distress, so that they can be referred for further counselling and therapy (Dean, 1987; Ramírez et al., 1993). This would imply a focus on individuals, with an emphasis on creating behaviour change or strengthening personal capacity. These are midstream interventions. Other types of intervention, such as immunotherapy to enhance the functioning of the immune system response against the tumour, work at the biological level. These types of interventions target cellular mechanisms and can be classed as downstream. Another, and yet often overlooked, way of tackling psychosocially mediated health outcomes would be to consider public policies that can redistribute wealth so that there are fewer low-income people. This upstream approach would allow more people to have the opportunities to live and work in conditions that are better for their overall health and well-being.

## Materialist

Materialist explanations of health inequalities posit that the availability of resources at the micro- (such as income) or macro-level (such as social safety net) create structural forces that shape individual agency. For cancer, the lack of material resources directly influences cancer risk (Hiatt & Breen, 2008), results in a poorer quality of life (Fenn et al., 2014), and leads to a higher rate of cancer-related mortality (Booth et al., 2010).

How does this occur? In the simplest of explanations, low-income groups participate less frequently in cancer screening because they lack awareness of such programs and have difficulty in arranging transportation or child care so they can utilize the service (Canadian Partnership Against Cancer, 2014). In addition, the lack of a national program to cover prescription medications implies that each province in Canada has its own rules and regulations regarding coverage for cancer drugs (Chafe et al., 2011). This inherently implies that some people will struggle to access curative therapy. The absence of public policies that support good and stable working conditions (Reeder-Hayes, Wheeler, & Mayer, 2015) is also problematic, as cancer patients can struggle to maintain employment (Bradley et al., 2008), resulting in financial hardship and even loss of employment-based health insurance.

Women are more likely to be working in precarious jobs, with few or no benefits (Bezanson, 2006). The situation is worse for women of colour, as they are more likely than white women to be underemployed, underpaid, and discriminated against (McGibbon & McPherson, 2011). Given that care-giving is highly gendered, women are likely to find themselves in the unpaid role of social reproduction (Luxton, 2006) and juggling competing household financial, physical, and emotional needs.

The lack of transportation or availability of child care has been directly reported as a hindrance to the utilization of mammography for breast cancer screening (Douglas, Waller, Duffy, & Wardle, 2015). But out-of-pocket expenses that are related to access to cancer care include an array of other costs such as parking fees, food, accommodation, prescription drug coverage, family care, rehabilitation, home nursing, and medical devices (Longo & Bereza, 2011). Breast cancer patients are more likely than patients with other cancers to report these costs as unmanageable (Longo & Bereza, 2011). Some patients even report having to prioritize needs and rationing money between food, medicines, and transportation (Sinding, 2010). Some women find themselves struggling to continue work despite increasing nausea and fatigue (Sinding, 2010). Lower income, lack of health insurance and prescription drug coverage, or high levels of insurance co-payment have all been associated with poorer compliance to anti-cancer therapy (Taylor, 2014). This in turn can influence long-term disease-free survival (Partridge, 2006).

Strategies to mitigate health inequalities that are materially based can focus on improving access to health care and prescription drug coverage. Some of these are geared to enhancing the ability of people with low resources to reach healthcare institutions and can include subsidies for parking or reimbursement of travel costs. Strategies also include providing financial coverage for anti-cancer therapy, although these are almost always means-tested and include a percentage of copayment (Cancer Care Ontario, 2017). Because the target of these interventions is individuals, this approach is distinctly midstream.

An upstream approach to tackling material-based health inequalities is to improve the quality and distribution of the social determinants of health so that cancer patients can have better living and working conditions (Sayani, 2017). Altering the way in which the social determinants of health are structured, however, will require a political commitment to challenge the organization of global economic forces and neo-liberal capitalism (Bryant, Raphael, Schrecker, & Labonte, 2011; Navarro, 1999; Raphael, 2012).

## Life Course

Life-course explanations of health inequalities posit that past historical events leave a permanent imprint on the body and through this process influence risk, vulnerability to disease, opportunity to access care, and ultimately individual health outcomes. We have already discussed how certain risk factors for cancer, such as smoking and alcohol consumption, are heavily social class-based. However, individuals from lower social classes experience a broad array of lifestyle and environmental exposures that can increase their likelihood of getting cancer and reduce their chances of recovery. Fruit and vegetable intake, for example, is important in cancer prevention (Su et al., 2010). However, food insecurity is prevalent among the poor, and they are also the least likely to consume adequate amounts of the essential nutrients found in such foods (Di Noia & Byrd-Bredbenner, 2014).

On a similar note, exposure to air pollutants, toxic wastes, and ionizing radiation are all associated with an elevated cancer risk (Kogevinas, Pearce, Susser, & Boffetta, 1997). Individuals from lower social classes have higher degrees of exposure to these environmental toxins, because they are more likely to be living in neighbourhoods that contain the sources of such pollution (Kogevinas et al., 1997). Occupational exposure to carcinogens is responsible for between 2% and 8% of all cancers (Purdue, Hutchings, Rushton, & Silverman, 2015). Not surprisingly, these cancers are concentrated in the lower social classes, particularly manual labourers (Ramsay et al., 2014). There is also evidence that links the higher incidence of cancer-causing chronic infections among the lower social classes (Kogevinas et al., 1997). This includes bacteria such as helicobacter pylori (causing stomach cancer) and viruses such as hepatitis B and C (causing hepatocellular carcinoma) and human papilloma virus (causing cervical cancer).

Breast cancer occurs through a multistage process of tumour development, whereby spontaneous and environmentally induced alterations in the breast tissue trigger the progression of normal cells to precancerous lesions, cancer, and then metastasis (Institute of Medicine, 2012). The changes occurring at the genetic, epigenetic, and cellular level affect hormonal and immune reactions that regulate tumour biology and clinical behaviour. Many of these processes are part of a chain reaction of complex phenomena, and it is difficult to narrow down etiology to a single environmental exposure or biological response (Institute of Medicine, 2012).

Some studies have helped us understand correlations between exposure over the life course and breast cancer risk. For example, smoking (Terry & Rohan, 2002) and alcohol consumption (Berkey et al., 2010) are both associated with a higher risk of developing cancer. Exposure to gamma radiation or occupational hazards such as night-shift work have also been found to increase the risk of breast cancer (Weiderpass, Meo, & Vainio, 2011). On the contrary, a diet rich in fresh fruits and fibre is protective against breast cancer (Su et al., 2010). Social class differences are also clearly apparent for the most aggressive phenotype of breast cancer, called Triple Negative Breast Cancer (TNBC; Hyslop, Michael, Avery, & Rui, 2013). This type of breast cancer has a distinctly poor prognosis and is found to occur more commonly in those with lower socio-economic status and minority population groups (Hyslop et al., 2013).

Lifestyle-based interventions focus on modifying risk through influencing individual health behaviours (a midstream approach). These strategies are now known to be the least effective in influencing health outcomes (Scott-Samuel & Smith, 2015). On the contrary, these approaches are more likely to increase levels of stress and guilt as the health behaviours are structured by social class rather than personal choice (Daykin & Naidoo, 1995). Downstream measures are focused on cellular physiology, and the identification and treatment of biological pathways that can hinder tumour growth and encourage tumour regression. Successful examples of these include Tamoxifen and Her2/neu. Upstream approaches intervene at the political or economic level and aim to restructure how patterns of risk and exposure are shaped by social circumstance (Smith, 2015). This can include enhancing the social determinants of health, such as public policies that reduce exposure to occupational hazards. Policies can also focus further upstream to redistribute wealth and reduce inequalities across the social classes.

## THE UPSTREAM, MIDSTREAM, AND DOWNSTREAM OF CANCER

It is now well recognized in public health promotion practice that a focus on individuals and their personal risk factors is important, but not sufficient to reduce inequalities in health (Carey, Malbon, Crammond, Pescud, & Baker, 2017; Popay, Whitehead, & Hunter, 2010). Emphasis is increasingly placed on improving the upstream determinants of health, which are the political and economic drivers of social inequalities that underpin all health inequalities (Raphael, 2009). Models of health promotion and determinants of health therefore categorize interventions and/or approaches to health inequalities as being distinctly upstream, midstream, or downstream, depending on the locus of action (Gehlert et al., 2008; National Collaborating Centre for Determinants of Health, 2014; Raphael, 2016; Smith, 2015; Turrell et al., 1999; Williams, Costa, Odunlami, & Mohammed, 2008).

To facilitate a more nuanced understanding of cancer risk, management, and outcomes, however, these health promotion models need to be adapted to one of disease management. This will allow us to ask more refined questions, focus on our areas of expertise, and yet enable us to keep the "big picture" of cancer inequalities in mind (see the third box in Figure 7.1).

For cancer, it is important to understand the downstream cellular mechanisms and pathways that trigger cancer growth and enable metastasis. These discoveries have led to vast leaps in tumour therapy, such that many cancers now have a good prognosis.

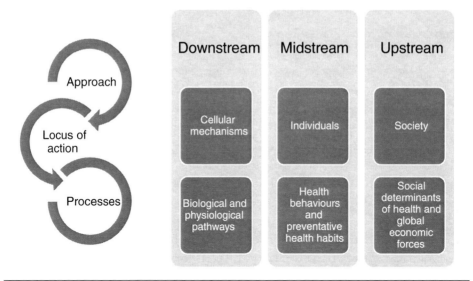

**Figure 7.1:** The Upstream, Midstream, and Downstream of Disease Management for Inequalities in Health

However, if we consider inequalities in cancer outcomes, some downstream questions remain unanswered. We are aware of physiological and biological predispositions to disease in the lower social classes. Yet how do these influence cancer occurrence and severity? Are therapies equally effective across all social classes? Why is it that tumours at a similar stage can have distinctly poorer outcomes in the socially deprived? Is this mediated at the cellular level, and, if so, is there a supplemental therapy that can be devised? While these are all important questions that must be answered, it is equally important that we do not veer away from the recognition that cellular processes, which are a result of social inequalities, require societal reform that cannot be rectified by treatment at the cellular level.

A midstream approach to the management of cancer is focused on the individual. Typically, these include health promotion practices that encourage a modification of risky lifestyle behaviours and participation in preventative health services, such as screening and vaccination. Midstream approaches to reduce cancer inequalities typically intervene by identifying priority populations that need social or welfare support to access therapy and avail of health services. While these interventions are useful in the short-term, it is important to realize that this approach is analogous to applying bandages to the injured. The bandage does nothing to prevent the injury and does little to promote recovery.

An upstream approach to managing inequalities in cancer risk and outcomes is focused on the living and working conditions of citizens and cancer patients. This approach is cognizant that social stratification creates an unequal allocation of resources and, as a result, mediates differences in cancer risk, outcomes, and mortality. From an upstream perspective, it is important to improve the quality and distribution of the social determinants of health. It is through this process that the living and working conditions of cancer patients can be improved and social inequalities in cancer-related health outcomes can be redressed. An upstream approach also entails that cancer care workers are aware of global economic forces and neo-liberal policies that create social stratification, as these processes directly influence how successfully care is received by cancer patients and their families.

## THE WAY FORWARD

While the focus of this chapter has been to draw out the links between social class and health inequalities using cancer as an example, you will find that many of the theoretical underpinnings and concepts can be applied to almost any illness. Social class is a strong determinant of opportunities and life chances. This happens through the mediation of risk, ability to seek care, and the ongoing sustainability of health-promoting resources over the lifespan. I encourage you to think critically about these issues as you carve a niche in future health services.

## CRITICAL THINKING QUESTIONS

1.  Why is there differential access to anti-cancer drugs across Canada? How can this influence social class differences in health outcomes?
2.  How can we reduce cancer risk across the population? In which ways would an upstream approach to prevention differ from midstream and/or downstream interventions?
3.  How do you think social class differences will influence risk, morbidity, and mortality for other non-communicable chronic illnesses such as heart disease, stroke, and diabetes?

## FURTHER READINGS

Bartley, M. (2016). *Health inequality: An introduction to theories, concepts, and methods* (2nd ed.). Cambridge: Polity Press.
This book provides a key to understanding the four most widely accepted theories of what lies behind inequality in health: behavioural, psychosocial, material, and life-course approaches.

Grabb, E. G. (2007). *Theories of social inequality* (5th ed.). Toronto: Harcourt Canada.
This volume provides a thorough explanation of the social construction of inequality based on a solid grounding in the work of the major classical theorists, such as Karl Marx, Max Weber, and Emile Durkheim, among others.

Sayani, A. (2017). Socially based inequities in breast cancer care: Intersections of the social determinants of health and the cancer care continuum. *Women's Health in Urban Life, 13*(1). Retrieved from https://ojs.scholarsportal.info/uoit/index.php/whul/article/view/2

This paper describes the ramifications of spending cuts and social structural inequality on the cancer care trajectory. By using the example of breast cancer care, it advances the discussion of how power, resources, and opportunities create gendered social inequality, and the implications of such "structures of constraint" for women experiencing cancer.

Sayani, A. (2018). Inequities in genetic testing for hereditary breast cancer: Implications for public health practice. *Journal of Community Genetics*, 1–5.
This paper explores the intersections of social identity with the social determinants of health, and how together they influence access to genetic screening for hereditary breast cancer. Implications for public health practice in recognizing and ameliorating these differences are presented.

Wright, E. (2015). *Understanding class.* New York: Verso.
Erik Wright interrogates the divergent meanings of this fundamental concept in order to develop a more integrated framework of class analysis. Beginning with the treatment of class in Marx and Weber, and proceeding through the writings of Charles Tilly, Thomas Piketty, Guy Standing, and others, it provides a compelling view of how to think about the complexity of class in the world today.

## RELEVANT WEBSITES

### *Health Reports*
https://www150.statcan.gc.ca/n1/en/catalogue/82-003-X
   *Health Reports* is a peer-reviewed journal of population health and health services research. It is designed for a broad audience that includes health professionals, researchers, policy-makers, and the general public, and publishes articles of wide interest that contain original and timely analyses of national or provincial/territorial surveys or administrative databases.

### The Equality Trust
https://www.equalitytrust.org.uk/
   The Equality Trust is a registered charity that works to improve quality of life in the U.K. by reducing economic and social inequality. The organization campaigns for changes that will have significant impact in reducing inequality and advocate a range of policies that can reduce inequality at a national, local, and individual level.

### Canadian Centre for Policy Alternatives (CCPA)—Inequality and Poverty
https://www.policyalternatives.ca/issues/inequality-and-poverty
   Inequality and poverty are at the heart of much of the CCPA's work. In particular, the Growing Gap project takes an in-depth look at one of the biggest challenges of our time: worsening income and wealth inequality in Canada.

**The Townsend Centre for International Poverty Research**

https://www.bristol.ac.uk/poverty/

The Townsend Centre for International Poverty Research is dedicated to multidisciplinary research on poverty in both the industrialized and the developing worlds. Its work focuses on defining and measuring poverty, poverty and social exclusion, and health inequalities.

**What Are the Determinants of Health and Why Do They Matter So Much?**

https://www.youtube.com/watch?v=tLHCy2k5xa4&t=631s

Narrative story-telling is used to describe how the social determinants of health influence access to care and ultimately influence health outcomes, with a particular emphasis on the cancer continuum of care.

## GLOSSARY

**Socio-economic status:** An aggregate term used to operationalize concepts of social class into a metric or measurement for purposes of a research study and/or hypothesis. Frequently, measures that indicate material resources (such as income and education) or prestige (such as occupational rank) are used as a proxy to socio-economic status (Krieger, 2001).

**Social gradient:** A term that describes the differences in health observed between different groups of people based on their socio-economic status. Generally, individuals who have a lower socio-economic status also have poorer health indicators. As the socio-economic status of individuals improve, health indicators also improve, such that those people at the top of the gradient are those that have the highest socio-economic means and the best health indicators (Eikemo & Bambra, 2008).

**Social location:** The rank order an individual occupies on a hierarchical ladder of power, privilege, and prestige, also referred to as social position. Many elements work in tandem, or intersect, to influence social location. These include material and social resources such as wealth and income, gender, age, religious affiliation, and mental or physical disability (Anderson, 2011).

**Social inequality:** A term used to describe the unequal distribution of power, privilege, and prestige across a society. Inherently, individuals who occupy positions of social advantage by virtue of their personal wealth and credentials are more able to access resources and services (Grabb, 2002), thereby creating further differentiation between social classes.

**Social stratification:** The hierarchical ordering of people based on their position in society, determined by their level of power, prestige, and privilege. When social inequality becomes systematically entrenched in a society, such that it is institutionalized into policies and procedures that continue to differentiate between social classes, it is called social stratification (McMullin & Davies, 2010).

## REFERENCES

Anderson, E. (2011). *Feminist epistemology and philosophy of science.* Retrieved April 30, 2015, from http://plato.stanford.edu/archives/spr2011/entries/feminism-epistemology/

Bartley, M. (2004). *Health inequality: An introduction to concepts, theories and methods.* Cambridge: Polity Press.

Bartley, M. (2016). *Health inequality: An introduction to concepts, theories and methods.* Cambridge: Polity Press.

Ben-Shlomo, Y., & Kuh, D. (2002). A life course approach to chronic disease epidemiology: Conceptual models, empirical challenges and interdisciplinary perspectives. *International Journal of Epidemiology, 31*(2), 285–293. doi:10.1093/ije/31.2.285

Berkey, C. S., Willett, W. C., Frazier, A. L., Rosner, B., Tamimi, R. M., Rockett, H. R. H., & Colditz, G. A. (2010). Prospective study of adolescent alcohol consumption and risk of benign breast disease in young women. *Pediatrics, 125*(5), e1081–e1087. doi:10.1542/peds.2009-2347

Bezanson, K. (2006). *Gender, the state, and social reproduction: Household insecurity in neo-liberal times.* Toronto: University of Toronto Press.

Blane, D. (2005). The life course, the social gradient, and health. In M. Marmot & R. Wilkinson (Eds.), *Social determinants of health* (pp. 54–77). Oxford: Oxford University Press.

Booth, C. M., Li, G., Zhang-Salomons, J., & Mackillop, W. J. (2010). The impact of socioeconomic status on stage of cancer at diagnosis and survival. *Cancer, 116*(17), 4160–4167. doi:10.1002/cncr.25427

Bourdieu, P. (1973). Cultural reproduction and social reproduction. In R. Brown (Ed.), *Knowledge, education and cultural change* (pp. 71–84). Abingdon, U.K.: Taylor & Francis.

Bradley, C. J., Yabroff, K. R., Dahman, B., Feuer, E. J., Mariotto, A., & Brown, M. L. (2008). Productivity costs of cancer mortality in the United States: 2000–2020. *Journal of the National Cancer Institute, 100*(24), 1763–1770. doi:1093/jnci/djn384

Bryant, T., Raphael, D., Schrecker, T., & Labonte, R. (2011). Canada: A land of missed opportunity for addressing the social determinants of health. *Health Policy (Amsterdam, Netherlands), 101*(1), 44–58. doi:10.1016/j.healthpol.2010.08.022

Canadian Cancer Research Alliance. (2017). Cancer research investment in 2015. Retrieved from https://www.ccra-acrc.ca/index.php/about-us/news-and-announcements/338-cancer-research-investment-in-2015

Canadian Cancer Society's Advisory Committee on Cancer Statistics. (2017). *Canadian cancer statistics 2017.* Retrieved from http://www.cancer.ca/~/media/cancer.ca/CW/cancer%20information/cancer%20101/Canadian%20cancer%20statistics/Canadian-Cancer-Statistics-2017-EN.pdf?la=en

Canadian Cancer Statistics Advisory Committee. (2018). *Canadian cancer statistics 2018.* Retrieved from http://www.cancer.ca/~/media/cancer.ca/CW/cancer%20information/cancer%20101/Canadian%20cancer%20statistics/Canadian-Cancer-Statistics-2018-EN.pdf?la=en

Canadian Partnership Against Cancer. (2012). *Breast cancer control in Canada: A system performance special focus report.* Retrieved from https://s22457.pcdn.co/wp-content/uploads/2019/01/Breast-cancer-control-EN.pdf

Canadian Partnership Against Cancer. (2014). *Examining disparities in cancer control : A system performance special focus report.* Retrieved from https://s22457.pcdn.co/wp-content/uploads/2019/01/Examining-disparities-in-cancer-control-EN.pdf

Canadian Partnership Against Cancer. (2015). Cancer screening in Canada: An overview of screening participation for breast, cervical and colorectal cancer. Retrieved from https://s22457.pcdn.co/wp-content/uploads/2019/01/Breast-Cervical-Colorectal-Screening-Participate-2015-EN.pdf

Cancer Care Ontario. (n.d.). My CancerIQ. Retrieved February 28, 2018, from https://www.mycanceriq.ca/

Cancer Care Ontario. (2017, June 28). Provincial drug reimbursement programs. Retrieved August 21, 2018, from https://www.cancercareontario.ca/en/cancer-care-ontario/programs/provincial-drug-reimbursement

Carey, G., Malbon, E., Crammond, B., Pescud, M., & Baker, P. (2017). Can the sociology of social problems help us to understand and manage "lifestyle drift"? *Health Promotion International, 32*(4), 755–761. doi:10.1093/heapro/dav116

Cassel, J. (1976). The contribution of the social environment to host resistance: The Fourth Wade Hampton Frost Lecture. *American Journal of Epidemiology, 104*(2), 107–123. doi:10.1093/oxfordjournals.aje.a112281

Chafe, R., Culyer, A., Dobrow, M., Coyte, P. C., Sawka, C., O'Reilly, S., … Sullivan, T. (2011). Access to cancer drugs in Canada: Looking beyond coverage decisions. *Healthcare Policy, 6*(3), 27–36. doi:10.12927/hcpol.2011.22177

Coburn, D. (2000). Income inequality, social cohesion and the health status of populations: The role of neo-liberalism. *Social Science & Medicine (1982), 51*(1), 135–146. doi:10.1016/S0277-9536(99)00445-1

Coburn, D. (2004). Beyond the income inequality hypothesis: Class, neo-liberalism, and health inequalities. *Social Science & Medicine, 58*(1), 41–56. doi:10.1016/S0277-9536(03)00159-X

Crompton, R. (2008). *Class and stratification* (3rd ed.). Cambridge: Polity Press.

Crompton, R. (2010). Class and employment. *Work, Employment and Society, 24*(1), 9–26. doi:10.1177/0950017009353667

Daykin, N., & Naidoo, J. (1995). Feminist critiques of health promotion. In R. Bunton, S. Nettleton, & R. Burrows (Eds.), *The sociology of health promotion: Critical analyses of consumption, lifestyle and risk* (pp. 59–69). London: Routledge.

de Oliveira, C., Weir, S., Rangrej, J., Krahn, M. D., Mittmann, N., Hoch, J. S., … Peacock, S. (2018). The economic burden of cancer care in Canada: A population-based cost study. *Canadian Medical Association Journal Open, 6*(1), e1–e10. doi:10.9778/cmajo.20170144

Dean, C. (1987). Psychiatric morbidity following mastectomy: Preoperative predictors and types of illness. *Journal of Psychosomatic Research, 31*(3), 385–392. doi:10.1016/0022-3999(87)90059-6

Di Noia, J., & Byrd-Bredbenner, C. (2014). Determinants of fruit and vegetable intake in low-income children and adolescents. *Nutrition Reviews, 72*(9), 575–590. doi:10.1111/nure.12126

Diez Roux, A. V., Merkin, S. S., Arnett, D., Chambless, L., Massing, M., Nieto, F. J., … Watson, R. L. (2001). Neighborhood of residence and incidence of coronary heart disease. *The New England Journal of Medicine, 345*(2), 99–106. doi:10.1056/NEJM200107123450205

Dinca-Panaitescu, M., Dinca-Panaitescu, S., Raphael, D., Bryant, T., Pilkington, B., & Daiski, I. (2012). The dynamics of the relationship between diabetes incidence and low income: Longitudinal results from Canada's National Population Health Survey. *Maturitas, 72*(3), 229–235. doi:10.1016/j.maturitas.2012.03.017

Douglas, E., Waller, J., Duffy, S. W., & Wardle, J. (2015). Socioeconomic inequalities in breast and cervical screening coverage in England: Are we closing the gap? *Journal of Medical Screening, 23*(2), 98–103. doi:10.1177/0969141315600192

Edwards, B. K., Brown, M. L., Wingo, P. A., Howe, H. L., Ward, E., Ries, L. A. G., … Pickle, L. W. (2005). Annual report to the nation on the status of cancer, 1975–2002, featuring population-based trends in cancer treatment. *Journal of the National Cancer Institute, 97*(19), 1407–1427. doi:10.1093/jnci/dji289

Eikemo, T. A., & Bambra, C. (2008). The welfare state: A glossary for public health. *Journal of Epidemiology and Community Health, 62*(1), 3–6.

Engels, F. (1987). *The condition of the working class in England*. New York: Penguin Classics. Originally published 1845.

Esping-Andersen, G. (1990). The three political economies of the welfare state. *International Journal of Sociology, 20*(3), 92–123. doi:10.1080/15579336.1990.11770001

Fenn, K. M., Evans, S. B., McCorkle, R., DiGiovanna, M. P., Pusztai, L., Sanft, T., … Chagpar, A. B. (2014). Impact of financial burden of cancer on survivors' quality of life. *Journal of Oncology Practice, 10*(5), 332–338. doi:10.1200/JOP.2013.001322

Fournier, A., Santos, G. D., Guillas, G., Bertsch, J., Duclos, M., Boutron-Ruault, M.-C., … Mesrine, S. (2014). Recent recreational physical activity and breast cancer risk in postmenopausal women in the E3N cohort. *Cancer Epidemiology, Biomarkers & Prevention, 23*(9), 1893–1902. doi:10.1158/1055-9965.EPI-14-0150

Gehlert, S., Sohmer, D., Sacks, T., Mininger, C., McClintock, M., & Olopade, O. (2008). Targeting health disparities: A model linking upstream determinants to downstream interventions. *Health Affairs, 27*(2), 339–349. doi:10.1377/hlthaff.27.2.339

Gerend, M. A., & Pai, M. (2008). Social determinants of black-white disparities in breast cancer mortality: A review. *Cancer Epidemiology, Biomarkers & Prevention, 17*(11), 2913–2923. doi:10.1158/1055-9965.EPI-07-0633

Gomaa, N., Nicolau, B., Siddiqi, A., Tenenbaum, H., Glogauer, M., & Quiñonez, C. (2017). How does the social "get under the gums"? The role of socio-economic position in the oral-systemic health link. *Canadian Journal of Public Health, 108*(3), e224–e228. doi:10.17269/cjph.108.5930

Grabb, E. (2002). *Theories of social inequality*. Toronto: Harcourt Canada.

Groome, P. A., Schulze, K. M., Keller, S., & Mackillop, W. J. (2008). Demographic differences between cancer survivors and those who die quickly of their disease. *Clinical Oncology, 20*(8), 647–656. doi:10.1016/j.clon.2008.05.006

Hart, C. L., Hole, D. J., Gillis, C. R., Smith, G. D., Watt, G. C., & Hawthorne, V. M. (2001). Social class differences in lung cancer mortality: Risk factor explanations using two Scottish cohort studies. *International Journal of Epidemiology, 30*(2), 268–274. doi:10.1093/ije/30.2.268

Harwood, J., & Sparks, L. (2003). Social identity and health: An intergroup communication approach to cancer. *Health Communication, 15*(2), 145–159. doi:10.1207/S15327027HC1502_3

Hiatt, R. A., & Breen, N. (2008). The social determinants of cancer: A challenge for transdisciplinary science. *American Journal of Preventive Medicine, 35*(2 Suppl.), s141–s150. doi:10.1016/j.amepre.2008.05.006

Holford, T. R., Cronin, K. A., Mariotto, A. B., & Feuer, E. J. (2006). Changing patterns in breast cancer incidence trends. *Journal of the National Cancer Institute. Monographs,* (36), 19–25. doi:10.1093/jncimonographs/lgj016

Hyslop, T., Michael, Y., Avery, T., & Rui, H. (2013). Population and target considerations for triple-negative breast cancer clinical trials. *Biomarkers in Medicine, 7*(1), 11–21. doi:10.2217/bmm.12.114

Institute of Medicine. (2012). Examining mechanisms of breast cancer over the life course: Implications for risk. In *Breast cancer and the environment: A life course approach* (pp. 239–281). Washington, DC: The National Academies Press.

Kogevinas, M., Pearce, N., Susser, M., & Boffetta, P. (1997). *Social inequalities and cancer.* Oxford: International Agency for Research on Cancer.

Krieger, N. A. (2001). A glossary of social epidemiology. *Journal of Epidemiology and Community Health, 55*(10), 693–700.

Krieger, N., Williams, D. R., & Moss, N. E. (1997). Measuring social class in US public health research: Concepts, methodologies, and guidelines. *Annual Review of Public Health, 18*(1), 341–378. doi:10.1146/annurev.publhealth.18.1.341

Lemstra, M., Rogers, M., & Moraros, J. (2015). Income and heart disease: Neglected risk factor. *Canadian Family Physician, 61*(8), 698–704.

Longo, C. J., & Bereza, B. G. (2011). A comparative analysis of monthly out-of-pocket costs for patients with breast cancer as compared with other common cancers in Ontario, Canada. *Current Oncology, 18*(1), e1–e8. doi:10.3747/co.v18i1.681

Luxton, M. (2006). Feminist political economy in Canada and the politics of social reproduction. In K. Bezanson & M. Luxton (Eds.), *Social reproduction* (pp. 11–44). Montreal: McGill-Queen's University Press.

Macdonald, D. (2018). *Born to win: Wealth concentration in Canada since 1999.* Canadian Centre for Policy Alternatives. Retrieved from https://www.policyalternatives.ca/sites/default/files/uploads/publications/National%20Office/2018/07/Born%20to%20Win.pdf

Macintyre, S. (1997). The Black Report and beyond: What are the issues? *Social Science & Medicine, 44*(6), 723–745. doi:10.1016/S0277-9536(96)00183-9

Mackillop, W. J., Zhang-Salomons, J., Groome, P. A., Paszat, L., & Holowaty, E. (1997). Socioeconomic status and cancer survival in Ontario. *Journal of Clinical Oncology*, *15*(4), 1680–1689. doi:10.1200/JCO.1997.15.4.1680

Macleod, U., Ross, S., Fallowfield, L., & Watt, G. C. M. (2004). Anxiety and support in breast cancer: Is this different for affluent and deprived women? A questionnaire study. *British Journal of Cancer*, *91*(5), 879–883. doi:10.1038/sj.bjc.6602072

Marchildon, G. (2013). *Health systems in transition: Canada* (2nd ed.). Toronto: University of Toronto Press.

Marmot, M., & Wilkinson, R. G. (2001). Psychosocial and material pathways in the relation between income and health: A response to Lynch et al. *BMJ: British Medical Journal*, *322*(7296), 1233–1236. doi:/10.1136/bmj.322.7296.1233

Maruti, S. S., Willett, W. C., Feskanich, D., Rosner, B., & Colditz, G. A. (2008). A prospective study of age-specific physical activity and premenopausal breast cancer. *Journal of the National Cancer Institute*, *100*(10), 728–737. doi:10.1093/jnci/djn135

Marx, K., & Engels, F. (2011). *The German Ideology*. New Castle, DE: Martino Fine Books. Originally published 1846.

Marx, K. (1974). *Das Kapital: A critique of political economy* (Reprint edition). Washington, DC.: Gateway Editions.

McCartney, G., Bartley, M., Dundas, R., Katikireddi, S. V., Mitchell, R., Popham, F., … Wami, W. (2018). Theorising social class and its application to the study of health inequalities. *SSM - Population Health*. doi:10.1016/j.ssmph.2018.10.015

McCartney, G., Collins, C., & Mackenzie, M. (2013). What (or who) causes health inequalities: Theories, evidence and implications? *Health Policy*, *113*(3), 221–227. doi:10.1016/j.healthpol.2013.05.021

McEwen, B. S. (1998). Protective and damaging effects of stress mediators. *New England Journal of Medicine*, *338*(3), 171–179. doi:10.1056/NEJM199801153380307

McGibbon, E., & McPherson, C. (2011). Applying intersectionality & complexity theory to address the social determinants of women's health. *Women's Health and Urban Life*, *10*(1), 59–86.

McMullin, J., & Davies, L. (2010). Social class and health inequalities. In T. Bryant, D. Raphael, & M. Rioux (Eds.), *Staying alive: Critical perspectives on health, illness, and care* (2nd ed., pp. 181–204). Toronto: Canadian Scholars' Press.

Meng, L., Maskarinec, G., & Wilkens, L. (1997). Ethnic differences and factors related to breast cancer survival in Hawaii. *International Journal of Epidemiology*, *26*(6), 1151–1158. doi:10.1093/ije/26.6.1151

Muntaner, C., Borrell, C., Ng, E., Chung, H., Espelt, A., Rodriguez-Sanz, M., … O'Campo, P. (2011). Politics, welfare regimes, and population health: Controversies and evidence. *Sociology of Health & Illness*, *33*(6), 946–964. doi:10.1111/j.1467-9566.2011.01339.x

Muntaner, C., Borrell, C., Vanroelen, C., Chung, H., Benach, J., Kim, I. H., & Ng, E. (2010). Employment relations, social class and health: A review and analysis of conceptual and measurement alternatives. *Social Science & Medicine (1982)*, *71*(12), 2130–2140. doi:10.1016/j. socscimed.2010.09.038

Muntaner, C., Eaton, W. W., & Diala, C. C. (2000). Social inequalities in mental health: A review of concepts and underlying assumptions. *Health*, *4*(1), 89–113. doi:10.1177/136345930000400105

National Collaborating Centre for Determinants of Health. (2014). *Let's talk: Moving upstream*. Antigonish, NS: National Collaborating Centre for Determinants of Health, St. Francis Xavier University. Retrieved from http://nccdh.ca/images/uploads/ Moving_Upstream_Final_En.pdf

Navarro, V. (1999). Health and equity in the world in the era of "globalization." *International Journal of Health Services: Planning, Administration, Evaluation*, *29*(2), 215–226. doi:10.2190/ MQPT-RLTH-KUPJ-2FQP

Navarro, V. (2007). Neoliberalism as a class ideology; or, the political causes of the growth of inequalities. *International Journal of Health Services: Planning, Administration, Evaluation*, *37*(1), 47–62. doi:10.2190/AP65-X154-4513-R520

Navarro, V. (2009). What we mean by social determinants of health. *International Journal of Health Services: Planning, Administration, Evaluation*, *39*(3), 423–441. doi:10.2190/HS.39.3.a

Neuhouser, M. L., Aragaki, A. K., Prentice, R. L., Manson, J. E., Chlebowski, R., Carty, C. L., & Anderson, G. L. (2015). Overweight, obesity, and postmenopausal invasive breast cancer risk: A secondary analysis of the women's health initiative randomized clinical trials. *JAMA Oncology*, *1*(5), 611–621. doi:10.1001/jamaoncol.2015.1546

Øversveen, E., Rydland, H. T., Bambra, C., & Eikemo, T. A. (2017). Rethinking the relationship between socio-economic status and health: Making the case for sociological theory in health inequality research. *Scandinavian Journal of Public Health*, *45*(2), 103–112. doi:10.1177/1403494816686711

Partridge, A. H. (2006). Non-adherence to endocrine therapy for breast cancer. *Annals of Oncology*, *17*(2), 183–184. doi:10.1093/annonc/mdj141

Pay Equity Commission. (2011). *What is the gender wage gap?* Retrieved from http://www. payequity.gov.on.ca/en/GWG/Pages/what_is_GWG.aspx

Peto, R., Darby, S., Deo, H., Silcocks, P., Whitley, E., & Doll, R. (2000). Smoking, smoking cessation, and lung cancer in the UK since 1950: Combination of national statistics with two case-control studies. *British Medical Journal Clinical Research*, *321*(7257), 323–329. doi:10.1136/bmj.321.7257.323

Popay, J., Whitehead, M., & Hunter, D. J. (2010). Injustice is killing people on a large scale—but what is to be done about it? *Journal of Public Health*, *32*(2), 148–149. doi:10.1093/pubmed/ fdq029

Prince, S. A., Kristjansson, E. A., Russell, K., Billette, J.-M., Sawada, M. C., Ali, A., … Prud'homme, D. (2012). Relationships between neighborhoods, physical activity, and obesity: A multilevel analysis of a large Canadian city. *Obesity*, *20*(10), 2093–2100. doi:10.1038/oby.2011.392

Purdue, M. P., Hutchings, S. J., Rushton, L., & Silverman, D. T. (2015). The proportion of cancer attributable to occupational exposures. *Annals of Epidemiology*, *25*(3), 188–192. doi:10.1016/j.annepidem.2014.11.009

Ramírez, A. J., Pinder, K. L., Black, M. E., Richards, M. A., Gregory, W. M., & Rubens, R. D. (1993). Psychiatric disorder in patients with advanced breast cancer: Prevalence and associated factors. *European Journal of Cancer*, *29*(4), 524–527. https://doi.org/10.1016/S0959-8049(05)80144-3

Ramsay, S. E., Morris, R. W., Whincup, P. H., Papacosta, A. O., Lennon, L. T., & Wannamethee, S. G. (2014). Time trends in socioeconomic inequalities in cancer mortality: Results from a 35 year prospective study in British men. *BMC Cancer*, *14*(1), 474. doi:10.1186/1471-2407-14-474

Raphael, D. (2007). Making sense of poverty: Social inequality and social exclusion. In D. Raphael (Ed.), *Poverty and policy in Canada: Implications for health and quality of life* (pp. 85–115). Toronto: Canadian Scholars' Press.

Raphael, D. (2009). Reducing social and health inequalities requires building social and political movements. *Humanity & Society*, *33*(1–2), 145–165. doi:10.1177/016059760903300109

Raphael, D. (2018). Narrative review of affinities and differences between the social determinants of oral and general health in Canada: Establishing a common agenda. *Journal of Public Health*, fdy152. doi:10.1093/pubmed/fdy15

Raphael, D. (Ed.). (2012). *Tackling health inequalities: Lessons from international experiences.* Toronto: Canadian Scholars' Press.

Raphael, D. (Ed.). (2016). *Social determinants of health: Canadian perspectives* (3rd ed.). Toronto: Canadian Scholars' Press.

Raphael, D., & Bryant, T. (2006). Maintaining population health in a period of welfare state decline: Political economy as the missing dimension in health promotion theory and practice. *Global Health Promotion*, *13*(4), 236–242. doi:10.1177/175797590601300402

Reeder-Hayes, K. E., Wheeler, S. B., & Mayer, D. K. (2015). Health disparities across the breast cancer continuum. *Seminars in Oncology Nursing*, *31*(2), 170–177. doi:10.1016/j.soncn.2015.02.005

Savage, M. (2015). *A Pelican introduction: Social class in the 21st Century* (U.K. ed.). London: Pelican Books.

Sayani, A. (2017). Socially-based inequities in breast cancer care: Intersections of the social determinants of health and the cancer care continuum. *Women's Health & Urban Life: An International and Interdisciplinary Journal*, *13*(1), 24–36. Retrieved from https://ojs.scholarsportal.info/uoit/index.php/whul/article/view/2

Scambler, G. (2012). Health inequalities. *Sociology of Health & Illness*, *34*(1), 130–146. doi:10.1111/j.1467-9566.2011.01387.x

Scott-Samuel, A., & Smith, K. E. (2015). Fantasy paradigms of health inequalities: Utopian thinking? *Social Theory & Health*, *13*(3–4), 418–436. doi:10.1057/sth.2015.12

Sinding, C. (2010). Using institutional ethnography to understand the production of health care disparities. *Qualitative Health Research*, *20*(12), 1656–1663. doi:10.1177/1049732310377452

Smith, H., & Ley, D. (2008). Even in Canada? The multiscalar construction and experience of concentrated immigrant poverty in gateway cities. *Annals of the Association of American Geographers*, *98*(3), 686–713. doi:10.1080/00045600802104509

Smith, V. C. (2015). Upstream or downstream? *The Medical Journal of Australia*, *203*(10), 412–413. doi:10.5694/mja15.00718

Statistics Canada. (2017a, September 13). Census in brief: Children living in low-income households. Retrieved August 11, 2018, from https://www12.statcan.gc.ca/census-recensement/2016/as-sa/98-200-x/2016012/98-200-x2016012-eng.cfm

Statistics Canada. (2017b, September 13). Income in Canada, 2016 Census of Population. Retrieved August 10, 2018, from https://www150.statcan.gc.ca/n1/pub/11-627-m/11-627-m2017026-eng.htm

Su, X., Tamimi, R. M., Collins, L. C., Baer, H. J., Cho, E., Sampson, L., … Colditz, G. A. (2010). Intake of fiber and nuts during adolescence and incidence of proliferative benign breast disease. *Cancer Causes & Control*, *21*(7), 1033–1046. doi:10.1007/s10552-010-9532-7

Taylor, D. W. (2014). Benefits outweigh costs in universal healthcare: Business case for reimbursement of take-home cancer medicines in Ontario and Atlantic Canada. *American Journal of Medicine and Medical Sciences, 4*(4), 126–138.

Terry, P. D., & Rohan, T. E. (2002). Cigarette smoking and the risk of breast cancer in women: A review of the literature. *Cancer Epidemiology, Biomarkers & Prevention*, *11*(10), 953–971.

Townsend, P., Davidson, N., & Whitehead, M. (Eds.). (1999). *Inequalities in health: The Black Report and the Health Divide.* London: Penguin.

Turrell, G., Oldenburg, B., McGuffog, I., & Dent, R. (1999). *Socioeconomic determinants of health: Towards a national research program and a policy and intervention agenda.* Brisbane, QLD: Queensland University of Technology, School of Public Health, Centre for Public Health Research.

Virchow, R. (1985). Report on the typhus epidemic in Upper Silesia. In L. J. Rather (Ed.), *Collected essays by Rudolph Virchow on public health and epidemiology, Volume 1* (pp. 205–319). Canton, MA: Science History Publications. Originally published 1848.

Watson, M., Haviland, J. S., Greer, S., Davidson, J., & Bliss, J. M. (1999). Influence of psychological response on survival in breast cancer: A population-based cohort study. *The Lancet, 354*(9187), 1331–1336. doi:10.1016/S0140-6736(98)11392-2

Weber, M. (2013). *Economy and Society.* G. Roth & C. Wittich (Eds.). Berkeley: University of California Press. Originally published 1978.

Weiderpass, E., Meo, M., & Vainio, H. (2011). Risk factors for breast cancer, including occupational exposures. *Safety and Health at Work*, *2*(1), 1–8. doi:10.5491/SHAW.2011.2.1.1

Wilkinson, R. G. (1997). Socioeconomic determinants of health. Health inequalities: Relative or absolute material standards? *British Medical Journal*, *314*(7080), 591–595. doi:10.1136/bmj.314.7080.591

Wilkinson, R. G. (1999a). Health, hierarchy, and social anxiety. *Annals of the New York Academy of Sciences*, *896*(1), 48–63. doi:10.1111/j.1749-6632.1999.tb08104.x

Wilkinson, R. G. (1999b). Income inequality, social cohesion, and health: Clarifying the theory—A reply to Muntaner and Lynch. *International Journal of Health Services, 29*(3), 525–543. doi:10.2190/3QXP-4N6T-N0QG-ECXP

Wilkinson, R. G., & Pickett, K. E. (2006). Income inequality and population health: A review and explanation of the evidence. *Social Science & Medicine, 62*(7), 1768–1784. doi:10.1016/j.socscimed.2005.08.036

Wilkinson, R. G., & Pickett, K. E. (2010). *The spirit level: Why greater equality makes societies stronger*. New York: Bloomsbury Publishing.

Williams, D. R., Costa, M. V., Odunlami, A. O., & Mohammed, S. A. (2008). Moving upstream: How interventions that address the social determinants of health can improve health and reduce disparities. *Journal of Public Health Management and Practice, 14*(6), S8–S17. doi:10.1097/01.PHH.0000338382.36695.42

Woods, L. M., Rachet, B., & Coleman, M. P. (2006). Origins of socio-economic inequalities in cancer survival: A review. *Annals of Oncology: Official Journal of the European Society for Medical Oncology/ESMO, 17*(1), 5–19. doi:10.1093/annonc/mdj007

World Health Organization. (2010). A conceptual framework for action on the social determinants of health. Retrieved from http://www.who.int/social_determinants/publications/9789241500852/en/

Wright, E. O. (Ed.). (2005). *Approaches to class analysis*. Cambridge: Cambridge University Press.

# CHAPTER 8

## Shifting Vulnerabilities: Gender, Ethnicity/Race, and Health Inequities in Canada[1]

*Ann Pederson and Stefanie Machado*

## INTRODUCTION

The WHO Commission on Social Determinants of Health (CSDH; 2008) argued that health emerges in daily living conditions, which are shaped by inequitable access to power, money, and resources. Gender and ethnicity/race are among the factors that influence access to power, money, and other resources and, therefore, are important determinants of health. Ten years after the CSDH reported, analysts are declaring that its ambitions have not been met and issues of gender and ethnicity/race inequities remain critical problems across the globe. Rasanathan (2018, p. 1176), for example, suggests, "there has not been widespread policy uptake of [the Commission's] recommendations to improve daily living conditions, tackle the inequitable distribution of power, money, and resources, and monitor both inequities and the impact of policies to address them …" in part because "powerful actors actively work against reducing health inequities when it threatens their political and economic interests." This analysis suggests that challenging gender inequality and ethnic/racial inequities may be regarded as potentially socially disruptive and controversial.

Adopting the understanding from Grotti Malakasis, Quagliariello, and Sahraoui (2018) that vulnerability and resilience are not fixed states but rather shifting characteristics dependent upon the context in which people live their lives, in this chapter we examine how vulnerability and resilience emerge "in the context of specific social and historical relations" (Butler, Gambetti, & Sabsay, 2016, p. 4) of gender and ethnicity/race among im/migrant and Indigenous women and girls in Canada. Rather than characterizing particular populations of women as inherently vulnerable, we build on Fineman's (2008) notion that vulnerability is the essential human condition, because as material, embodied beings, humans are collectively and individually subject to injury, harm, and dependency throughout the life course. Instead of seeing vulnerability as exceptional, we should recognize, for example, that infants are born dependent on other humans for sustenance, safety, and support, and that illness, change, and decline are inevitable aspects of human experience. Fineman also contends that resilience, through which individuals and communities overcome or are sustained despite their vulnerability, is influenced by one's ability to garner resources—monetary, cognitive, social, legal, etc.—to manage. But as with the determinants of health, both vulnerability and resilience are unevenly distributed in a given social group. And as gender and ethnicity/race shape experiences of vulnerability and resilience, the specific features of a given situation or population and its actual experiences of vulnerability and resilience should therefore be documented.

By examining how gender and ethnicity/race shape the health of im/migrant and Indigenous women and girls, we seek to identify the commonalities as well as differences in how their respective social locations and positioning contribute to health and access to health care. While both populations have distinct experiences and histories, in many instances they share experiences of racialization, discrimination, dislocation, and marginalization. Our aim is to uncover and describe these processes and suggest means of reducing their adverse effects.

With respect to creating change, the CSDH recommended "political empowerment" to address the health challenges that arise from gender and ethnicity/race inequities by deliberately creating structures and opportunities for inclusion and giving voice to those who are marginalized and excluded. To enhance gender equality, we suggest that this may be achieved in health care, in part, through gender-transformative interventions, which focus on addressing gender inequity as part of health promotion, and ensuring that health care is trauma-informed and culturally safe. And, in health care and beyond, reducing vulnerability and fostering resilience involve engaging Indigenous and im/migrant women in determining acceptable and appropriate services, interventions, and supports.

## FRAMING THE DISCUSSION

Given the importance of social position and context in experiences of vulnerability and resilience, we suggest that it is important to understand some aspects of us as authors, as well as some key concepts germane to the discussion of gender, ethnicity/race, and health.

### Positioning Ourselves

We approach this analysis as a dialogue between feminist researchers and program developers from distinct backgrounds and generations.

#### *Stefanie Machado*

Migration has always played and continues to play a powerful role in my life. My great-grandfather migrated from India to Burma for employment, and my grandfather fled back to India due to political conflict in the 1940s. My parents migrated to the United Arab Emirates from India in 1990 for better economic opportunities. I identify as an immigrant woman of Indian origin who was born and raised in Abu Dhabi. At the age of 18,

I migrated to Canada to pursue post-secondary education, first landing as an international university student and gaining permanent residency status shortly after.

When I first moved to Canada, I belonged to a community of international students who reciprocally shared migration experiences, including relevant challenges and supports that impacted health. With lived experiences of structural barriers to accessing sexual and reproductive health (SRH) care, difficulties navigating the Canadian health system, and challenges fitting into Western ideals and norms, I realized that I did not face these issues alone. Other young immigrants faced similar health-related hurdles, in addition to issues faced by many populations in Canada, such as long wait times in hospitals and challenges related to health insurance coverage.

Therefore, through my lived and living experiences, I have had a range of experiences where gender, ethnicity/race, and health intersect to influence my access to care, sexual health, and mental health outcomes. However, through valuable connections and relationships with other young immigrant men and women who share similar, yet diverse, experiences, I have also developed and learned coping mechanisms and strategies for resiliency.

### Ann Pederson

I too am a product of im/migration. My father's parents each came from a different part of Scandinavia (Norway and Finland) but met on Canada's west coast in the 1920s. My father was born in Vancouver, as was I. My mother was evacuated to Canada during World War II and, though she returned to Britain immediately following the war, she eventually immigrated back to the west coast to pursue post-secondary education.

My father's health was always precarious, as he had survived numerous childhood illnesses in the period before antibiotics were available. Rheumatic fever left him with permanent heart damage. My mother suffered from depression, and both my parents were challenged by anxiety and the stresses of finite financial resources with which to raise four children in the 1960s. My parents died comparatively young, at 70 and 73, respectively. Their relatively premature deaths reflect their specific life experiences as well as developments in health care.

As a well-educated white woman, I presumably have access to the best of care, yet I too have experienced both privileges and challenges in accessing health services, especially mental health care and SRH services. I've had to endure absurd remarks from clinicians, such as one surgeon who said that gallbladders were his way of paying for his children's university education, and I've experienced extreme kindness from physiotherapists, podiatrists, and dentists.

I recognized when my mother was in an intensive care unit that my family was regarded as a "model" family because we deferred to medical authority, asked medically informed questions, participated in research, and came in small numbers. I witnessed overt racism as other families were chastised for coming in large numbers, staying continuously, and asking to visit their family member persistently. Yet I wished there had been more than the five of us to pay witness to my mother's grievous state.

In my work in women's health, I continue to seek ways to redress the inequities in access and outcomes for girls, women, and their families, using what privilege I have to open doors, and hoping that my humanity is attuned to recognizing disadvantage in its many forms. And I am paying attention to my status as a member of settler society, something that I was not educated about until mid-life.

We have had profoundly different life journeys and experiences, which inform our shared interest in issues of gender and race/ethnicity, but as individuals from different generations and ethnic/race backgrounds, we do not claim to be able to fully speak of the experiences of the other.

## Notes on Terminology

A few core terms are central to the arguments explored in this chapter, including gender, sex, ethnicity, race, Aboriginal, Indigenous, im/migrant, and intersectionality. This section explains and illustrates these terms.

### Gender/Sex

It is common in the health field to distinguish between the concepts of "sex" and "gender." "Sex" is generally understood to refer to biological aspects of being male or female. While sex is perhaps most visible in terms of the reproductive organs, there are other underlying physiological processes and anatomical features that are typically different in males and females, such as hormone patterns, fat distribution, and metabolism. "Gender," on the other hand, refers to the social attributes commonly ascribed to males or females to create the categories of "men" and "women." All societies are organized in ways that reflect constructions of women and men as different kinds of people, with respective roles, responsibilities, and opportunities, including access to resources and benefits. As a social construct, particular expressions and understandings of gender can vary over time and place and among communities. Behaviours, customs, roles, and practices are flexible and more variable across societies than the sex-related hormonal, anatomical, or physiological processes that typically characterize male and female bodies.

Marmot (2007, p. 1155), former head of the CSDH, said that

> The differential status of men and women in almost every society is perhaps the most pervasive and entrenched inequity. As such, the relation between the sexes represents as pressing a societal issue for health as the social gradient itself.

In saying this, Marmot was referring to what many call "gender relations," which involve relations between people of different genders (Health Canada, 2000), including the relative power of individuals and groups. Legal codes that frame social relationships—such as marriage, divorce, common-law relationships, and child custody—are important expressions of gender relations and shape, among other things, individuals' access to or responsibility for employment, education, income, housing, child care, inheritances, pensions, and other social benefits. This is evident, for example, in earlier structures and economic supports for newborn child care, which was typically organized to support women to take care of infants. Today's system of parental benefits in Canada, however, offers some flexibility for sharing of child care between biological, adoptive, or legally recognized parents caring for a newborn or newly adopted child or children. Maternity benefits offer support to both biological and surrogate mothers who are pregnant or have recently given birth. This set of options is very recent and reflects contemporary understandings of gender relations that recognize various possible arrangements for caring for (and carers of) children.

It is important to mention that discussions of gender and health need not only be about women and girls—although they still bear the greatest burdens of gender-based inequalities—but can also be about men and boys. A recent editorial in *The Lancet* (2018) argued, for example, that rigid gender norms, such as notions of masculinity being about self-control and being physically tough and vigorous, are increasingly understood to put men and boys at risk for poor health by encouraging them to suppress feelings, ignore symptoms, or engage in risk-taking. However, though we recognize that gender and health is not synonymous with women and girls, in this chapter, we focus on gender and gender relations in relation to the health of Indigenous and im/migrant women and girls.

### Ethnicity/Race

"Ethnicity" and "race" are two terms that are sometimes conflated. Ethnicity is generally understood as the state of belonging to a social group with shared national or cultural traditions, whereas race is more commonly associated with variations in external appearance among humans. Indeed, Krieger (2003) states that: "Myriad epidemiological studies continue to treat 'race' as a purely biological (i.e., genetic) variable or seek to explain racial/ethnic disparities in health absent consideration of the effects of racism on health" (p. 195). We take the stance, however, that neither ethnicity nor race offers much explanatory power when it comes to understanding the lives and health of individuals and groups. Instead, we are interested in processes of racialization, whereby ethnic or racial identities are ascribed/assigned to a group that does not identify itself as such. "Racialization" is a term that considers how groups of individuals come to be treated as inferior to the dominant group (Allahar & Côté, 1998). As such, racialization, as a construct, serves as a bridge between discrimination and its effects upon those who are discriminated. Because "race" is a social rather than biological construct, so too are the attributes assigned to people in the process of racialization. Racialization is not reserved for im/migrant people only, though. Ascribing characteristics to a group on the basis of their assumed "race" commonly affects various non-dominant, non-White groups in Canada, including Indigenous women and girls.

### Aboriginal/Indigenous

Aboriginal people are the indigenous inhabitants of Canada prior to contact from Europeans. Today, Canada recognizes three distinct groups of Indigenous peoples—First

Nations, Inuit, and Métis—each of whom has a distinct history, relationship to government, and experiences of health, but none of these groups are homogenous (Royal Commission on Aboriginal Peoples, 1996). In this chapter, we use the words "Aboriginal" and "Indigenous" interchangeably. This is modelled after a recent report from the National Collaborating Centre for Aboriginal Health (Odulaja & Halseth, 2018), which uses both terms to refer to First Nations, Inuit, and Métis peoples collectively.

### Im/migrant People

The International Organization for Migration (2018b) defines a migrant as "any person who is moving or has moved across an international border or within a State away from his/her habitual place of residence, regardless of (1) the person's legal status; (2) whether the movement is voluntary or involuntary; (3) what the causes for the movement are; or (4) what the length of the stay is." We use the term "im/migrants" to include immigrants, who intentionally leave their home country or country of origin to *settle* in another country, as well as migrants, who move within a country or across borders, but not necessarily with the intention of settling (International Rescue Committee, 2018). We use the term "im/migrants" to also include diverse populations, including refugees, asylum seekers, economic migrants, and undocumented people who have entered Canada recently or who have been living in the country long term, but recognize that diverse experiences and health outcomes are faced both within and between these heterogeneous populations.

### Intersectionality

In this chapter, we are examining gender and ethnicity/race together to understand how they mutually influence the health of im/migrant and Aboriginal women. Such an approach is an example of intersectional theorizing. Intersectional theory suggests that we need to move beyond seeing ourselves and others as single points in some specific set of dichotomies and rather think of ourselves and others as existing at the intersection of multiple identities, all of which influence one another and together shape experiences of self and other (Reid, Pederson, & Dupéré, 2012). We are particularly interested, in this discussion, in how gender and ethnicity/race intersect in the lives of im/migrant and Indigenous women and girls. As the poem in Box 8.2 suggests, it is powerful to understand the experience of people from not only one lens, such as gender, but through the simultaneous experience of two or more—in our case, from the simultaneous experience of being girls and women who either have lived as members of a society affected by contact with Europeans and its subsequent social, economic, and political impact or have experienced migration and settlement.

## Theoretical Foundations

As already noted, this chapter is also informed by writings on vulnerability and resilience. We chose this approach because it reframes the origins of vulnerability and also points to the possibilities that arise from resilience.

---

**Box 8.1:** Key Migration Terminology in Canada

---

**Refugee**—a person who is forced to flee from persecution (Canadian Council for Refugees, n.d.).

**Asylum seeker**—a person who seeks safety from persecution or serious harm in a country other than his or her own (International Organization for Migration, 2015).

**Refugee claimant**—a person who has made a claim for protection as a refugee (Canadian Council for Refugees, n.d.).

**Resettled refugee**—a refugee who has been offered a permanent home in a country while still outside that country (Canadian Council for Refugees, n.d.). Under the Government-Assisted Refugees (GAR) Program, refugees are referred to Canada for resettlement by the United Nations Refugee Agency (UNHCR) or another referral organization (International Organization for Migration, 2015).

**Protected person**—according to Canada's *Immigration and Refugee Protection Act*, a person who has been determined by Canada to be either (a) a Convention Refugee or (b) a person in need of protection (Canadian Council for Refugees, n.d.).

**Permanent resident**—a person who has been granted permanent resident status in Canada. The person may have come to Canada as an immigrant or as a refugee (Canadian Council for Refugees, n.d.).

**Temporary resident**—a person who has permission to remain in Canada on a temporary basis (the main categories are students, temporary workers, and visitors; Canadian Council for Refugees, n.d.).

**Person without status/undocumented**—a person who has not been granted permission to stay in the country, or has overstayed their visa. The term can cover a refugee claimant who is refused refugee status but has not removed from Canada because of a situation of generalized risk in the country of origin. The term "undocumented" can refer to refugees or immigrants who lack identity documents from their country of origin (Canadian Council for Refugees, n.d.).

---

As Fineman (2008, p. 8) has observed, vulnerability in the public health sense is "typically associated with victimhood, deprivation, dependency, or pathology," and the term is sometimes used to refer to people living in poverty or living with particular diseases, or those who are supported by state institutions and care facilities. Yet instead of seeing vulnerability as a fixed attribute of individuals or groups, Grotti et al. (2018) suggest that "(v)ulnerability is socially produced, through people's locations in hierarchical social orders and power relations and effects" (p. 2). Fineman (2008) argues that "(b)ecause we are positioned differently within a web of economic and institutional relationships, our vulnerabilities range in magnitude and potential at the individual level" (p. 10). While tracing the experiences of pregnant migrant women to Europe, for example, Grotti et al.

**Box 8.2:** An Example of Intersectionality

I am not just woman. I am a Mohawk woman. It is not solely my gender through which I first experience the world, it is my culture (and/or race) that precedes my gender. Actually if I am the object of some form of discrimination, it is very difficult for me to separate what happens to me because of my gender and what happens to me because of my race and culture. My world is not experienced in a linear and compartmentalized way. I experience the world simultaneously as Mohawk and as woman. It seems as though I cannot repeat this message too many times. To artificially separate my gender from my race and culture forces me to deny the way I experience the world. Such denial has devastating effects on Aboriginal constructions of reality (Monture-Angus, 1995, pp. 177–178).

(2018) observed that whether healthy or not, pregnant women were deemed "vulnerable" and fast-tracked into health care and social protection immediately, while other migrants were not. The healthcare system thus became a source of interpretation regarding different migrants' relative needs and a pathway through which individuals and families could navigate the complexities of migration. Recognizing that "vulnerability" is not a given but rather conferred in part by those with power—including those in health care—offers promise for understanding the specific social and historical relations of gender and ethnicity/race that shape individual and group health and access to health care.

## THE INTERSECTION OF GENDER, ETHNICITY/RACE, AND HEALTH

We suggest that gender, ethnicity/race, and health intersect to influence health and social outcomes for different populations in different ways. While these outcomes are sometimes positive, certain populations often bear the burden of unjust experiences due to various social and structural factors. One of these populations is im/migrants in Canada; another is the Indigenous people who reside in the land area today known as Canada.

### Im/migrant Populations

Rates of im/migration in Canada, particularly among women, have tripled over recent years, likely due to forced migration and family separations in the United States (Toughill, 2018) and political unrest in countries in the Middle East and Central America (Schwartz, 2015).

#### Population Profile

In 2011, im/migrants in Canada represented 20.6% of the country's total population, over 50% of whom were women between the ages of 25 and 54 and primarily residing in

Ontario, Quebec, British Columbia, and Alberta (Statistics Canada, 2015). Since 2011, these numbers have risen, with rapidly increasing rates of migration due to political conflict and violence in countries in the Middle Eastern and Central American regions. This is evident through increased numbers of asylum seekers and refugees migrating to Canada from Iraq, Syria, and Colombia since 2005 (Schwartz, 2015). In addition to these rates, the Canadian government planned to admit 310,000 new permanent residents in 2018, and projected that this number would increase to 350,000 by 2020 (Immigration, Refugees and Citizenship Canada, 2018).

Women and girls have accounted for, and continue to account for, a large percentage of the total im/migrant population in Canada, with over 3 million im/migrant women living in Canada in 2011 and accounting for approximately 21% of the total female population (Immigration, Refugees and Citizenship Canada, 2018). With numbers steadily increasing, it is projected that by 2031 there could be over 11 million im/migrants residing in the country, over 50% of whom would be women and girls of reproductive age and from visible minorities (Statistics Canada, 2015).

Canada places an increased focus on economic growth and skilled employment, appropriately matching the steady increase in the number of permanent residents in the country, most of whom have arrived from the Philippines, India, and Syria (Government of Canada, 2017). Additionally, political conflict, violence, and severe discrimination against marginalized populations (e.g., LGBT people) in many parts of the world have led to exponential increases in the admission of refugees in Canada, exceeding planned targets (Government of Canada, 2017).

While the Canadian government implements and provides a number of resettlement programs for im/migrants, as well as culturally appropriate and tailored training for service providers, im/migrants face important and varying challenges in accessing these services. For example, research demonstrates that in Canada, key barriers faced by im/migrant women include language differences (e.g., lack of translation services), difficulty navigating the healthcare system (e.g., limited health insurance coverage), migratory factors (e.g., precarious legal status), and negative experiences with service providers (e.g., discriminatory attitudes; Chang, Hall, Campbell, & Lee, 2018). However, social support (e.g., family and friends) and supportive health professionals have facilitated access (Chang et al., 2018; Grewal, Bhagat, & Balneaves, 2008; Winn, Hetherington, & Tough, 2018). Programs and services that include gender-specific considerations and incorporate a focus on women (e.g., support services for women experiencing gender-based violence and sexual assault; Immigration, Refugees and Citizenship Canada, 2018), are examples of important efforts to improve im/migrant women's health in Canada.

In addition to gendered differences in accessing services during the resettlement process, there has historically been and continues to be a significant employment wage gap between men and women, regardless of the type of im/migrant population (e.g., economic migrants or refugees). Im/migrant men typically obtain higher earnings than their female counterparts (Government of Canada, 2017). As well, although rates of educational attainment among im/migrant women are increasing, they continue to have lower levels of education than men. Im/migrant women are less likely to receive a university-level education, while their male counterparts are more likely to obtain a degree at the master's or doctoral level (Government of Canada, 2017). This is closely connected to the increased likelihood of im/migrant women in Canada obtaining employment within the informal sector (e.g., domestic services and entertainment), which is often lower-paying and not subject to strict regulations (Statistics Canada, 2017), and thus limits their safety and protection. As well, due to stigmatization and racialization, im/migrants in general are exposed to poor and unsafe working conditions and fewer job opportunities that provide a living wage (Statistics Canada, 2017).

The rising number of im/migrants in Canada, and the stark differences in characteristics between and within populations, plays an important role in their health status and outcomes. Factors such as access to settlement services, employment, income, and education are important determinants that intersect with structural and social issues commonly faced by im/migrant men and women, including discrimination, stigmatization, and social exclusion, to influence their health and access to care. Importantly, these influences and subsequent results are also gendered, and im/migrant women typically face more severe health and non-health-related challenges in navigating through issues and building a safe and accepting home in Canada.

### *Health Status of Im/migrants in Canada*

While many im/migrants arrive in Canada in good health, evidence indicates that, over time, their health status declines and becomes equivalent to their Canadian counterparts (Gushulak, Pottie, Roberts, Torres, & DesMeules, 2011; Vang, Sigouin, Flenon, & Gagnon, 2017). However, the "Healthy Immigrant Effect" and this average profile of im/migrant health does not capture unique structural vulnerabilities and barriers to optimal health faced by im/migrant populations. Additionally, it ignores the diverse migratory, health, and social experiences of individuals arriving in Canada, particularly in recent years when the country has witnessed the arrival of significant numbers of asylum seekers and refugees.

The diversity between and among im/migrants is immense, with experiences and health status varying across the life course and based on factors such as the type of im/migrant population (e.g., asylum seekers, refugees, undocumented, or economic migrants), type of migration (e.g., international or internal), age and duration of migration, time spent in the destination country and country of origin, and reasons for migration. For example, undocumented im/migrants are often unable to access health services due to a lack of health insurance and the constant fear and possibility of deportation and family separation during any interaction with government or legal officials (Alaggia, Regehr, & Rishchynski, 2009). Additionally, many im/migrant women experiencing intimate partner violence rarely report or discuss their experiences and continue to stay in abusive relationships due to the risk of disclosing their undocumented status (Alaggia et al., 2009).

In contrast, economic migrants typically arrive in Canada with appropriate documentation, the means to secure employment and housing, and the resources required to obtain adequate health insurance.

The health of im/migrants and their access to care, like many marginalized populations, are deeply shaped by the social determinants of health; more specifically, the health of im/migrant men and women is shaped by diverse experiences faced during the different phases of the migration process, including the pre-migration phase in the country of origin, travel and transit, the destination phase, and sometimes return to the country of origin (International Organization for Migration, 2018a). Some of the determinants of migrant health that directly influence the health and well-being of im/migrant populations include, but are not limited to, legal status, immigration policies, pre-migration trauma, and access to services during the migratory journey (International Organization for Migration, 2018a). Legal status, in particular, is an important determinant of im/migrants' access to care, as those who are undocumented often do not seek or are unable to access appropriate care due to fear of deportation, family separation, or other legal charges; there is a lack of legislation ensuring access to care for im/migrant populations, regardless of legal status. For example, many health providers will refuse to serve clients who lack documentation and may be required by their healthcare institution to report undocumented patients.

Throughout the migration journey, health changes among im/migrant populations are commonly seen through mental health outcomes. Negative mental health outcomes such as anxiety, postpartum depression, and post-traumatic stress disorder (PTSD) among im/migrants often centre around the stress of being in a new country, pre-migration trauma, and a lack of access to appropriate care (Guruge & Butt, 2015).

In addition to traumatic events during the pre-migration stage, such as political violence and war, and experiences during travel, such as sexual violence and family separation, mental illnesses during post-migration are often determined by income, experiences of discrimination and racialization, age of migration, and time spent in Canada (Hilario, Oliffe, Wong, Browne, & Johnson, 2015). Vang et al. (2017) and Kalich, Heinemann, and Ghahari (2016) review and outline mental health issues faced by im/migrant populations across the life course and in the post-migration phase, and further explain some of the barriers faced in accessing mental health care. These include language, a lack of information and knowledge about available services, negative interactions with service providers (e.g., stigmatizing attitudes), financial barriers (e.g., perceived costs associated with accessing care), and long wait times in hospitals.

Additional barriers to accessing SRH care are commonly faced by im/migrant women across the life course and throughout the migration journey. For example, im/migrant women have limited access to SRH care when the migration journey involves travelling for long distances, often by foot, across international borders, while facing potential danger (e.g., gender-based violence). For example, in addition to sexual assault commonly faced by im/migrant women during pre-migration, travel, and post-migration, LGBT im/migrants placed in detention centres often face severe discrimination and violence (Hananel, 2018), with little to no access to safety and care. Additionally, young im/migrant women and girls face are particularly vulnerable during migration. Evidence on the health of younger im/migrant women and girls in Canada is limited, and additional research is required to build a more comprehensive understanding of their SRH needs and realities. Importantly, there are complex intersections between the social determinants of migrant health, gender, and ethnicity/race that shape these structural vulnerabilities, inequities, and health outcomes amongst im/migrants—and this is most commonly seen through the poor SRH outcomes, challenges, and barriers to care faced by im/migrant women.

### *Intersection of Gender, Ethnicity/Race, and Health in Im/migrant Women's Lives*

The intersections between migration, health, ethnicity/race, and gender are complex yet important, and while a focus on men is important, im/migrant women are disproportionately affected by SRH inequities. Health transitions and outcomes vary by ethnicity/race and gender, socio-economic status, and contextual factors (De Maio, 2010); and, structural and social issues, including discrimination, stigmatization, and social exclusion often exacerbate health and gender-related inequities faced by im/migrant women.

Although the majority of evidence we have detailed in this area is based in Canada, evidence from other settings suggests that im/migrant women are at risk for poorer health outcomes than men; this relates to their increased exposure and risk of gender-based and intimate partner violence, sexual assault, and sexually transmitted infections (STIs), which are often a result of stereotypical gender roles; discrimination and marginalization; unequal gendered power dynamics; poor access to SRH care; and limited economic resources. Evidence indicates that SRH issues and inequities faced by im/migrant women vary across the life course and across the different stages of migration. During pre-migration, women may be fleeing from situations of severe sexual violence, with a lack of access to SRH support; however, during the post-migration or destination stage, im/migrant women may have increased access to SRH services (e.g., maternity care, breast and cervical cancer screening), but may continue to face challenges, including racialization, limited health insurance coverage, or precarious legal status. As well, during travel and transit, women may temporarily reside in unfamiliar settings with limited social support and little knowledge of available resources and services to support themselves and their families. Limited research on this subject in Canada, and even less that incorporates such diversity across the migration journey, poses challenges to gaining a comprehensive understanding of the broader SRH needs of and inequities faced by diverse im/migrant women populations.

Importantly, the experiences of im/migrants across the migration journey are gendered. For example, women im/migrants often face severe gender-based violence throughout the journey. Although many flee their country of origin to escape this form of abuse, violent attacks often continue during travel and post-migration, where im/migrants without appropriate documentation are left unprotected, and many lack adequate resources.

Intimate partner violence is also common across the stages of migration due to unequal gendered power dynamics, with male partners often being the main source of income and holding significant power over their female partner (Alaggia et al., 2009; Guruge & Humphreys, 2009). In addition to the trauma of experiencing such violence, experiences of family separation, deportation, and other legal actions (Ochoa & Sampalis, 2014) also increase im/migrant women's vulnerability to mental health issues and risk decreasing their resources, particularly for those who are dependent on a male partner.

Women's stereotypical gender roles also play an important role in the health and well-being of im/migrants. With an increased focus on the health and protection of their family and children, im/migrant women are often unable to prioritize their own health, seek appropriate care for optimal health and well-being, or fully engage in community programs and services to better their post-migration experiences (Alaggia et al., 2009). In such cases, im/migrant women experience a double (and often triple) burden, holding the responsibility of caring for children, the household, and often generating an income. This is particularly problematic, as im/migrant women require diverse healthcare services, including, but not limited to, screening (e.g., breast/cervical cancer, HIV/AIDS, STIs), treatment (e.g., anti-retroviral therapy), contraception (e.g., condoms, birth control pills, IUD), mental health services (e.g., counselling due to gender-based violence, post-partum depression, poor working conditions), maternity care (e.g., breastfeeding information, perinatal care), and SRH education (e.g., safe sex practices, screening guidelines and procedures).

In addition to the gendered power dynamics and roles that im/migrant women face, various structural barriers related to Canada's healthcare system prevent women from appropriately accessing SRH care. Across different provinces, im/migrant women often do not access SRH care due to stigma, discrimination, and racism (Higginbottom et al., 2016; O'Mahony, Donnelly, Raffin Bouchal, & Este, 2013; Ochoa & Sampalis, 2014); a lack of social and/or emotional support (Chang et al., 2018; Higginbottom et al., 2015; Ochoa & Sampalis, 2014); migration-related factors such as language barriers and an undocumented legal status (Chang et al., 2018; Higginbottom et al., 2015; Merry, Gagnon, Kalim, & Bouris, 2011; Ochoa & Sampalis, 2014; Peláez, Hendricks, Merry, & Gagnon, 2017); difficulties in navigating the healthcare system (Higginbottom et al., 2016; Peláez, Hendricks, Merry, & Gagnon, 2017); negative experiences with healthcare providers (Chang et al., 2018); and a lack of information on available health services (Higginbottom et al., 2016; Hippman et al., 2016; Vahabi & Lofters, 2016).

The social determinants of migrant health therefore clearly demonstrate gender as a cross-cutting theme (International Organization for Migration, 2018b); importantly, ethnicity/race is an additional factor and theme that plays a vital role in the health of im/migrant women and their intersecting categories of identity. For example, im/migrants that belong to minority groups often experience discrimination, stigmatization, and violence, as well as poorer health outcomes as a result of barriers to accessing various types of care. When considering both gender and ethnicity/race as intersecting and influencing factors, many im/migrant women in Canada who are visible minorities face a double burden—the burden of belonging to an ethnicity/race that faces societal discrimination as well as the burden of being a woman, a concept highlighted by Gupta (2000).

## Indigenous Women

A gender, ethnicity/race, and health lens highlights how colonization generates particular vulnerabilities for Indigenous women (and girls).

### *Population Profile*

According to the 2016 Census, there were 1,673,785 Aboriginal people in Canada, including 977,230 First Nations people, 587,545 Métis, and 65,025 Inuit (Statistics Canada, 2017). The Aboriginal population is young and growing: The average age is just over 32 years, which is nearly 10 years younger than the non-Aboriginal population, and the population grew 42.5% in the decade from 2006–2016 (Statistics Canada, 2017).

A statistical profile generated from the 2011 National Household Survey focused specifically on First Nations, Métis, and Inuit women reported that there were 718,500 Aboriginal women and girls in Canada at the time, about 4% of the total female Canadian population (Statistics Canada, 2016).

About half of Aboriginal women aged 25–64 surveyed reported some form of post-secondary education; 12% had a university degree. This compares to two-thirds of non-Aboriginal women of the same age range having some post-secondary qualification and 28% having a university degree. Yet Aboriginal women were more likely to have a university degree than Aboriginal men (12% versus 7%). Educational levels are increasing among younger Aboriginal women in all three Aboriginal groups. Among younger Aboriginal women, 14% had a university degree. Looking at the other end of the educational spectrum, among Aboriginal girls who did not complete secondary school, the most common reasons for leaving school were pregnancy or to care for their own children. Nearly 40% of Inuit women and 25% of off-reserve first Nations and Métis women gave these reasons. Aboriginal men who left school cited, in contrast, "a desire to work, money problems, school problems, and lack of interest" (Statistics Canada, 2016, p. 17).

Aboriginal women were less likely to be employed than non-Aboriginal women, and the median income of Aboriginal women was lower than for their non-Aboriginal counterparts by $5,500, and $3,600 lower than that of Aboriginal men (Statistics Canada, 2016). Both employment rates and income increased with educational attainment, however.

### *Health Status of Indigenous Women in Canada*

Reading and Wien (2009) identified proximal, intermediate, and distal determinants of Aboriginal health.

> Proximal determinants are conditions that directly influence the four dimensions of Indigenous well-being (physical, mental, emotional and spiritual), such as health behaviors like smoking, alcohol abuse, lack of exercise and diet; elements

of the physical environment such as housing, water supply, geographic location; as well as socio-economic factors like employment, income, education and food security … (as cited in Odulaja & Halseth, 2018, p. 12)

Intermediate determinants are more removed from individual health practices and living conditions and include the healthcare and educational systems, community resources, cultural continuity, and environmental stewardship, which together produce the proximal determinants.

Finally, distal determinants are the least visible but perhaps the most profound and include colonialism, racism and social exclusion, and self-determination. With regard to the health of Indigenous women, Halseth (2013, p. 5) argues that gender can be considered a distal determinant of health "because of the way it interacts with other determinants at all three levels" to create the conditions of women's health. Halseth (2013) specifically suggests that Aboriginal women may face discrimination based on gender, as well as class and race, that leads to "material, social and health inequities that can marginalize women" (p. 5).

---

**Box 8.3:** Some Aspects of Indigenous Women's Health

- Aboriginal women are less likely that either non-Aboriginal women or Aboriginal men to report their health as excellent or very good, and Aboriginal women aged 15 and over are more likely than non-Aboriginal women to report being diagnosed with at least one chronic condition.
- Among the most commonly reported chronic conditions, the rates for arthritis, hypertension, asthma, and mood or anxiety disorders were all higher among Aboriginal women.
- Reported rates of activity limitation due to disability were also higher among Aboriginal women, and the difference in rates increased with age.
- Though more than half of Aboriginal women living off-reserve reported excellent or very good mental health, this was far lower than among non-Aboriginal women, of whom 72% made the same claim.
- Almost a quarter of Aboriginal women over age 18 report having had suicidal thoughts, compared to 12% of the non-Aboriginal female population.
- Over 20% of Aboriginal women reported living with food insecurity compared to 8% of non-Aboriginal women.
- And compared to non-Aboriginal women, Aboriginal women in Canada are at a higher risk of experiencing violence.

*Source:* Statistics Canada. (2016). First Nations, Inuit and Metis women. *Women in Canada: A gender-based statistical report* (7th ed.). Ottawa: Author. Statistics Canada Publication 89-503-X.

Numerous studies report significantly poorer health among Indigenous women than their non-Indigenous counterparts. One such indicator is the maternal mortality rate, which serves as a proxy for women's living conditions and access to antenatal healthcare services (Sharma et al., 2016). Though maternal mortality is a rare event in Canada, recent data nevertheless indicate that Indigenous women face double the risk of maternal mortality as the general Canadian population (Sharma et al., 2016).

Halseth (2013) has documented lower life expectancy and poorer self-reported health among Aboriginal women as compared to non-Indigenous women. She also notes that prevalence rates for type 2 diabetes have been increasing rapidly and are alarmingly high among Indigenous women of childbearing age. Though difficult to track, some studies also suggest that cervical cancer is a problem among Aboriginal women, possibly reflecting lower participation in screening programs, as well as tobacco use (a risk factor for many cancers, including cervical). Other pressing health issues for Aboriginal women are HIV/AIDS and hepatitis C infection and care and relationship violence, including intimate partner violence and sexual assault.

Though data on the extent and nature of violence against Indigenous women are limited, various surveys, police reports, and studies suggest that Indigenous women experience much higher rates of violence, including intimate partner violence and sexual assault, than non-Indigenous women—as much as 3.5 times higher (Amnesty International, 2009). As long as three decades ago, the Ontario Native Women's Association argued that "it is not possible to find an Aboriginal woman whose life has not been affected in some way by family violence. Either as a child witnessing spousal assault, as a child victim herself, as an adult victim of a husband or boyfriend's violence, or as a grandmother who witnesses the physical and emotional scars of her daughter or granddaughter's beatings: we are all victims of violent family situations" (Ontario Native Women's Association, 1989, p. iii). Indeed, though they are but a fraction of the female population in Canada, Aboriginal women disproportionately experience physical violence, including sexual assault, relationship violence, homicide, and other intentional injuries, as well as psychological and sexual abuse (Adelson, 2005; Halseth, 2013). "Many Aboriginal women and girls … live

**Box 8.4:** Monitoring Maternal Morbidity and Mortality in Canada

Canada is now embarking on efforts to create a national reporting framework for maternal morbidity and mortality with British Columbia, Alberta, Nova Scotia, and Ontario, initiating a pilot project to create a minimal set of indicators for this critical issue. Assuming that the data include Indigenous identity as a demographic characteristic, this project should help highlight this serious discrepancy in health outcome and seek its remediation. For a discussion of the importance of surveillance of maternal morbidity and mortality in Canada, see Society of Obstetricians and Gynaecologists of Canada (2018).

each day under the threat of interpersonal violence and its myriad consequences" (Patrick, 2016, p. E78).

A report of a recent systematic review on the perspective of Indigenous women themselves regarding their health identified the key contributors to women's health outcomes as (1) the availability of healthcare resources, (2) the extent to which healthcare services consider the socio-economic or lifestyle barriers that affect Indigenous women's health, and (3) the impact of colonization on interactions with healthcare providers (Sheppard et al., 2017).

### *Intersection of Gender, Ethnicity/Race, and Health in Indigenous Women's Lives*

If the health status of Indigenous people in Canada is the sum total of their individual and collective experiences, it is increasingly argued that the most important influence on their health has been contact with Europeans (starting in the 17th century) and their subsequent colonization (Health Council of Canada, 2005; Royal Commission on Aboriginal Peoples, 1996). Historic records indicate that Aboriginal peoples were in good health at the time of contact but that colonization and numerous policies "eroded the traditional way of life for many Aboriginal persons … [which] has had a negative impact on the health and well-being of individuals, their families and communities" (Health Council of Canada, 2005, p. 3). This is because "colonialism is not simply an historic event, but continues to manifest in the present day through various political and social policies and institutional racism," such that it is understood that colonialism is "the root of all causes of ill health for Indigenous peoples, resulting in a loss of land, culture, language, family values and spirituality, which contributes to despondency, loss of self-esteem, and loss of pride in cultural identity" (Odulaja & Halseth, 2018, p. 13).

---

**Box 8.5:** Colonial Policy and Indigenous People in Canada

According to an international consortium of researchers in Canada and Australia,

> Various historical events associated with colonial policies have impacted Indigenous Canadians negatively, including the destruction of lands which are vital to Indigenous ways of life, forced placement and separation from families through residential schooling, marginalization of languages and spiritual beliefs, assaults on dignity and autonomy through the introduction of assimilation policies, and multiple forms of racial discrimination. Many Indigenous people who experienced colonialism have suffered from trauma and the resulting effects of the trauma, such as mental illness, anxiety, depression, suicide, violence, low self-esteem, anger, feelings of hopelessness, challenges in recognizing and expressing emotions and sexual, alcohol and drug-related vulnerabilities. (Sharma et al., 2016, p. 335)

**Box 8.6:** Missing and Murdered Indigenous Women in Canada

Canada's federal government established a national inquiry into missing and murdered Indigenous women and girls in 2015 as one response to a call to action from the Truth and Reconciliation Commission (Patrick, 2016) as well as many advocates, such as the Native Women's Association of Canada, who had been tracking the names and identities of missing and murdered women. At the time of writing, the National Inquiry into Missing and Murdered Indigenous Women and Girls (MMIWG) had not released its final report; however, its interim report (MMIWG, 2017) documents the findings of its three-year process of listening to individuals, families, and communities about their experiences. The MMIWG has adopted Indigenous methods for its work as a deliberate strategy to "affirm the resistance and resurgence of Indigenous women and girls, including LGBTQ2S people" (p. 5). By mid-fall 2018, the MMIWG had heard from 1,273 families and survivors through hearings and received 340 expressions in the form of art (http://www.mmiwg-ffada.ca/media/). This process, though not yet complete, is a historic opportunity in Canada to learn the truth about the extent and nature of violence in the lives of Indigenous women and girls. Already, it is clear that there have been gaps in data, unsolved crimes, and broken lives at a scale that is entirely disproportionate to the size of the population of Indigenous women and girls. As the interim report states, "Simply being Indigenous and female is a risk" (MMIWG, 2017, p. 8).

For example, in accounting for the high rates of violence that Indigenous women and girls experience, analysts return again and again to the damage to gender relations wrought by colonization (Adelson, 2005; Amnesty International, 2009): "The implementation of colonialism, which combined patriarchal practices with racism, shaped institutions, laws, legislation, and policies that have had a long-lasting negative effect on Indigenous women's health" (Kubik, Bourassa, & Hampton, 2009, pp. 26–27). Thus the determinants of health intersect in the lives of Indigenous girls and women through gender relations, which limit gender equality and girls' and women's value, independence, and opportunities (Halseth, 2013). Actions to enhance the status of girls and women legally, politically, socially, economically, and culturally are therefore likely to also enhance their health.

## ANALYSIS: DIFFERENT ORIGINS, SHARED EXPERIENCES

In this chapter, we have examined the mechanics of gender, ethnicity/race, and health among im/migrant and Indigenous women. Though both im/migrant and Indigenous women are diverse, and so we must be cautious about generalizing, it is evident that some women in both groups experience racialization and both race- and gender-based discrimination. There is also evidence that health care is a setting in which racism occurs and where individuals from both groups may experience barriers to care and poorer health outcomes than non-immigrant and non-Aboriginal women. Both groups are at risk of gender-based violence, including during their reproductive years, and both women and children may suffer from violence within the home. On average, the Aboriginal population is younger than the median age of non-Aboriginal Canadians and, similarly, many im/migrants are of childbearing age. Access to culturally appropriate reproductive health care may therefore be a shared need.

Researchers who have looked at how to improve the healthcare experiences of Indigenous and im/migrant populations point to the critical necessity of including members of the population in planning, designing, and implementing interventions. This is an ethical, efficient, and effective strategy. Care needs to be not only accessible but also culturally safe, as defined by those who use the services. Clinicians providing services need to be trained in cultural humility and cultural safety as foundational skills for improving health equity (EQUIP Health Care, 2017). Because providers cannot expect to know everything about a person in advance, they need to adopt a stance of cultural humility and ask respectfully for the patient to lead them to understanding. Given the specific health needs of some members of each population, a combination of universal and tailored services (proportionate universalism) is likely necessary to address both common and distinct needs. Recognizing that there are proximal, intermediate, and distal determinants of health, interventions of different types are needed at different levels. Finally, given that gender and ethnicity/race can be sources of discrimination on their own or combined, interventions are needed to reduce the biases associated with each.

By outlining the different sources of barriers to health and well-being for im/migrant and Indigenous women, it becomes clear that vulnerability arises out of social and historic conditions—conditions that can be altered. This can be a powerful insight if public health proponents, researchers, and policy-makers recognize this mutability and move away from notions that vulnerability is a fixed characteristic of certain individuals and/or collectivities.

## STRATEGIES TO ADDRESS GENDER, ETHNICITY/RACE AS DETERMINANTS OF HEALTH

Tackling the determinants of gender-based and ethnicity/race inequities requires actions that change the cultural fabric, some of which can be done through small-scale efforts, while others will require grand gestures and transformations. We therefore want to acknowledge at the outset that, particularly with respect to improving the health of Indigenous women and girls (as well as men and boys), actions associated with Canada's commitments to Truth and Reconciliation will be required:

> It's clear that a common web—woven of a legacy of colonization and cultural genocide, and a cumulative history of societal neglect, discrimination and

injustice—underlies both endemic interpersonal violence and health disparities in Canada's Indigenous populations. There is no conversation to be had about one without a conversation about the other—if the aim is healing—because the root causes are the same. (Patrick, 2016, p. E78)

According to a recent report released by the National Collaborating Centre for Aboriginal Health (Odulaja & Halseth, 2018, p. 4), the global Sustainable Development Goals (SDG) "agenda comes at a potential turning point for Indigenous peoples in Canada, who have long experienced socio-economic marginalization and poorer health outcomes than non-Indigenous Canadians." Because the SDGs include issues that both low- and high-income countries need to tackle to be sustainable, centred around the three pillars of sustainability (poverty eradication, economic growth, and environmental protection), they offer direction, potential leverage, and international accountability for improving the conditions for everyday living and health for Indigenous people (Odulaja & Halseth, 2018, p. 4).

Changes within systems, including health care, are also required and can serve to address both gender and ethnicity/race. Here we highlight two approaches. In her plenary address at the XIIIth International AIDS Conference, Gupta (2000) provided important perspectives on addressing unequal gendered power dynamics and imbalances and the SRH of women, both of which are key underlying components of the intersections between gender, ethnicity/race, and the health of im/migrant and Indigenous women in Canada. She discussed the importance of engaging in open discussions around gender and power, and the possibility for these discussions to positively influence the health and well-being of women. As is typical of the public health realm, she argued that these power imbalances have historically been examined from a biomedical perspective, and urged an immediate shift in perspective to a larger focus on the sexual health and well-being of women—inclusive of their SRH rights and safety. Gupta (2000) also encouraged the immediate use of the limited evidence that currently exists on addressing gendered power dynamics, avoiding the standard call for additional research and evidence in order to take action. Lastly, she pushed for the implementation of interventions that, at the very least, do not necessarily directly address the deeply entrenched gendered issues faced by men and women, but that avoid perpetuating ideas of men as violent perpetrators and women as powerless victims.

Greaves, Pederson, and Poole (2014) also provide important directions in addressing the needs and health of im/migrant women through a unique lens and focus on the physical activity uptake of im/migrant women through structured programs. They emphasize the provision of space for im/migrants, particularly women, to act as champions and leaders, providing opportunities for them to take control of their own health and well-being. They also demonstrate the important need to understand and address barriers to accessing programs and services, recognizing the complexity of these challenges within and between im/migrant populations. Importantly, the authors highlight the need for consulting and learning from im/migrant women, and engaging them throughout the program planning process; they emphasize that this point must also be extended to policy development and implementation—after all, im/migrant women are the experts on their own needs. These directions are critical to highlighting the diversity and heterogeneity amongst im/migrant populations.

## Gender-Transformative Health Promotion

The emergence of HIV/AIDS in the 1980s heightened attention to SRH interventions that could engage those affected with health services and/or prevent new infections. In the quest for such interventions, Gupta (2000) famously argued that "to effectively address the intersection between HIV/AIDS and gender and sexuality requires that interventions should, at the very least, not reinforce damaging gender and sexual stereotypes" (p. 8). She went on to describe a continuum of actions that could ignore, accommodate, or transform gender relations and their role in the HIV/AIDs epidemic. Since then, this approach has been incorporated into SRH interventions in many ways, including in programming that aims to reduce gender-based violence through challenging gender stereotypes of masculinity and femininity. Through interventions that address health and safety issues by transforming gender relations, this programming addresses health and gender inequalities simultaneously.

Canadian scholars have extended the framework of gender-transformative interventions to other health concerns (Pederson, Greaves, & Poole, 2015; Pederson et al., 2010), notably tobacco use (Bottorff et al., 2006; Greaves, 2014). The power of this approach is that interventions recognize and address how gender relations shape risk, limit access, and/or frame a health issue and then seek to challenge and reframe so as not to reinforce stereotypes or practices that limit women's or men's capacity for acting on their health.

The significance of gender-transformative interventions is that they call on those working in the health field to explicitly account for the contribution of gender as a determinant of health within whatever issue is under consideration. Theoretically, gender-transformative approaches can be applied to any aspect of gender relations that affects health and hence can be a valuable approach to addressing a wide range of gender norms, recognizing that there is no single, fixed expression of gender or only one form of gender relations. Indeed, it is the very flexibility of gender norms that makes them mutable, as can be seen in the shift in gender patterns of employment in many countries. Yet, while the proportion of women in the workplace in Canada, for example, has grown over the past four decades, there remains a gender wage gap (Canadian Women's Foundation, 2018) and gender segregation in the workforce (Statistics Canada, 2017), and women have not achieved parity in public roles and leadership positions (World Economic Forum, 2017). Only one woman, Jeanne Sauvé, has ever served as the Speaker in the House of Commons (she was chosen in 1980).

## Equitable Health Services

Another approach that can help address the inequities arising from the intersections of gender, ethnicity, and health has been articulated by the scholars associated with Equiphealthcare.ca. Through studies in primary and emergency care settings, this team has developed a framework to support healthcare providers and systems to support equity for all. A framework generated from their studies identifies trauma- and violence-informed care, culturally safe care, and harm reduction as the three key dimensions of equity-oriented care (EQUIP Health Care, 2017).

### *Trauma- and Violence-Informed Care*

Sometimes referred to as trauma- and violence-informed practice (TVIP; to recognize the "art" of this approach), trauma- and violence-informed care is coming to be recognized as a way to ensure that all who seek health services experience emotional and psychosocial safety. TVIP involves recognizing that trauma is commonplace and that anyone who comes for health care has experienced trauma. TVIP therefore seeks to avoid re-traumatizing patients while supporting patient safety (physical, emotional, spiritual, and mental), choice, and control. The goal of TVIP is not to offer healing per se; it is not trauma care. Rather, the aim is to acknowledge and assist with the impacts that trauma experiences can have on patients that may lead them to be cautious about approaching healthcare providers, uncomfortable with the probing questions that sometimes accompany healthcare diagnostics, or reluctant to have certain physical examinations. TVIP shifts the frame of thinking about patients in terms of what is wrong with them to what

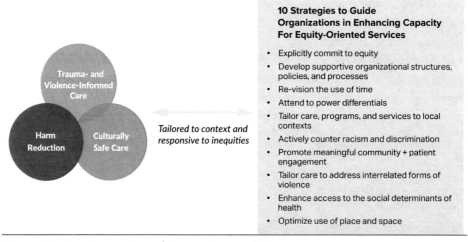

**Figure 8.1:** Key Dimensions of Equity-Oriented Care

*Source:* Browne, A. J., Varcoe, C., Ford-Gilboe, M., Wathen, C. N., Smye, V., Jackson, B. E., . . . Blanchet Garneau, A. (2018). Disruption as opportunity: Impacts of an organizational health equity intervention in primary care clinics. *International Journal for Equity in Health, 17*(1), 154. doi: 10.1186/s12939-018-0820-2

has happened to them, thus enabling healthcare providers to approach interaction more compassionately and responsibly.

In addition, TVIP recognizes that violence is ubiquitous, especially gender-based violence. Gender-based violence (GBV) is violence perpetrated as a result of someone's gender identity, gender expression, or perceived gender (Status of Women Canada, 2018). GBV can involve physical violence; sexual violence (e.g., sexual exploitation, rape, child sexual abuse); emotional and/or psychological violence (i.e., intimidation); financial abuse; online harassment; and structural or systemic violence (Status of Women Canada, 2018). In recent years, there has been a call for improving the healthcare response to gender-based violence, particularly sexual assault and relationship violence. Notably, pregnancy is a time when GBV can escalate, but there can also be increased contact with healthcare providers. Accordingly, perinatal healthcare providers are urged to familiarize themselves with the signs and symptoms of gender-based violence and to develop skills to have safe conversations with patients about it and refer them to specialized anti-violence workers. In British Columbia, an online course was recently created to support this effort (see http://www.bcwomens.ca/health-professionals/professional-resources/addressing-gender-based-violence/gender-based-violence-learning-series), and similar efforts are underway around the globe (see, for example, World Health Organization, 2017).

### Cultural Humility and Cultural Safety
First articulated in New Zealand by Māori nurses, cultural safety has today become an explicit commitment of health services in some parts of Canada. In British Columbia, peak or key organizations have signed a Declaration of Commitment to Cultural Safety and Humility in recognition of the importance of creating the conditions within health services for First Nations and Aboriginal individuals and communities to feel recognized, safe, and supported for who they are and what they bring to a healthcare encounter (see First Nations Health Authority, 2017).

To facilitate cultural safety and humility for Indigenous patients and families, staff of the Provincial Health Services Authority created a facilitated program to educate healthcare providers and others working in health services about the history and impact of colonization in Canada, particularly the contribution of such practices as residential schools, Indigenous hospitals, and the removal of children from Aboriginal families. This explicitly anti-racist program—the San'yas Indigenous Cultural Safety Training—has been underway for several years. Though it originated in B.C., the program is now being adapted and facilitated across the country. In Ontario, for example, there is now an Indigenous Cultural Safety (ICS) program available province-wide (http://soahac.on.ca/ics-training/), and there is a National Indigenous Cultural Safety Learning Series available across the country (http://soahac.on.ca/national-ics-webinar-learning-series/).

A core principle of the ICS approach is that making health services culturally safe for Indigenous people will make them safe for everyone. Extending this principle, another team in B.C. has created a tool to help healthcare providers see how embracing a cultural humility approach and applying the basic tenets of health literacy can help to improve communication and understanding between providers, clients, and families (see http://culturallyconnected.ca).

### Harm Reduction

The third dimension of equity-oriented care is harm reduction. In the current opioid crisis—but also long before it—reducing the risks associated with substance use, particularly injection drug use, is a critical way to save lives and reduce the harms associated with the practice. In practical terms, harm reduction can be understood as a set of support services and practices "to empower and support people to be safer and healthier" (see https://towardtheheart.com/about). These may involve initiatives to supply and recover needles used to inject drugs; offering substitutes for street drugs, such as methadone for heroin; establishing safe injection/overdose prevention sites; financing and training people to use naloxone to reverse an overdose (so-called take-home naloxone); and peer supports to monitor, assist, and support drug users.

Harm reduction aims to reduce both short- and long-term risks associated with substance use. And while it is most often thought of with respect to drug use and raises images of injection drug use, the principles are also used to reduce the very real harms of alcohol use (think of the low-risk drinking guidelines) and in ongoing research into the effects of caffeine consumption and now cannabis. Translated into a focus on the harms associated with substance use rather than the user of the substance, harm reduction is potentially destigmatizing as well as life-saving. As such, it can help address some of the gendered and racialized aspects of substance use, whether for the perinatal substance use population, tobacco or cannabis smokers, or injection drug users.

## CONCLUSIONS

Im/migrant and Indigenous women and girls have both been labelled as members of vulnerable populations in Canadian public health discourse. We have tried to illustrate that the health of im/migrant and Indigenous women is deeply influenced by the intersection of gender and ethnicity/race in both individual and collective lives. Fostering gender equality and eliminating racism could have profound effects on the lives and health of Indigenous and im/migrant women.

We need to broaden the categories of women's health concerns to include issues that are relevant to diverse groups of women. Existing studies of im/migrant women's health, particularly review papers, for example, have largely focused on HIV, mental, reproductive and maternal health, and access to testing; however, a more comprehensive, gender-focused review is required to understand the broader SRH needs of and inequities faced by im/migrant women (e.g., gender-based violence). As well, few studies that examined the SRH experiences of international migrant women from childhood to adulthood show differences in SRH inequities and well-being across the life course, indicating that the use of life-course approaches in im/migrant health research is critical to understanding the health needs and addressing challenges faced by younger im/migrant women and girls. Similarly, the SRH needs of im/migrants vary according to the stage, type, and duration of migration, little of which is explained in the literature. Most studies have focused on the SRH needs of im/migrant women before and after migration, and few have considered the influence of time spent in the home country and destination country on SRH outcomes and challenges.

We also need to continue to learn about the experiences of diverse groups of Aboriginal women in Canada in relation to health and well-being. The historic and contemporary differences between First Nations, Inuit, and Métis women generate different health potentials and constraints. Ideally, such research will involve Indigenous women and their allies to document how not only the distinct experiences of the three groups of women but also how different generations of women and girls are faring with respect to their physical, mental, emotional, and spiritual health, using methods aligned with Indigenous knowledge and priorities. Analyses need to be conducted at multiple levels to capture the dynamics of structural as well as individual factors as they relate to health in order for us to fully account for the operation of gender and ethnicity/race in their lives.

We suggest that attention to the conditions that generate resilience and not just vulnerability would also be welcomed by both im/migrant and Indigenous women. Such work should entail efforts to promote gender equality and eliminate racialization, both of which are distal determinants of health for im/migrant and Indigenous women.

## CRITICAL THINKING QUESTIONS

1. What are the potential consequences of ignoring issues of gender and ethnicity/race in health policy-making and research?
2. To what extent and in what ways is racial discrimination a current topic of discussion among policy-makers, the media, and the public at large?
3. What are some of the political, economic, and social barriers to health and well-being that racialized groups experience in Canada? What can be done to help remove these barriers? Are these experiences the same for women and men?

## FURTHER READINGS

Brown, V. B. (2018). *Through a trauma lens: Transforming health and behavioral systems.* New York: Routledge.
Trauma-informed practice is increasingly recognized as a foundation for high-quality health care. Written by Vivian Brown, a psychologist with four decades of experience designing, implementing, and evaluating community-based, integrated services for people with co-occurring disorders, particularly mental health, substance use, and trauma,

this volume illustrates successful examples of trauma-informed services with case studies and interviews.

Krieger, N. (2005). Embodiment: A conceptual glossary for epidemiology. *Journal of Epidemiology and Community Health, 59*, 350–355. doi:10.1136/jech.2004.024562

In this article, Nancy Krieger explains the concept of embodiment and its relevance for epidemiological research. She illustrates how social conditions leave marks upon the human body and argues that an embodied approach to understanding racism versus race as determinants of health "promotes testing hypotheses to ascertain if ... observed disparities are a biological expression of racial discrimination, past and present," whereas a "disembodied and decontextualized approach promulgates research focused on detrimental genes and/or 'lifestyles'" (p. 350).

Metcalfe-Chenail, D. (Ed.). (2016). *In this together: Fifteen stories of truth & reconciliation*. Victoria, B.C.: Brindle & Glass Publishing.

This edited collection is among the books recommended by the Edmonton-based Reconciliation in Solidary Edmonton (RISE) Book Club. Bringing together multiple voices, the text offers first-hand reflections on the meaning and experience of reconciliation efforts from both Indigenous and non-Indigenous contributors across Canada. This book helps us understand reconciliation as an active process of individuals as well as collectives.

Raphael, D. (Ed). (2017). *Immigration, public policy, and health: Newcomer experiences in developed nations*. Toronto: Canadian Scholars' Press.

From the editor: The origins of this volume are found in my experience of living in a city where over 50% of the population have emigrated from other nations. In the particular case of Toronto, most of this emigration over the last 30 years has come from the developing world and consists of people of colour. Despite admission requirements that immigrants be well-educated and trained, these groups are struggling to make ends meet. I am intrigued that Canada has acquired a reputation for welcoming immigrants but at the same time appears to do little to prevent this group of people from experiencing poverty and unemployment rates that are usually double those of people born in Canada. These rates not only depict a troubling image of quality of life for these new Canadians but are portents of health problems, as they are important social determinants of health. And there is evidence that the health of recent immigrants of colour to Canada shows significant declines over time.

## RELEVANT WEBSITES

**Centre of Excellence for Women's Health**

http://bccewh.bc.ca/2014/02/trauma-informed-practice-guide/

British Columbia's Trauma-Informed Practice (TIP) Guide was developed collaboratively to support the application of trauma-informed principles into practice and policy, by clinics, agencies, and groups assisting clients with mental health and substance use concerns in British Columbia.

### Caring for Kids New to Canada

https://www.kidsnewtocanada.ca/

Developed by the Canadian Paediatric Society, this site offers support to health professionals working with immigrant and refugee children and youth. See, in particular, the resources on cultural competence, cultural humility, and cultural safety.

### Clayman Institute for Gender Research

https://gender.stanford.edu/news-publications/gender-news/kimberl-crenshaw-delivers-
     exceptional-jing-lyman-lecture

This blog post captures the remarks of Kimberlé Crenshaw, developer of the concept of intersectionality, from her October 2017 lecture, part of the ongoing outreach and educational activities of the Clayman Institute for Gender Research at Stanford University. Crenshaw illustrated the persistent erasure and exclusion of black women, even in discussions of police brutality in the United States, and introduced the #SayHerName campaign, which invites us to identify and recognize black women affected by police violence.

### Culturally Connected

https://culturallyconnected.ca/

Developed by BC Children's and BC Women's Hospitals, both part of the Provincial Health Services Authority in British Columbia, this resource illustrates how the approaches of cultural humility and health literacy complement each other in supporting healthcare providers in working with diverse clients and families. The site includes video-based case studies and a set of fundamental practices, as well as tools and resources to support professional practice.

### National Collaborating Centre for Aboriginal Health (NCCAH)

https://www.ccnsa-nccah.ca/en/

The NCCAH was established in 2005 by the Public Health Agency of Canada to support public health practice in Canada. To date, the NCCAH has focused on the social determinants of Indigenous health and child and youth health. The NCCAH offers published resources as well as videos, webinars, and podcasts on numerous topics. They have three fact sheets on Indigenous health that should be required reading for everyone in public health in Canada.

### Native Women's Association of Canada (NWAC)

http://www.nwac.ca/

The Native Women's Association of Canada is founded on the collective goal to enhance, promote, and foster the social, economic, cultural, and political well-being of First Nations and Métis women within First Nation, Métis, and Canadian societies. NWAC is an aggregate of 13 Native women's organizations from across Canada and was incorporated as a non-profit organization in 1974. It aims to collectively recognize, respect, promote, defend, and enhance Native ancestral laws, spiritual beliefs, language, and traditions given by the Creator. The NWAC has important resources related to Missing and Murdered Indigenous Women and Girls and fact sheets on the root causes of violence against Aboriginal women in Canada that recognize the impact of colonization.

### Ontario Native Women's Association (ONWA) Missing and Murdered Indigenous Women

http://mmiwontario.ca/

The ONWA released a Missing Person tool kit in 2014 to assist people to take action in the event that someone goes missing. Specifically, it provides a step-by-step guide on how to report a missing adult or child, what to expect from law enforcement and social services, and how to cope, including strategies for self-care in the context of such a crisis. There are suggestions for how to use social media to support a search, pages to record a detailed description of the missing person, and spaces to note a physical, emotional, spiritual, and mental health plan for oneself.

### Manitoba Trauma Information and Education Centre

http://trauma-informed.ca/

A source of information and resources on trauma and trauma-informed practice, including trauma and First Nations people.

### World Health Organization

http://www.who.int/social_determinants/en/
http://www.who.int/gender-equity-rights/understanding/gender-definition/en/
http://www.who.int/news-room/facts-in-pictures/detail/health-inequities-and-their-causes
http://www.who.int/reproductivehealth/topics/violence/en/

Some key pages of the World Health Organization website that are relevant to discussions of social determinants in general but also specifically to gender and issues such as gender-based violence.

## GLOSSARY

**Aboriginal:** Aboriginal people are the indigenous inhabitants of Canada prior to contact from Europeans. Today, Canada recognizes three distinct groups of Indigenous peoples—First Nations, Inuit, and Métis—each of which has a distinct history, relationship to government, and experiences of health. These three groups are tremendously diverse, for example, with respect to language, practices, history, and relationship to particular land (or not).

**Gender:** Refers to the socially constructed roles, rights, responsibilities, possibilities, and limitations that, in a given society, are assigned to men and women—in other words, to what is considered "masculine" and "feminine" in a given time and place.

**Racism:** A set of beliefs that asserts the natural superiority of one racial group over another at the individual but also the institutional level. In one sense, racism refers to the belief that biology rather than culture is the primary determinant of group attitudes and actions. Racism goes beyond ideology; it involves discriminatory practices that protect and maintain the position of certain groups and sustain the inferior position of others (www.canadaimmigrants.com/glossary).

**Sex:** The biological and physiological characteristics of male and female animals: genitalia, reproductive organs, chromosomal complement, hormonal environment, etc.

**Sexism:** A form of discrimination. It is set of beliefs that asserts the superiority of one sex over another and can be expressed individually or institutionally. That is, individual people may express beliefs that one sex or the other is more suited for certain tasks or societal roles than the other. Sexism may also be expressed through procedures and assumptions that permeate organizations, legislation, and the law and that again assume that one sex or the other is naturally suited or capable or likely to perform certain roles and hold certain responsibilities as opposed to seeing people of either sex as possessing a diverse range of abilities. Sexism may reflect a limited appreciation of the extent to which differences between the sexes have been socially constructed and are often arbitrarily exaggerated through social codes, custom, and historical practices.

## NOTE

1. We acknowledge that this title was inspired by our reading of Grotti et al.'s compelling analysis of reproductive health care among migrants to Europe. See Grotti, V., Malakasis, C., Quagliariello, C., & Sahraoui, N. (2018). Shifting vulnerabilities: Gender and reproductive care on the migrant trail to Europe. *Comparative Migration Studies, 6*(1), 1–18. doi: 10.1186/s40878-018-0089-z

## REFERENCES

Adelson, N. (2005). The embodiment of inequity: Health disparities in Aboriginal Canada. *Canadian Journal of Public Health/Revue Canadienne de Sante'e Publique, 96*(Suppl. 2), S45–S61.

Alaggia, R., Regehr, C., & Rishchynski, G. (2009). Intimate partner violence and immigration laws in Canada: How far have we come? *International Journal of Law and Psychiatry, 32*(6), 335–341. doi:10.1016/j.ijlp.2009.09.001

Allahar, A., & Côté, J. E. (1998). *Richer and poorer: The structure of inequality in Canada*. Toronto: James Lorimer & Company.

Amnesty International. (2009). *No more stolen sisters: The need for a comprehensive response to discrimination and violence against Indigenous women in Canada.* London: Amnesty International

Bottorff, J. L., Kalaw, C., Johnson, J. L., Stewart, M., Greaves, L., & Carey, J. (2006). Couple dynamics during women's tobacco reduction in pregnancy and postpartum. *Nicotine & Tobacco Research, 8*(4), 499–509. doi:10.1080/14622200600789551

Butler, J., Gambetti, Z., & Sabsay, L. (Eds.). (2016). *Vulnerability in resistance.* Durham, NC: Duke University Press.

Canadian Council for Refugees. (n.d.). Talking about refugees and immigrants: A glossary of terms. Retrieved January 27, 2019, from https://ccrweb.ca/sites/ccrweb.ca/files/static-files/glossary.PDF

Canadian Women's Foundation. (2018). The facts about the gender wage gap in Canada. Retrieved October 30, 2018, from https://www.canadianwomen.org/the-facts/the-wage-gap/

Chang, S. H.-C., Hall, W. A., Campbell, S., & Lee, L. (2018). Experiences of Chinese immigrant women following "Zuo Yue Zi" in British Columbia. *Journal of Clinical Nursing, 27*(7–8), e1385–e1394. doi:10.1111/jocn.14236

Commission on Social Determinants of Health. (2008). *Closing the gap in a generation: Health equity through action on the social determinants of health.* Geneva, Switzerland: World Health Organization.

De Maio, F. G. (2010). Immigration as pathogenic: A systematic review of the health of immigrants to Canada. *International journal for equity in health, 9*(1), 27. doi:10.1186/1475-9276-9-27

EQUIP Health Care. (2017). Key dimensions of equity-oriented care: 10 strategies to guide organizations in enhancing capacity for equity-oriented health care. Retrieved from www.equiphealthcare.ca

Fineman, M. A. (2008). The vulnerable subject: Anchoring equality in the human condition. *Yale Journal of Law & Feminism, 20*(1), 1–23.

First Nations Health Authority. (2017). *Declaration of commitment on cultural safety and humility in health services.*

Government of Canada. (2017). *2017 Annual report to Parliament on immigration.* Retrieved October 20, 2018, from https://www.canada.ca/en/immigration-refugees-citizenship/corporate/publications-manuals/annual-report-parliament-immigration-2017.html

Greaves, L. (2014). Can tobacco control be transformative? Reducing gender inequity and tobacco use among vulnerable populations. *International Journal of Environmental Research and Public Health, 11*(1), 792–803. doi:10.3390/ijerph110100792

Greaves, L., Pederson, A., & Poole, N. (Eds.). (2014). *Making it better: Gender transformative health promotion.* Toronto: Canadian Scholars' Press.

Grewal, S. K., Bhagat, R., & Balneaves, L. G. (2008). Perinatal beliefs and practices of immigrant punjabi women living in Canada. *Journal of Obstetric, Gynecologic & Neonatal Nursing, 37*(3), 290–300. doi:10.1111/j.1552-6909.2008.00234.x

Grotti, V., Malakasis, C., Quagliariello, C., & Sahraoui, N. (2018). Shifting vulnerabilities: Gender and reproductive care on the migrant trail to Europe. *Comparative Migration Studies, 6*(23), 1–18. doi:10.1186/s40878-018-0089-z

Gupta, G. R. (2000). Gender, sexuality and HIV/AIDS: The what, the why and the how. *Canadian HIV/AIDS Policy Law Review, 5*(4), 86–93.

Guruge, S., & Butt, H. (2015). A scoping review of mental health issues and concerns among immigrant and refugee youth in Canada: Looking back, moving forward. *Canadian Journal of Public Health/Revue canadienne de santé publique, 106*(2), e72–e78. doi:10.17269/cjph.106.4588

Guruge, S., & Humphreys, J. (2009). Barriers affecting access to and use of formal social supports among abused immigrant women. *Canadian Journal of Nursing Research, 41*(3), 64–84.

Gushulak, B. D., Pottie, K., Roberts, J. H., Torres, S., & DesMeules, M. (2011). Migration and health in Canada: Health in the global village. *Canadian Medical Association Journal, 183*(12), e952–e958. doi:10.1503/cmaj.090287

Halseth, R. (2013). Aboriginal women in Canada: Gender, socio-economic determinants of health, and initiatives to close the wellness-gap. Prince George, BC: National Collaborating Centre for Aboriginal Health.

Hananel, S. (2018). LGBT immigrants in detention centers at severe risk of sexual abuse, CAP analysis says. Center for American Progress. Retrieved from https://www.americanprogress.org/press/release/2018/05/30/451380/release-lgbt-immigrants-detention-centers-severe-risk-sexual-abuse-cap-analysis-says/

Health Canada. (2000). *Reducing health inequalities: Implications for interventions.* Retrieved July 2002 from http://www.hc-sc.gc.ca/hppb/phdd/resources/red_inadequecies.htm

Health Council of Canada. (2005). *The health status of Canada's First Nations, Métis and Inuit peoples: A background paper to accompany health care renewal in Canada: Accelerating change.* Retrieved from http://publications.gc.ca/pub?id=9.696760&sl=0

Higginbottom, G. M., Safipour, J., Yohani, S., O'Brien, B., Mumtaz, Z., & Paton, P. (2015). An ethnographic study of communication challenges in maternity care for immigrant women in rural Alberta. *Midwifery, 31*(2), 297–304. doi:10.1016/j.midw.2014.09.009

Higginbottom, G. M., Safipour, J., Yohani, S., O'Brien, B., Mumtaz, Z., Paton, P., … Barolia, R. (2016). An ethnographic investigation of the maternity healthcare experience of immigrants in rural and urban Alberta, Canada. *BMC Pregnancy and Childbirth, 16*, 1–15. doi:10.1186/s12884-015-0773-z

Hilario, C. T., Oliffe, J. L., Wong, J. P.-H., Browne, A. J., & Johnson, J. L. (2015). Migration and young people's mental health in Canada: A scoping review. *Journal of Mental Health, 24*(6), 414–422. doi:10.3109/09638237.2015.1078881

Hippman, C., Moshrefzadeh, A., Lohn, Z., Hodgson, Z. G., Dewar, K., Lam, M., … Kwong, J. (2016). Breast cancer and mammography screening: Knowledge, beliefs and predictors for Asian immigrant women attending a specialized clinic in British Columbia, Canada. *Journal of Immigrant and Minority Health, 18*(6), 1441–1448.

Immigration, Refugees and Citizenship Canada. (2018). Immigration, Refugees and Citizenship Canada: Departmental plan 2018–2019. Retrieved October 20, 2018, from https://www.canada.ca/content/dam/ircc/migration/ircc/english/pdf/pub/dp-pm-2018-2019-eng.pdf

International Organization for Migration. (2015). Key migration terms. Retrieved January 27, 2019, from https://www.iom.int/key-migration-terms

International Organization for Migration. (2018a). Social determinants of migrant health. Retrieved October 30, 2018, from https://www.iom.int/social-determinants-migrant-health

International Organization for Migration. (2018b). Who is a migrant? Retrieved October 31, 2018, from https://www.iom.int/who-is-a-migrant

International Rescue Committee. (2018). Migrants, asylum seekers, refugees and immigrants: What's the difference? Retrieved October 30, 2018, from https://www.rescue.org/article/migrants-asylum-seekers-refugees-and-immigrants-whats-difference

Kalich, A., Heinemann, L., & Ghahari, S. (2016). A scoping review of immigrant experience of health care access barriers in Canada. *Journal of Immigrant and Minority Health, 18*(3), 697–709. doi:10.1007/s10903-015-0237-6

Krieger, N. (2003). Does racism harm health? Did child abuse exist before 1962? On explicit questions, critical science, and current controversies: An ecosocial perspective. *American Journal of Public Health, 93*(2), 194–199.

Kubik, W., Bourassa, C., & Hampton, M. (2009). Stolen sisters, second class citizens, poor health: The legacy of colonization in Canada. *Humanity & Society, 33*(1–2), 18–34. doi:10.1177/016059760903300103

*The Lancet*. (2018). Gender and health are also about boys and men. *The Lancet, 392*(10143), 188. doi:10.1016/S0140-6736(18)31610-6

Marmot, M. (2007). Achieving health equity: From root causes to fair outcomes. *The Lancet, 370*(9593), 1153–1163. doi:10.1016/S0140-6736(07)61385-3

Merry, L. A., Gagnon, A. J., Kalim, N., & Bouris, S. S. (2011). Refugee claimant women and barriers to health and social services post-birth. *Canadian Journal of Public Health, 102*(4), 286–290.

Monture-Angus, P. (1995). *Thunder in my soul: A Mohawk woman speaks*. Winnipeg: Fernwood.

National Inquiry into Missing and Murdered Indigenous Women and Girls. (2017). *Our women and girls are sacred*. Ottawa: Author.

O'Mahony, J. M., Donnelly, T. T., Raffin Bouchal, S., & Este, D. (2013). Cultural background and socioeconomic influence of immigrant and refugee women coping with postpartum depression. *Journal of Immigrant & Minority Health, 15*(2), 300–314. doi:10.1007/s10903-012-9663-x

Ochoa, S. C., & Sampalis, J. (2014). Risk perception and vulnerability to STIs and HIV/AIDS among immigrant Latin-American women in Canada. *Culture, Health & Sexuality, 16*(4), 412–425. doi:10.1080/13691058.2014.884632

Odulaja, O. O., & Halseth, R. (2018). *The United Nations Sustainable Development Goals and Indigenous Peoples in Canada*. Prince George, BC: National Collaborating Centre for Aboriginal Health.

Ontario Native Women's Association. (1989). *Breaking free: A proposal for change to Aboriginal family violence*. Thunder Bay, ON: Author.

Patrick, K. (2016). Not just justice: Inquiry into missing and murdered Aboriginal women needs public health input from the start. *Canadian Medical Association Journal, 188*(5), e78–e79. doi: 10.1503/cmaj.160117.

Pederson, A., Greaves, L., & Poole, N. (2015). Gender-transformative health promotion for women: A framework for action. *Health Promotion International, 30*(1), 140–150. doi:10.1093/heapro/dau083

Pederson, A., Ponic, P. L., Greaves, L., Mills, S., Christilaw, J. E., Frisby, W., … Young, L. (2010). Igniting an agenda for health promotion for women: Critical perspectives, evidence-based practice and innovative knowledge translation. *Canadian Journal of Public Health, 101*(3), 259–261.

Peláez, S., Hendricks, K. N., Merry, L. A., & Gagnon, A. J. (2017). Challenges newly-arrived migrant women in Montreal face when needing maternity care: Health care professionals' perspectives. *Globalization and Health, 13*(1), 5. doi:10.1186/s12992-016-0229-x

Rasanathan, K. (2018). 10 years after the Commission on Social Determinants of Health: Social injustice is still killing on a grand scale. *The Lancet, 392*(10154), 1176–1177. doi:10.1016/S0140-6736(18)32069-5

Reading, C. L., & Wien, F. (2009). *Health inequalities and the social determinants of Aboriginal peoples' health*. Prince George, BC: National Collaborating Centre for Aboriginal Health.

Reid, C., Pederson, A., & Dupéré, S. (2012). Addressing diversity and inequities in health promotion: The implications of intersectional theory. In I. Rootman, S. Dupéré, A. Pederson, & M. O'Neill (Eds.), *Health promotion in Canada: Critical perspectives on practice* (3rd ed., pp. 54–66). Toronto: Canadian Scholars' Press.

Royal Commission on Aboriginal Peoples. (1996). *Report of the Royal Commission on Aboriginal Peoples: Volume 1: Looking forward, looking back*. Ottawa: Indian and Northern Affairs Canada.

Schwartz, D. (2015). Canada's refugees: Where thy come from by the numbers. *CBC News*. Retrieved from https://www.cbc.ca/news/canada/canada-refugees-1.3239460

Sharma, S., Kolahdooz, F., Launier, K., Nader, F., June Yi, K., Baker, P., & Vallianatos, H. (2016). Canadian Indigenous women's perspectives of maternal health and health care services: A systematic review. *Diversity and Equality in Health and Care, 13*(5), 334–348. doi:10.21767/2049-5471.100073

Sheppard, A. J., Shapiro, G. D., Bushnik, T., Wilkins, R., Perry, S., Kaufman, J. S., & Yang, S. (2017). Birth outcomes among First Nations, Inuit and Métis populations. *Health Reports, 28*(11), 11–16.

Society of Obstetricians and Gynaecologists of Canada. (2018). *Working towards a national Canadian surveillance system to reduce maternal mortality and morbidity*. Ottawa: Author.

Statistics Canada. (2015). Immigrant women. *Women in Canada: A gender-based statistical report* (7th ed.). Ottawa: Author. Statistics Canada Publication 89-503-X.

Statistics Canada. (2016). First Nations, Inuit and Metis women. *Women in Canada: A gender-based statistical report* (7th ed.). Ottawa: Author. Statistics Canada Publication 89-503-X.

Statistics Canada. (2017). The Aboriginal population in Canada, 2016 Census of Population. Retrieved October 27, 2018, from https://www150.statcan.gc.ca/n1/pub/11-627-m/11-627-m2017027-eng.htm

Statistics Canada. (2017). Women and paid work. *Women in Canada: A gender-based statistical report* (7th ed.). Ottawa: Author. Statistics Canada Publication 89-503-X. Retrieved October 30, 2018, from https://www150.statcan.gc.ca/n1/pub/89-503-x/2015001/article/14694-eng.htm

Status of Women Canada. (2018). About gender-based violence. Retrieved October 31, 2018, from https://www.swc-cfc.gc.ca/violence/strategy-strategie/gbv-vfs-en.html

Toughill, K. (2018). Chaos coming to Canada after U.S. decision on refugees. *The Conversation.* Retrieved from https://theconversation.com/chaos-coming-to-canada-after-u-s-decision-on-refugees-98233

Vahabi, M., & Lofters, A. (2016). Muslim immigrant women's views on cervical cancer screening and HPV self-sampling in Ontario, Canada. *BMC Public Health, 16*(1), 868. doi:10.1186/s12889-016-3564-1

Vang, Z. M., Sigouin, J., Flenon, A., & Gagnon, A. (2017). Are immigrants healthier than native-born Canadians? A systematic review of the healthy immigrant effect in Canada. *Ethnicity & Health, 22*(3), 209–241. doi:10.1080/13557858.2016.1246518

Winn, A., Hetherington, E., & Tough, S. (2018). Caring for pregnant refugee women in a turbulent policy landscape: Perspectives of health care professionals in Calgary, Alberta. *International Journal for Equity in Health, 17*(1), 91–14. doi:10.1186/s12939-018-0801-5

World Economic Forum. (2017). The global gender gap report 2017. Retrieved October 30, 2018, from https://www.weforum.org/reports/the-global-gender-gap-report-2017

World Health Organization. (2017). *Strengthening health systems to respond to women subjected to intimate partner violence or sexual violence: A manual for health managers.* Geneva: Author.

# CHAPTER 9

## Politics, Public Policy, and Population Health

*Toba Bryant*

## INTRODUCTION

Social determinants of health such as income and its distribution, the availability and affordability of housing and food, stability and quality of employment, and the provision of health and social services profoundly influence health. Governments' public policy decisions influence the quality of these social determinants of health. These public policy decisions are themselves shaped by political, economic, and social forces within jurisdictions that privilege some approaches while excluding others.

This chapter explores why some jurisdictions implement public policies that support the social determinants of health and others do not. To do so, it examines the political, economic, and social forces that shape public policy in Canada and other nations with similar traditions, such as the United States (U.S.) and the United Kingdom (U.K.). Sweden and Norway are used as comparison nations, since they have very well-developed welfare states. A central argument of this chapter is that government actions in public policy domains that are not usually considered as health-related strongly influence the health and well-being of populations. Canadian policy-making is compared to other nations on the basis of its potential to create health-enhancing environments. The chapter will also examine austerity and its impact on the health of populations.

## WHAT IS PUBLIC POLICY?

At a minimum, public policy is decisions made by governments. The following definition of public policy considers what governments do to address problems and the values that guide problem definition and solution:

> Public policy is a course of action or inaction chosen by public authorities to address a given problem or interrelated set of problems. Policy is a course of action that is anchored in a set of values regarding appropriate public goals and

a set of beliefs about the best way of achieving those goals. The idea of public policy assumes that an issue is no longer a private affair. (Wolf, 2005)

Esping-Andersen (2002) argues that a primary concern of modern welfare states such as Canada is to provide sufficient economic resources to support citizens across the lifespan. Changes in the occupational structure of post-industrial societies require the accumulation of "cognitive and social capital" among citizens. It is especially important to provide children with these assets: "Since it is well established that the ability and motivation to learn in the first place depends on the economic and social conditions of childhood, policies that aim to safeguard child welfare must be regarded as an investment on par with and, perhaps, more urgent than educational investments" (Esping-Anderson, 2002, p. 9). These assets provide intellectual and social flexibility that support learning new skills and adaptation to changing work environments. Economies also benefit by having women in the workplace and providing training opportunities to assist workers in coping with changing employment situations.

These key public policy issues show similarities with population health formulations that emphasize the accumulation of health assets across the lifespan. In particular, Shaw and colleagues (1999) emphasize the importance of societal supports for significant transitions across the lifespan such as entering and leaving school, gaining and possibly losing employment, and entering retirement. These supports include provision of income and employment security, equitable distribution of resources, and educational and training opportunities across the lifespan. How can we evaluate whether nations are committed to such goals? What indicators of healthy public policy are available? What do these indicators tell us about the ideology of governments and public policy?

Political economy conceives politics and economics as related to each other and to societal functioning (see Chapter 3). Political economists examine a variety of indicators that reflect government commitments to achieve a well-functioning economy and a vibrant and healthy society. These measures include government transfer of resources from general revenues to citizens in the forms of cash benefits, provision of health and social services, and employment, educational, and family supports. A number of indicators of such commitments are explored in the following sections.

There are a variety of explanations as to how such commitments come about. Some argue that these commitments reflect the capacity of progressive political forces such as "left political parties" and working-class power to influence the policy change process. Others examine the influence of civil society and the extent to which political and cultural traditions support equitable approaches to governance. The elements outlined above—the role of the state, the balance between the market and political forces, and civil society—all contribute to understanding how public policy is made. One important indicator of the general shape of public policy is the extent to which nations collect and then distribute resources among the population.

## OVERALL SPENDING ON TRANSFERS

The Organisation for Economic Co-operation and Development (OECD) regularly provides indicators of government operations, including provision of supports and services (OECD, 2016). An especially important indicator is government transfers. Transfers refer to governments using fiscal resources that are generated by the economy and distributing them to the population as services, monetary supports, or investments in social infrastructure. Such infrastructure includes education, employment training, social assistance or welfare payments, family supports, pensions, health and social services, and other benefits. These are important determinants of the health of the population (Raphael, 2016).

Figure 9.1 shows that among the developed nations of the OECD, average public social expenditure was 21% of GDP in 2016 (OECD, 2018b). Public social spending in 2015 ranged from 17% of GDP to almost 28% in some countries. This reflects a rather large variation among countries, with Sweden (27%) ranking among the highest public social spenders. Canada's spending, at 17.2% of GDP, is well below the OECD average in 2015. The U.S. spends 19%, the U.K., 21.5%, and Norway, 24% of GDP (OECD, 2018b).

Table 9.1 shows two broad domains of total public social transfers total and cash transfers. It also shows specific areas such as spending on health, old age (mainly pensions), family, and incapacity or disability. Canada is well below the OECD average in total, cash, and all the specific types of benefits.

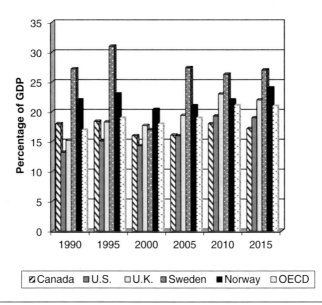

**Figure 9.1:** Overall Public Social Expenditure, 1990–2015, as a Percentage of GDP

*Source:* OECD. (2018). Social Expenditure Database. Retrieved October 12, 2018, from http://www.oecd.org/Index.aspx?datasetcode=SOCX_AGG

Health refers to public spending on healthcare services for the population. The U.S. does not provide universal healthcare coverage. U.S. health spending presented in Table 9.1 is for two publicly funded healthcare programs in the U.S. that cover low-income Americans: seniors and people with disabilities. In other words, health care is targeted to specific populations. In 2010, former President Barack Obama signed the *Patient Protection and Affordable Care Act* into law. The Act extends Medicaid coverage to approximately 15 million people. It universalizes access to health insurance by requiring all citizens to purchase health insurance—usually private insurance (Hall & Lord, 2014; Rosenbaum, 2011). The specific features of this legislation are examined in more detail in Chapter 10. Canada, the U.K., Sweden, and Norway offer government-operated programs for all, although the U.K. also has a separate for-profit healthcare stream. Even with its limited coverage, U.S. public health spending exceeds that of the other comparison countries. State-funded health care in all the other comparison nations ensures universal access to healthcare services and programs for all their citizens at much less cost than is the case for the U.S., where private care constitutes an additional 9% of GDP to the 8% spent in public funds.

Old age refers primarily to government payments to citizens upon retirement from paid employment. Employers can also provide pensions that employees pay into while they are employed. The U.S. spends about 1% more of GDP on public pension programs than Canada does. During the second term of George Bush's presidency, there were attempts underway to privatize—and, some argue, subsequently destroy—the U.S. pension program known as Social Security. President Barack Obama opposed privatization of

**Table 9.1:** Public Social Spending as a Percentage of GDP, 2016 or Most Recent Year

| Country | Total[1] | Cash[2] | Health[3] | Old Age[4] | Family[5] | Incapacity[6] |
|---|---|---|---|---|---|---|
| Canada | 17.2 | 9.8 | 7.1 | 4.6 | 0.96 | 0.9 |
| United States | 19.3 | 14.7 | 8.0 | 6.9 | 0.09 | 4.4 |
| United Kingdom | 21.5 | 10.3 | 7.1 | 6.1 | 2.2 | 5.6 |
| Sweden | 27.0 | 14.5 | 6.6 | 7.7 | 1.4 | 2.4 |
| Norway | 25.1 | 10.9 | 5.5 | 5.8 | 1.2 | 1.3 |
| OECD average | 21.0 | 11.6 | 6.0 | 8.2 | 2.0 | 2.3 |

*Sources:* Adapted from (1) OECD. (2016). Social Expenditure Database. Retrieved from http://stats.oecd.org/Index.aspx?datasetcode=SOCX_AGG; (2) OECD. (2018). *Social benefits to households (indicator).* doi:10.1787/423105c6-en; (3) OECD. (2018). *Health spending (indicator).* doi: 10.1787/8643de7e-en; (4) OECD. (2018). *Pension spending (indicator).* doi:10.1787/a041f4ef-en; (5) OECD. (2018). *Family benefits public spending (indicator).* doi:10.1787/8e8b3273-en; (6) OECD. (2018). *Public spending on incapacity (indicator).* doi:10.1787/f35b71ed-en

pensions. He argued that the financing of the program could be secured with some modifications. As of 2019, Republican members of the U.S. Congress were considering cuts to Social Security and Medicare to reduce a budget deficit apparently of their own making. President Donald Trump's position on Social Security is unclear. This tepid support in the U.S. for critical social programs reflects an extreme exemplar of a liberal welfare state.

As noted, among rich countries, the U.S. is the only one that does not provide universal health care to its citizens and systematically attempts to privatize social programs. In these non-healthcare areas, Sweden's and Norway's spending far exceed spending in Canada, the U.S., and the U.K. Sweden, Norway, and other Nordic countries have very different orientations toward social protection compared to Anglo-Saxon nations. Sweden's welfare states is one of the oldest, having begun building its state programs in the 1920s (Burström, Diderichsen, Östlin, & Östergren, 2002). Many Western countries, including Canada, the U.S., and the U.K., developed their welfare states after the Second World War (Teeple, 2000).

Many factors influence the development of public policy orientations. Social spending can be highly contentious in Canada and is especially so in the U.S. This is exemplified by Republicans' proposed cuts to Social Security and Medicare. Political dynamics such as government ideology and public attitudes toward those in need are significant determinants of the generosity of social spending. Ruling governments' ideologies can be assessed in terms of the level of commitment to income redistribution from higher- to lower-income groups and the provision of programs to support citizens in major life activities and transitions.

As an illustration of the role governments play in promoting health and well-being, consider the incidence of poverty before and after government programs and benefits are applied. The most recent poverty rates before taxes and transfers in 2015—primarily income earned as part of employment—was 29.5% for the U.K.; 24.9% for Sweden; 26.6% for the U.S.; 25.3% for Canada; and 24.9% for Norway (OECD, 2017). After benefits were applied, however, Sweden's rate fell to 9.1%; Norway's to 7%; Canada's to 14.2%; the U.K. to 11.1%; and the U.S. to 17.8%. Clearly, market forces by themselves without government intervention cannot be an effective approach to poverty reduction.

These poverty rates reflect the different orientations of these countries toward income distribution and poverty reduction. The U.S., with its market orientation to social welfare, has the highest poverty rates among the five countries. Canada is not far behind at 14.2%. Canada has made progress in reducing poverty among some groups, particularly the elderly. Poverty among non-elderly households, especially those with children, continues to be high. Since the mid-1980s, however, Canadian governments have emphasized deficit reduction. This approach has led to reduced social spending by both the federal and provincial governments. Why is there such variation in governments' willingness to reduce poverty?

Sweden and Norway have a political ethos of supporting their populations and undertaking measures to improve and maintain population health (Swedish National Institute of Public Health, 2003). Indeed, in April 2018, the Swedish government introduced a new public health bill entitled *Good and Equitable Public Health* in the Riksdag. The primary aim of public health policy there is to have a greater emphasis on achieving equitable health throughout the population, with an overriding aim to reduce avoidable health inequalities within a generation (Government Offices of Sweden, 2018). The policy identifies eight target areas, including early life conditions, education and training, working conditions, and income and employment opportunities, among others.

As we will see, Norway and Sweden represent what are called social democratic welfare states. These states have a commitment to reducing poverty and income inequality. Although these welfare states reduced social spending in some areas during the 1990s, Sweden and Norway have maintained among the highest public social spending compared to other Western nations (Figure 9.1). According to the OECD (2018c), virtually all Nordic countries—Denmark, Finland, Norway, and Sweden—have "below-average" poverty rates. Nordic countries seem to be more committed to improving and maintaining public health and well-being.

The U.S. and Canada have what is called a residual approach to social welfare and service provision. This is a situation where responsibility for well-being falls largely on individuals. When the individual encounters difficulties, it is expected that families and, if necessary, community-based agencies will provide support (Esping-Andersen, 1990, 1999). This approach has been found to result in considerably higher poverty rates compared to countries where there is a commitment to public service provision.

## POVERTY RATES AS AN INDICATOR OF PROGRESSIVE PUBLIC POLICY

As noted, an essential indicator of the general approach to public policy is the extent to which nations are committed to reducing the incidence of poverty. Poverty profoundly affects health and well-being and, at the very least, sets individuals upon disadvantageous health and educational trajectories (Auger, Raynault, Lessard, & Choinière, 2004; Pickett & Wilkinson, 2015). Poverty reduction is essential for the accumulation of cognitive and social capital, essential for an informed and productive workforce (Esping-Andersen, 2002). Where does Canada stand on this indicator of commitment to its citizenry?

The Luxembourg Income Study (LIS) provides income and demographic information on households in over 25 nations from 1967 to the present. Table 9.2 shows that using the commonly accepted international indicator of poverty as receiving income less than half the median population income—an indicator of ability to participate in a normal way in society—Canada has lower rates than the U.S. and the U.K but higher rates than Norway and Sweden. The poverty rates for Norway and Sweden, however, are rather higher than was the case as presented in the previous edition of this volume.

**Table 9.2:** Rates of Poverty for Various Age Groups in Canada, the U.S., the U.K., Sweden, and Norway, 2017

| Country | Overall | Children | Elderly |
|---|---|---|---|
| Canada | 12.4 | 14.2 | 7.4 |
| United States | 17.8 | 20.9 | 22.9 |
| United Kingdom | 11.1 | 11.8 | 14.2 |
| Sweden | 9.1 | 8.9 | 11.0 |
| Norway | 8.2 | 7.7 | 4.4 |

*Source:* Adapted from OECD. (2019). Poverty rate (indicator). doi: 10.1787/0fe1315d-en

The different poverty rates of these countries reflect different orientations to social provision. In a sense, these nations represent profoundly different manifestations of what is normally termed the welfare state. All developed nations have some form of welfare state. In capitalist economies, the welfare state is defined as one that uses government or state power to modify the influence of market forces in at least three ways:

- guarantees individuals and families a minimum income irrespective of the market value of their work or property
- narrows the extent of insecurity by enabling individuals and families to meet certain social contingencies such as sickness, old age, and unemployment, which lead otherwise to individual and family crises
- ensures that all citizens—without distinction of status or class—are offered the best standards available in relation to a certain agreed range of social services (Briggs, 1961)

What kind of welfare state does Canada have? Is it well developed or underdeveloped as compared to other modern industrialized nations? Earlier, data on social spending were provided for the five nations of Canada, the U.S., the U.K., Norway, and Sweden. Following were these data for all members of the OECD as of 2015.

In the most recent comparative OECD assessment of social spending in 35 countries, Canada ranks near the bottom. "Total public social expenditure" is defined in the OECD research as public and private institutions' provision of benefits to, and financial contributions targeted at, households and individuals in order to provide support during circumstances that adversely affect their welfare.

## Box 9.1: Canada's Total Social Spending Compared to Other Western Nations

Canada's social spending has been falling dramatically. In its most recent comparative assessment of social spending in 35 countries, Canada ranks near the bottom. In addition, Canada's spending levels in 2015 were 10.2% of GDP on health care and 17.2% of GDP on social services. Total gross social spending in Canada fell to 19.6%, down from the level of 20.4% of GDP in 2005.

"Total public social expenditure" is defined in the OECD research as public and private institutions' provision of benefits to, and financial contributions targeted at, households and individuals in order to provide support during circumstances that adversely affect their welfare.

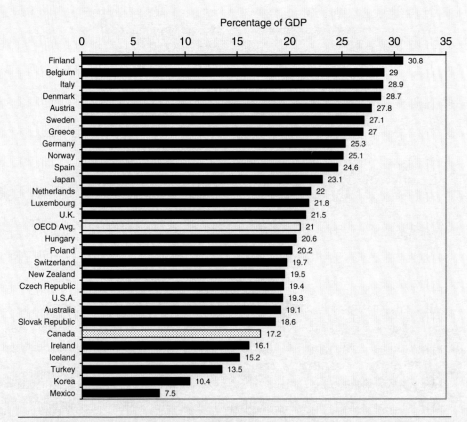

**Figure 9.2:** Total Public Social Expenditure as Percentage of GDP, 2016

*Source:* Adapted from OECD. (2018). Social Expenditure Database. Retrieved from http://stats.oecd.org/Index.aspx?datasetcode=SOCX_AGG

These benefits can be cash transfers, or can be the direct (in kind) provision of goods and services. Tax system benefits are included. It is "net," meaning after tax (the benefits an individual or household receives minus any tax they pay on the benefits).

The aim is to provide a comparable measure for that part of an economy's domestic production that is allocated to people in need of social benefits. It is an indicator of the share of resources a nation devoted to meeting social need in 2015 (the latest available data).

Canada, therefore, can do better. The problem is not one of Canada doing too much for its citizens and thereby potentially affecting the country's competitive situation. Too much has been stripped from one group of Canadians—lower-income households. The burden of fighting the deficit has not been equally shared.

Work on the form that welfare states can take reveals that Canada is seen—consistent with the findings presented above—as having a relatively weak welfare state, showing more similarities with the U.S. than with many European nations.

## WELFARE STATES AND PUBLIC POLICY

A variety of theoretical frameworks have been devised to understand how public policy components fit together to define a specific type of welfare state. Esping-Andersen (1990, 1999) devised a typology of capitalist welfare states that has generated much attention and research. Social democratic, liberal, and conservative welfare states form a continuum of government support to citizens, ranging from high government intervention welfare systems in the social democratic countries to residual welfare systems as seen in liberal nations. Conservative nations fall midway between these others in service provision and citizen supports.

Sweden and Norway are representative of social democratic welfare states, while the U.S., the U.K., and Canada are liberal welfare states. The level of welfare-oriented policies in Canada represents both its similarities to the other liberal nations, as well as its placement within the liberal cluster. While Canada frequently appears to be very different from the U.S. in its policies, in comparison, it is closer to the U.S. in its welfare provisions than it is to social democratic and conservative nations such as France and Germany.

Conservative welfare states such as France, Germany, and Italy tie benefits to one's occupation and earnings, and tend to stratify citizens rather than promote equality. There is less effort to support families or women. The vast majority of benefits are earnings-related and contributory rather than universal entitlements as is the case with social democratic nations.

Esping-Andersen (1990) defines the liberal welfare state as involving means-tested assistance, modest universal transfers, and modest social-insurance plans. Means testing refers to benefits in the liberal welfare state being primarily geared to low-income groups. Social assistance is limited by traditional, liberal work-ethic attitudes that stigmatize the needy and attribute failure to the individual rather than to society. Liberal nations limit welfare benefits since it is believed that generous benefits lead to a preference for welfare dependency rather than gainful employment.

The nature of benefits in liberal nations results from an implicit—and frequently explicit—view that low-income or poor people are poor due to moral failings. This individualistic view fails to acknowledge the structural causes of low income, such as high unemployment rates, which have plagued all OECD countries since the 1980s. Such a view also fails to acknowledge the role poor material conditions of life play in contributing to poor educational and social development in deprived communities. Differences in the form the welfare state takes should be related to overall population health, and indeed there is evidence to this effect.

Other welfare state typologies have been devised. For example, Olsen (2002) describes the categorical welfare state, which simply divides welfare states into one of two categories: residual or institutional welfare states (Olsen, 2002). It was devised to capture the qualitative dimensions of welfare states. Residual welfare states are consistent with Esping-Andersen's liberal welfare state cluster. Such welfare states provide minimal support to families and individuals. They are less comprehensive, comprising a limited range of social supports that are generally targeted to families and individuals in need. Such programs meet only the immediate needs of applicants. In contrast, the institutional welfare state is more generous, providing a range of social welfare measures and income-replacement programs. A limitation of this dichotomous typology is that, with its broad categorizations, it may obscure significant differences between welfare states (Olsen, 2002).

Arts and Gelissen (2001) consolidate the different welfare state typologies devised to challenge Esping-Andersen's typology. Most still retain the original clusters of Esping-Andersen's model. Additional categories have been proposed, such as one for the Latin welfare states of Portugal, Spain, Italy, and Greece (Bonoli, 1997; Saint-Arnaud & Bernard, 2003). This category was created because this type of welfare regime is unique to the countries of Southern Europe (e.g., Spain, Greece, Italy, and Portugal). The Latin welfare state emphasizes the principle of solidarity, similar to conservative welfare states in Esping-Andersen's typology. Family has a central function in contribution to the material well-being of households in Latin regimes. Esping-Andersen (1990) classified these welfare states as underdeveloped conservative welfare regimes.

Another category proposed is Antipodean to capture the unique features of Australia's and New Zealand's welfare states (Castles, 1998). It has been argued that Australia and New Zealand have a more specific and comprehensive approach to social protection compared to the liberal cluster in Esping-Andersen's typology.

The three clusters of Esping-Andersen's original formulation are generally retained. Canada and the United States are still included in the liberal cluster, given their social and health spending as percentages of GDP. Health researchers have used Esping-Andersen's formulation to compare population health profiles of countries. As Arts and Gelissen (2001) argue, however, more theorizing on welfare states is needed to advance the understanding of the welfare state and the forms it can assume.

## WELFARE STATES AND POPULATION HEALTH PROFILES

Navarro and Shi (2002) drew upon Esping-Andersen's insights to identify nations governed predominantly from 1945 to 1980 by social democratic (Sweden, Finland, Norway, Denmark, and Austria), Christian democratic (Belgium, Netherlands, Germany, France, Italy, and Switzerland), or Anglo-Saxon liberal political parties (Canada, Ireland, the U.K., and the U.S.). They then compared these nations on a range of political, economic, and population health indicators.

The social democratic regimes presented higher levels of union density—that is, a greater proportion of workers belong to organized labour unions (Navarro & Shi, 2002). Social democratic regimes also had higher levels of social security and public employment expenditures. Between 1960 and 1990, these regimes had the highest public healthcare expenditures, and the most extensive healthcare coverage of citizens. These nations implemented full employment strategies, attained high rates of female employment, and showed the lowest levels of income inequality and poverty rates. Social democratic nations also had the lowest percentage of national income derived from capital investment and the largest from wages, indicating less wealth accumulation by those already wealthy. On a key indicator of population health—infant mortality—these countries had the lowest rates from 1960 to 1996.

The conservative/Christian democratic regimes were second to the social democratic regimes in public healthcare expenditures (Navarro & Shi, 2002). These countries had lower public healthcare coverage of citizens, but higher levels than the liberal regimes. A smaller proportion of the working-age population was employed by governments, and a lower proportion of women were employed overall compared to the social democratic regimes. Christian democratic countries had high income inequalities compared to social democratic countries. This is due to more favourable treatment of wealth and investments and the lower redistributive effect of the state.

Anglo-Saxon liberal political economies had the lowest healthcare expenditures and the lowest coverage by public medical care (Navarro & Shi, 2002). They had greater incidence of low-wage earnings, higher income inequalities, and the highest poverty rates. These economies derived the greatest proportion of income from capital investment rather than wages. These liberal countries had the lowest improvement rates in infant mortality rates from 1960 to 1996.

Recent work by Raphael (2011) shows the differences among countries using Esping-Andersen's typology of liberal, social democratic, conservative, and Latin welfare states. Not surprisingly, he found that liberal or social democratic welfare states tended to make explicit commitments to the provision of the prerequisites of health (Raphael, 2013). Yet, despite these commitments, liberal welfare states lag behind social democratic and conservative welfare states in instituting public policies that deliver higher-quality and equitable distribution of the social determinants of health. Latin welfare states tend to show little commitment to providing the social determinants of health. As a result, there is minimal public policy activity to promote health.

Clearly, then, politics influence public policy and population health. What are the specific forces that determine the trajectory that a nation takes in its establishment of a welfare state? Esping-Andersen (1999) argues that unique historical and cultural forces set a nation on a general path. For the Nordic nations, the advanced welfare state developed as a result of alliances established between workers and farmers, supported by the presence of electoral democracy that applied proportional representation (Esping-Andersen, 1985). In Canada such alliances have rarely existed. Failure to develop these political alliances is responsible, in part, for Canada's relatively weak welfare state. In addition, Canada's welfare state appears to be under even further threat. We now turn to these threats.

## POLITICAL, ECONOMIC, AND SOCIAL FORCES THAT SHAPE PUBLIC POLICY IN LIBERAL ECONOMIES

Within the typology of welfare states, there is room for national variation. Both global and national political, economic, and social forces influence public policy and the shape of the welfare state in Canada. Within the Canadian system, these dynamics include political ideologies of the government of the day and competing interests. The rise of neo-liberalism has influenced welfare state policies in Canada. Coburn (2000) defines neo-liberalism as a political ideology that is committed to a market economy as the best allocator of resources and wealth in a society. It perceives individuals as motivated by material and economic concerns. Competition is considered the primary market instrument for innovations. Moreover, neo-liberal adherents argue that an unfettered market ensures economic development and a fair distribution of resources.

Considering that Canada is already identified as a liberal political economy within Esping-Andersen's typology, it may be especially susceptible to neo-liberal ideology (see Vandenbroucke [2002] for a discussion of European Union resistance to neo-liberal influences). And many have argued that this has been the case. Indeed, as Swank (1998) argues:

> Where institutions of collective interest representation—social corporatism and inclusive electoral institutions—are strong, where authority is concentrated, and where the welfare state is based on the principle of universalism, the effects of international capital mobility are absent, or they are positive in the sense that they suggest economic and political interests opposed to neo-liberal reforms … have been successful in defending the welfare state. (p. 44)

Much has been written about neo-liberalism as the dominant political ideology in post-industrial capitalism. *Neo* means new, and *liberalism* refers to freedom from government (McGregor, 2001). Markets are central to neo-liberalism and offer the preferred means to organize human interaction and activities (Schrecker & Bambra, 2015). Markets are preferred because they can produce efficient outcomes and increase welfare. The responsibility of the state is to facilitate efficient functioning of markets.

Neo-liberalism is now the dominant political ideology around the world. Some describe it as a "hegemonic paradigm," attributing its dominance to its flexibility and tractability (Cerny, 2014). It thrives in a socio-economic environment in which material conditions and ideas are in flux. The lack of an alternative paradigm seems to lend legitimacy to neo-liberalism.

Teeple (2000) provides a well-developed analysis of the role neo-liberalism has played in the decline of Canada's welfare state. Neo-liberalism serves as a justification for increasing economic globalization and concentrating wealth and power to increase corporate profits. For Teeple, the unrestrained economic power of private property has eroded the post–Second World War welfare state that supported redistribution of wealth and the provision of strong health and social services. The rise of neo-liberalism in liberal political economies (e.g., Thatcherism in the United Kingdom, Reaganism in the United States, and Mulroneyism in Canada) has created increased income inequalities and weakened social provision. Certainly, policies followed by Finance Minister Paul Martin during the 1990s reflect both a neo-liberal approach and a distinct threat to the Canadian welfare state (Scarth, 2004).

## AUSTERITY AND NEO-LIBERALISM: IMPACT ON THE WELFARE STATE AND HEALTH INEQUALITIES

The growth of the welfare state in Canada levelled off in the early 1980s. Since 1990, there has been a drastic decline in public expenditures in support of a variety of welfare state policies (Stanford, 2004, 2015). Following the financial crisis in 2008, a number of countries shifted to austerity policies. Austerity refers to measures that cut state spending in order to reduce debt and deficits and end recessions (Stanford, 2015). Austerity measures have increased insecurity and health inequalities, especially with aggressive monetary policy to control inflation. These actions can prolong an economic downturn. This is attributed to aggressive monetary policy. For example, central banks may raise interest rates too high and too quickly to control inflation. Such actions slow the economy too much.

Some countries in the European Union cut public spending on health, most notably Greece (Quaglio, Karapiperis, Van Woensel, Arnold, & McDaid, 2013). Public health spending in that country fell from 9.8% of GDP pre-crisis to 6% post-crisis. Other countries, such as Romania, Slovenia, and the United Kingdom, froze or decreased wages and/ or eliminated posts or did not replace them. Some countries also introduced user fees to conform with austerity requirements (Schrecker & Bambra, 2015; Stuckler & Basu,

2013). The health implications of these measures include increased mental health problems (e.g., suicidal behaviour) and chronic physical health issues (e.g., heart disease, type 2 diabetes).

Austerity increased poverty and widened the gap between income groups (Stuckler & Basu, 2013). It led to worse population health, especially for those at the lower end of the income distribution. Austerity is driven by political ideology of governments, specifically neo-liberalism.

## ANALYSIS AND IMPLICATIONS

Canada has a relatively weak welfare state compared to other nations, and even this state is under threat. What do we know about the determinants of a strong welfare state that can assist those wishing to resist these threats and strengthen public policy in the service of health?

The role of politics and political parties is central to understanding the level of commitment to the welfare state. In particular, the influence of "left political parties" is important to the development of the welfare state and its maintenance in the post-industrial capitalist era. These parties support redistribution of wealth and advocate for universal social and health programs. Rainwater and Smeeding (2003) used data from the Luxembourg Income Study to consider the role that left representation played in reducing child poverty. The proportion of left cabinet share is associated with the size of the welfare state.

A systematic review on the relationship between political characteristics and population health outcomes found that political characteristics were strongly associated with a number of population health indicators, including life expectancy, infant mortality (Barnish, Tørnes, & Nelson-Horne, 2018). Of 102 studies on welfare state comprehensiveness, 17 studies on political traditions found a positive association between comprehensive welfare state support and left-of-centre political traditions.

One important process that has assisted left political parties in having influence is proportional representation in elections. Esping-Andersen (1985) identifies proportional representation as essential to the development of the Nordic welfare state. Electoral systems also influence outcomes. Indeed, countries with majoritarian or first-past-the-post electoral systems—as in Canada—are more likely to elect conservative governments, or larger traditional political parties (Döring & Manow, 2017). In contrast, countries with proportional representation tend to produce more varied outcomes in which left-of-centre parties are more likely to gain seats in the national or regional legislatures. It is noteworthy that, in the 2015 general election in Canada, Justin Trudeau promised electoral reform but then backtracked, claiming that the Canadian electorate was not ready for it. It might well be argued that he was reluctant to change an electoral system that gave him a large majority government.

Importantly, proportional representation had been on the public policy agenda nationally and provincially. In British Columbia, New Brunswick, and Ontario, governments initiated processes of electoral reform. However, in the provincial election in Ontario in 2007, the electorate rejected the model of proportional representation recommended by a citizen advisory committee. The B.C. government recently held a referendum on proportional representation (Elections BC, 2018). It was also defeated.

If proportional representation were to be implemented in Canada, this would provide strong support for strengthening the welfare state and bringing in health-supportive public policies. In a sense, governments would be in a permanent minority government situation, a situation that has been associated with progressive public policy in Canada at both the federal and provincial levels.

## LABOUR UNION AND LABOUR DENSITY

The strength of labour is an important determinant of the strength of the welfare state. In particular, class structure and union density are important. In Chapter 3, it was shown that greater union membership is related to lower poverty rates.

Navarro and colleagues (2003) found that left party governance correlates strongly with unionization rates, and that both are associated with strong welfare states and numerous indicators of health. In the U.S., unionization and the ability to organize is weakly supported and actively opposed (Zweig, 2004). Union power is somewhat greater in Canada but also has been under some attack. These findings beg the question as to whose interests are served by discouraging unionization and the development of institutions that serve the interests of the working class. Research into population health seldom considers the implications of such forces on population health and well-being, particularly of the groups that are least well-off as a result. The diverse social conditions of Canada, the U.S., the U.K., and Sweden reflect differing political dynamics that influence social spending.

## APPLICATION TO SPECIFIC CANADIAN PUBLIC POLICY DOMAINS

Canada is placed within the liberal type of welfare state. Although Canadian governments tend to play to the political centre, they have implemented many neo-liberal policies in recent years. This became particularly apparent during the 1990s in housing, early childhood education and care, social assistance, and labour policy as the federal and provincial governments reduced social spending in all of these areas (Figure 9.3). Government spending—most of which goes to assist the average Canadian—is now at levels not seen since the early 1970s. The most severe cuts came during the Liberal government during the early 1990s. There was an increase in response to the severe 2008 recession, but now spending levels are again declining.

*Housing*: Walks and Clifford (2015) show how Canadian housing policy reflects a unique mix of financialization under capitalism, shaped by the organization of mortgage markets and the state role in the process of securitization. Securitization is central

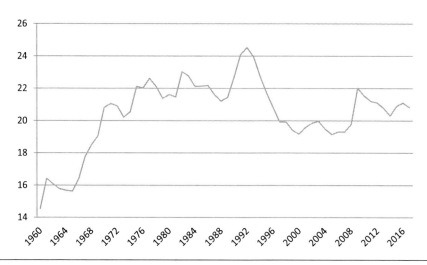

**Figure 9.3:** Government Spending as a Function of GDP, Canada, 1960–2017

*Source:* World Bank. (2019). Canada: Government spending, percent of GDP. Retrieved from https://www. theglobaleconomy.com/Canada/Government_size/

to the neo-liberalization of housing policy. The state role involves insuring, directing, and financing residential mortgage-supported securities that shore up and justify the federal shift from social rental housing provision to private sector dominance in this sector. Hulchanski (2003) showed how both federal and provincial governments—with the exception of Quebec—stopped providing affordable housing. In Ontario, Canada's largest province, social housing starts declined from 15,000 social housing starts in 1970 to none in 1998. Not surprisingly, there is a crisis in homelessness across Canada. Comprehensive overviews of housing policy and its effects upon health are available (Bryant, 2004, 2016; Bryant & Shapcott, 2016; Shapcott, 2004).

*Early childhood education and care (ECEC)*: Early childhood education and care is a patchwork of for-profit and non-profit programs across Canada (Friendly, 2004, 2016). ECEC provides a number of social benefits (Akbari & McCuaig, 2017). These include job creation, in addition to enabling parents to work and upgrade skills. These programs also reduce reliance on income support programs. Although Canadian provinces and territories have increased their ECEC spending by about $1 billion, this falls well below the average for OECD countries of 5% to 6% of GDP (Akbari & McCuaig, 2017). In Canada, 3% is the highest percentage achieved by a province. Ontario and Quebec surpassed this spending benchmark. An increase in spending is expected in 2018, when the provinces and territories contribute to the federal transfers.

There is pressure to establish a national child care program, but there has been little discussion about establishing the foundations for a national system of early learning and child care. Canada lags behind many countries in this area, although the U.S. appears to be an exceptionally poor provider of family supports (see Box 9.2).

## Box 9.2: U.S. Family Policy in International Perspective

Research Finds U.S. Lags Far behind Scores of Countries Globally in Guaranteeing Working Conditions That Support Working Families

For immediate release: Wednesday, June 16, 2004

Boston, MA—A new report of research on 168 countries led by Jody Heymann, Associate Professor of Society, Health and Human Development at the Harvard School of Public Health (HSPH), finds that working conditions in the United States that support working families lag far behind scores of other countries. The report, *The Work, Family and Equity Index*: *Where Does the United States Stand Globally?* is being released today in Washington, DC.

Among the report's findings:

- More than 160 countries offer guaranteed paid leave to women in connection with childbirth. The U.S. does not.
- The only other industrialized country which does not have paid maternity or parental leave for women, Australia, guarantees a full year of unpaid leave to all women in the country. The Family Medical Leave Act in the U.S. provides only 12 weeks of unpaid leave to approximately half of mothers and nothing for the remainder.
- 45 countries ensure that fathers either receive paid paternity leave or have a right to paid paternity leave. The U.S. does not guarantee either.
- At least 96 countries around the world in all geographic regions and at all economic levels provide for paid annual leave. The U.S. does not ensure paid annual leave.
- 76 countries guarantee working mothers the right to breastfeed. The U.S. does not protect the ability of working mothers to breastfeed, despite its importance to the health of baby and mother alike.
- 139 countries mandate paid sick leave. 117 of these countries ensure at least one week. The U.S. does not guarantee even one day leave for illness.

"The United States trails enormously far behind the rest of the world when it comes to legislation to protect the health and welfare of working families. Scores of countries guarantee paid leave for new mothers and fathers, the opportunity to breastfeed, sick leave, and some minimum annual leave that can be spent with children, elderly parents or other family members. The United States guarantees none of these to working Americans or their families." Jody Heymann explained, "This is only the beginning of the list. Protections against extreme work hours or weeks with no breaks are among the other areas where the U.S. lags. Moreover, we have fallen behind when it comes to services for pre-school and school age children, as well as in working conditions. The costs are enormous to the health and welfare of children, the disabled and elderly, and the working adults who care for them."

*Source:* Harvard School of Public Health. (2004). Press release. Retrieved from http://archive.sph. harvard.edu/press-releases/archives/2004-releases/press06162004.html

*Social assistance*: Social assistance or welfare programs are administered by the provincial and territorial governments in Canada. Canada falls behind most other OECD countries in this area. Canadian governments have been slower than Western European governments to upgrade or improve spending on social assistance.

*Labour policy*: Active labour policy consists of formal classroom training; on-the-job training programs; subsidies to private-sector employers; job-search assistance (e.g., job clubs, individual counselling, etc.); special training programs for youth (e.g., training, employment subsidies, direct job-creation measures); and direct job creation for adult workers. Nations use such programs to eradicate high and persistent unemployment and reduce low pay and poverty among the working-age population. Canada's active labour market policies in 2015 comprised on average 0.24% of GDP, compared to Sweden's 1.27%, Norway's 0.52%, the U.K.'s 0.23%, and the U.S.'s 0.10% of GDP (OECD, 2018a). Sweden and Norway's more generous labour market policies provide more extensive job training and retraining for older workers. These are key areas for promoting the cognitive and social skills necessary for Canada and other welfare states to provide healthy economic and social conditions.

These policy issues are important to Canadians' health and well-being and should be debated and acted upon. A minority government situation—that is, no one party can govern without the consent of one or other parties in Parliament—may increase sensitivity to these issues. The issues discussed in this chapter should be included in any national debate about the future of Canadian public policy.

## CONCLUSIONS

There is little consideration given to public policy in the population health literature. Political economy approaches focus on how the market and economics, political ideology, and other dynamics are integrally related and influence the nature of public policy. These are not preordained or natural processes, but socially determined by politics and the power of groups that strive to influence government decisions to achieve policy objectives.

Spending on health and social programs can be politically contentious, yet in the end determine citizens' health and well-being. Moreover, political economy approaches can identify interests that benefit from low social spending and how these interests operate through the political system to influence public decision-making on these issues. Political ideology profoundly influences income redistribution and the policies that affect income, social, and health inequalities.

However, there has been little consideration of these concepts in population health research and discussion. There is a need to move away from biomedical and epidemiological models to consider the influence of political ideology, social organization, and economic infrastructure to understand how economic and social inequalities lead to health inequalities. Directing the health sector's gaze to broader political and economic factors may be the most effective means of improving population health and reducing inequalities in health.

## CRITICAL THINKING QUESTIONS

1.  Prior to reading this chapter, what were your views concerning the extent of poverty in Canada? Did you feel that Canada was doing a good or a poor job in addressing the issue? What is the effect on public perceptions and public policy-making of having the U.S., with its very high poverty rates, as a neighbour?
2.  What are some political, social, and economic barriers to having progressive social policies such those seen in Sweden implemented in Canada?
3.  Why are Canadian families not lobbying for family-friendly policies? Why aren't Canadian workers pressuring governments for active labour market policies, such as increased job training for youth and retraining for older workers?
4.  To what extent is proportional representation an issue in Canada? What are the barriers to implementing it in Canada? How can proportional representation be placed on the public policy agenda in Canada?
5.  How much influence does the labour movement have in making Canadian public policy? What are your views concerning the role that organized labour could play in making public policy? Would you personally benefit from increased labour influence? Why or why not?

## FURTHER READINGS

Alesina, A., & Glaeser, E. L. (2004). *Fighting poverty in the U.S. and Europe: A world of difference*. Oxford: Oxford University Press.
The authors provide an analysis of how differing historical traditions and political and social structures explain differences between American and European approaches to fighting poverty. Their presentations include data from Canada, in addition to the U.S. and Europe.

Esping-Andersen, G. (1990). *The three worlds of welfare capitalism*. Princeton, NJ: Princeton University Press.
Esping-Andersen, G. (1999). *Social foundations of postindustrial economies*. Toronto: Oxford University Press.
These books provide a typology of Western welfare states that takes into account a range of social policies and links these with variations in the historical development of Western countries. The author describes how profound differences among liberal (e.g., the U.S., Canada, and the U.K.), conservative (e.g., Germany, France, and Italy), and social democratic (e.g., Sweden, Norway, and Denmark) political economies translate into widely differing lived experiences among citizens of these nations.

Esping-Andersen, G. (Ed.). (2002). *Why we need a new welfare state*. Oxford: Oxford University Press.

Contributors argue that welfare states need to consider issues of social inclusion and justice. The volume focuses on four social domains: (1) the aged and transition to retirement; (2) welfare issues related to changes in working life; (3) risks and needs that arise in households, especially in families with young children; and (4) the challenges of creating gender equality.

Rainwater, L., & Smeeding, T. M. (2003). *Poor kids in a rich country: America's children in comparative perspective.* New York: Russell Sage Foundation.
The authors consider why poverty rates are so high in the U.S. By comparing the situation of American children in low-income families with their counterparts in Western Europe, Australia, and Canada, they provide a detailed perspective on the dynamics of child poverty in developed nations.

Schrecker, T., & Bambra, C. (2015). *How politics makes us sick: Neoliberal epidemics.* Basingstoke, U.K.: Palgrave Macmillan.
This text is essential reading on the health effects of austerity and neo-liberalism. The authors call for political action to address health inequalities and other effects of austerity and neo-liberalism.

## RELEVANT WEBSITES

### Economic and Social National Data Rates and Rankings
http://dataranking.com/exp.cgi?LG=e
Kenji Suzuki, of the European Institute of Japanese Studies at the Stockholm School of Economics, maintains a current repository of a wide range of national data. The site provides rates and rankings for each nation compared to the world, developed nations, continents, etc.

### Human Development Reports
http://hdr.undp.org/
The UN's Human Development Report was launched in 1990 with the goal of placing people at the centre of the development process in terms of economic debate, policy, and advocacy. The Human Development Reports provide current information on a range of development topics.

### Institute for Research on Public Policy (IRPP)
www.irpp.org/
IRPP's mission is to assist Canadians in making more effective policy choices. Their research aims to enhance the quality of the debate on the issues related to economic performance, social progress, and sound democratic governance.

**Luxembourg Income Studies (LIS)**

www.lisdatacenter.org/working-papers/

The Luxembourg Income Studies provide working papers on a range of issues related to income and other indicators. The working papers can be downloaded from this site.

**Organisation for Economic Co-operation and Development (OECD)**

www.oecd.org

This site provides a wealth of reports, publications, and statistics about every aspect of society in modern industrialized states. Many of its contents are free or available electronically through your local university's library.

## GLOSSARY

**Active labour policy:** A government's policies and programs developed to create or maintain jobs for all workers. Employment measures for workers with disabilities range from sheltered workshops and other job-creation measures in regular public service and public works projects (i.e., building and highway construction). It also covers subsidies to private business to hire new employees or extend seasonal work throughout the year; apprenticeship training, on-the-job training and retraining, and work-study programs to ease transition from school to employment; and job-transition training for workers facing layoffs.

**Family policy:** Policies and programs designed to provide a secure growing environment for children and to ensure that parents have the material and psychological supports for rearing children. Through these policies, usually involving various forms of financial support and the system of child care, society compensates citizens for some of the costs borne by families with children.

**Gross domestic product (GDP):** The total market value of all goods and services produced in a country in a given year. It is equal to total consumer, investment, and government spending, plus the value of exports, minus the value of imports.

**Left political parties:** Political parties that support the redistribution of wealth by way of income support and publicly funded programs for individuals with disabilities, and families and individuals with low income. Strongly aligned with the labour movement, they also advocate for policies to support workers and other policy initiatives that reduce social and health inequalities in a population. The New Democrats in Canada, the Social Democrats in Sweden, and the Labour Party in the U.K. are considered left parties. The U.S. does not have a politically relevant left party.

**Proportional representation:** A variety of systems used for electing a legislature in which the number of seats a party wins is more or less proportional to the percentage of popular votes cast. This is in contrast to the first-past-the-post approach, in which the party candidate with the most votes in each constituency wins the seat. Proportional representation is the norm in most European nations. It is seen as contributing to the influence of left parties on progressive legislation in many modern welfare states.

## REFERENCES

Akbari, E., & McCuaig, K. (2017). *Early childhood education report 2017.* Toronto: Atkinson Centre for Society and Child Development/University of Toronto.

Arts, W., & Gelissen, J. (2001). Welfare states, solidarity, and justice principles: Does the type really matter? *ACTA Sociologica, 44*(4), 283–299. https://doi.org/10.1177/000169930104400401

Auger, N., Raynault, M., Lessard, R., & Choinière, R. (2004). Income and health in Canada. In D. Raphael (Ed.), *Social determinants of health: Canadian perspectives* (pp. 39–52). Toronto: Canadian Scholars' Press.

Barnish, M., Tørnes, M., & Nelson-Horne, B. (2018). How much evidence is there that political factors are related to population health outcomes? An internationally comparative systematic review. *BMJ Open, 8*(10), [e020886]. https://doi.org/10.1136/bmjopen-2017-020886

Bonoli, G. (1997). Classifying welfare states: A two-dimensional approach. *Journal of Social Policy, 26*(3), 351–372.

Briggs, A. (1961). The welfare state in historical perspective. *European Journal of Sociology, 2*(2), 251–258.

Bryant, T. (2004). Housing and health. In D. Raphael (Ed.), *Social determinants of health: Canadian perspectives* (pp. 217–232). Toronto: Canadian Scholars' Press.

Bryant, T. (2016). Housing and health. In D. Raphael (Ed.), *Social determinants of health: Canadian perspectives* (3rd ed., pp. 360–383). Toronto: Canadian Scholars' Press.

Bryant, T., & Shapcott, M. (2016). Housing. In D. Raphael (Ed.), *Social determinants of health: Canadian perspectives* (3rd ed., pp. 343–359). Toronto: Canadian Scholars' Press.

Burström, B., Diderichsen, F., Östlin, P., & Östergren, P. P. (2002). Sweden. In J. Mackenbach & M. Bakker (Eds.), *Reducing inequalities in health: A European perspective* (pp. 274–283). London: Routledge.

Castles, F. G. (1998). *Comparative public policy: Patterns of post-war transformation.* Cheltenham, U.K.: Edward Elgar.

Cerny, P. G. (2014). Globalization and the resilience of neoliberalism. *Critical Policy Studies, 8*(3), 359–362. https://doi.org/10.1080/19460171.2014.944370

Coburn, D. (2000). Income inequality, social cohesion, and the health status of populations: The role of neoliberalism. *Social Science & Medicine, 51*(1), 135–146.

Döring, H., & Manow, P. (2017). Is proportional representation more favourable to the left? Electoral rules and their impact on elections, parliaments and the formation of cabinets. *British Journal of Political Science, 47*(1), 149–164. https://doi.org/10.1017/S0007123415000290

Elections BC. (2018). 2018 referendum on electoral reform. Retrieved from https://elections.bc.ca/referendum/

Esping-Andersen, G. (1985). *Politics against markets: The social democratic road to power.* Princeton, NJ: Princeton University Press.

Esping-Andersen, G. (1990). *The three worlds of welfare capitalism.* Princeton, NJ: Princeton University Press.

Esping-Andersen, G. (1999). *Social foundations of postindustrial economies.* New York: Oxford University Press.

Esping-Andersen, G. (Ed.). (2002). *Why we need a new welfare state.* Oxford: Oxford University Press.

Friendly, M. (2004). Early childhood education and care. In D. Raphael (Ed.), *Social determinants of health: Canadian perspectives* (pp. 109–123). Toronto: Canadian Scholars' Press.

Friendly, M. (2016). Early childhood education and care as a social determinant of health. In D. Raphael (Ed.), *Social determinants of health: Canadian perspectives* (pp. 192–217). Toronto: Canadian Scholars' Press.

Government Offices of Sweden. (2018). Public health policy to be more equitable. Retrieved from https://www.government.se/articles/2018/05/public-health-policy-to-be-more-equitable/

Hall, M. A., & Lord, R. 2014. Obamacare: What the Affordable Care Act means for patients and physicians. *British Medical Journal, 349*, g5376. https://doi.org/10.1136/bmj.g5376

Hulchanski, J. D. (2003). *Housing policy for tomorrow's cities.* Ottawa: Canadian Policy Research Networks Inc. Retrieved from http://www.urbancentre.utoronto.ca/pdfs/researchassociates/Hulchanski_Housing-Policy-C.pdf

McGregor, S. (2001). Neoliberalism and health care. *International Journal of Consumer Studies, 25*(2), 82–89. https://doi.org/10.1111/j.1470-6431.2001.00183.x

Navarro, V., Borrell, C., Benach, J., Muntaner, C., Quiroga, A., Rodrigues-Sanz, M., … Pasarin, M. I. (2003). The importance of the political and the social in explaining mortality differentials among the countries of the OECD, 1950–1998. *International Journal of Health Services, 33*, 419–94. doi:10.2190/R7GE-8DWK-YY6C-183U

Navarro, V., & Shi, L. (2002). The political context of social inequalities and health. In V. Navarro (Ed.), *The political economy of social inequalities: Consequences for health and quality of life* (pp. 403–418). Amityville, NY: Baywood.

Olsen, G. (2002). *The politics of the welfare state: Canada, Sweden, and the United States.* Don Mills, ON: Oxford University Press.

Organisation for Economic Co-operation and Development. (2016). *Society at a glance 2016: OECD social indicators.* doi:10.1787/9789264261488-en

Organisation for Economic Co-operation and Development. (2017). Income distribution and poverty database.

Organisation for Economic Co-operation and Development. (2018a). *Active labour market policies: Connecting people with jobs.* Retrieved from http://www.oecd.org/employment/activation.htm

Organisation for Economic Co-operation and Development. (2018b). *Social spending.* Paris: Author.

Organisation for Economic Co-operation and Development. (Ed.). (2018c). *Income distribution and poverty* (vol. 2018). Paris: Author.

Pickett, K. E., & Wilkinson, R. G. (2015). Income inequality and health: A causal review. *Social Science & Medicine, 128*, 316–326. doi:10.1016/j.socscimed.2014.12.031

Quaglio, G. L., Karapiperis, T., Van Woensel, L., Arnold, E., & McDaid, D. (2013). Austerity and health in Europe. *Health Policy, 113*(1–2), 13–19. doi:10.1016/j.healthpol.2013.09.005

Rainwater, L., & Smeeding, T. M. (2003). *Poor kids in a rich country: America's children in comparative perspective.* New York: Russell Sage Foundation.

Raphael, D. (2011). Canadian public policy and poverty in international perspective. In D. Raphael (Ed.), *Poverty in Canada: Implications for health and quality of life* (pp. 374–405). Toronto: Canadian Scholars' Press.

Raphael, D. (2013). The political economy of health promotion: Part 1, national commitments to provision of the prerequisites of health. *Health Promotion International, 28*(1), 95–111. doi:10.1093/heapro/dar084

Raphael, D. (Ed.). (2016). *Social determinants of health: Canadian perspectives* (3rd ed.). Toronto: Canadian Scholars' Press.

Rosenbaum, S. (2011). The Patient Protection and Affordable Care Act: Implications for public health policy and practice. *Public Health Reports, 126*(1), 130–135. doi:10.1177/003335491112600118

Saint-Arnaud, S., & Bernard, P. (2003). Convergence or resilience? A hierarchial cluster analysis of the welfare regimes in advanced countries. *Current Sociology, 51*(5), 499–527. doi:10.1177/00113921030515004

Scarth, T. (Ed.). (2004). *Hell and high water: An assessment of Paul Martin's record and implications for the future.* Ottawa: Canadian Centre for Policy Alternatives.

Schrecker, T., & Bambra, C. (2015). *How politics makes us sick: Neoliberal epidemics.* Basingstoke, U.K.: Palgrave Macmillan.

Shapcott, M. (2004). Housing. In D. Raphael (Ed.), *Social determinants of health: Canadian perspectives* (pp. 201–215). Toronto: Canadian Scholars' Press.

Shaw, M., Dorling, D., Gordon, D., & Smith, G. D. (1999). *The widening gap: Health inequalities and policy in Britain.* Bristol, U.K.: Policy Press.

Stanford, J. (2004). Paul Martin, the deficit, and the debt: Taking another look. In T. Scarth (Ed.), *Hell and high water: An assessment of Paul Martin's record and implications for the future* (pp. 31–54). Ottawa: Canadian Centre for Policy Alternatives.

Stanford, J. (2015). *Economics for everyone: A short guide to the economics of capitalism* (2nd ed.). Ottawa: Canadian Centre for Policy Alternatives.

Stuckler, D., & Basu, S. (2013). *The body economic: Why austerity kills. Recessions, budget battles, and the politics of life and death.* Toronto: HarperCollins.

Swank, D. (1998). *Global capital, democracy, and the welfare state: Why political institutions are so important in shaping the domestic response to internationalization.* Berkeley: University of California Press.

Swedish National Institute of Public Health. (2003). *Sweden's new public health policy.* Retrieved from https://www.drugsandalcohol.ie/5868/1/Sweden_new_public_health_policy_2003.pdf

Teeple, G. (2000). *Globalization and the decline of social reform: Into the twenty-first century* (2nd ed.). Aurora, ON: Garamond.

Vandenbrucke, F. (2002). Foreword. In G. Esping-Andersen (Ed.), *Why we need a new welfare state* (pp. viii–xxvi). New York: Oxford University Press.

Walks, A., & Clifford, B. (2015). The political economy of mortgage securitization and the neoliberalization of housing policy in Canada. *Environment and Planning A: Economy and Space, 47*(8), 1624–1642.

Wolf, R. (2005). What is public policy? *Alberta Health Watch.* Retrieved from http://albertahealthwatch.ca/policy_and_practice.php

Zweig, M. (Ed.). (2004). *What's class got to do with it?: American society in the twenty-first century.* Ithaca, NY: Cornell University Press.

# PART III

## CANADA'S HEALTHCARE SYSTEM

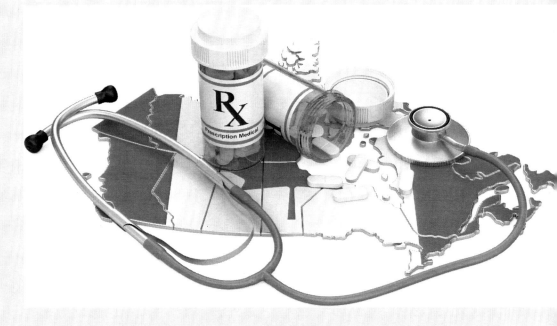

One of the most commented upon differences between Canada and the U.S. is that every Canadian is entitled to doctor and hospital care, while many Americans are subject to bankruptcy and destitution if they become ill. Indeed, the healthcare system in Canada is typically considered the "crown jewel" of Canada's welfare state. These differences in approaches to health care between Canada and the U.S. are of relatively recent origin, however, and reflect different political dynamics in these two nations.

Not surprisingly, healthcare policy is a dominant feature of ongoing public debate and governmental concern in both Canada and the U.S., and the recent decade has seen ongoing attempts to reform and modernize both healthcare systems to meet changing needs and priorities. Central to these attempts at reform are issues of public versus private financing and public versus for-profit healthcare services.

Any understanding of the evolution and future of health care in Canada must consider issues of power and influence. What political and economic forces led to the development of the Canadian healthcare system? How are these forces influencing the current attempts at reform? How do political, economic, and other forces influence the organization and delivery of health care and the responsibilities of various healthcare professionals within this system?

This section considers the history of health care in Canada and how Canada's healthcare system came about. It explores its similarities with—and differences from—the U.S. healthcare system and the forces that led to these differences. Current trends in reform are examined, and issues that will determine its future direction are outlined. Running through all of these issues are questions about public versus private financing and public versus private healthcare services.

In Chapter 10, Georgina Feldberg, Robert Vipond, and Toba Bryant review the history of health care in Canada. They identify the key populations, patterns of illness, institutions, and funding mechanisms that have shaped the evolution of Canadian health care. They show how, until relatively recently, the healthcare systems of Canada and the U.S. were similar, as were the health profiles of the two nations. They then examine the divergence of healthcare approaches in Canada and the U.S. and the health consequences of those differences. Included in this examination are the political developments that led to universal access to health care in Canada and the population-based Medicare and Medicaid programs in the U.S. Some of the powerful economic and political forces that continue to influence these developments, such as recent fiscal crises, are outlined. They also consider the changes that have occurred in both Canada and the U.S. in recent years that may erode access to healthcare services.

In Chapter 11, Mary Wiktorowicz and Michelle Wyndham-West outline some of the key aspects of healthcare systems in Canada and the U.S. They trace very recent developments in healthcare reform in both nations and identify the political, economic, and social forces driving such developments. They also consider lessons that can be learned from other nations and the unique features of change that have occurred in Canada and the U.S. Political structures of Canada and the U.S. are seen as key determinants of whether legislation to reform healthcare systems is successful or not. Some of the key dimensions considered in examination of these healthcare systems are public versus private financing of health care and public versus private delivery of health care. In Canada, concerns with regionalization or jurisdictional organization of health care and integration of services are emerging as key planning issues.

In Chapter 12, Ivy Lynn Bourgeault reviews the development and division of responsibilities in the healthcare system. She highlights the gendered nature of the division of labour and how this has led to the devaluing of the healthcare professions dominated by women, with a particular focus on nursing. Bourgeault is also concerned with how the healthcare division of labour has been differentially affected by recent reforms such as managed care and the privatization of some services. She describes the development of managed care and raises critical questions about this approach. She also examines how increasing privatization of the system is affecting those in various healthcare professions.

# CHAPTER 10

## Cracks in the Foundation: The Origins and Development of the Canadian and American Healthcare Systems

*Georgina Feldberg, Robert Vipond, and Toba Bryant*

## INTRODUCTION

In a CBC online poll, conducted in the fall of 2004, Canadians registered their pride in Canada's healthcare system by naming Tommy Douglas, the father of medicare, the "greatest Canadian" of all time. Almost simultaneously, the Supreme Court of Canada ruled that "the Canada Health Act and the relevant [provincial] legislation do not promise that any Canadian will receive funding for all medically required treatments" (Supreme Court of Canada, 2004). The Court's language, part of its decision on payment for autism treatments, startled many. The decision shook Canadians' pride in a universal, publicly funded system that we believe is comprehensive, serves the needs of all, and distinguishes us from our American neighbours. It seemed to undermine what former Minister of Health Monique Bégin (1988) called "Canada's right to health." Faced with change, we have come to expect that services will increase to meet new needs, whether through the inclusion of ever-expanding medical and surgical interventions or, as in the case of autism treatments, with an acknowledgement of the social determinants of health that extends healthcare funding into non-traditional domains.

As Canadians confront unwelcome challenges to health care, they regularly invoke "history"—the Canadian tradition—to provide a clear set of standards or ideals by which change can be judged. History is used to justify our expectations and, most regularly, to distinguish what is truly Canadian from American ways and practices that do not measure up to our social commitments. However, what is called history is often actually nostalgia, a constructed memory of better ways and better times that glosses over problems, conflicts, and inconsistencies. Despite affirmations of difference, Canada and the U.S. share markedly similar healthcare pasts. Until late in the 20th century, the evolution of healing methods, the design of healthcare institutions and funding systems, and patterns of illness closely paralleled one another. Those similarities suggest that some of the disturbing changes in the Canadian healthcare system do not represent new "Americanization" but, rather, cracks in the historical foundation of Canada's healthcare system. In this chapter, we expose those cracks so that history can be used to outline a path for change rather than to lament a paradise lost.

## THE DEMOGRAPHIC AND SOCIAL ORIGINS OF NORTH AMERICAN HEALTH AND HEALTH CARE (1700–1900)

The marked similarities in the evolution of health care in English Canada[1] and the United States reflect other shared traditions that shape and intersect with health, disease, and healing. Because the two young, industrialized nations were both originally colonies of England, they have common political, cultural, and economic heritages. Both operate under a federal system in which responsibility for health care is split between national and local levels of government and in which the welfare state reflects the dominance of a liberal political tradition. Both nations were built by immigrants; their populations are a mix of Indigenous, European, Asian, Central and South American, and African descendants. Their populations are sparse and spread over similar geographies, large expanses of land that cover diverse climates and terrains. Both built capitalist economies whose growth centred on the creation of transcontinental markets and that are now deeply integrated with each other.

The history of health care in North America begins with the informal healing traditions that emerged in the pre-colonial and colonial periods and predominated until the late 19th century. Prior to the 20th century, few Canadians would have visited a doctor or a hospital. McGill College granted "Canada's" first medical degree in 1833, and both European and locally trained physicians practiced in Upper and Lower Canada (now Ontario and Quebec), but their practices were limited and located primarily in cities. Hospitals, which had strong ties to religious orders, were institutions for the destitute and dying (Connor, 2000). Most Canadians, especially those living outside of cities, relied on informal healing traditions, such as herbalism and midwifery, that had both Indigenous (or local) and European origins. Prior to the arrival of British and French settlers, a range of First Nations practiced herbalism. Teas, smoke, and tinctures (made from the fruit, leaves, berries, or bark of local grasses, plants, and trees) provided remedies for the respiratory, digestive, and skin conditions most common during this period. European colonists similarly relied on herbal and botanical remedies. Though the European preparations were initially distinct, with time the imported and local traditions mixed (Crellin, 1994; Kelm, 1998).

Science, licensing, and regulation were not part of the early healing traditions. Herbalists, midwives, and other healers learned through apprenticeship. Lore, tradition, and reputation ensured the integrity of their healing practices, but there were few formal rules for education or accreditation. The lack of formal regulation allowed for diverse and widespread participation in healing practices that were often informal or rooted in the domestic economy. There were expert herbalists, but mothers regularly taught their daughters how to grow and brew common and essential remedies, recipes that they included in

**Box 10.1:** Canadian Timeline

| | |
|---|---|
| 1400–1850 | Contact between European and Indigenous populations creates new diseases and patterns of spread |
| 1867 | *British North America Act* |
| 1882 | Robert Koch identifies the *tubercle bacillus* |
| 1912 | Lloyd George introduces the *Insurance Act* in Great Britain |
| 1939–1945 | Second World War |
| 1945 | Early attempts at health insurance in Canada and the U.S. |
| 1957 | *Hospital and Diagnostic Services Act* (Canada) |
| 1962 | Saskatchewan doctors' strike |
| 1965 | U.S. Medicare/Medicaid |
| 1967 | *Medical Care Act* (Canada) |
| 1984 | *Canada Health Act* |

family cookbooks. Women regularly gave birth at home, assisted by their family, neighbours, or the local midwife (Biggs, 1983; Mitchinson, 2002).

The *British North America (BNA) Act* (1867), which shaped the constitutional framework of the Canadian federation, reflected contemporary experiences with disease and the relative unimportance of what we now call scientific medicine. Prior to Confederation, Canadians regularly confronted infections and epidemic diseases that had huge social and economic costs. Tuberculosis, typhoid, cholera, and smallpox—the most common infections—decimated Indigenous populations. They disrupted trade, killed young productive citizens, and caused disability that shortened working lives. Throughout the 19th century, most American and Canadian physicians ascribed these diseases to filth and decay rather than germs. Building on the "sanitary ideal" that had developed in Britain, they argued the need for city planning and development that would reduce garbage, promote clean water, and ensure the proper design of communities (Cassel, 1994; MacDougall, 1990). The structures of Canadian government that the *BNA Act* created reflected both the immediacy of health hazards posed by infections and the state of health knowledge. The *BNA Act* split jurisdiction for health care between the federal government and the provinces. Recognizing the economic significance of infections and their implications for trade and the military, the Act assigned to the federal government responsibility for quarantines and marine hospitals. Recognizing that most other interventions against infection (e.g., sanitation) took place at the local level, it implicitly assigned the remaining responsibility for health to provinces and cities. The Act created a relationship between the control of infections, public health, and the state, but it largely ignored curative medicine.

What is now called modern or allopathic biomedicine came into dominance during the late 19th century and changed the structure and delivery of North American health care. In 1882, the German physician Robert Koch provoked a "bacteriologic, immunologic, and chemotherapeutic" revolution when he isolated the bacterium that caused tuberculosis. Koch's postulates allowed physicians and public health departments to focus their attention on the microbes that caused diseases, rather than on the social and physical conditions in which they bred. While some historians argue that many physicians never lost sight of the social and other factors that made individuals vulnerable to bacteria (Feldberg, 1995; Leavitt, 1992), North American medicine nonetheless changed dramatically after 1900. Medical education and research became increasingly scientific and institutional. Healthcare professions became increasingly regulated and stratified by race, class, and gender; male and class dominance emerged in medical practice. Hospitals became centres of care.

## Box 10.2: The Bacteriologic Revolution and the Transformation of Health Care

Prior to the late 19th century, physicians and public health authorities understood that diseases could be spread from person to person. However, they attributed infections to filth and dirt, bad air, smells, and unsanitary conditions, and they believed that behavioural and environmental change were most effective in preventing the spread of diseases.

In 1882, the German physician Robert Koch isolated the bacterium that caused tuberculosis (TB). Using what became known as Koch's postulates, Koch established a causal relationship between bacterial infection and disease. First, Koch isolated bacteria from the blood of a diseased animal. He grew the microbes in a petri dish, injected them back into animals, and observed that these animals developed all the signs and symptoms of the original disease. He then drew blood from the sick animals and showed that he could isolate the same microbes in it.

Koch's work is thought to have inspired a revolution that transformed both the theory and practice of public health. It allowed physicians to focus on controlling bacteria rather than behaviours. It paved the way for the development of antibiotics and vaccines that would treat or prevent infections. By the middle of the 20th century, physicians and pharmaceutical manufacturers had capitalized on the knowledge that bacteria caused infections, and they believed that they had successfully eradicated many infectious diseases.

The bacteriologic revolution was never conceptually or practically complete. Even at its height many physicians continued to recognize that when healthy women and men were exposed to bacteria, they did not always fall ill. Because a healthy host seemed to resist infection, they argued that individuals who ate correctly, slept well, worked and played in moderation, and lived in clean and well-ventilated houses could avoid falling ill. Newly emerging infections, such as SARS and BSE, have also challenged public confidence in the bacteriologic revolution.

By the early decades of the 20th century, North Americans recognized the need to reshape and regulate medical practice. As rigid standards for medical training and licensing emerged, medical schools, which had previously existed informally or independently, sought affiliation with universities. Women, who had played significant roles in informal caregiving, were now excluded from education and practice and sought access to formal medical education. Some of Canada's earliest women physicians went to the U.S. to study. Others founded independent women's medical colleges. Still others demanded access to existing schools and programs.

It is important to note that these changes in medical training and practice affected Canada and the United States in broadly similar ways. In 1910, Abraham Flexner undertook a review of medical schools in the United States and Canada designed to standardize and improve education and care. Canada was included in Flexner's review because of long-standing medical exchanges between the two nations. Like many others, Emily Stowe, Canada's first woman doctor, travelled to the U.S. to study medicine. Leaders of Canadian medicine and nursing, such as Frank Rattray Lillie, William Osler, and Isabel Maitland Stewart, left Canada for the U.S., where they played key roles in education, practice, and research. Philanthropic and voluntary associations, such as the National Tuberculosis Association, spanned both countries. The Rockefeller Foundation, a prominent American funding agency, founded and intellectually shaped public health programs at Ontario and Quebec universities.

Throughout the early decades of the 20th century, a market for health care and a basket of medical services that North Americans sought access to emerged. Instead of relying on informal healing traditions and public health interventions, Americans and Canadians sought the expertise and technology of physicians and hospitals. The ability to pay for these services consequently became paramount, as did the relationship of curative medicine to the state.

## INSURING HEALTH (1900–1980)

Differences in health insurance coverage represent the great divide between Canada and the U.S., yet Canada and U.S. also share early traditions of healthcare insurance. Prior to 1900, when hospitals were primarily institutes for the dying and destitute and medicines were compounded locally, health care was limited and cheap. Professionalism and science combined to make health care more necessary and more costly. By the end of the First World War, most European nations, including England, had recognized a public need for access to hospital and medical care and established some form of government-administered health insurance. Canada and the United States had not. Between 1912 and 1929, American physicians were "almost persuaded" (Numbers, 1978). Despite strong ties with Britain, Canadian doctors avoided and resisted discussions of national health insurance. In 1912, after British Prime Minister Lloyd George introduced his *Insurance Act*, an entry in the *Canadian Medical Association Journal* warned that government insurance plans would undermine the spirit of charity in medicine, turn physicians into civil servants, and create a culture of private practice. The Depression cast national health insurance in a different light. Physicians' medical practices declined during the 1930s, and they struggled to earn a living by bartering services for goods. In this climate of economic crisis, existing insurance plans—offered by benevolent associations, religious orders, or insurance providers—either failed or proved inadequate. Medical associations consequently began to lobby for government health plans that would ensure access to care and payment to care providers. In 1934, the Canadian Medical Association (CMA) accused provincial and municipal governments of failing to provide necessary medical care for the indigent and unemployed, and it proposed the remedy of "state health insurance." As late as 1943, a strong majority of physicians who belonged to the CMA continued to support this position (Bothwell & English, 1976).

Following the Second World War, plans for national health insurance emerged in both Canada and the United States. In 1945, Prime Minister William Lyon Mackenzie King introduced his plan for national health insurance to the Dominion-Provincial Conference on Reconstruction. Mere months later, President Harry S. Truman presented an ambitious plan for universal health insurance to Congress. Both plans failed. Fears of socialism and government encroachment on individual liberties blocked Truman's efforts (Kooijman, 1999). The bickering over provincial–federal jurisdiction that has come to characterize discussions of health reform proved the Canadian obstacle; several Canadian provinces rejected King's plans for a national health insurance scheme on grounds that it encroached on provincial jurisdiction in health (Tuohy, 1999).

Early plans for national health insurance failed, but during the 1950s, government spending on health care nonetheless increased in both Canada and the U.S. Setting what might be seen as a pattern, Ottawa approved new expenditures for hospital construction throughout the decade. The United States Congress made extensive investments in medical research, medical education, and hospital construction during the same period. In short, both countries invested heavily in medical education, research, and hospitals, but neither moved to ensure broad access to medical services.

The growth of hospitals, their emergence as treatment centres, and the escalating costs of hospital care prompted the need for broader insurance coverage. In 1957, Canada responded to an emerging crisis by implementing the *Hospital and Diagnostic Services Act*. This plan made coverage of hospital services more readily and widely available, but even then, only half of Canadians had coverage for any other kind of expense. Patterns of coverage were similar in the United States, where employment-based and veterans' plans provided coverage for many families, and Blue Cross emerged as a major hospital insurance provider. In both countries, about 60% of services were covered, but disparities were huge. Over 90% of those Americans who worked in the highly unionized manufacturing sector had extensive coverage, but only 40% of farm workers had any. First Nations communities, women, and immigrants were underserved in both countries. Urban–rural and regional disparities were also great (Starr, 1982).

The struggle to instate health insurance as a democratic right of citizenship took real shape in 1961 when Premier Tommy Douglas, a Baptist minister and leader of Saskatchewan's social democratic government, introduced a comprehensive medical insurance plan in the province. By the 1960s, medicine had become lucrative, and the CMA members who had supported national or public health insurance plans no longer needed government funding. They prospered financially, and they commanded considerable respect from their patients and communities. Hence, Saskatchewan's physicians now staunchly opposed Douglas's efforts. The Saskatchewan medicare plan, which culminated in the historic doctors' strike of 1962, fundamentally shaped the structure and tensions of Canadian health care by institutionalizing the model of private practice/public payment. In introducing medicare, the Douglas government committed itself to creating a system that was "acceptable both to those providing the service and those receiving it" (Naylor, 1986, p. 182). On the one hand, the Saskatchewan plan promised all citizens, regardless of financial circumstances, a comprehensive system of medical services that was financed through taxes and administered publicly. On the other, the Saskatchewan plan acknowledged the powerful interests of physicians. From the outset, the Douglas plan rejected European models that paid physicians by capitation (the number of patients listed in their practice) or salary in favour of the traditional fee-for-service model of payment. Physicians continued to practice as individuals and to bill by service, but the government, rather than the individual patient or an insurance company, now paid the bill.

Saskatchewan's plan became the inspiration for Canada's national health insurance program, known as medicare. It put into place the guiding principles of the 1967 *Medical Care Act*: universality (all citizens are entitled to health coverage), comprehensiveness (all "medically necessary" services are covered), and portability (all Canadian citizens and permanent residents are entitled to care regardless of where in Canada they live or travel). By 1972, when the Yukon introduced its medical services insurance plan, medicare was in place throughout Canada.

The implementation of national health insurance seemed to distinguish Canada and the U.S. starkly. However, the differences were not initially very great. Throughout the 1960s and 1970s, the U.S. government also implemented programs that made health services available to a broader public. The U.S. focused its efforts on vulnerable populations. The *Migrant Health Act* of 1962 and President Lyndon B. Johnson's "War on Poverty" provided U.S. federal funding for rural health clinics, maternal and child health programs, community mental health services, and neighbourhood health centres. In 1965, amendments to the *Social Security Act* established Medicare and Medicaid, which extended coverage to the elderly and the poor. Medicare, a national program with uniform standards for eligibility and benefits, covered all hospital and some physician costs for Americans over 65 and some people with disabilities. Medicaid, a joint federal–state program, provided federal grants to the states to reimburse doctors and hospitals that cared for medical indigents and people on welfare.

Costs, coverage, and health status did not differ significantly north and south of the Canada–U.S. border either. In 1971, the U.S. and Canada spent essentially the same percentage of their gross national product on health care—7.6% and 7.4%, respectively—and the vast majority of citizens had access to some medical services. In 1976, nearly 90% of Americans had either public or private health insurance, a rate not so very different from Canada. Throughout the first half of the 20th century, mortality and morbidity from the leading causes of death—infectious diseases, like tuberculosis—were similar in Canada and the U.S. Thereafter, key health status indicators, such as infant and maternal mortality, remained comparable. In 1940, maternal mortality, calculated as maternal deaths per 100,000 live births, stood at 400 in Canada and 376 in the U.S. After 1950, infant and maternal mortality rates declined significantly, and by 1960 maternal deaths in both countries had decreased by half to about 200. During the next two decades, they fell to less than 10 per 100,000 (United States Bureau of the Census, 1975, p. 109).

## Box 10.3: Measuring the Impacts of Medical Interventions

During the 20th century, national and international health agencies regularly used a series of indicators to measure the effectiveness of medical and public health interventions. Because public health interventions originally developed in Europe as part of mercantilist assumptions about the economic benefits of a strong population, many indicators focused on population growth. Life expectancy (the number of years men or women could expect to live to) was one indicator. National rates of maternal and infant mortality also became common measures of the success of healthcare systems. Maternal mortality is the number of women who die in childbirth; infant mortality is the number of children under one year of age who die. Reducing maternal and infant mortality was a key health goal of the early healthcare policy reforms. Reductions in maternal and infant mortality were taken as signs that medical and technological interventions into birth had been successful. They were seen as evidence that medical "advances" had reduced infections associated with birth and early childhood and that those medical procedures had been made widely available.

There are two problems with historical mortality indicators. First, national averages hide significant race and class differences. It is important to note that in both Canada and the U.S., the average rates do not expose the significant death rates in Native, African-American, Hispanic, and other minority populations. For example, in Canada, rates of maternal and infant mortality have traditionally been, and continue to be, much higher in northern First Nations communities than in the rest of the country. In the U.S., minority populations similarly have higher rates of maternal and infant mortality. Second, statistics are difficult to keep when births occur outside hospitals. Most important, while reductions in mortality are often attributed to medical intervention, changes may actually reflect social and economic changes.

# CHANGES IN HEALTH, CHANGES IN COVERAGE (1984–2000)

The *Canada Health Act* of 1984 changed the delivery of health care and marked a point of significant departure between Canada and the U.S. Canada's national health plan insured services. The United States had chosen instead to insure populations. By the 1980s, inequities resulting from both approaches were apparent. Canada's *Medical Care Act* (1967) had allowed for private billing above the medicare cap. This included provincial premiums and co-payments for specialist services. In particular, obstetricians and gynecologists could bill patients above the approved government rate, and this "extra billing" reduced access to care. Canadians living in remote areas, women, and minorities were differentially disadvantaged by the premiums and co-payments that national health insurance allowed.

In the U.S., Medicare and Medicaid covered less than half the medical expenses of senior citizens and one-third of health costs for the poor. Like private insurance plans, Medicare limited coverage of hospital stays to a set number of days, and it paid only part of approved physicians' fees or other forms of out-patient care. Recipients were responsible for the remaining charges, and many purchased supplementary private insurance to help cover the extra costs. Seniors who could not afford the co-payment required by Medicare, either because they were already poor or because a long illness had drained their bank accounts, often found themselves on Medicaid. Because Medicaid was funded out of general revenues at both the state and federal levels, the base coverage from state to state was uneven. Moreover, Medicaid carried a stigma of welfare or public assistance.

The *Canada Health Act* of 1984 strengthened Canada's commitment to universal health insurance by prohibiting premiums and extra billing. It ensured that virtually all Canadians had access to medical services. In contrast, public and private commitments to health insurance declined in the U.S. In 1988, 13% of Americans under 65 had no private or public health insurance. The number of Americans without health insurance rose dramatically thereafter. Drastic reductions in funding for Medicare and Medicaid were one source of decreased coverage. The rising costs of health benefits eroded pre-tax corporate profits, so that many companies reduced health insurance coverage. As a result, employees paid greater percentages of premiums and costs. The percentage of Americans with no insurance coverage also increased because of corporate restructuring; full-time staff were replaced by part-time employees who had no entitlement to benefits. By 1992, the number of Americans who were not insured had risen to 38.9 million, or 17.4% of the population under 65. Another 40 million were underinsured. Health care even began to seem unaffordable to middle-class Americans, many of whom worried that they might have financial difficulty paying for the costs of a major illness (Tuohy, 1999).

Key health status indicators began to reflect these national differences in access to health care. Maternal mortality once again provides an example. Dramatic declines in maternal mortality, often attributed to increased and improved access to medical care, occurred in both the U.S. and Canada between 1900 and 1980. However, between 1982 and

1999, there was no further decline in maternal mortality in the U.S. By 1990, the U.S. rate of 12/100,000 was double the Canadian rate of 6/100,000 (World Health Organization, 1996). The difference in rates reflected the ability of young and indigent mothers to access appropriate medical care. It also reflected different levels of access to social and economic resources that are key to health.

The *Canada Health Act* was passed during a period of broad, global rethinking of health care and the determinants of health. The change in name, from the *Medical Care Act* to the *Canada Health Act*, reflected this new approach. Four sources of discontent affected the ways in which this rethinking occurred in Canada and the U.S.: (1) apparent increases in the costs of healthcare spending; (2) changing patterns of disease that drew attention to the limitation of existing insurance plans; (3) a commitment to alternative forms of service delivery; and (4) populist critiques of scientific medicine that intersected with a consumer rights and activist agenda. This latter stream included critics who saw the value of medical interventions, but wanted relief from unnecessary medical procedures and other abuses of medical power; it also included those who questioned the priority given to biomedicine and looked for extra-medical alternatives.

At the end of the 1980s, Canada spent only 8.6% of its GNP on health care, while in the United States, spending had risen to 11.4%. But by the 1990s, some Canadian health economists also sounded the alarm over rising healthcare expenditures: the portion of GNP spent on healthcare had jumped by 10%. As the North American medical system grew more expensive, escalating costs seemed to present a crisis. Subsequent studies would attribute the apparent rise in Canadian healthcare spending to a decline in the economy as a whole, rather than an absolute rise in healthcare expenditures, but physicians, politicians, economists, and the public all worried that costs were spiralling out of control while the quality of care declined (Tuohy, 1999).

Some responded to the apparent fiscal crisis by focusing on excesses in "consumer demand." Seeking culprits, American politicians and physicians blamed Medicare and Medicaid, which, having finally made medical services accessible to senior citizens and the poor, achieved their objectives of democratizing use. When Medicare or Medicaid coverage made it possible for Americans to visit physicians, the number of office visits often increased in the covered populations. One study suggested that, in 1964, poor Americans went to the doctor 20% *less* often than more affluent Americans; 10 years later, they visited the doctor 18% *more often* (Starr, 1982). Canadians, like Ontario Premier Mike Harris, also blamed "consumer abuse" of the system. Others focused on the "supply side" of the equation. When the Canada Health and Social Transfer (CHST) reduced federal transfer payments, Manitoba, Ontario, and other provinces imposed caps on the amount physicians could bill in any given year, and hence on the numbers of patients they could see. Doctors and administrators tried to cut spending by restructuring the hospital system in ways that would reduce expenditures on costly hospital services and shift care into the community. Many provinces delisted services they considered non-essential (like in vitro fertilization and cosmetic surgery) from compulsory coverage. Provincial leaders with strained budgets questioned whether new immigrants, especially those with pre-existing chronic illness, should be eligible for healthcare benefits. These changes intensified regional, economic, and gender-based disparities in access to care. Canadians living in small towns, rural areas, and the North complained about the concentration of new technology in large cities. Increasing numbers of homeless Canadians found themselves without adequate access to care.

Other "reformers" seized the opportunity to develop new options for financing and delivering medical care. They critiqued fee-for-service and other payment schemes that created incentives for the use of costly services, and they proposed alternatives, like the health maintenance organizations (HMOs). First introduced in the 1970s, HMOs and their Canadian counterpart, the health service organization (HSO), initially promised to provide integrated care at lower cost. Prepaid a fixed sum per patient, administrators received bonuses for keeping costs low and patients out of hospitals. Many provinces took part in the experiment in group practice. Quebec led the way with local community health centres, and English Canada introduced a range of alternative forms of service delivery, community health centres among them.

HMOs, HSOs, and other alternative delivery plans also promised to broaden health coverage. Panic over rising costs hijacked the healthcare debate, and the intensity of concerns about financing drew attention away from more fundamental questions about the definitions of health and health care. After 1950, infectious diseases declined in North America. Tuberculosis, which had been the "costliest of communicable diseases" and "the leading cause of death," all but disappeared from view. Chronic diseases—heart disease, cancer, diabetes, and depression—replaced infections as the leading causes of North American deaths.

As Canadians reflected on their healthcare system, many critics noted that healthcare services needed to shift to prevent and accommodate new conditions. They drew attention to the interconnections between poverty, life experience, and disease. They drew distinctions between preventive public health and medical care; they argued for public investment in health rather than health care.

Proposals for new forms of service delivery attempted to address some of these concerns about the limits to modern medicine. HMOs in the U.S., for example, provided

**Table 10.1:** Changes in Mortality, 1900–1975, Deaths per 100,000

| Year | Tuberculosis | Heart Disease | Cancers |
|------|-------------|---------------|---------|
| 1900 | 194 | 137 | 64 |
| 1950 | 30 | 322 | 135 |
| 1975 | 3.9 | 1,037 | 351 |

Source: United States Bureau of the Census. (1975). *Historical statistics of the United States: Colonial times to 1970.* Washington, DC: Government Printing Office.

an opportunity to change both the kind of care that was delivered and the way it was delivered. Attractive to those who sought to reduce costs, HMOs also had appeal across the political spectrum because prepaid group practices seemed to provide an opportunity to achieve "equity and access" (Fein, 1972). They combatted the focus on physicians and the limitations of solo practice. Early models, such as the Harvard Community Health Plan, appealed to the progressive left because they integrated the services of a range of healthcare providers. In Canada, HSOs and *centres locaux de santé communitaire* (CLSCs) also found support because they improved access to health services and broadened the scope of care. The *Medical Services Act*, as reflected in its title, provided payment only for medical services that *physicians* delivered. HSOs and CLSCs finessed these limitations. They encouraged physicians to work in groups with other practitioners (such as massage therapists or psychologists) whose services were not included in the medicare basket. The HSO paid physicians a salary or capitation fee, rather than the approved fee for service, and any savings could be used to publicly finance non-medical services. The new practices also shifted the site of integrated care from hospital to community.

HMOs became symbols of the chaotic American medical scene, "managed care," and consumer discontent. In the U.S., they shifted the "problem" from overmedicalization to undertreatment, yet undertreatment is a problem only if tests and prescriptions are actually necessary. As proponents have noted, HMOs can lack the incentive to overtreat and emphasize and encourage preventive health measures, such as Pap smears. They rely on family physicians or nurse practitioners, who use fewer tests and less invasive procedures than specialists. In many HMOs, for example, nurse-midwives, rather than obstetricians, deliver babies in normal births.

HMOs, HSOs, and other alternative forms of service delivery helped to reduce healthcare costs, promised to enhance access to care, and broadened the meaning of care. Despite this, they addressed only part of the problem. As the government of Canada renewed its commitment to universal coverage for medical care, increasing numbers of historians, demographers, and epidemiologists challenged the relationship between medicine and health. Thomas McKeown's (1980) *The Role of Medicine* questioned whether medicine had improved the health of Europeans and attributed increasing longevity and declining mortality to improvements in the standard of living. National governments, led by the World Health Organization (1978), affirmed that health was more than the absence of disease. At Alma Ata, they affirmed the importance of economic and social determinants of health. The re-emergence of tuberculosis and other infections drew attention to historical patterns of disease and disease control and shaped a challenge to the premises of the bacteriologic revolution. Physicians, they found, had rarely focused narrowly on the bacterial causes of disease; they had regularly argued that these diseases were due in large part to "social misery." Epidemiologic and other analyses consistently showed a correlation between social spending and health status, so that Nordic and Northern European countries had the best indicators.

North American health policy did not always heed this new emphasis on health or these new directions in health research. The *Canada Health Act* changed the parameters of funding and language, but it did not change the emphasis or direction of spending. Rather than integrating social and health spending, when Canadian governments reframed and reviewed healthcare financing during the 1990s, they repeatedly revised funding formulas to divorce social spending from healthcare spending. The separation of funding envelopes for health, education, and welfare allowed spending on medical care to increase and investment in health—education, work, and housing that increase health status—to decrease.

## RECENT DEVELOPMENTS IN HEALTH CARE

Throughout the second decade of the 21st century, Canadians have faced increasing problems with equity, access, and quality of care. Declining federal transfers to provincial and territorial healthcare plans, block funding for health and social programs, and the steady reduction of federal contributions to provincial and territorial healthcare plans have reduced services and forced provincial and territorial governments to bear a larger share of healthcare costs that rise each year (Armstrong & Armstrong, 2003).

Reduced federal transfers, alongside ever-increasing healthcare costs, have led provincial governments to consider a range of market mechanisms that they hope will reduce healthcare spending. These include public–private partnerships (P3s) to build hospitals and other social service infrastructures, and expanding the role the private sector plays in financing and delivering healthcare services. Provincial governments have delisted prescription medications previously covered by provincial drug formularies, transferred services to the home or community (outside the funded hospital system), and introduced user fees for some healthcare services that were previously insured under provincial healthcare plans. Ontario, for example, eliminated coverage for eye examinations. These changes have all been justified as ensuring the financial sustainability of the healthcare system (Butler, 2017; Canadian Union of Public Employees, 2017; Flood, 2006).

In marked contrast to the United States, where the election of President Obama in 2008 provoked comprehensive debate about the public financing and delivery of health care, during this first decade of the 21st century, the Canadian debate has become increasingly narrow. Canadian healthcare reform has concentrated on a limited range of issues, such as the delivery of care and wait times (Rachlis, 2004). Public policy-makers have focused on the efficiency advantages of increased commercialization of health care, even though the evidence to date shows that allowing private providers to deliver health care neither reduces wait times in the public system nor provides better quality care.

As noted in Chapter 9, former President Barack Obama signed the *The Patient Protection and Affordable Care Act* into law on March 23, 2010 (Hall & Lord, 2014). The Act changed the American healthcare landscape, but it did not create a universal healthcare system as exists in Canada and other countries. It universalized access to healthcare services but did nothing about excessive co-payments or limits on insurance. It did not remove the for-profit aspects of health insurance. This legislation is considered among the most contentious since the Civil Rights era in the U.S. It was devised as a middle-ground solution that retains private health insurance for most American citizens but changes the market to promote rather than weaken policy goals (Hall & Lord, 2014).

Anything perceived as related to socialism, such as proposals to implement a single-payer system, are rejected outright in the U.S. As long as this is the case, the U.S. will likely continue to outspend nations with universal health care. The latest data from the Organisation for Economic Co-operation and Development (OECD) shows that the U.S. continues to outspend other countries on health. In 2016, the U.S. spent 17% of GDP on health care, compared to 11% of GDP in comparable countries (Sawyer & Cox, 2018). On average, the U.S. spends $10,224 U.S. on health per person, compared to approximately $5,280 U.S. per person in comparable OECD countries.

Canadian medicare is also undergoing changes that threaten equitable access to health care, a cornerstone of the system. During the 2015 federal general election campaign, the Liberal Party promised to renegotiate the 2004 *Health Accord*, the 10-year plan to strengthen the healthcare system. Since its election, however, the majority Liberal government has not renegotiated the 2004 accord.

Instead, the federal government has negotiated bilateral agreements with all the provinces except Manitoba. These agreements lock in the Harper cutbacks of increases at 3% per year with some additional funds for home care and mental health of approximately $11 billion over a 10-year period. Advocacy groups have raised concerns about the implications for healthcare service provision, particularly the impact of under-resourcing. The bilateral agreements do not include investment for enforcement of the *Canada Health Act*. This raises fears about a potential shift toward further privatization, extra-billing by physicians, and two-tiered health care that will lead to inequitable access to healthcare services.

A considerable body of research evidence from countries that have adopted a two-tiered system suggests that those waiting for care in the public system cannot afford private care; that a parallel private healthcare system would draw resources, particularly human health resources, away from the public system; and that the private sector can provide powerful incentives for physicians and allied health professions to leave the public system (Flood, Stabile, & Kontic, 2005). There are no assurances that equity, access, or quality would increase were Canada to replace its historical tradition of "private practice, public payment" with a system in which private payment played a greater part (Laugesen, 2005).

Finally, the issue of Canada's healthcare system not covering prescription drugs outside of hospital has again raised the importance of pharmacare as a necessary component of Canada's healthcare system. While the benefits of such a program are widely recognized, governments continue to be reluctant to institute such a program (Canadian Medical Association, 2016).

## CONCLUSIONS

Saskatchewan's celebrated public health insurance plan provided the model for Canadian medicare. It also set some of the cracks in Canada's healthcare foundation. It provided the model for private practice–public payment, which has challenged the very existence of Canadian medicare; it reinforced battles over provincial and federal jurisdiction; and it set the framework for an insurance scheme in which medicine and medical care dominated.

Canada's national medicare plan did much to address who paid for medical services, but it did little to change the delivery of services. Canadian doctors remained in private practice and billed medicare for a set fee per service. To an important extent, then, the founders of medicare, first in Saskatchewan, then nationally, built a tension into the healthcare system between the egalitarian ends (universal and accessible medical services) and the market-based means (delivery by physicians in private practice). Defenders of medicare worry that the establishment of a parallel system of private clinics in provinces like Alberta will create a two-tiered healthcare system in which wealthier citizens will have preferential access to treatment. It is important to realize that this challenge feeds off the original compromises that created room, within Canada's healthcare system, for wealth-maximizing private practice.

This fee structure was determined by negotiations between doctors and each province. The national health insurance system was financed partly by the federal government, but since the Canadian constitution assigns responsibility for health care to the provinces, medicare is administered at the provincial level. From the start, hospitals and physicians were also the backbone of the system. Until 1984, when the *Canada Health Act* prohibited extra billing, co-payments, in the form of provincial premiums, were allowed, and specialists, including obstetricians and gynecologists, were permitted to bill patients above the government rate. As in the United States, hospitals rather than community clinics remained the site of most healthcare delivery.

The original medicare plan, incubated in Saskatchewan and then appropriated nationally, is often used as an example of what is good about federalism. Yet it is also clear that the peculiar division of jurisdiction in the Canadian federation—in which the federal government has the dominant fiscal capacity while the provinces possess most of the constitutional authority to deliver programs—has created a policy environment in which discord and competition are endemic. More than this, the disconnect between payment (Ottawa) and delivery (provinces) of social programs has made it extremely difficult to imagine how the two levels of government would work together to accomplish what the Nordic countries have done—namely, to seriously frame programs that go beyond medical services and address the social determinants of health.

The Supreme Court of Canada's decision regarding autism treatments points to a third crack in the foundation of Canada's healthcare system. Canadians enjoy a publicly funded health insurance scheme, in which eligibility is universal and not predicated on income, marriage, or employment. However, the emphasis on medical care restricts the range of services covered. Ironically, midwifery is not covered under Canada's universal health system. Legalized only in 1994 in Ontario and Alberta, coverage for midwifery remains outside the public financing system of many provinces. Similarly, alternative health services—including counselling, chiropractic, naturopathic therapy, homeopathic therapy, and hydrotherapy—available through many private insurers in the United States, are not made publicly available to Canadians.

More critically, a range of health-promoting services fall outside of the domain of both federal and provincial health departments. New patterns of mortality and morbidity have created new needs and expectations, not all of which are or can be met by our current system. The limitations reflect our history. The *BNA Act* initially made public health interventions the domain of the state; it overlooked private practice and curative medicine. The reforms of the 1960s addressed the new status of biomedicine and brought physicians and treatment into public financing plans. However, as those reforms took place, patterns of disease shifted. The new diseases, often labelled lifestyle diseases, are actually diseases of circumstance. They reflect living conditions, poverty, and access to housing and income. For historical reasons, Canada has not integrated these social and economic domains into the modern organization or financing of health.

## CRITICAL THINKING QUESTIONS

1. What distinguished the delivery of health care in the periods before and after 1900?
2. In what three ways were healthcare systems in the U.S. and Canada similar before 1980?
3. Saskatchewan's experiment in publicly funded health insurance laid the foundation for Canadian medicare. What principles did the Saskatchewan model establish?
4. What are three foundational cracks in Canada's national health insurance plan?
5. How did the *Medical Care Act* enhance health care in Canada, and how did it compromise the achievement of health?

## FURTHER READINGS

Feldberg, G., Ladd-Taylor, M., Li, A., & McPherson, K. (2003). *Women, health, and nation: Canada and the U.S. since 1945*. Montreal and Kingston: McGill-Queen's University Press.
Changes in the financing and delivery of health care had special implications for women. The introduction to this collection outlines the diverging and converging histories of health and health care in Canada and the U.S. The essays explore the ways in which women promoted and were affected by changes in the financing and delivery of health care.

McKeown, T. (1976). *The modern rise of population*. New York: Academic Press.
This classic work challenges the received wisdom that European population growth was the result of medical "advances," such as the conquest of infectious disease. McKeown was one of the first to suggest that social and economic factors played a critical role.

Naylor, C. D. (1986). *Private practice, public payment: Canadian medicine and the politics of health insurance, 1911–1966*. Montreal and Kingston: McGill-Queen's University Press.

An outline of the development of publicly funded health insurance in Canada, this book describes and explains the tensions built into the medicare system. It underscores the ways in which fee-for-service models threaten universal health insurance.

Naylor, C. D. (2003). *Learning from SARS: Renewal of public health in Canada, a report of the National Advisory Committee on SARS*. Ottawa: National Advisory Committee on SARS and Public Health.
A report to Health Canada, this document outlines the history of public health initiatives and points to the ways in which historical patterns shape current health responses.

Tuohy, C. H. (1999). *Accidental logics: The dynamics of change in the health care arena in the United States, Britain, and Canada*. New York and Oxford: Oxford University Press.
An analysis of the compounded financial crises facing the healthcare systems in Canada, the United States, and Britain, this book shows how different "accidents" of history have shaped the dilemmas facing the healthcare systems in the three countries.

## RELEVANT WEBSITES

### Health Council of Canada
www.healthcouncilcanada.ca

No longer being funded by the Government of Canada, the Health Council of Canada fostered accountability and transparency by assessing progress in improving the quality, effectiveness, and sustainability of the healthcare system. Archived publications, videos, news, and events, as well as external links, are all posted on the site.

### Statistics Canada
https://www150.statcan.gc.ca/n1/en/subjects/Health

This Statistics Canada website contains historical health statistics for Canada that can be used to track patterns of health and disease.

### U.S. Census Bureau
www2.census.gov/prod2/statcomp

This U.S. government website contains historical statistics for the United States from the 1700s onward. It can be used to track changes in health and disease.

### The Tommy Douglas Webpage
https://sites.google.com/site/tommydouglaswebpage/about-tommy-douglas

This website chronicles the achievements of Tommy Douglas, the father of Canadian medicare. It provides sections on his life as a minister, his political career, and his interest in medicare.

**World Health Organization**
www.who.int
This website for the World Health Organization includes historical disease and health statistics, along with declarations about health services and healthcare interventions.

## GLOSSARY

**Alternative service delivery:** A general term used to refer to the organization and payment of medical services. It includes group practices, such as health maintenance organizations (HMOs), health service organizations (HSOs), or *centres locaux de santé communitaire* (CLSCs). It is designed to reduce healthcare spending, ensure continuity of care, and extend coverage to a wider range of services. More recently, it has been associated with efforts to contain costs and reduce the quality of care.

**Canada Health Act (1984):** The CHA supplanted the *Medical Care Act* as the foundation of the Canadian medicare system. In particular, the CHA reinforced the principles of Canadian medicare by penalizing provinces financially if they allowed physicians to extra bill—that is, charge patients over and above the amount paid by the government for their services.

**Canada Health and Social Transfer (CHST):** The CHST is a block funding arrangement that was introduced in the federal budget in 1995. It replaced the Established Programs Financing (EPF) and the Canada Assistance Plan (CAP). Through fiscal years 1996–97 and 1997–98, total CHST was capped at $26.9 billion and $25.1 billion, respectively. As a result of the 2003 First Ministers' Accord on Health Care renewal, the CHST was restructured to establish a separate Canada Health Transfer and Canada Social Transfer. The intention was to enhance transparency and accountability.

**Medical Care Act (1967):** The act of Parliament that enshrined a national program of hospital and medical insurance on the "Saskatchewan model." The Act established joint responsibility for the delivery of health care in Canada, with the federal government providing funding and the provincial governments responsible for delivering health care. By 1972, the *Medical Care Act* was in place across the country in 10 provinces and two territories.

**Medicare:** In both Canada (medicare) and the United States (Medicare), a government-funded program of health insurance. In Canada, medicare is defined by the hospital and medical services that are provided. In the United States, Medicare is delimited by the population it serves, specifically the elderly.

## NOTE

1.  The evolution of health care and healing in Quebec has distinctive characteristics that are beyond the scope of this chapter.

## REFERENCES

Armstrong, H., & Armstrong, P. 2003. *Wasting away: The undermining of Canadian health care.* Toronto: Oxford University Press.

Bégin, M. (1988). *Medicare: Canada's right to health.* Montreal: Optimum Publishing International.

Biggs, C. L. (1983). The case of the missing midwives: A history of midwifery in Ontario from 1795–1900. *Ontario History, 75*(1), 21–36.

Bothwell, R.S., & English, J. (1976). Pragmatic physicians: Canadian medicine, and healthcare insurance, 1910–1945. *University of Western Ontario Medical Journal, 47*(3), 14–17.

Butler, M. (2017). Health accord loss means a new decade of our public health care being underfunded. *The Council of Canadians.* Retrieved from https://canadians.org/blog/health-accord-loss-means-new-decade-our-public-health-care-being-underfunded

Canadian Medical Association. (2016). *National pharmacare in Canada: Getting there from here.* Ottawa: Author.

Canadian Union of Public Employees. (2017). Health care—why bilateral deals are a problem. Retrieved from https://cupe.ca/health-care-why-bilateral-deals-are-a-problem

Cassel, J. (1994). Public health in Canada. In D. Porter (Ed.), *The history of public health and the modern state* (pp. 276–312). Leiden: Rodopi.

Connor, J. T. H. (2000). *Doing good: The life of Toronto's general hospital.* Toronto: University of Toronto Press.

Crellin, J. K. (1994). *Home medicine: The Newfoundland experience.* Montreal: McGill-Queen's University Press.

Fein, R. (1972). On achieving access and equity in healthcare. *Milbank Memorial Fund Quarterly, 50*(4), 157–190.

Feldberg, G. D. (1995). *Disease and class: Tuberculosis and the shaping of modern North American society.* New Brunswick, NJ: Rutgers University Press.

Flood, C. M. (Ed.). (2006). *Just medicare: What's in, what's out, how we decide.* Toronto: University of Toronto Press.

Flood, C. M., Stabile, M., & Kontic, S. (2005). The evidence on waiting, dying, and two-tier systems. In C. M. Flood, K. Roach, & L. Sossin (Eds.), *Access to care, access to justice: The legal debate over private health insurance in Canada* (pp. 296–320). Toronto: University of Toronto Press.

Hall, M. A., & Lord, R. (2014). Obamacare: What the *Affordable Care Act* means for patients and physicians. *British Medical Journal, 349*, g5376. doi:10.1136/bmj.g5376.

Kelm, M. (1998). *Colonizing bodies: Aboriginal health and healing in British Columbia, 1900–1950.* Vancouver: UBC Press.

Kooijman, J. (1999). *And the pursuit of national health: The incremental strategy toward national health insurance.* Atlanta, GA: Rodopoi.

Laugesen, M. J. (2005). Why some market reforms lack legitimacy in health care. *Journal of Health Politics, Policy, and Law, 30*(6), 1065–1108. doi: 10.1215/03616878-30-6-1065

Leavitt, J. W. (1992). Typhoid Mary strikes back: Bacteriological theory and practice in early twentieth-century public health. *Isis, 83*(4), 608–629.

MacDougall, H. (1990). *Activists and advocates: Toronto's health department, 1883–1983.* Toronto: Dundurn Press.

McKeown, T. (1980). *The role of medicine: Dream, mirage, or nemesis?* Princeton, NJ: Princeton University Press.

Mitchinson, W. (2002). *Giving birth in Canada, 1900–1950.* Toronto: University of Toronto Press.

Naylor, C. D. (1986). *Private practice, public payment: Canadian medicine and the politics of health insurance, 1911–1966.* Montreal: McGill-Queen's University Press.

Numbers, R. L. (1978). *Almost persuaded: American physicians and compulsory health insurance 1912–1920.* Baltimore: Johns Hopkins University Press.

Rachlis, M. (2004). *Prescription for excellence: How innovation is saving Canada's health care system.* Toronto: HarperCollins.

Sawyer, B., & Cox, C. (2018). How does health spending in the U.S. compare to other countries? *Peterson Center on Health Care and Kaiser Family Foundation.* Retrieved from https://www.healthsystemtracker.org/chart-collection/health-spending-u-s-compare-countries/#item-relative-size-wealth-u-s-spends-disproportionate-amount-health

Starr, P. (1982). *The social transformation of American medicine: The rise of a sovereign profession and the making of a vast industry.* New York: Basic Books.

Supreme Court of Canada. (2004). *Auton (Guardian ad litem of) v. British Columbia (Attorney General).* Ottawa: Supreme Court of Canada. Retrieved from https://scc-csc.lexum.com/scc-csc/scc-csc/en/item/2195/index.do

Tuohy, C. H. (1999). *Accidental logics: The dynamics of change in the health care arena in the United States, Britain, and Canada.* New York: Oxford University Press.

United States Bureau of the Census. (1975). *Historical statistics of the United States: Colonial times to 1970.* Washington, DC: Government Printing Office.

World Health Organization. (1978). *Declaration of Alma Ata.* Retrieved from www/who.int

World Health Organization. (1996). *Revised 1990 estimates of maternal mortality.* Geneva: World Health Organization.

# CHAPTER 11

## Evolution of Healthcare Policy: Deconstructing Divergent Approaches

*Mary E. Wiktorowicz and Michelle Wyndham-West*

## INTRODUCTION

The healthcare systems in Canada and the United States have evolved along different paths. In this chapter, we explore the manner in which political and economic forces have shaped the divergence in healthcare systems, along with recent reforms. Lessons from developments in other nations are considered, and unique aspects of change in Canada and the U.S. are examined for their impact upon the health of citizens. Recent developments in medicare in Canada and the introduction of the *Patient Protection and Affordable Care Act of 2010* (ACA) in the U.S. are of special interest.

At the close of the 20th century, the healthcare systems in Canada and the United States were founded on different ideological premises and political authority, and these forces continue to shape their evolution. Canada and the U.S.'s responses to the challenges of access to and escalating costs of health care have, in turn, led them to embrace different approaches with some similarities. With respect to approaches to achieve "integrated health systems," similar examples can be found in both nations. At the same time, the strategies adopted to address issues of pharmaceutical cost and access demonstrate divergent paths. In exploring the most important aspects of policy convergence and divergence that Canada and the U.S. have adopted toward their healthcare sectors, we consider how the different political systems in each state have shaped recent restructuring efforts, and how international systems of care have informed the directions taken.

## DIVERGING PREMISES FOR HEALTHCARE SYSTEMS

The legislative and political structures that guide democratic reform in Canada and the U.S. shape their approaches to social policy, and the healthcare sector represents one of the most significant areas of divergence, even with the introduction of the ACA in the U.S. Several political and historical forces have influenced the design and delivery of health care in Canada and the United States, which we explore through the lenses of ideological perspective, political authority, including legislative agendas, and modes of financing and delivery.

## Ideological Perspective

Most countries have common goals regarding health care that include:

- *Social protection*: Enable those with fewer resources to access health care.
- *Redistribution*: Redistribute healthcare costs among individuals, employers, and society.
- *Efficiency*: Ensure efficiency in the production and consumption of health services.

At the same time, the high cost of health care has made the development and reform of national healthcare systems highly politicized. How health care is organized and funded fuels many debates within each nation. These debates stem from different opinions about the role of government in health care, which arise from different values and national traditions. These, in turn, shape the insurance systems and administrative processes through which health professionals deliver services.

Health care in the U.S. is primarily based on a system of private health insurance. Public health insurance for people on social security (aged 65 and older), referred to as Medicare, and on social assistance, referred to as Medicaid, is also in place. Access to health care for the remainder of the population is through private insurance, which can be a benefit of employment, or through other benefit plans, such as those for veterans through Veterans Affairs. The introduction of the ACA reduced the number of uninsured individuals—from 45 million who lacked insurance prior to the ACA to 23 million—bringing the U.S. "halfway" to universal coverage (Hall, 2011, p. 522). There are, however, several million individuals who are underinsured, such that their health insurance plan does not cover all the healthcare services they require. The ACA is currently under threat as the Trump administration tries to implement "repeal and replace" (Roubein, 2017, p. 1), which is intended to claw back fundamental elements of the ACA. By contrast, Canada has a universal system of public health insurance, in which provincial public insurance plans develop contracts with private healthcare institutions, such as hospitals and health practitioners, to deliver care to the population. The differences in the two healthcare systems have evolved as a result of different ideological conceptions and political institutional processes through which legislation is developed (Maioni, 1998; Tuohy, 1999).

In many ways, national health insurance symbolizes the great divide between liberalism and socialism, the free market and the planned economy (see Box 11.1). Such principles are deeply rooted within each nation. For example, the Canadian constitution is based on such principles as "peace, order, and good government." By contrast, the American constitution emphasizes "life, liberty, and the pursuit of happiness."

**Box 11.1:** Liberalism and Socialism

Liberalism comes from the word *libre*, and emphasizes the following:
- *Personal freedom*: Absence of coercion; individuals can pursue their own interests.
- *Limited government*: Government acts only as an umpire to enforce the rules of society needed to sustain a free market. The limits on government are defined in the constitution, which clarifies the government's jurisdiction in different areas.
- *Equality of right*: Everyone must abide by the same rules. Reform Liberals redefined the notion of equality to equality of opportunity. Reform Liberals consider the positive role of the state in promoting individuals' potential.
- *Consent of the governed*: Elections.

Alternatively, socialism is motivated by a dislike of the consequences of the market economy that are inherent in the liberal vision. Instead, socialism:
- Emphasizes assets are owned by the community, while benefits are distributed to all, not just select private owners.
- Aspires to a higher degree of "equality of result."
- Works toward political gradualism. The goal is to make the state more politically accountable. (MacLean & Wood, 2002, p. 57)

In most industrialized nations, public health insurance has been adopted at least partially to address the market failure in the health sector (see Box 11.2), and societal judgments concerning equitable access to necessary care irrespective of ability to pay and differences in "need." Such a perspective reflects Rawls's (1971) *A Theory of Justice*, which suggests that those who design social systems put themselves behind a "veil of ignorance," where their position in the resulting distribution is unknown. Under these circumstances, most individuals would have *social primary goods distributed equally* to preserve the dignity of all individuals, but still allow social and economic inequalities if they worked to everyone's advantage. The driving force of publicly operated health systems is to extend coverage based on social justice. As Stone (1988) suggests, "the pattern of public needs is the signature of a society. In its definition of public needs, a society says what it means to be human and to have dignity in that culture" (p. 81). Such ideologies can be referred to as dominant ideas that prevail within a society at a given time (Doern & Phidd, 1988; Dyson, 1980; Simeon, 1976). While dominant ideas are important, they are only one factor in the constellation of political dynamics that shape health policy in each nation.

## Political Institutions and Historical Perspective

Political and historical forces shaped the different paths that Canada and the U.S. took in developing their healthcare systems, which influenced their subsequent reforms. Although

**Box 11.2:** Market Failure: A Rationale for Government Intervention

**Free market:**
Liberal economists believe public welfare is promoted by a competitive market through the so-called invisible hand: People's utility-maximizing behaviour and firms' profit-maximizing behaviour will, through the "invisible hand," lead to an optimal distribution of goods.

*But economic reality differs from the assumptions of the competitive model:*
Efficient outcomes are not always promoted by the market, leading to market failures, which provide the economic rationale for government intervention.

**The market fails for such public goods as:**
- primary and secondary education
- health care
  Society benefits from an educated population whose healthcare needs are addressed. The market does not, however, distribute these on a universal basis, which provides the rationale for government involvement (Weimer & Vining, 1989).

health care emerged as a political issue in both nations as early as the 1930s, it was not until the 1960s that the basis of each system was formulated through their respective legislative processes.

In the U.S., policy reforms based on new laws must be passed by a majority of the elected members in both the Senate and House of Representatives, and receive the support of the president, representing three potential levels of veto.

Since regions across the U.S. are well represented in the Senate (each state has two seats) and the House of Representatives (seats are assigned based on population), there are only two major political parties: Republicans and Democrats. Health reformers in the Democratic Party who proposed universal health care were forced to modify and dilute their plans to appeal to a broad coalition of groups (such as the unions and the labour movement) that the Democratic Party represents. This forced the Democrats to abandon many of the tenets on which their proposal for healthcare reform was based, as they would otherwise risk losing the support of key groups. Even if the Democrats succeeded in attaining consensus within their party, an additional hurdle remained. The absence of party discipline in the Senate and House of Representatives—where members of a political party are not required to vote for the measures their party proposes—means there was no assurance that all Democratic members would vote for the legislation.

Moreover, several interest groups, such as the American Medical Association and private health insurance companies, oppose legislation that would change the conditions under which they practice. Such interest groups and the lobbyists they employ seek to influence elected members of the Senate, the House of Representatives, and the president to oppose the proposed changes. Introducing legislation that would change how health professionals practice and how insurance companies conduct their business, and increase the level of taxes that citizens pay to support a program of national healthcare insurance, therefore faces enormous challenges (Maioni, 1998), as was evidenced with the introduction of the ACA in 2010.

Additional factors that influenced the policy trajectory toward employer-sponsored health insurance in the 1950s included the labour movement's shift to collective bargaining rather than national politics to gain health insurance, the business community's preference for offering fringe benefits instead of supporting government-run health insurance, and tax reform (enshrined in legislation) that excluded employer-paid premiums from employees' taxable income and subsidized employer-sponsored health insurance, which became the primary health insurance system in the U.S. (Hacker, 2002). As a result, advocates of national health insurance shifted their focus from the general population to those who were largely excluded from the workforce: the elderly and low-income people. The public health insurance system was thus targeted to people not expected to work and designed around a private but tax-subsidized insurance system for employees and their families. Employer-sponsored insurance, however, excludes large numbers of low- and modest-income workers (Feder, 2004).

In contrast, passing legislation concerning universal public health insurance in the Canadian Parliament faced fewer obstacles for three reasons. First, Canadian political parties adhere to the concept of party discipline; members of a party generally support the legislation proposed by members of their party. Second, when a political party governs the House of Commons, its members comprise the executive: the prime minister and a select group of ministers referred to as the Cabinet. The fusion between the governing party and the executive means that interest groups such as the Canadian Medical Association (CMA), which opposed the legislation enshrining public health insurance, had few alternate avenues through which they could influence the legislative process. Such was the case when the CMA attempted to block the *Medical Care Act* in 1967.

A third factor that supported the introduction of innovations in Canada was the absence of a system of regional representation, which led to the establishment of a third party. Although representation in Parliament is based on population distribution, the Senate lacks a formal system of regional representation. Regional interests thus have more incentive to develop political parties outside the two major parties (Liberals and Conservatives) as a vehicle to assert their voice in federal policy. Western-based parties, such as the Canadian Commonwealth Federation (CCF), which later evolved into the New Democratic Party (NDP), thus played a decisive role in changing the political landscape by introducing policy proposals that would not have otherwise been raised by the two main traditional parties.

The CCF in Saskatchewan adopted medicare, which provided the impetus for a legislative proposal for universal health insurance at the national level. The establishment of the CCF created a channel through which the populist Western movement could advance its interests and counter the medical lobby, reshaping the debate on public health insurance. The Canada–U.S. comparison reflects important contrasts between the multiple points of access for influence and veto inherent in the American separation of powers, and the consolidated power of the Canadian parliamentary system, in which executive and legislative powers are effectively fused (Maioni, 1998).

Once a health system was adopted in Canada and the U.S., a series of interest groups (the medical profession, private insurance companies, allied health professionals) and organizational constructs became entrenched within each national system, making the ability to change course through subsequent reforms much more difficult. President Clinton's 1993 attempt to achieve universal health insurance through legislative reform, for example, failed to gain support. Instead, reforms in the U.S. and Canadian healthcare systems reflect logical progressions of the organizational dynamics on which they were founded (Tuohy, 1999). In the U.S., private insurance companies that deliver employee-sponsored health care resisted further government involvement. Private insurers also diminished the autonomy of the medical profession by placing limits on the types of treatments covered, which effectively restricted how physicians could practice. Once the elderly and the poor were covered through Medicare and Medicaid, subsidization of health insurance for the economically disadvantaged became a political challenge as any new measures would financially disrupt the insured population (Feder, 2004). Innovations in health care instead occurred through private insurers' organizational delivery systems.

In Canada, despite considerable "restructuring" and realignment of the hospital sector within each province, the medical profession maintains its clinical autonomy, even though fiscal pressures have led the government to tame the medical profession's entrepreneurial discretion (Tuohy, 1999). Canadian health reform has instead occurred through regionalization of provincial healthcare systems. Alberta and New Brunswick, however, amalgamated their health regions into one and two health authorities, respectively.

Although attempts to expand private healthcare delivery have largely been resisted, they continue nevertheless. An example is the *Chaoulli* case in Quebec, challenging the constitutional validity of Quebec legislation—that also exists in five other provinces—that prohibits private insurance for publicly insured hospital and physician services. Such legislation makes it difficult for a parallel private health system to exist in these provinces. Given lengthy wait lists for medical procedures, the Supreme Court of Canada ruled that this Quebec law violates guarantees in the *Quebec Charter of Human Rights and Freedoms*. Importantly, the Supreme Court's decision did not apply to the Canadian *Charter*, such that it does not affect other provinces with similar legislation (Flood & Xavier, 2008).

The Quebec government's response was to develop a White Paper. It also enacted Bill 33, which permitted private health insurance in three clinical areas. At the same time, it implemented a process to cap wait times in the public healthcare system in those three clinical areas, which reduced the incentive to purchase private insurance. Quebec's response was strategic in that it addressed the Supreme Court's decision while simultaneously taking measures to protect the publicly funded healthcare system. *Chaoulli* has, however, led to a range of claims concerning health care in other provinces based on *Charter* rights. Over time, conceptions of the right to health care have shifted from an emphasis on social solidarity to that of civil rights to access private health insurance (Bhatia, 2010). The case thus appears to have altered the terms of debate concerning private health care in Canada (Flood & Xavier, 2008).

Mental health care is another area of concern, for which funding has declined from 11% to 7% of healthcare spending from 1979 to 2017, respectively, in Canada. Following two waves of deinstitionalization in the 1960–1970s and 2000s, patients were shifted to the community without adequate supports, which fostered passive privatization. Wait lists for mental health care increased. One reason is that as the *Canada Health Act* (1984) is a spending statute, it excludes (1) the services provided by allied health professionals in community settings (unless permitted by a provincial government), and (2) psychiatric hospitals are excluded from the definition of hospitals covered by federal transfers. Provinces could underfund mental health care without being penalized through reductions in federal transfers (Bartram, 2017; Bartram & Lurie, 2017). Similar limitations for mental health care have occurred in the U.S., for example, through the absence of funding mechanisms for allied health professionals offering mental health care in Accountable Care Organizations (O'Donnell, Williams, Eisenberg, & Kilbourne, 2013). Funding mechanisms are thus a pivotal issue, as the next section explores.

## Organizational Design: Modes of Financing and Delivery

To better understand the distinctions between the Canadian and U.S. systems, we consider how national healthcare systems are organized by focusing on three dimensions referred to by economists as:

- *Financing*: How are healthcare services paid for: publicly or privately?
- *Delivery*: How are health services delivered: publicly or privately?
- *Allocation*: How are the funds allocated to service providers?

Healthcare services can be *financed* and *delivered* through either public or private means. *Allocation* refers to the way healthcare professionals are paid, including the kinds of incentives incorporated in different methods of payment. When referring to *financing* and *delivery*, there are strengths and weaknesses in having a publicly or privately financed and delivered healthcare system. The best way to demonstrate these is by exploring the approaches different nations have adopted, their comparative advantages and disadvantages, and the reforms used to address their weaknesses (Deber, 2004).

### *Financing: Insuring and Purchasing Healthcare Services*
Financing healthcare services includes a system of insurance to protect individuals from the risk and cost of falling ill and requiring costly healthcare services (diagnosis, treatment,

and rehabilitation). In a *publicly financed* healthcare system, all citizens contribute and pay into the health insurance system through their personal income and other taxes. Important advantages include: (1) spreading the risk of illness across the entire population so that insurance is affordable to all citizens, even those with greater risk of falling ill; (2) more effective cost control over healthcare services; and (3) universal coverage.

Since all citizens face the risk of becoming ill, most would rather pay into a system in which they are protected should they fall ill even if they are currently healthy. As such, in publicly insured systems, healthy individuals who do not require extensive healthcare services subsidize those who become ill and require treatment. In contrast, in a privately financed system individuals pay private insurance companies to insure them against the risk of illness and needing costly healthcare services. To ensure a high profit, private insurance companies are selective in choosing those whom they will insure by charging higher premiums to people with pre-existing illnesses. The cost of such high premiums effectively excludes those people who can't afford the premiums. People with a chronic condition such as diabetes or high blood pressure, or even a family history of an illness such as cancer must thus pay a higher premium, which may render the insurance unaffordable and leave them without coverage.

A second advantage of publicly financed systems is relative cost control over healthcare services. This is achieved because the government is the single purchaser of healthcare services, endowing it with *monopsony* power. It collects funds from the public and negotiates with healthcare providers on behalf of the public regarding the services to be offered and the remuneration that healthcare providers will receive. If healthcare professionals are not satisfied with the government's offer, their only recourse is to negotiate better terms or to go on strike by refusing to offer their services. The government is thus in a relatively strong position as it has the capacity to negotiate more advantageous terms on behalf of the entire population.

Germany and the Netherlands have healthcare systems that involve *private financing* through private insurance (sickness funds), as shown in Table 11.1. The effect has been that *private financing has led to risk shifting among insurers*. Private insurers have sought to enroll clients who are healthier, free of chronic conditions, and thus less expensive to care for. They have also discouraged clients with chronic conditions from enrolling in their insurance plans by charging them higher fees. The problem then becomes one of affordability. For the elderly and those with chronic conditions, attaining healthcare insurance has become increasingly expensive, and many are unable to afford it, leaving them without insurance.

The reforms Germany and the Netherlands have enacted to address this problem include government regulation of the sickness funds. Such insurance funds are prevented from excluding patients with chronic illness by ensuring the range of fees they charge are reasonable and that the risk is spread throughout the enrolled population. As a result, the sickness funds co-operate by using similar insurance criteria, and thereby operate as a quasi-single payer. A problem associated with privately financed systems is one of *cost control in the absence of monopsony*. If healthcare providers are not pleased with the

**Table 11.1:** International Healthcare Systems: Comparing Financing and Delivery

| Delivery | Financing | |
|---|---|---|
| | **Public** | **Private** |
| Public | Britain, Sweden: National Health Service | — |
| Private | Canada, France: public insurance system | Germany,* Netherlands, Switzerland,* U.S.: Private insurance |

*Note:* * Mixture of private insurance and government subsidy: Government regulates and subsidizes private mutual aid societies.

remuneration offered by one private insurance company, they can seek higher compensation from another company. As insurance companies seek to attract healthcare professionals through higher remuneration, the cost of providing health care rises. Private insurance thus does not offer effective cost control, and consumers face higher charges for the same kinds of healthcare services.

The third advantage of publicly financed systems is universality. Since the entire population contributes to the insurance plan, all citizens have access to it, even those who are least able to contribute. Public financing thus achieves equity across the population.

Critics of publicly financed systems, however, point to the waiting lists for diagnostic and treatment services, suggesting that if private financing were allowed, individuals could purchase private services to reduce their wait for healthcare services. A parallel private system exists in some publicly financed systems, such as in the United Kingdom and Australia. The problem with allowing a parallel private system is that many of the best healthcare professionals gravitate to its more lucrative remuneration. As found in Britain, the result is that people who can afford to pay privately move to the front of the queue, while the remainder of the population relying on the public system face an even lengthier wait as health professionals working in the private sector provide fewer services to the public system. As the private system does not provide comprehensive services, however, it still relies on the public national system. When private care expands, support for the public system diminishes since those who purchase private health care withdraw their support for the public system. Considerable inequities thus result from a parallel private system due to the deterioration in the public system.

France has a different system, where health care is publicly insured up to a certain point depending on the diagnosis (except for low-income people, who are fully insured), and where private insurance supplements the public insurance system. Public and private insurance thus cover the same health care. Private insurers are also regulated in the same manner as the public insurance system, and the reimbursement rules for healthcare providers are the same whether they are private not-for-profit or for-profit (Sandier, Paris, & Polton, 2004).

### Health Service Delivery: Public or Private

Publicly delivered healthcare services—where healthcare providers are considered employees of the state—have been found to result in less than optimal health care, as Britain and Sweden demonstrate. The disadvantage of public delivery is that the healthcare system's responsiveness to clients may be questionable in the absence of incentives in place. In contrast, with privately delivered healthcare services, if clients are not pleased with the quality of the service, or if the wait for services is too lengthy, they have the option of seeking health care elsewhere. In the case of a public provider, however, the usual market signal of consumers choosing to purchase care elsewhere is not available. In the case of health care, this is further complicated because of what economists refer to as "imperfect information": Medical care is complex and consumers cannot easily discern the quality of the services they receive, which is thus another form of market failure, nor are there obvious ways for the client to signal their dissatisfaction with the care received.

A distinction must also be made between *for-profit* and *not-for-profit* private delivery as *for-profit* delivery is more likely to lead to suboptimal care. The evidence is drawn from a study that compared for-profit and not-for-profit healthcare firms in the U.S. In comparing dialysis services for patients, for example, not-for-profit companies were more likely to send their patients for kidney transplant to alleviate their renal failure, which eliminated their need for dialysis. In contrast, the for-profit clinics were less likely to send their clients for renal transplant, leading their clients to be dependent on renal dialysis for the remainder of their lives (Devereaux et al., 2002). For-profit delivery is thus acceptable only when outcome standards can be clearly specified and monitored, which is difficult to attain for complex services such as health care (Deber, 2004). Private not-for-profit delivery is thus optimal.

Healthcare systems that include *public financing* and *public delivery* thus offer good cost control and good equity, but questionable client responsiveness. Reforms to address the suboptimal client responsiveness initially focused on internal markets to realign the incentives to provide quality service delivery, as shown in Box 11.3. These include the purchaser–provider split, where providers are required to compete for service delivery contracts. Under the purchaser–provider split, purchasers are responsible to the budgetary authority for cost control and to patients for the quality and accessibility of care. While the public financing component in these systems has largely remained, a measure of private delivery has been introduced. More recently in Britain, the *Health Act 2009* requires providers to submit a *Quality Account* annually that offers measures of the quality of the services (patient safety, the effectiveness of treatments patients receive, and patient feedback about the care provided), creating an incentive to enhance responsiveness to patient needs. The *Health and Social Care Act 2012* introduced amendments that require social indicators to be included within the measures collected (National Health Service, 2018).

The role of purchasers has also been enhanced in the U.S.'s managed care plans and selective contracting by insurers. While several countries used this model for the purchase of hospital services (Australia, Britain, New Zealand, Sweden, Italy, Portugal, and Greece), Britain and New Zealand experimented with using primary care doctors as purchasers.

In Britain, this involved general practitioners serving as fund holders who purchased specialist and hospital services on behalf of patients in their practice. Evidence suggests that such purchaser–provider arrangements had little effect in changing patterns of service delivery (Docteur & Oxley, 2003). As of 2013, Clinical Commissioning Groups (CCGs) have replaced primary care trusts as the commissioners of services funded by the National Health Service (NHS) in England and control about two-thirds of the NHS budget. Primary care practices must be a member of a CCG that commissions secondary and community care services for their local populations and supports quality improvement in general practice (Edwards & Naylor, 2013). Health and Wellbeing Boards (HWBs) comprised of local authorities were also established by the 2012 *Health and Social Care Act*. HWBs are intended to assess local needs to inform health and local authority social care commissioners, and to align strategic plans across diverse organizations to enhance their co-operation. The CCGs and HWBs collaborate to create health and social partnerships that collectively improve health outcomes and reduce inequalities (Coleman et al., 2014).

## Box 11.3: Planned Market Initiatives

Planned market initiatives reflect a set of conscious choices about how to introduce market-style incentives into existing allocation-based management structures. In other words, to promote efficiency, the government intercedes in a publicly insured healthcare system by introducing market-based tools to maximize social welfare. An example of the planned market approach is in the reforms adopted by Britain, shown below.

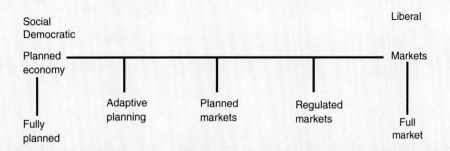

*Planned markets*: Intermediate position between command-and-control planning systems and pure market systems.

*Regulated markets*: State power limits certain socially disruptive behaviours that occurred previously.

*Planned market*: State uses select market instruments to achieve government policy objectives.

*Adaptive planning*: Management decentralized to regional planning bodies to enhance responsiveness to local needs. (Saltman & von Otter, 1992, p. 16)

### Britain's Internal Market: "Purchaser Split from Provider"

*Health authorities (100 regions)*: Given fixed budget to purchase hospital care.

*Hospitals (400) became providers*: Self-financing trusts compete for contracts.

*Fund-holding family practices (100s)*: Given budget to buy specialist client care.

*Specialist hospital doctors (providers)*: Work in public and private sector.

### Britain's Internal Market:

Did not significantly reduce costs except by cutting services

Doubled administrative costs

Did not improve hospital care; budget pressure took precedence over patient needs

Reduced patient choice of hospitals (GPs)

Created two- to three-tiered care

- Private care
- Fund-holding practices
- Non-fund-holding practices

### Problem: Waiting Lists

1. Hospital doctors on *minimum part-time* contract earn 90% of salary for half a week's work.
2. Hospital doctors can practice privately and earn as much or more from private practice.
3. Surgeons with the most private practice have the longest waiting lists.

### "New Labour" Reforms (2000)

1. Increased NHS spending (6% per annum)
2. Expanded number of doctors and nurses
3. Prohibited senior NHS doctors from private practice in the first seven years after appointment
4. Increased role for nurses
5. Contracts with private acute and long-term care facilities for National Health Service patient beds

In summary, for *financing* medically required services, the best approach is public financing as:

1. monopsony (single-payer) control over providers gives superior cost control
2. public financing avoids "cherry picking," whereas private insurers profit by refusing high-risk individuals

For *delivery* of medically required services, the best approach is private non-profit as:

1. public delivery can mean less responsiveness to clients; introducing incentives and organizational approaches to co-ordinate services can, however, optimize cost-efficiency and quality
2. for-profit delivery is acceptable only when outcome standards can be clearly specified and monitored, which is difficult to develop for health care as it is a complex service

The lesson for Canada from this international comparison is that the public system should increase incentives and foster health and social partnerships that enhance responsiveness and maintain confidence in care. Canadians should be cautious about allowing a parallel private system as it siphons off the best practitioners, increases waiting lists, and reduces support for the public system. A private system would rely on the public system, which would support the patients the private system does not treat and offer the full array of services the private system does not.

## RECENT REFORMS

### Medicare and Medicaid in the United States

Although the system of public health insurance in the U.S. has grown, the reforms have, historically, been modest. Medicare was expanded in 1972 to include people with end-stage renal disease and disabled beneficiaries of Social Security. Medicaid was first expanded to include children of lower-income employed parents, pregnant women in two-parent working families, and individuals with disabilities who could return to the workforce if provided with supports. A second phase of expansion in the 1980s and 1990s led to national income eligibility standards for children and pregnant women. The state Children's Health Insurance Program (CHIP) modestly increased the coverage for children in the late 1990s. *Medicaid* is thus largely geared toward low-income children and pregnant women. Although states have the option of covering both parents, in most states parents on minimum wage earn too much income to be eligible. Moreover, low-income people who are not parents of dependent children are not eligible for Medicaid (Feder, 2004).

Medicaid is jointly funded and administered by the federal and state governments. Federal funding of the program comes with minimum national standards and accountability for the open-ended federal dollars spent (states cover 23%–50% of Medicaid benefit costs). States are also given the flexibility to design their health service delivery systems according to local conditions, to set provider rates, and to impose cost-control mechanisms. States, however, vary in the proportion of the population they cover (from 28%–59% of the low-income uninsured among 13 states assessed) and benefits provided: from $7,749 per beneficiary in New York to $2,334 in California in 2001 (Mann & Westmoreland, 2004).

Some gradual expansion in the beneficiaries has occurred as states have the option of expanding their program to cover people in eligible groups at higher incomes, and most have done so for some groups of beneficiaries. Medicaid was also expanded to pay for vaccines for uninsured and underinsured children who are not Medicaid beneficiaries. States could also expand eligibility to uninsured women diagnosed with breast or cervical cancer in a program initiated in 2000 by the Centers for Disease Control and Prevention. Medicaid accounts for about 16% of state budgets, second only to education (Mann & Westmoreland, 2004).

Access to healthcare services under Medicaid also varies across states due to payment factors—low payment rates have in some cases compromised people's ability to access care. The breadth of services covered also varies. While Medicaid law requires states to offer nursing home services, home- and community-based long-term care services are not mandatory, and some states have not made them available as they believe they cannot afford their costs.

In terms of reforms, the federal government has made available "section 1115" waivers that allow states to use federal Medicaid funds in ways other than those specified in the legislation to promote research and demonstration projects. States have used the provisions of the waiver to expand coverage, however, or to introduce other programmatic and financial changes. The federal Medicaid matching rate was increased through legislation in 2003, temporarily shifting a greater proportion of its costs to the federal government, which assisted states in averting eligibility rollbacks and reductions in coverage and benefits. Nevertheless, Medicaid essentially functions as a high-risk pool, covering people with disabilities and chronic illnesses who would otherwise not have access to insurance. Increasing budget pressures, however, threaten the viability of many state Medicaid programs and suggest some future retrenchment. Medicaid is thus in need of reform as it has been extremely flexible, growing in response to myriad needs in an incremental, piecemeal manner, but without the benefit of system-wide planning (Mann & Westmoreland, 2004).

Medicare is also on the threshold of reform due to the rising cost of health care, and the rising proportion of the retired population. Problems, however, exist in the adequacy of its benefits. To provide some coverage for prescription drugs, the *Medicare Prescription Drug, Improvement, and Modernization Act* was enacted in 2003, and took effect in 2006. The federal government's coverage of healthcare expenses for Medicare beneficiaries averages about 60%. About 15% of Medicare beneficiaries are sufficiently impoverished to qualify for Medicaid benefits.

Medicare as a public subsidy program, however, enjoys universal popularity, but only as long as administrative agencies limit the extent to which individual choice is narrowed. Cost-control measures within public programs have thus been limited to restraining physician payments instead of curtailing clinical services (Vladeck, 2004).

## Challenges to Managed Care

In the U.S., managed care was developed by the private sector as an alternative to government regulation. When employers were faced with covering increasingly high health insurance premiums, they shifted their employees to managed care programs. Although managed care has achieved economic success, patients have become disaffected with such gatekeeping aspects as "utilization review," which curtails the medical services they receive. The advantages managed care offers in terms of lower inflation for medical costs have been outweighed by the disadvantages of such cost-cutting care to employees, who seek litigation where limitations in medical care lead to adverse health consequences. Managed care firms are thus moving from tightly managed to loosened utilization review, which, in turn, increases costs to employers. As a consequence, employees are being asked to pay a greater share of their health insurance premium.

## The *Patient Protection and Affordable Care Act* (ACA) of 2010

The ACA is a landmark bill that aims to expand health care to millions of uninsured or underinsured Americans, while maintaining the architecture of the country's healthcare system. As such, the ACA represents an intricate and continually evolving intergovernmental partnership that reflects the federalist approach to United States governmental structure. Like Medicaid and CHIP, which preceded the ACA and continue within the confines of the ACA, the ACA relies on the federal and state governments working together by sharing the costs of programs and on a mix of federal, state, and local administrators who implement the programs (Sparer, 2011).

In pursuing health reform, President Barack Obama and his administration "had to navigate difficult interest-group politics, respond to broad cultural concerns about the role of government, and overcome the checks and balances of America's political institutions that are designed to make it hard to enact major federal legislation" (Sparer, 2011, p. 463). In terms of interest groups, the Obama administration had to work with physician, hospital, pharmaceutical manufacturer, insurer, and employer representative groups, all of which have a vested interest in, and wish to shape, health reform. State governments also functioned as an effective interest group through organizations like the National Governors Association. The concept of state-based health insurance exchanges, instead of national or regional exchanges, was endorsed by the states, as was expanded federal funding to underpin health reform. Under Section 1321 in the ACA, the states must create state-based health insurance exchanges, which allow individuals and small businesses to compare and contrast plans available in their states and make applications for financial assistance, and serve as a mechanism through which to buy health insurance. The exchanges are designed to assist individuals who are not eligible for health insurance through an employer or another affiliation (Rodwin, 2011). It is important to emphasize that while the states do not represent homogenous views or health care and systems needs and goals, bloc representation can be an effective negotiating strategy when dealing with the federal government (Sparer, 2011).

Within the U.S. context, ideological conceptions and political institutional processes have, in the past, been thought to be an impediment to health reform. These ideological conceptions focus upon "the widely held view that the source of America's greatness is its grounding principles of individual rights, capitalism, and personal responsibility" (Sparer, 2011, p. 464). As a result, it has been thought that Americans are not keen to embrace group or communalistic approaches to government policy and programs. This is why healthcare reform with a focus on universal coverage has been framed as "socialist," which is thought to rely on too much governmental interference and lead to diluted standards of care (Sparer, 2011, p. 464). This ideological perception was countered by the Obama administration by superimposing the ACA on top of the existing healthcare infrastructure, instead of following a strategy to change the existing system. As Tuohy (2011) posits, "large-scale or rapid changes in overall health care frameworks are rare, because they require extraordinarily favourable conjunctions of institutional and political conditions" (p. 572). As a result, the ACA takes the form of a mosaic strategy to reform, as opposed to big-bang or blueprint approaches. Big-bang strategies take a sweeping and fast approach to reform; blueprint strategies follow a sweeping, but slow approach to reform; and mosaic strategies take the form of quickly implemented, smaller-scale change (Tuohy, 2011, p. 572). As such, the Obama administration attempted to refute the notion that the ACA was a "federal takeover" by following existing intergovernmental relationships and placing the new insurance exchanges under state control, as well as funnelling insurance expansion programs through state-administered Medicaid, instead of through the federally run Medicare program (Sparer, 2011, p. 465).

In keeping with the mosaic model, healthcare reform began with a set of eight narrow guiding "principles," which focused upon "protecting families' financial health," making "health coverage affordable, striving for universality of coverage," "providing portable coverage," allowing consumer choice, "invest[ing] in prevention and wellness," "improv[ing] patient safety and quality care," and ensuring "long-term fiscal sustainability" (*Politico*, 2009, p. 1). These principles were communicated to Congress in the February 2009 budget (*Politico*, 2009, p. 1). These eight principles were also set to function within the pre-existing employer-based framework and be implemented swiftly. In order to facilitate fast-paced adoption of the ACA, deadlines were set for congressional approvals. These deadlines included "'reconciliation instructions' in the budget resolution passed by Congress in April 2009, allowing the Democratic majority to circumvent a filibuster if agreement had not been reached in six months" (Tuohy, 2011, p. 574). The strategy for gathering consensus on healthcare reform, which has been and continues to be a contentious issue, was to demonstrate that universal coverage could be achieved in the United States without upending the existing system. As a result, reforms were proposed in the small-group and individual markets, as well as for the uninsured, by extending Medicaid programs, making subsidies available for the acquisition of private insurance and state-based health exchanges that worked to "manage competition among private insurers in the individual and small employer markets" (Tuohy, 2011, p. 574). During the legislative process, various proposals were presented and rescinded, but an important adjustment was the inclusion of a "scoring" system through which the legislation could be evaluated for is financial viability, which was one of the eight ACA guiding principles.

One of the most contentious aspects throughout the ACA's legislative development was its treatment of abortion. The ACA does not allow abortion to be covered by federal monies, except in cases protected by the Hyde Amendment, which provides exemptions in cases of rape and incest or when the woman's life is endangered. This provision allowed pro-life Democrats to support the ACA, and their backing was secured when President Obama promised to release an executive order reinforcing that federal funding would not be available for abortion in the ACA and through the proposed health exchanges, in accordance with the Hyde Amendment restrictions. President Obama signed the Executive Order 13535, entitled *Ensuring Enforcement and Implementation of Abortion Restrictions in the Patient and Affordable Care Act,* on March 29, 2010. The Executive Order also stipulated that federal monies could not be used for abortions, except in Hyde Amendment cases, delivered though community health centre programs (Executive Order 13535, 2010, p. 2).

Due to the mosaic strategy approach, the ACA is a complex and lengthy piece of legislation spanning 906 pages. The ACA has over 400 sections, a budget reconciliation act comprised of 38 sections, and the four-section 13535 Executive Order. Tuohy (2011) posits that "the Achilles heel of a mosaic approach is the very complexity and interdependence of its multiple provisions. The complexity, born of elite bargains, presents an enormous communications challenge in order to engage public understanding and solidify support" (p. 575). From an overarching perspective, as per Grogan (2017, pp. 987–989), the ACA thematically addresses the following with the goal of attaining health equity:

1. Title 1 of the ACA concentrates upon changes to the individual and group health insurance markets. This title addresses potential discrimination that is based upon race, ethnicity, gender, disability, or age.
2. Title II is focused upon the ameliorating access to Medicaid. This title highlights the aim of boosting maternal, infant, and early childhood home visiting programs designated for at-risk communities. This is meant to address health disparities.
3. Title III sets out policy and programs to raise the standard of health care in terms of efficacy and efficiency with the view of attaining health equity across population groupings and geographic areas. This title also outlines performance bonus payments for Medicare plans, which narrow health disparity gaps.

4. Title IV outlines the formation of the Prevention and Public Health Fund. This is an important inclusion as it creates the first federal dedicated funding line for public health. The fund focuses on curbing the spread of infectious disease and containing their outbreaks, as well as tobacco cessation, addressing obesity, and providing greater access to preventative services. Title IV focuses on creating healthy communities by addressing the social determinants of health, including social, economic, geographic, racial, and ethnic inequities.
5. Title V is centered upon strengthening the healthcare workforce with particular focus upon cultural sensitivity and public health training to address health disparities.
6. Title VI includes the creation of the Patient-Centered Outcomes Research Institute to monitor health outcomes and to improve care through evidence-based research.
7. Title VII addresses access to emerging medical technologies, particularly improving the availability of affordable medicines, devices, and therapies for children and underserviced communities.

Pragmatically, the ACA has been lauded for introducing the following measures:

1. Providing tax credits to low-income individuals who purchase health insurance (ACA, sec. 1401).
2. Regulating private health insurers by restricting insurance ratings to age, geographic area, family status, and whether or not an individual smokes or not only to reduce discrimination; guaranteeing individuals with pre-existing conditions can qualify for coverage; restricting lifetime and annual limits on coverage; and increasing the age dependents qualify for insurance to 26 years of age (ACA, sec. 2702, 2704, 2714).
3. Mandating small-group and individual health insurance must cover the 10 following essential health benefits: ambulatory care; emergency care; hospitalization; pregnancy/maternity/newborn care; mental health and substance abuse care; prescription drugs; rehabilitation services and devices; laboratory testing; preventative care and pediatric care, including dental and eye care (Government of the United States, 2018, p. 1; ACA, sec. 1302, 2707).

However, there are still health equity gaps in the ACA. Individuals not covered by the ACA include undocumented immigrants and legal immigrants who have not resided in the U.S. for five years, as it takes five years of residency to be eligible for Medicaid. Furthermore, the health exchanges regulate insurance purchased through this mechanism, but not employer or group-based insurance. As a result, if one obtains insurance outside an exchange, there is no guarantee that the insurance will be sufficient. As per Rodwin (2011), "employers can exclude coverage for any medical condition, cap spending per employee, and offer as *few* benefits as they wish" (p. 598, emphasis in original). Furthermore, low- and middle-income individuals often find it hard to afford health insurance payments, which have been rising since the ACA took effect. Lastly, low- and middle-income individuals are not always able to afford health insurance without expenditure caps, meaning they do not have limitless coverage. Therefore, low- and middle-income individuals can suffer financial hardship if catastrophic illness strikes and can become bankrupt (Rodwin, 2011, p. 598). As a result, the ACA has been described as a "halfway technology" (Oliver, 2011, p. 603) that is buttressing an uneven healthcare system with many fissures that are not likely to be rectified within a mosaic approach to reform.

The ACA is financed through annual fees on branded pharmaceutical manufacturers and importers, medical device manufacturers and importers, and health insurance providers (ACA: sec. 9008, 9009, 9010). The ACA also requires "an excise tax on high-cost employer sponsored health coverage" (sec. 9001), "an additional hospital insurance tax on high income taxpayers" (sec. 9015), and "excise tax on elective cosmetic procedures" (sec. 9017; US Government, 2010, p. 10). The financing mechanisms covered in the sections listed above have been criticized by the Republican Party and form a portion of the rationale behind President Trump's efforts to "repeal and replace" the ACA (Grogan, 2017, p. 989). It should also be noted, though, that the Trump administration opposes much of the ACA on ideological grounds, as the Republican Party holds the concepts of "individual rights, capitalism, and personal responsibility" (Sparer, 2011, p. 464) as important American values. These values, as expressed by President Trump and many Republicans, are important pillars for health reform and, as per their perspective, not reflected in the ACA. As a result, the Trump administration has dedicated efforts to repeal and replace the ACA.

### *Repealing and Replacing the* **Patient Protection and Affordable Care Act** *of 2010*

In order to repeal and replace the ACA, the Republicans created the *American Health Care Act* (AHCA), which passed the House of Representatives' Budget Committee in March 2017. However, the AHCA was pulled by Paul Ryan from the House of Representatives due to insufficient votes to pass the bill in late March 2017 (Roubein, 2017). The AHCA proposed to remove the individual mandate and subsidies for low-income individuals to make health insurance voluntary, with individuals purchasing insurance with the assistance of tax credits (Grogan, 2017, p. 989). The AHCA would also only increase federal Medicaid funding until the end of the year 2019, when it would be repealed. Upon repeal, Medicaid would be funded through a per capita cap, instead of the existing federal-state matching formula, which would be based on historical per-person expenditures. This would have resulted in fewer federal funds being funnelled via the states into Medicaid. Additionally, the tax on well-off Americans used to fund the ACA would have been repealed, and the Prevention and Public Health fund would have been disbanded (Grogan, 2017, p. 990). In April 2017, the House Freedom Caucus supported a revised bill, keeping afloat the repeal-and-replace movement. This revised AHCA allowed states to forgo insurance regulations. In May 2017, the ACA repeal bill was approved by the

House of Representatives in a narrow 217–213 vote. In June 2017, the Republican Party released another draft of their ACA repeal bill, called the *Better Care Reconciliation Act of 2017* (BRCA), which, according to the Congressional Budget Office (CBO), would have resulted in 15 million fewer individuals being insured than if the ACA remained. In July 2017, Republicans revised the bill further with an amendment from Senator Ted Cruz, which proposed that insurers do not have to sell health insurance plans that meet all of the ACA requirements if they sell ones that do incorporate ACA health insurance plan stipulations. In July 2017, Republican Senator John McCain returned to the Senate while ill with brain cancer to vote against the bill. On July 20, 2017, the Senate released its then-current BRCA version, without the Cruz amendment, and it was forwarded to the CBO for assessment. The CBO concluded that the BRCA version would substantially ease federal deficits, but result in more Americans without health insurance—up to a projected 21 million individuals by 2026. On July 25, 2017, the Republicans released a revised version of BRCA, which included the Cruz and Portman amendments. The Portman amendment increased Medicaid funding with the view of tackling the opioid addiction crisis. This version of BRCA did not pass the Senate (UCSF/UC Hastings Consortium on Law, Science and Health Policy, 2018, pp. 2–8; Roubein, 2017, pp. 1–3).

On July 26, 2017, the Senate introduced the *ObamaCare Repeal Reconciliation Act* (ORRA), which would essentially repeal the ACA without providing replacement measures. ORRA was not passed. On July 26, 2017, numerous bills focusing on ACA repeal and replace were introduced in the Senate, and none passed. On July 27, 2017, the proposed "Skinny Bill," or the *Health Care Freedom Act*, did not pass as Republican Senators McCain, Collins, and Murkowski voted against it, along with Democratic Senators. In September 2017, Republican Senators Graham and Cassidy prepared a new ACA repeal bill, which focused on giving states federal funding in the form of block grants, but it did not have sufficient Republican support in the Senate. On September 13, 2017, Senator Bernie Sanders introduced the *Medicare for All* bill, which proposed a Medicare-run healthcare system and would result in a single-payer system. On September 26, 2017, the Republicans decided to not have a vote on the Graham-Cassidy bill, thereby killing it. On October 12, 2017, President Trump signed an executive order that undermined the ACA by instructing federal departments to permit the sale of interstate plans. On October 12, 2017, President Trump terminated cost-sharing reductions (CSR) payments, stating that the payments were a "bailout" for the insurance industry (UCSF/UC Hastings Consortium on Law, Science and Health Policy, 2018, p. 2). A CSR allows individuals who purchase a silver health insurance plan to be eligible for reduced deductibles, co-pays, and co-insurance payments (HealthCare.gov, n.d.). As a result, 19 states filed an injunction to halt the payment cessation due to fears that the health insurance marketplaces would face disruption and uncertainty (UCSF/UC Hastings Consortium on Law, Science and Health Policy, 2018, pp. 2–8; Roubein, 2017, pp. 1–3).

On November 2, 2017, the Trump administration declared that it would move its focus away from repealing and replacing the ACA to tax reform. The subsequent *Individual*

*Tax Reform and Alternative Minimum Tax Act* (subsequently referred to as the *Tax Cut and Jobs Act*) removed the tax penalty for not having health insurance, thus repealing the ACA's individual mandate. On November 8, 2017, the CBO released its analysis of *Tax Cut and Jobs Act* and concluded that removing the individual mandate would save $338 billion over 10 years, but would result in 13 million more individuals without health insurance by 2027. On November 16, 2017, the *Tax Cut and Jobs Act* passed in the House of Representatives, and it was also approved in the Senate on December 7, 2017. A revised version of the *Tax Cut and Jobs Act* was then reconciled and passed in both Chambers of Congress on December 19, 2017; this version still repeals the individual mandate. On December 22, 2017, President Trump signed the *Tax Cut and Jobs Act* into law (UCSF/ UC Hastings Consortium on Law, Science and Health Policy, 2018, pp. 2–8; Roubein, 2017, pp. 1–3). The repeal-and-replace efforts by the Republicans did not garner enough consensus within their own party to be successful. As of May 2019, the Trump administration was still labouring to remove the ACA through indirect political maneuvering, as evidenced by the inclusion of a fundamental ACA provision in the *Tax Cut and Jobs Act*. This, ironically, is also a mosaic approach to reform, although a slow-paced strategy due to the lack of internal consensus within the Republican Party, that works within existing governmental architecture to produce the desired change.

## INTEGRATED HEALTH SYSTEMS: POLICY CONVERGENCE

Although Canada and the U.S. diverge in how health care is financed and delivered, some common strategies have begun to emerge in an effort to improve the integration of care. The concept of integrated delivery networks (IDNs), organized systems of care that reduce fragmentation among healthcare providers and promote greater continuity of care to enhance quality outcomes, is a common theme (Leatt, Pink, & Naylor, 1996). Such integrated systems are recognized as being particularly important for managing chronic illness by co-ordinating multiple health professionals with different specialties. The intent of IDNs is to bridge care at different levels—from prevention to acute, rehabilitative, and supportive home care—to ensure a seamless transition among the levels and to facilitate continuity of care. From an organizational perspective, this involves *integration and coordination* (Shortell, Gillies, Anderson, Erickson, & Mitchell, 2000).

Such *integration* has varying forms in Canada and the U.S. Similarities are reflected in the merger of hospitals and other healthcare organizations with various specialties that can together offer a broader continuum of health care. It can alternatively involve organizations developing contracts or memorandums of agreement to share client referrals and information. The organizational and political forces guiding such mergers, however, vary across the two nations.

In the U.S., *integration* was initially fostered through private health insurance companies and health maintenance organizations (HMOs) that contracted with an array of healthcare providers and organizations (hospitals, diagnostic clinics, and primary care clinics) to offer a comprehensive package of healthcare services. More recently, the Medicare Shared Savings Program (MSSP), a key provision of the ACA, enables the development of Accountable Care Organizations (ACOs) that facilitate care co-ordination across provider settings and link reimbursement to quality improvement for sub-populations of Medicare patients with chronic conditions. ACOs are formed through the patient-centred medical home (PCMH) model, in which continuous, anticipatory, team-based care is organized around patients to improve quality and outcomes (O'Donnell et al., 2013).

In Canada, *integration* has been guided largely through the process of regionalization. Regionalization involves the devolution of funding authority for healthcare services from a provincial Ministry of Health to a defined number of regional health authorities (RHAs). It also involves centralization at the local level through the integration of hospitals and other healthcare organizations under a regional board of governors and an overarching management structure (Kouri, 2002). In Ontario, such amalgamation of organizational boards has not occurred; instead Local Health Integration Network (LHIN) boards exist, in additional to organizational boards.

Some critics, however, caution that organizational integration and co-ordination are unable to address cost and quality concerns related to healthcare systems. Developing integrated organizations can, for example, be costly and require years before efficiencies are realized. Integration also involves such challenges as melding organizational cultures, developing new operating processes across several organizations, and attaining physician co-operation to refer their patients by using e-Referral platforms with centralized patient co-ordination, which is often difficult to achieve. Two types of care co-ordination programs have shown promise, focusing on (1) programs for patients with a particular chronic condition such as diabetes, and (2) case-management programs for patients with a complex set of conditions (Burns & Pauly, 2002). Such programs are aimed at improving co-ordination of care, addressing health issues before they become more serious, and reducing costly hospitalizations (Wagner, Davis, Schaefer, von Korff, & Austin, 1999; Weisner, Mertens, Parthasarathy, Moore, & Lu, 2001). Another means to achieve co-ordinated care is through an alliance of local organizations whose executive directors collaborate to achieve coordination (Wiktorowicz et al., 2010).

Information technology (IT) supports co-ordinated and integrated care as electronic medical records (EMRs) allow physicians and other health professionals to access patient information from a centralized medical record database through a communication network. Where providers use different information systems, information interfaces among organizations are required to access information across organizations.

Recentralization of healthcare authority has occurred. In 2009, the 12 Alberta health authorities joined to form Alberta Health Services (AHS). In New Brunswick, eight Regional Health Authorities were amalgamated into two (Regional Health Authority A and B). Despite the recentralization, the previous regionalization led to considerable progress in integrating and co-ordinating health and social services.

While there is some convergence between Canada and the United States in terms of moving toward more integrated and co-ordinated healthcare systems, divergence is, however, apparent with respect to access to pharmaceuticals, including the regulation of pharmaceutical prices.

## ACCESS TO PHARMACEUTICALS: HEALTH SYSTEM DIVERGENCE

Canada and the United States differ in their approaches to ensuring access to pharmaceuticals. In Canada, provincial public health insurance includes drug benefits that facilitate access to medications for people 65 years and over and those on social assistance. In some provinces, such as Quebec, the entire population has access to a subsidized drug benefit program, while other provinces such as Ontario make subsidized programs available to families with catastrophic drug costs and children and youth under 25 years. As of April 1, 2019, this program will only cover children and youth not covered by a private health plan. The remainder of the population attains access to drug insurance coverage largely through private employment benefit plans. This creates a problem for those employed in low-paying and part-time work, who do not normally gain access to such private insurance through employment and are forced to pay for the medications they require. This is a serious issue for people on a low income with a psychiatric history who require medications, but do not receive drug benefits from their employer or their provincial drug benefit plan, as it can compromise their health and well-being. Only New Brunswick offers drug benefits to low-income people with a psychiatric disability who are employed.

By contrast, Medicare in the U.S. did not include insurance for medications, which made the elderly population vulnerable, as most were unable to afford private insurance. An amendment to Medicare in 2006 subsidized about 50% of the costs of pharmaceuticals for seniors. The remainder of the population is expected to access coverage for pharmaceuticals through private insurance either through employment benefit plans or individually. Moreover, private insurance plans include variable coverage for pharmaceuticals, with co-payments often required even with insurance coverage. Uninsured Americans are, however, forced to pay for their medications. The ACA, however, narrows the Medicare Part D "doughnut hole," where individuals are caught between initial drug reimbursement levels and the catastrophic coverage levels, thereby incurring large prescription drug-related expenses (ACA, sec. 3302).

Another contrast between Canada and the U.S. concerns the regulation of pharmaceutical prices. In Canada, the prices of pharmaceuticals are regulated by the Patented Medicines Prices Review Board, which uses an index based on the average price of a specific product in seven industrialized nations, to set the price in Canada. If a new medicine provides a novel and effective therapy for a condition with few therapies available, it will be considered a breakthrough product and granted a higher price than other new products on the market that provide no new breakthrough in therapy. Once set, the prices of patented pharmaceuticals must not increase beyond the rate of inflation. Companies that do not adhere to such regulations must pay penalties. Price regulation in Canada is, however, becoming less effective in addressing access to medicines. For example, the cost of medications for the treatment of cancer is increasing, and provincial health insurers are becoming more selective as to which ones will be covered (Flood & Hardcastle, 2007).

In the United States, by contrast, pharmaceuticals are not subject to price regulation, though individual drug companies will negotiate bulk discounts for their products with large insurers and Veterans Affairs. Such divergent processes have resulted in price differentials of up to 50% less for medicines in Canada than in the U.S. These price differences have sparked a movement in Internet pharmacies, where Americans purchase their medicines in Canada. Cross-border purchase of drugs in Canada is allowed only if a Canadian physician writes the prescription. Internet pharmacies thus operate by having a Canadian physician review an American patient's file and issue a prescription for them. The Internet pharmacy business has grown in the order of $1 billion in trade per year. Such growth has led pharmaceutical firms to issue letters to provincial governments indicating they will limit supply of their drugs only to quantities sufficient for their population.

The reasons such differences exist can be partially attributed to the perspective in Canada that medicines are subject to market failure due to price inelasticity (see Box 11.4), and therefore their prices should be regulated to ensure access. In the U.S., different concepts of the market and political pressure from the patented pharmaceutical trade

---

**Box 11.4:** Market Failure and Pharmaceutical Price Regulation

One reason pharmaceutical prices are regulated in Canada is their price inelasticity. Price inelasticity refers to the concept that the demand for them is inelastic: If the price of these products rises sharply, most people will simply pay the extra cost because they require the product for health reasons. In time of need, the decision to purchase a medicine is insensitive to the cost of the product, even when a consumer pays directly. Since price competition for patented products does not exist, which normally decreases prices to competitive levels, profit-maximizing firms will charge prices that are too high and produce output levels that are too low from the allocational point of view (Brander, 1992). Since increasing the price of pharmaceuticals has little effect on their demand, consumers and the public bear the consequences of high prices (Wiktorowicz, 1995). In Canada, the Patented Medicines Prices Review Board regulates the prices of pharmaceuticals to ensure their accessibility to the population and to public drug benefit plans. In contrast, medicines whose patents have expired are subject to competition from generic product manufacturers, which drives down their prices. For this reason, Canada does not regulate the prices of generic products.

association, one of the most powerful groups, on members of Senate and the House of Representatives have ensured that pharmaceuticals are not subject to price regulation. Governments are under pressure to ensure a competitive private sector drives their economy (Hancher, 1990). An analysis of regulatory measures must thus consider the government's competing imperatives of ensuring access to health care and preserving market competition. The divergent balances struck in Canada and the U.S. reflect their differing perspectives on how to address these important issues.

# CONCLUSIONS

Canada has attained universal coverage and contained the costs of health care, even though mental health care historically has been less well funded than other areas, and timely access to care can be an issue. The U.S. has not achieved universal access to health care despite efforts under the ACA, and instead relies primarily on employer-based insurance coverage for its population under age 65, leaving approximately 23 million people without health insurance coverage. Although the ACA was passed in the U.S., it has not led to universal health insurance coverage, with vulnerable groups, such as undocumented immigrants and legal immigrants who have not resided in the U.S. for five years, being excluded. Additionally, health exchanges regulate insurance purchased through this mechanism, but not employer or group-based insurance, so if insurance is obtained outside an exchange, there is no guarantee that the insurance will meet an individual's health needs. Furthermore, low- and middle-income individuals have difficulty affording rising health insurance fees and are not necessarily able to purchase expensive health insurance without expenditure caps, meaning that they can become bankrupt if they fall ill. The repeal-and-replace movement also threatens the health equity measures in the ACA by eliminating the individual mandate (through the *Tax Cut and Jobs Act*), wishing to fund Medicaid through a per-person cap instead of existing federal-state matching formulas, which would lower federal funding to the states, to repeal the tax on wealthy Americans that is used to partially fund the ACA, and to forgo insurance regulations, meaning that insurance companies would not have to adhere to mandatory essential health benefits. Strong opposition to the ACA arises from private insurance companies and insured citizens who fear their level of choice or the quality of their healthcare plans will be diminished, as well as within the Republican repeal-and-replace movement. Despite the areas of convergence and divergence in the healthcare systems of Canada and the United States, ongoing challenges remain for both in terms of meeting public expectations within public and private budgetary constraints.

## CRITICAL THINKING QUESTIONS

1. On which aspects do liberalism and socialism differ?
2. Consider the different processes through which laws are passed in Canada and the U.S. Why is it more difficult to pass laws in general, and laws concerning health care in particular, in the U.S. than in Canada?

3.  In countries with a publicly insured universal healthcare system, what inequities result from allowing a parallel private system?
4.  Why is public financing considered the optimal form of healthcare financing? Why is the optimal mode of healthcare delivery considered to be private not-for-profit?
5.  What challenges are faced by American Medicare, Medicaid, and managed care?
6.  What are the strengths and weaknesses to the mosaic, big-bang, and blueprint strategies to health reform? Which approach is likely to be successful in bringing about health equity throughout the health reform process?

## FURTHER READINGS

Bartram, M., & Lurie, S. (2017). Closing the mental health gap: The long and winding road? *Canadian Journal of Community Mental Health, 36*(2), 5–18. doi:10.7870/cjcmh-2017-021
A historic analysis of the limitations for funding mental health care in Canada.

Feder, J. (2004). Crowd-out and the politics of health reform. *Journal of Law, Medicine, and Ethics, 32*(3), 461–464.
Judith Feder provides political and historical analysis of the resistance to universal public health insurance in the U.S. She provides a pithy analysis of the challenges to universal healthcare coverage in that country.

Maioni, A. (1998). *Parting at the crossroads: The emergence of health insurance in the United States and Canada.* Princeton, NJ: Princeton University Press.
The differences in the historical and political trajectories for the development of healthcare insurance in Canada and the U.S. are analyzed. Maioni's historical analysis also clarifies the differences in the political contexts of the two nations.

Tuohy, C. H. (1999). *Accidental logics: The dynamics of change in the health care arena in the United States, Britain, and Canada.* New York: Oxford University Press.
A comparative political analysis that draws on the theory of path dependency to clarify how past choices in the development of health insurance in U.S., Canada, and Britain shape these nations' responses to current challenge of escalating costs. It provides an understanding of the forces leading to change in different national contexts.

Tuohy, C. H. (2011). American reform in comparative perspective: Big bang, blueprint, or mosaic? *Journal of Health Politics, Policy and Law, 36*(3), 571–576.
A political analysis of American healthcare policy reform focusing on the ACA.

---

## RELEVANT WEBSITES

### Centers for Medicare and Medicaid Services
www.cms.hhs.gov/
   Provides information on changing provisions in the benefit plans associated with the U.S.'s Medicare and Medicaid programs. Links to related research and information sites on Medicare and Medicaid are also included.

### Kaiser Family Foundation
www.kff.org
   The Kaiser Family Foundation provides analysis of managed care. It also provides access to papers offering evidence-based analysis of different types of healthcare plans in the U.S.

### Organisation of Economic Co-operation and Development (OECD)
www.oecd.org
   The OECD website provides access to their overviews of national healthcare systems, as well as analysis of national healthcare systems from a comparative perspective.

### *The Patient Protection and Affordable Care Act* of 2010
https://www.gpo.gov/fdsys/pkg/PLAW-111publ148/pdf/PLAW-111publ148.pdf
   This website provides the full text of the ACA.

### WHO Regional Office for Europe on Behalf of the European Observatory on Health Systems and Policies
www.euro.who.int/document/e83126.pdf
   The European Observatory provides in-depth analysis of national healthcare systems from both individual nations and comparative perspectives.

---

## GLOSSARY

**Case manager:** A nurse, doctor, or social worker who works with patients, providers, and insurers to co-ordinate all services deemed necessary to provide the patient with a plan of medically necessary and appropriate health care.

**Health maintenance organization (HMO):** An entity that provides or arranges for coverage of health services needed by members for a fixed, prepaid premium.

**Integrated delivery systems:** Organized systems of health care that reduce fragmentation among healthcare providers and promote greater continuity of care to enhance quality outcomes.

**Managed healthcare plan:** An arrangement that integrates financing and management with the delivery of healthcare services to an enrolled population. It employs or contracts with an organized system of providers who deliver services and frequently share financial risk.

**Utilization review:** A formal review of utilization for appropriateness of healthcare services delivered to a member on a prospective, concurrent, or retrospective basis.

## REFERENCES

Bartram, M. (2017). Making the most of the federal investment of $5 billion for mental health. *Canadian Medical Association Journal, 189*(44), e1360–e1363. doi:10.1503/cmaj.170738

Bartram, M. & Lurie, S. (2017). Closing the mental health gap: The long and winding road? *Canadian Journal of Community Mental Health, 36*(2), 5–18. doi:10.7870/cjcmh-2017-021

Bhatia, V. (2010). Social rights, civil rights and health reform in Canada. *Governance, 23*(1), 37–58. doi:10.1111/j.1468-0491.2009.01466.x

Brander, J. (1992). *Government policy toward business* (2nd ed.). Toronto: Butterworths Canada.

Burns, L., & Pauly, M. V. (2002). Integrated delivery networks: A detour on the road to integrated health care? *Health Affairs, 21*(4), 128–143. doi:10.1377/hlthaff.21.4.128

Coleman, A., Checkland, K., Segar, J., McDermott, I., Harrison, S., & Peckham, S. (2014). Joining it up? Health and wellbeing boards in English local governance: Evidence from clinical commissioning groups and shadow health and wellbeing boards. *Local Government Studies, 40*(4), pp. 560–580. doi:10.1080/03003930.2013.841578

Deber, R. B. (2004). Delivering health care: Public, not-for-profit, or private? In G. P. Marchildon, T. McIntosh, & Forest, P.-G., *The fiscal sustainability of health care in Canada* (pp. 233–296). Toronto: University of Toronto Press.

Devereaux, P. J., Schünemann, H. J., Ravindran, N., Bhandari, M., Garg, A. X., Choi, P.T., … Guyatt, G. H. (2002). Comparison of mortality between private for-profit and private not-for-profit hemodialysis centers: A systematic review and meta-analysis. *JAMA, 288*(19), 2449–2457. doi:10.1001/jama.288.19.2449

Docteur, E., & Oxley, H. (2003). Health-care systems: Lessons from the reform experience. *OECD Health Working Papers, 9*. Retrieved from www.oecd.org/dataoecd/5/53/22364122.pdf

Doern, G. B., & Phidd, R. W. (1988). *Canadian public policy: Ideas, structure, process.* Scarborough, ON: Nelson Canada.

Dyson, K. P. (1980). *The state tradition in Western Europe.* Oxford: Basil Blackwell.

Edwards, N., & Naylor, C. (2013). Commissioning. Still as many questions as answers about CCGs. *Health Service Journal, 123*(6335), 19–21.

Executive Order 13535. (2010, March 24). Ensuring enforcement and implementation of abortion restrictions in the *Patient and Affordable Care Act.* Retrieved from https://obamawhitehouse.

archives.gov/the-press-office/executive-order-patient-protection-and-affordable-care-acts-consistency-with-longst

Feder, J. (2004). Crowd-out and the politics of health reform. *Journal of Law, Medicine, & Ethics, 32*(3), 461–464. doi:10.1111/j.1748-720X.2004.tb00158.x

Flood, C., & Hardcastle, L. (2007). *The private sale of cancer drugs in Ontario's public hospitals: Tough issues at the public/private interface in health care.* Montreal: McGill Health Law Publication.

Flood, C., & Xavier, S. (2008). Health care rights in Canada: The Chaoulli legacy. *Medicine and Law, 27*(3), 617–644.

Government of the United States. (2018). *What marketplace health insurance plans cover.* Washington, DC: Author.

HealthCare.gov. (n.d.). *Cost sharing reductions.* Washington, DC: U.S. Centers for Medicare & Medicaid Services.

Grogan, C. (2017). How the ACA addressed health equity and what repeal would mean. *Journal of Health Politics, Policy and Law, 42*(5), 985–993. doi:10.1215/03616878-3940508

Hacker, J. (2002). *The divided welfare state.* New York: Cambridge University Press.

Hancher, L. (1990). *Regulating for competition: Government, law, and the pharmaceutical industry in the United Kingdom and France.* Oxford: Clarendon Press.

Hall, M. (2011). Getting to universal coverage with better safety-net programs for the uninsured. *Journal of Health Politics, Policy and Law, 36*(3), 521–526. doi:10.1215/03616878-1271198

Kouri, D. (2002). Is regionalization working? *Canadian Healthcare Manager.*

Leatt, P., Pink, G. H., & Naylor, C. D. (1996). Integrated delivery systems: Has their time come in Canada? *Canadian Medical Association Journal, 154*(6), 803–809.

MacLean, G. A., & Wood, D. R. (2002). *Introduction to politics: Power, participation, and the distribution of wealth.* Toronto: Pearson Education Canada.

Maioni, A. (1998). *Parting at the crossroads: The emergence of health insurance in the United States and Canada.* Princeton, NJ: Princeton University Press.

Mann, C., & Westmoreland, T. (2004). Attending to Medicaid. *The Journal of Law, Medicine, & Ethics, 32*(3), 416–425. doi:10.1111/j.1748-720X.2004.tb00152.x

National Health Service. (2018). About quality accounts. Retrieved from https://www.nhs.uk/aboutNHSChoices/professionals/healthandcareprofessionals/quality-accounts/Pages/about-quality-accounts.aspx

O'Donnell, A. N., Williams, B. C., Eisenberg, D., & Kilbourne, A. M. (2013). Mental health in ACOs: Missed opportunities and low hanging fruit. *The American Journal of Managed Care, 19*(3), 180–184.

Oliver, T. (2011). Health care reform as a halfway technology. *Journal of Health Politics, Policy and Law 36*(3), 603–609.

*Politico.* (2009, February 26).Obama-care 101: The president's 8 principles. Retrieved from https://www.politico.com/story/2009/02/obama-care-101-the-presidents-8-principles-019362

Rawls, J. (1971). *A theory of justice.* Cambridge, MA: Harvard University Press.

Rodwin, M. A. (2011). Why we need health care reform now. *Journal of Health Politics, Policy and Law, 36*(3), 597–601. doi:10.1215/03616878-1271324

Roubein, R. (2017, September 26). Timeline: The GOP's failed effort to repeal ObamaCare. *The Hill*. Retrieved from https://thehill.com/policy/healthcare/other/352587-timeline-the-gop-effort-to-repeal-and-replace-obamacare

Saltman, R. B., & von Otter, C. (1992). *Planned markets and public competition: Strategic reform in Northern European health systems*. London: Open University Press.

Sandier, S., Paris, V., & Polton, D. (2004). *Health care systems in transition: France*. Copenhagen: WHO Regional Office for Europe on behalf of the European Observatory on Health Systems and Policies. Retrieved from www.euro.who.int/document/e83126.pdf

Shortell, S. M., Gillies, R. R., Anderson, D. A., Erickson, K. M., & Mitchell, J. B. (2000). *Remaking health care in America: The evolution of organized delivery systems* (2nd ed.). San Francisco: Jossey-Bass.

Simeon, R. (1976). Studying public policy. *Canadian Journal of Political Science, 9*(4), 548–580. doi:10.1017/S000842390004470X

Sparer, M. (2011). Federalism and the Patient Protection and Affordable Care Act of 2010: The Founding Fathers would not be surprised. *Journal of Health Politics, Policy and Law, 36*(3), 461–468. doi:10.1215/03616878-1271099

Stone, D. A. (1988). *Policy paradox and political reason*. Glenview, IL: Scott Foresman.

Tuohy, C. H. (1999). *Accidental logics: The dynamics of change in the health care arena in the United States, Britain, and Canada*. New York: Oxford University Press.

Tuohy, C. H. (2011). American reform in comparative perspective: Big bang, blueprint, or mosaic? *Journal of Health Politics, Policy and Law, 36*(3), 571–576. doi:10.1215/03616878-1271279

UCSF/UC Hastings Consortium on Law, Science and Health Policy. (2018). *Health reform tracker: ACA repeal and replace efforts timeline 2017*. Retrieved from http://www.healthreformtracker.org/ahca-timeline/

US Government. (2010). *The Patient Protection and Affordable Care Act of 2010*. Retrieved from https://www.gpo.gov/fdsys/pkg/PLAW-111publ148/pdf/PLAW-111publ148.pdf

Vladeck, B. C. (2004). The struggle for the soul of Medicare. *The Journal of Law, Medicine, & Ethics, 32*(3), 410–415. doi:10.1111/j.1748-720X.2004.tb00151.x

Wagner, E. H., Davis, C., Schaefer, J., von Korff, M., & Austin, B. (1999). A survey of leading chronic disease management programs: Are they consistent with the literature? *Managed Care Quarterly, 7*(3), 56–66.

Weimer, D. L., & Vining, A. R. (1989). *Policy analysis, concepts, and practice*. Englewood Cliffs, NJ: Prentice-Hall.

Weisner, C., Mertens, J., Parthasarathy, S., Moore, C., & Lu, Y. (2001). Integrating primary medical care with addiction treatment: A randomized controlled trial. *JAMA, 286*(14), 1715–1723. doi:10.1001/jama.286.14.1715

Wiktorowicz, M. (1995). Regulating biotechnology: A rational-political model of policy development." PhD thesis, University of Toronto.

Wiktorowicz, M., Fleury, M.-J., Adair, C. E., Lesage, A., Goldner, E., & Peters, S. (2010). Mental health network governance: Comparative analysis across Canadian regions. *International Journal of Integrated Health, 10*(4), 1–14. doi:10.5334/ijic.525

# CHAPTER 12

## The Provision of Care: Professions, Politics, and Profit

*Ivy Lynn Bourgeault*

## INTRODUCTION

The National Film Board documentary *Bitter Medicine* (1983), which details the birth of medicare in Saskatchewan, describes the key outcome of the struggle for Canadian health care as the coverage of those healthcare services deemed most expensive—hospitals and physicians. It is not surprising, therefore, that rising costs of health care have become a problem, and that hospitals and physicians have been the primary target of efforts to control costs. In the first part of this chapter, I address which healthcare providers are called upon to provide what sorts of care, including how this has evolved historically. This is followed by a discussion of how the healthcare division of labour is managed, and the impact of cost controls on both who provides care and what care they provide.

But it is not only that the most expensive services are covered, but that they continue to be provided largely in privately owned facilities. Naylor (1986) described this situation in medicine as public payment for private practice. Many advocates of further privatization of the Canadian healthcare system emphasize that our system is already based on private delivery. Indeed, the continuity of private provision of healthcare services in Canada has made it vulnerable not only to increased privatization—much of which has been insidious—but also to the intrusion of for-profit care models and motives. These are addressed directly in the second part of this chapter.

Many of the policies to curb rising healthcare costs and the expansion of private, for-profit provision have been imported from the United States, a much more expensive (per capita) and highly privatized system. In light of this, it is imperative to look at the dynamics of professions, profit, and care in Canada in this comparative context. In addition to drawing upon a comparative lens, this chapter will take a critical perspective by teasing apart the rhetoric from the reality, exposing the broader structural forces that impinge upon the provision of care, and emphasizing the impact that gender has played on these processes.

# EVOLUTION OF THE HEALTHCARE DIVISION OF LABOUR

As noted in this volume's historical essay by Feldberg, Vipond, and Bryant (Chapter 9), the healthcare systems—and, by extension, the *healthcare divisions of labour*—in Canada and the United States developed along very similar lines. The provision of care was initially quite eclectic, including care by Indigenous healers, then by religious orders (usually nuns working as nurses) with arrival of settlers, barber surgeons, and various forms of midwives (Connor, 1989; Laforce, 1990; Mason, 1988). There were large differences between urban centres in Upper and Lower Canada and the "Western Territories," the latter being largely either self-sufficient or reliant on lay models of care. Lay or self-provision of care also reflected class and urban and rural differences as well (Mason, 1988). Waves of immigration brought healthcare providers trained in other jurisdictions, some of whom initially practiced only in their cultural communities, but later among the larger population (Biggs, 2004). Local educational and training programs were established beginning with the first medical school in Montreal in 1824 and the first nursing school in St. Catharines, Ontario, in 1874 (Coburn, 1988; Coburn, Torrance, & Kaufert, 1983). These developments increased not only the numbers but also, in some areas, the competition among healthcare providers.

Due to a variety of factors, the medical profession emerged as the dominant health occupation in Canada in the late 19th and early 20th centuries, consolidating its power between the First World War and the Saskatchewan doctors' strike of 1962 (Coburn et al., 1983). Its dominance was attained first by establishing powerful professional organizations that successfully lobbied for protective legislation to place limits on who would be officially allowed to practice medicine. These organizations and their leaders also began to exert control over the production of medical knowledge and, by extension, entrance to medical schools and who would ultimately practice as physicians. It was particularly critical that the profession began to appeal to elite members of society to support overall lobbying efforts. Perhaps most critically, the medical profession sought sponsorship by state officials and wealthy patrons. This was most clearly exemplified in the Carnegie Foundation sponsorship of medical school reform in the U.S. and Canada in the early 20th century through the Flexner Report.[1]

One of the key consequences of the strategies to achieve medical dominance has been the gendered exclusion and segregation of the healthcare division of labour assigning a secondary status to women.[2] Historically, gender was used as an exclusionary criterion by the medical profession in its quest for professional status. This began with the efforts to exclude women from medical school and, failing that, from medical practice and/or hospital admitting privileges. Prior to the mid-20th century, only a handful of women under the most unusual circumstances managed to receive medical training in Canada (Strong-Boag, 1979). Even when female students were admitted, they were made to feel very uncomfortable, there was a lack of female role models, and many experienced subtle and not-so-subtle gender and sexual harassment.

**Box 12.1:** Types of Healthcare Providers

Wardwell (1981) and Willis (1989) both define the three different kinds of professions in terms of their relationship to the dominant medical profession:
- *ancillary or subordinate professions* that are different as ... under the direct control of supervision by medicine
- *limited professions* that are defined as ... practicing independently of medicine but with a limited scope of practice (in terms of patient or treatment modality)
- *marginal or excluded professions*, which are defined as ... practicing outside of the mainstream medical system and denied official legitimacy

Women's involvement in the healthcare division of labour was largely channelled into support occupations—such as nursing, dental hygiene, and dental assistant work—with limited scopes of practice, lower status, and little autonomy (Adams & Bourgeault, 2004; Valentine, 1996). Indeed, female-dominated professions have been regarded by some as achieving only "semi-professional" (Etzioni, 1969) or subordinate (Willis, 1989) status, often functioning only under the direct supervision of more powerful professions dominated by men (see Box 12.1). Thus, while women make up the bulk of healthcare providers, their employment is not evenly distributed across healthcare provider groups.

Some female professions, such as midwifery, were excluded altogether from many segments of the Canadian healthcare division of labour. Indeed, another consequence of medicine's quest for dominance has been the exclusion of healthcare provider groups altogether. In addition to midwifery, many provider groups that are now considered to be complementary or alternative medical practitioners—such as homeopaths and herbalists—were also excluded from the Canadian healthcare landscape (Connor, 1994).

When the efforts arose to reshape the healthcare division of labour following the inception of medicare, the various professional groups were at very different starting points. Medical dominance, as Coburn et al. (1983) argue, was beginning to decline. The status of largely female health professions, such as nursing, was just beginning to climb, propelled in part by the women's movement and labour movements. Despite these shifts in power, which have continued to evolve, medicare legislation has structurally embedded medical dominance into the fabric of the health system (Bourgeault & Mulvale, 2006).

## REFORMS DIRECTED TOWARD WHO PROVIDES CARE

All professions are subject to a process *of rationalization*, which focuses on the most efficient use of healthcare resources, or the assignment of tasks to the "most appropriate" professional. Two key issues involved in the rationalization process include a focus on *flexibility* and the ability to respond to shortages and surpluses through the substitution of health labour. The second and, some would argue, primary, concern is with *keeping costs low* so that the least expensive worker performs tasks at the lowest unit cost. These issues have led to some dramatic changes in *who* does *what* in the provision of health care.

One element of efforts to rationalize the healthcare division of labour is health workforce planning. This involves preparing, regulating, deploying, and assigning tasks to people who work in health care. The key questions posed include:

- What types of workers should exist?
- What will each type of worker do? And what is the distribution of labour across worker groups?
- What training and educational requirements are required for these workers to accomplish their tasks?

When medicare came into effect, several provincial governments sponsored reviews of the healthcare division of labour. Many of these addressed the key problems of the supply, mix, and distribution of healthcare providers (see Box 12.2). In Ontario, this was accomplished by the Ontario Committee of the Healing Arts, which was struck in 1966. In its 1970 report to the provincial government, the committee made several recommendations, some of which addressed increasing medical school enrollment, whereas others addressed the issue of expanding the scope of practice of such professions as nurse-midwives and nurse practitioners. It is important to note that these recommendations were made in a context of a perceived physician shortage. Although nurse practitioners experienced a short-lived surge of interest in the early 1970s (Angus & Bourgeault, 1999), nurse-midwifery failed to capture enough political support at that time to become more fully integrated into the publicly funded healthcare system (Bourgeault, 2005b).

Little changed in the ensuing 10 years, until the Ontario government appointed a Health Professions Legislation Review (HPLR) in 1982 to respond to various pressures

## Box 12.2: Health Human Resource Issues

Health human resources, or what is more recently referred to as health workforce issues, addresses three basic problems:

- *Problems with supply*: The numbers of healthcare professionals providing services to a population
- *Problems with mix*: The relative numbers of healthcare professionals providing various types of specialty services
- *Problems with distribution*: The location or deployment of healthcare professionals across geographic areas

for change in the way health professions were regulated. The mandate of the HPLR was to make recommendations to the minister of health in the form of draft legislation with respect to which health professions should be regulated and a new structure for the legislation governing the health professions in the province (HPLR, 1989). Although the primary objective of the review was to design a new regulatory framework that would more effectively advance and protect the public interest, it also attempted to increase the flexibility of the healthcare division of labour through this framework. The way this was to be achieved was by regulating healthcare providers through a model of controlled acts rather than through exclusive scopes of practice. Some of the controlled acts included in the initial legislation were:

- communicating a diagnosis
- performing a procedure on tissue below the dermis
- administering a substance by injection or inhalation
- applying or ordering the application of a form of energy (e.g., X-rays)

One or more professions are allowed to undertake particular controlled acts, or elements of a controlled act, allowing for overlapping scopes of practice. For example, both midwives and physicians are able to manage labour or deliver a baby, another one of the controlled acts under this legislation, but midwives are limited to labour and deliveries that are considered low risk.

This attempt to increase the flexibility of the healthcare division of labour was not simply an Ontario phenomenon. Similar legislation exists in British Columbia. Further, the 1991 report by health economists Morris Barer and Greg Stoddart for the federal/provincial/territorial ministers of health also addressed the issue of eliminating exclusive scopes of practice and replacing these with a more circumscribed set of controlled acts and reserved titles through legislation similar to the HPLR recommendations (Barer & Stoddart, 1991; Scully, 1999). Several of these recommendations were directed toward managing what was at the time perceived to be an oversupply of physicians. In addition to recommending strategies to curb the medical workforce, the report also addressed the mix of providers, particularly in primary care. A key recommendation addressed the expanded use of primary care nurse practitioners.

Primary care has historically been the most highly sought after and fiercely defended of all healthcare domains. More recently, however, general medical practice has become less attractive (Cesa & Larente, 2004). In Canada in the 1990s, for example, whereas family physicians made up approximately 48% of practicing physicians, less than 40% of new practice entrants chose family medicine (Hawley, 2004; Kralj, 1999), although there has been a more recent small reversal of this declining trend.[3] In the U.S., this is even lower, with some states having only 11% of their complement of physicians in family practice. This has created a strong impetus for the expansion of a variety of both medical and non-medical primary care providers (see Box 12.3) in order to meet patient needs.

**Box 12.3:** The Primary Healthcare Division of Labour in Canada and the U.S.

| Canada | United States |
|---|---|
| Family physicians<br>Primary care specialists<br>Gynecologists for women<br>Internists for men<br>Pediatricians for children<br>Primary care nurse practitioners<br>Physician assistants | Family physicians<br>Primary care specialists<br>Gynecologists for women<br>Internists for men<br>Pediatricians for children<br>Nurse practitioners<br>Physician assistants |

- *Nurse practitioners* are advanced practice nurses who provide a broad range of healthcare services, including: taking the patient's history, performing a physical exam, and ordering appropriate laboratory tests and procedures; diagnosing, treating, and managing acute and chronic diseases; providing prescriptions and co-ordinating referrals; and promoting healthy activities in collaboration with the patient (www.nlm.nih.gov/medlineplus/ency/article/001934.htm).
- *Physician assistants* are healthcare professionals licensed to practice medicine with physician supervision. Common services provided by a PA include taking medical histories and performing physical examinations; ordering and interpreting lab tests; diagnosing and treating illnesses; assisting in surgery; prescribing and/or dispensing medication; and counselling patients (www.asapa.org/page/PA).

But this begs the question as to whether non-physician primary care providers are alternatives to medical providers or complementary. Both perspectives are evident in the Canadian context. Prior to the Barer-Stoddart report, Lomas and Stoddart (1985) estimated that between 20% and 32% of general practitioners in Ontario could be replaced by a nurse practitioner. A complementary approach, however, is most salient, particularly at the political level. For example, one family physician who has worked extensively with NPs notes:

> The family practice and nursing models should mesh very nicely to fulfil the demand that NPs' strengths in patient education, counselling and health promotion be linked with family physicians' strengths in diagnosis, treatment and prevention of disease. (Way, quoted in Birenbaum, 1994, p. 77)

Representatives from medical associations have been more forceful, stating that "physicians cannot be expected to accept the proposal to create another health care provider when that creation is based on their own devaluation" (Boadway, quoted in Birenbaum, 1994, p. 77).

The trend toward expanding the deployment and scope of practice of nurse practitioners has an interesting gender dimension because most tend to be female. Some have argued that the reasoning behind the notion that non-physician providers are cheaper than physicians can be related to societal notions of skill, which have been argued to be inherently gendered. For example, the delegation of technical skills to women has long been justified on the basis of driving down the cost of labour (Wajcman, 1991), and female health professions are no exception to this phenomenon. Historically, the poorly rewarded work of nurses, for example, was viewed as a natural extension of the caring services that women provided for their families in the private sphere; it was therefore not seen as the product of rigorous training (Coburn, 1988; Kazanjian, 1993). But the notion that people are paid on the basis of their skills obscures the very nature of skilled work as a socially defined and socially evaluated set of characteristics that varies according to the gender, race, and power of workers, as well as with historical and economic context (Gaskell, 1986). Specifically, female healthcare providers operate within a social system of health care that devalues their skills and knowledge.

In part because of this devaluation of nursing work, the nursing profession has also been subjected to similar kinds of "substitution," as have primary care providers (Bourgeault, 2005a). Given that the nursing workforce is one of the primary budgetary items for hospitals, they are clearly targeted for cost-cutting measures in times of fiscal restraint. As a direct result of hospital cost cutting, the nursing profession has experienced a dramatic loss of jobs and replacement of RNs by lesser-trained nursing staff. Concurrent with these changes, more full-time positions have been converted to part-time as a means of increasing the flexibility of the nursing workforce. Nursing layoffs have been exacerbated by the trend toward the replacement of RNs with registered practical nurses (RPNs) and other unregulated care providers, such as personal support workers (PSWs). For example, in the mid-1990s, one hospital in Toronto replaced almost 100 full-time RN jobs with RPNs and unregulated generic healthcare workers, who, with as little as three weeks of on-the-job training, were being assigned direct patient care. Similar policies have also been implemented in American hospitals with little evidence to support the substitution.

Provincial nursing organizations in Canada have responded to these initiatives with strong opposition. They argue that the increased acuity of patients in hospitals and the decreased length of hospital stays require nurses with a higher rather than a lower level of knowledge, and a broader range of skills and competency. The cost-effectiveness of replacing RNs has also been called into question by several studies suggesting the opposite (Aiken et al., 2005; Norrish & Rundall, 2001). They claim that it is a misconception that RNs are too expensive and, moreover, that it is illogical to blame nurses' present situation on their previously successful negotiations for a fair wage.

So there have been a variety of policies directed toward the rationalization of the healthcare division of labour, most of which address the supply and, to a lesser extent, the mix aspects of the situation. Far less attention has been paid to the consideration of the needs that this supply is supposed to meet. Tomblin Murphy et al. (2003), for example, argue that:

> Decisions about the level and deployment of health human resources are often made in response to short-term financial pressures as opposed to evidence of the effect healthcare staff have on health outcomes … while the stated goal of health human resources planning is to match human resources to *need* for services, decisions on how to allocate healthcare staff are primarily based on *demand* for services. (p. 1)

Newer approaches to health workforce planning highlight the importance of taking a broader perspective. O'Brien-Pallas, Tomblin, Birch, and Baumann (2001) present a broad conceptual framework for making sound health workforce decisions that highlights the importance of population health needs; how supply, production, financial, and management factors should all feed into planning and forecasting; and how utilization should be measured in terms of health outcomes, provider outcomes (such as workload and prevention of burnout), and system outcomes to ensure an efficient and effective mix of health workers. We have built upon this model to consider not only the focus on population needs–based planning elements, but also how the deployment of the health workforce should feed back into the planning process (Bourgeault, Demers, & Bray, 2015; see Figure 12.1). This better addresses the key health workforce issues of supply, distribution, and mix of services to meet population health needs.

### A Revised Health Workforce Planning and Deployment Framework

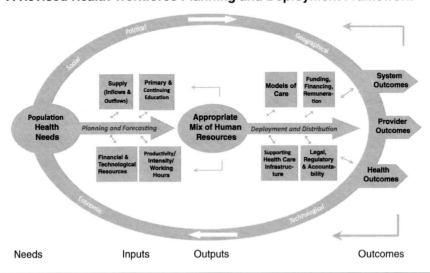

**Figure 12.1:** Conceptual Framework for Understanding Health Human Resources

*Source:* Bourgeault, I. L., Demers, C., & Bray, E. (2015). The need for a pan-Canadian health human resources strategy and coordinated action plan. In S. Carson, K. Nossal, & J. Dixon (Eds.), *Toward a healthcare strategy for Canadians*. Montreal: McGill-Queen's University Press.

# REFORMS DIRECTED TOWARD THE HOW AND THE WHAT: MANAGING CARE AND LEAN

Reforms have not only focused on who is providing care. Policies have also been developed and implemented regarding what or how care is to be provided. Care is increasingly managed, and those doing the managing have changed. This is where we see a strong influence of U.S. policies aimed at making health care more efficient and cost-effective. More recently, Lean, a production-line discipline, has been applied to reduce waste and improve health system quality in a number of provinces (Marchildon, 2013; see Box 12.4).

The increasing management of health care is not a particularly new phenomenon. Initially, when the government decided to fund health care in Canada, it agreed to pay the full costs incurred by hospitals and physicians, less a small administrative fee. This situation did not last for long. In 1978, the federal government began to set limits on healthcare spending, because the costs of providing health care far outstripped indicators of economic growth. This resulted in a cascade of economic constraints that have trickled down from provincial governments to hospitals to the day-to-day practices of healthcare providers.

Reforms to the hospital sector have included shorter hospital stays, more out-patient services and day surgery, deinstitutionalization more generally, cutting beds and staff, contracting out services, and increased standardization of care through protocols. Such reforms focus primarily on getting people out of healthcare institutions or not letting them enter in the first place (or delaying them from accessing care). But reforms focus not only on utilization. Many are focused on rationalizing the organization of healthcare work. This includes such policies as total quality management, patient-focused care, and other models developed in the for-profit, goods-producing sector, which have had a negative impact on hospital-based work, particularly nursing

---

**Box 12.4:** A Brief Description of Lean

---

Originating as a production-line discipline (sometimes known as the "Toyota Production System" or TPS), the term Lean eventually embraced process improvements involving inventory management (Just-In Time [JIT] and Kanban, a signalling process to support JIT), waste reduction (5S), and quality improvement techniques (Six Sigma). Since the mid-1990s, Lean ideas began to be exported to sectors beyond manufacturing, including health care (Brandao de Souza, 2009). In particular, the Virginia Mason Medical Center's application of Lean "became the catalyst for Lean healthcare" in other health systems, particularly in the United States and the United Kingdom (Wood, 2012, p. 28).

---

*Source:* Marchildon, G. (2013). Implementing lean health reforms in Saskatchewan. *Health Reform Observer—Observatoire des Réformes de Santé, 1*(1), 2. doi:10.13162/hro-ors.01.01.01

(Armstrong & Armstrong, 2002). For example, Armstrong and Armstrong (2002) argue that although the total quality approach is portrayed as building on and strengthening nurses' approach to care, the consequences of these reforms have been an increasing fragmentation and quantification of nursing work, that is, focusing on quantity rather than quality of care. They describe further that "care disappears, in part because it is less visible and easy to measure, in part because it is mainly done by women. … Meanwhile, work for providers becomes more intensive, less satisfying, and less secure" (Armstrong & Armstrong, 2002, p. 226).

The origin of many of these new managerial strategies can be traced to the United States. Similar to Canada, the management of health care in the United States has also emerged slowly in the last couple of decades so as to reduce unneeded services and constrain cost (Mechanic, 2004). The most recent umbrella term used for a wide range of largely market-based organizational forms to the allocation of care is "managed care." Managed care has a variety of definitions, but usually involves:

> The provision of health services through a single point of entry and formal enrollment where patient care is managed to ensure an emphasis on quality preventive and primary care, a reduction in inappropriate use of services, control of costs, and management of risk.[4]

Its origins can be drawn from industry-based health programs where companies contract with physicians to provide basic medical care for their employees through a capitation arrangement (Mechanic, 2004). In the last two decades, both private and public healthcare providers have incorporated various aspects of managed care. Further, although many managed care organizations were largely non-profit organizations in the early 1980s, by the end of that decade, more than two-thirds of them were for-profit (Armstrong et al., 2000). Not surprisingly, the for-profit organizations have become powerful voices in setting the American healthcare agenda.

Based on some key indicators, some could say that managed care has been successful in containing healthcare costs, but as Mechanic (2004) notes, "Many of the cost reductions came by negotiating, some would say dictating, lower rates of reimbursement for hospitals, doctors, other professionals, and a variety of ancillary services" (p. 77). Indeed, a constant state of negotiation is a salient theme in how healthcare providers in the U.S. view managed care. Physicians and nurses tell of an increasing burden of negotiating care for patients—particularly textually mediated negotiations—as the access to and amount of care are increasingly limited through managed care policies (Bourgeault et al., 2004). Providers particularly complain about the myriad of plans and insurers they need to negotiate with; constantly changing criteria for inclusions and exclusions; equally changing drug formularies; and changing networks of decision makers. The amount of time devoted to negotiating care is also salient in Canada, particularly where the hospital sector has been restructured through mergers and closures. Healthcare providers in the U.S., however, have been particularly concerned about the audience for negotiations—which in their case are insurers as opposed to other care providers, as is the case in Canada—and the purpose of the negotiations—securing payment and not just care.

Managed care is ultimately a means of rationing care both in terms of access and amount (Bourgeault et al., 2001). As Mechanic (2004) states, "managed care ... was rationing in your face" (p. 77). Access is clearly rationed in the U.S., with more than 44 million Americans without any healthcare insurance (Garfield, Orgera, & Damico, 2019). Access is not so much denied in the Canadian context—due in large part to its publicly funded healthcare system—as it is delayed through the waiting lists for particular procedures. Many more similarities are revealed when we examine how the amount of care is rationed in the U.S. and Canada. Various tools, such as policies that mandate shorter times for hospital stays and increase the number of patients for which healthcare providers are responsible, have been adopted on both sides of the border, with the criteria for adoption being based more on their ability to control costs than evidence of improved quality.

## THE PRIVATIZATION AND PROFITIZATION OF CARE

Many of the practices of managed care and Lean management strategies result in an insidious *privatization* of health care (see Box 12.5). According to Armstrong et al. (2003), privatization can take many forms, including: the introduction of for-profit practices into public systems of provision; the replacement of public payment for services with private payment, whether directly by individuals or through private insurance; the shift from publicly funded services to private, for-profit provision; and the transfer of work—primarily care work—to the home, where the responsibility is disproportionately borne by women working without pay. This latter, more invisible form of privatization is particularly problematic because women are increasingly involved in paid employment, and hence are not readily available to care for sick relatives. If they do take on care, both their paid work and their unpaid caring work are compromised. This can in turn result in greater stress and negative health consequences for the provider and often also greater risks for those being cared for, who may not be receiving the most appropriate care. There is also the added burden of greater financial costs for the entire household.

Although some argue that the only conceivable solution to rising costs in health care and other public services is thought to be further market penetration and the adoption of more for-profit practices, Armstrong et al. (2003) argue that mixing public and private, for-profit partnerships squeezes out public values and practices. What are left are corporate, for-profit values and methods combined with limited choice. In its worst form, it substitutes profit maximization for essential care, it can limit access to critically needed services, it can deliver substandard services to consumers, and/or it can set inadequate reimbursement rates for care providers.[5] Further, what is lost is "the efficiency of a public system, the social solidarity created by shared responsibility and rights and the democratic accountability that is possible in a public system" (Armstrong et al., 2003, p. 16).

**Box 12.5:** The Case against Privatization

---

Armstrong et al. (1999) highlight at least three major differences between healthcare delivery and goods production, differences that raise significant questions about how appropriate market-based techniques are for the provision of health care.

First, care providers assume and demand autonomy in making decisions based on their assessments of complex individual needs. This is particularly the case with doctors, who determine many of the healthcare expenditures. In contrast, *strategies in the for-profit sector assume and demand managerial control over processes and decision-making.*

A second major difference between the two sectors relates to sales. *In the for-profit sector, selling more is critical to maintaining profit growth.* Customers are encouraged to spend and use more. In healthcare reform, however, the stated purpose is to spend and use less. Utilization reviews are intended to reduce the number of procedures and processes to lower costs and improve care.

This is related to a third major difference between healthcare delivery and for-profit production. *Customer choice is defined as a primary basis for competition in the market,* but many patients lack the knowledge, the capacity, or the time to decide among alternatives. In other words, many are not in a position to exercise the choice that is seen as a fundamental basis for efficiency in for-profit settings. This unpredictability makes care delivery less amenable than goods production to managerial planning and costing based on assumptions about regularity and uniformity among products.

## CONCLUSIONS

At the outset of this chapter, I intended to shed some light on how the healthcare division of labour in Canada developed, how it has evolved, and how it has been differentially affected by recent reforms that have increasingly managed care. The management strategies we have examined here address not only who provides care in terms of health human resources, but also how that care is provided. The critical perspective taken in this examination should not be viewed as a general unquestioning criticism of all forms of healthcare reforms. Rather, this perspective, I hope, helps to reveal what some of the consequences of these reforms—both intended and unintended—have been for the people who provide care within our healthcare system.

## CRITICAL THINKING QUESTIONS

1.  How has the rationalization of the healthcare division of labour differentially affected the medical profession versus predominantly female health professions such as nursing?
2.  Why do you think so many health human resource policies deal with the issue of *supply*?
3.  What is the difference between *rationalizing* and *rationing* when it comes to health care?
4.  What might be some of the problems in transferring policies created to solve problems in the American healthcare system to Canada?
5.  What is the impact of the profit motive on the provision of health care in Canada and the United States?

## FURTHER READINGS

Armstrong, P., Armstrong, H., Bourgeault, I. L., Choinière, J., Lexchin, J., Mykhalovskiy, E., Peters, S., & White, J. (2003). Market principles, business practices, and health care: Comparing the U.S. and Canadian experiences. *International Journal of Canadian Studies, 28*, 13–38.
This article provides a critical comparison of the provision of care in Canada and the United States.

Bourgeault, I. L. (2015). Magali Safarti-Larson & Anne Witz on the professionalization of medicine, class and gender. In F. Collyer (Ed.), *The Palgrave handbook on social theory on health and medicine* (p. 520–534). Basingstoke, U.K.: Palgrave Macmillan.
This chapter explores the theoretical approaches described by Magali Safarti-Larson and separately by Anne Witz, both of which advanced sociology of profession approaches.

Bourgeault, I. L., & Barer, M. (2012). The case for a pan-Canadian health workforce observatory: Moving from crisis management to future planning, now. In N. Roos, S. M. Singer, K. O'Grady, C. Tapp, & S. Turczak (Eds.), *Canadian health policy in the news: Why evidence matters* (p. 361–363). Evidence Network eBook. Retrieved from http://umanitoba.ca/outreach/evidencenetwork/wp-content/uploads/2012/12/Canadian-Health-Policy-in-the-News_DEC-10_12.pdf
This op-ed provides an overview of the need for some form of co-ordinated health workforce agency.

Bourgeault, I. L., Demers, C., & Bray, E. (2015). The need for a pan-Canadian health human resources strategy. In S. Carson, K. Nossal, & J. Dixon (Eds.), *Toward a healthcare strategy for Canadians*. Montreal: McGill-Queen's University Press.
This chapter outlines the history of health workforce planning, policy, and management in Canada and makes a case for the need for a health workforce strategy.

Bourgeault, I. L., & Merritt, K. (2015). Deploying health human resources: Scopes of practice, skill-mix and shifting tasks in the provision of health care. In E. Kuhlmann, R. H. Blank, I. L. Bourgeault, & C. Wendt (Eds.), *The Palgrave international handbook of healthcare policy and governance*. Basingstoke, U.K.: Palgrave Macmillan.
This chapter provides an overview of the scoping review undertaken on behalf of the Canadian Academy of Health Sciences, along with an updated version of the conceptual model included therein.

## RELEVANT WEBSITES

### Canadian Health Workforce Network (CHWN)

https://www.hhr-rhs.ca/

CHWN is the recently rebranded Canadian Health Human Resources Network, which was established with development funds from Health Canada and the Canadian Institutes of Health Research. It is comprised of national experts, researchers, and policy-makers involved/interested in health human resource research, policy, and/or planning.

### Canadian Institute for Health Information (CIHI)

https://www.cihi.ca/en

CIHI is an independent, not-for-profit organization that provides essential information on Canada's health systems and the health of Canadians. It collects, compiles, and reports on data on the health workforce across Canada.

### Health Canada: Health Human Resources Strategy

https://www.canada.ca/en/health-canada/services/health-care-system/health-human-resources/strategy.html

Health Canada and its partners are pursuing a range of targeted strategies over the short term, designed to increase supply, make more effective use of the workforce's skills, and provide the ongoing support and education to promote high-quality care and effective HHR planning, thus optimizing the Canadian health workforce.

### Human Resources for Health

www.human-resources-health.com/home/

This is an open-access, peer-reviewed, online journal covering all aspects of planning, producing, and managing the health workforce—all those who provide health services worldwide.

### International Health Workforce Collaborative (IHWC)

https://ihwc.royalcollege.ca/

The IHWC was initiated in 1996 (as the International Medical Workforce Collaborative) by an informal group of health economists, representatives of medical organizations, and government officials from the United States, United Kingdom, and Canada who agreed there would be some value in organizing an international invitational conference to discuss physician workforce issues. Australia joined in 1997. The partners have met every 12 to 18 months since 1996.

## GLOSSARY

**Managed care:** The provision of health services through a single point of entry and formal enrollment where patient care is managed to ensure an emphasis on quality preventive and primary care, a reduction in inappropriate use of services, control of costs, and management of risk. It does so by closely monitoring and controlling the decisions of healthcare providers.

**Privatization:** The process of transferring property from public ownership to private ownership and/or transferring the management of a service or activity from the government to the private sector.

**Profitization:** A form of privatization that gives primacy to profit ahead of individual and community need.

**Rationalization:** In the context of the healthcare division of labour, the process of assigning tasks to the "most appropriate" healthcare provider and an overall focus on the most efficient use of healthcare human resources, with the implicit or explicit purpose of controlling rising healthcare costs. Rationalization is the organization of a business according to scientific principles of management in order to increase efficiency.

**Rationing:** The process of apportioning care according to some plan; rationing of care comes in a variety of forms, including more implicit, upstream forms of rationing, or *macro*-allocation, which includes government policy, funding decisions, and distribution of services; and the more explicit, downstream rationing, or *micro*-allocation, which occurs at patients' bedsides.

## NOTES

1.  Although no medical schools in Canada were closed as a result of this review, several schools in the U.S. were recommended for closure, primarily those for women and ethnic and visible minorities.

2.  It is important to note that there were also racial dimensions to the exclusion of particular forms of care (e.g., Indigenous healers), which, albeit important, are beyond the scope of this discussion here, which is focused on the evolving "official" healthcare division of labour.

3.  The terms "general practitioners," "family physicians," and "primary care physicians" are treated synonymously here, although there are some distinctions between entry to practice requirements for each of these.

4.  Retrieved from www3.uta.edu/sswtech/sapvc/information/teens13_15/Teens_(ages13-15)_Glossary.htm

5. Catholic Charities USA. (2000). The profitization of social services: Where do
   we set limits on a market-driven social service system? Retrieved from www.
   catholiccharitiesusa.org/news/opinion/2000/profitization.htm

## REFERENCES

Adams, T. L., & Bourgeault, I. L. (2004). Feminism and women's health professions in Ontario. *Women's Health, 38*(4), 73–90. doi:10.1300/J013v38n04_05

Aiken, L. H., Clarke, S. P., Sloane, D. M., Sochalski, J. A., Busse, R., Clarke, H., … Shamian, J. (2001). Nurses' reports on hospital are in five countries: The ways in which nurses' work is structured have left nurses among the least satisfied workers, and the problem is getting worse. *Health Affairs, 20*(3), 43–53. doi:10.1377/hlthaff.20.3.43

Angus, J., & Bourgeault, I. L. (1999). Medical dominance, gender, and the state: The nurse practitioner initiative in Ontario. *Health and Canadian society, 5*(1), 55–81.

Armstrong, P., & Armstrong, H. (2002). *Wasting away: The undermining of Canadian health care.* Toronto: Oxford University Press.

Armstrong, P., Armstrong, H., Bourgeault, I. L., Choinière, J., Lexchin, J., Mykhalovskiy, E., … White, J. (2003). Market principles, business practices, and health care: Comparing the U.S. and Canadian experiences. *International Journal of Canadian Studies, 28*, 13–38.

Armstrong, P., Armstrong, H., Bourgeault, I. L., Choinière, J., Mykhalovskiy, E., & White, J. (1999). *Managed care: The experience of nurses in California.* Sacramento: California Nurses Union.

Armstrong, P., Armstrong, H., Bourgeault, I. L., Mykhalovskiy, E., & White, J. (Eds.). (2000). *Heal thyself: Managing health care reform.* Aurora: Garamond.

Barer, M. L., & Stoddart, G. L. (1991). *Toward integrated medical resource policies for Canada.* Winnipeg: Manitoba Ministry of Health.

Biggs, C. L. (2004). Rethinking the history of midwifery in Canada. In I. L. Bourgeault, C. Benoit, & R. E. Davis-Floyd (Eds.), *Reconceiving midwifery* (pp. 17–45). Montreal: McGill-Queen's University Press.

Birenbaum, R. (1994). Nurse practitioners and physicians: Competition or collaboration? *Canadian Medical Association Journal, 151*(1), 76–78.

Bourgeault, I. L. (2005a). Gendered professionalization strategies and the rationalization of health care: Midwifery, nurse practitioners, and hospital nurse staffing in Ontario, Canada. *Knowledge, Work and Society, 3*(1), 25–52.

Bourgeault, I. L. (2005b). *Push! The struggle for midwifery in Ontario.* Montreal: McGill-Queen's University Press.

Bourgeault, I. L., Armstrong, P., Armstrong, H., Choinière, J., Lexchin, J., Mykhalovskiy, E., … White, J. (2001). The everyday experiences of implicit rationing: Comparing the voices of nurses in California and British Columbia. *Sociology of Health and Illness, 23*(5), 633–653. doi:10.1111/1467-9566.00269

Bourgeault, I. L., Demers, C., & Bray, E. (2015). The need for a pan-Canadian health human resources strategy. In A. S. Carson, K. R. Nossal, & J. Dixon, (Eds.), *Toward a healthcare strategy for Canadians* (pp. 87–110). Montreal: McGill-Queen's University Press.

Bourgeault, I. L., Lindsay, S., Mykahalovskiy, E., Armstrong, P., Armstrong, H., Choinière, J., ... White, J. (2004). At first you will not succeed: Negotiating care in the context of health reform. *Research in the Sociology of Health Care, 22*, 261–276.

Bourgeault, I. L., & Mulvale, G. (2006). Collaborative health care teams in Canada and the U.S.: Confronting the structural embeddedness of medical dominance. *Health Sociology Review on Medical Dominance, 15*(5), 481–495. doi:10.5172/hesr.2006.15.5.481

Brandao de Souza, L. (2009). Trends and approaches in lean healthcare. *Leadership in health services, 22*(2), 121–39. doi:10.1108/17511870910953788

Cesa, F., & Larente, S. (2004). Work force shortages: A question of supply and demand. *Health Policy Research Bulletin, 8*, 12–16.

Coburn, D. (1988). The development of Canadian nursing: Professionalization and proletarianization. *International Journal of Health Services, 18*(3), 437–456. doi:10.2190/1BDV-P7FN-9NWF-VKVR

Coburn, D., Torrance, G. M., & Kaufert, J. M. (1983). Medical dominance in Canada in historical perspective: The rise and fall of medicine? *International Journal of Health Services, 13*(3), 407–432. doi:10.2190/D94Q-0F9Y-VYQH-PX2V

Coburn, J. (1987). "I see and am silent": A short history of nursing in Ontario 1850–1930. In D. Coburn, C. D'Arcy, G. Torrance, & P. New (Eds.), *Health and Canadian society* (2nd ed., pp. 441–462). Markham, ON: Fitzhenry and Whiteside.

Connor, J. T. H. (1989). *Minority medicine in Ontario, 1795–1903: A study of medical pluralism and its decline.* PhD dissertation, University of Waterloo.

Connor, J. T. H. (1994). "Larger fish to catch here than midwives": Midwifery and the medical profession in nineteenth-century Ontario. In D. Dodd & D. Gorham (Eds.), *Caring and curing: Historical perspectives on women and healing in Canada* (pp. 103–134). Ottawa: University of Ottawa Press.

Etzioni, A. (Ed.). (1969). *The semi-professions and their organization: Teachers, nurses, and social workers.* New York: Free Press.

Garfield, R., Orgera, K., & Damico, A. (2019). *The uninsured and the ACA: A primer — Key facts about health insurance and the uninsured amidst changes to the Affordable Care Act.* Washington, D.C.: Kaiser Family Foundation.

Gaskell, J. (1986). Conceptions of skill and the work of women: Some historical and political issues. In R. Hamilton & M. Barrett (Eds.), *The politics of diversity: Feminism, Marxism and nationalism* (pp. 361–380). London: Verso.

Hawley, G. (2004). Canada's health care workers: A snapshot. *Health Polity Research Bulletin, 8*, 8–11.

Health Professions Legislation Review. (1989). *Striking a balance.* Toronto: Queen's Park Printers.

Kazanjian, A. (1993). Health-manpower planning or gender relations? The obvious and the oblique. In E. Riska & K. Wegar (Eds.), *Gender, work and medicine: Women and the medical division of labour* (pp. 147–171). Newbury Park, CA: Sage.

Kralj, B. (1999). Physician human resources in Ontario: A looming crisis. *Ontario Medical Review, 66*(4), 16–20.

Laforce, H. (1990). The different stages of the elimination of midwives in Quebec. In K. Arnup, A. Levesque, & R. Roach Pierson (Eds.), *Delivering motherhood: Maternal ideologies and practices in the 19th and 20th Centuries* (pp. 36–50). New York: Routledge.

Lomas, J., & Stoddart, G. (1985). Estimates of the potential impact of nurse practitioners on future requirements for physicians in office-based general practice. *Canadian Journal of Public Health, 76*(2), 119–123.

Marchildon, G. (2013). Implementing lean health reforms in Saskatchewan. *Health Reform Observer, 1*(1), Article 1. doi:10.13162/hro-ors.01.01.01

Mason, J. (1988). Midwifery in Canada. In S. Kitzinger (Ed.), *The midwife challenge* (pp. 99–133). London: Pandora.

Mechanic, D. (2004). The rise and fall of managed care. *Journal of Health and Social Behavior, 45*(Extra Issue), 76–86.

National Film Board of Canada. (1983). *Bitter medicine: The birth of medicare.* Tom Shandel (Director); G. Johnson & T. Shandel (Producers).

Naylor, C. D. (1986). *Private practice, public payment: Canadian medicine and the politics of health insurance, 1911–1966.* Montreal: McGill-Queen's University Press.

Norrish, B. R., & Rundall, T. G. (2001). Hospital restructuring and the work of registered nurses. *The Milbank Quarterly, 79*(1), 55–79. doi:10.1111/1468-0009.00196

O'Brien-Pallas, L., Tomblin, M. G., Birch, S., & Baumann, A. (2001). Framework for analyzing health human resources. In *Canadian institute for health information. Future development of information to support the management of nursing resources: Recommendations.* Ottawa: Canadian Institute for Health Information.

Scully, H. (1999). Building on one of the best delivery systems in the world. *Healthcare Papers, 1*(1), 23–32.

Strong-Boag, V. (1979). Canada's women doctors: Feminism constrained. In L. Kealey (Ed.), *A not unreasonable claim: Women and reform in Canada* (pp. 109–129). Toronto: Women's Press.

Tomblin Murphy, G., O'Brien-Pallas, L., Alksnis, C., Birch, S., Kephart, G., Pennock, M., … Wang, S. (2003). *Health human resources planning: An examination of relationships among nursing service utilization, an estimate of population health and overall health status outcomes in the province of Ontario.* Canadian Health Services Research Foundation. Retrieved from https://www.cfhi-fcass.ca/SearchResultsNews/03-11-01/92fbedf4-4b7e-4ad9-ae3a-90614d4b72fa.aspx

Valentine, P. E. (1996). Nursing: A ghettoized profession relegated to women's sphere. *International Journal of Nursing Studies, 33*(1), 98–106. doi:10.1016/0020-7489(95)00037-2

Wajcman, J. (1991). Patriarchy, technology, and conceptions of skill. *Work and Occupations, 18*(1), 29–45. doi:10.1177/0730888491018001002

Wardwell, W. I. (1981). Chiropractors: Challengers of medical dominance. *Research in the Sociology of Health Care, 2,* 207–250.

Willis, E. (1989). *Medical dominance: The division of labour in the Australian health care system* (rev. 2nd ed.). Sydney: George Allen and Unwin.

Wood, D. (2012). Taking the pulse of lean healthcare. *Healthcare Quarterly, 15*(4), 27–33.

# PART IV

## CRITICAL ISSUES IN HEALTH, ILLNESS, AND HEALTH CARE

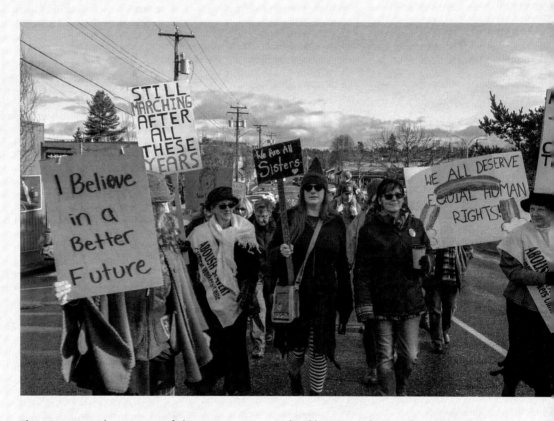

This section explores some of the current issues in health care. Politicians and the public usually define a healthcare crisis in terms of long waiting lists for treatment or a shortage of general practitioners in either urban or rural areas. While these are important issues, also of importance are more difficult-to-define issues of how and why different groups are treated differently by the healthcare system, how healthcare professionals and the public understand illness and disability, and the appropriate and most effective response to such issues.

Also of great importance is the role that political and economic forces play in the treatment of disease and illness. The issue of pharmaceuticals—the drugs used to treat illness and disease—is a potent example of such influences. And the understandings that citizens have concerning the sources of health and disease are critical in that they both reflect and contribute to the emphasis societies place on providing living conditions that support health versus emphasis upon curative medical care provided by healthcare professionals. The chapters in this section address these issues and illustrate the value of each of the broad approaches to understanding health, illness, and health care in Canadian society.

In Chapter 13, Pat Armstrong explores the centrality of gender to understanding and delivering health care. The centrality of gender recognizes women as the primary caregivers both within their families and in the healthcare system. She illustrates this concept with nurses' experiences as workers and caregivers. She also examines gender as a determinant of health and why health and health care are women's issues. It is also important to consider differences among women. She explores the differences in healthcare treatments administered to men and women, differences in symptoms, experiences, and outcomes. Armstrong identifies the gaps in understanding that result from failing to apply a gendered analysis to healthcare issues.

In Chapter 14, Marcia Rioux and Tamara Daly examine different theoretical approaches to understanding disability and illness and how social structures determine how professionals and the public construct disability. In particular, they discuss how women experience disability as a phenomenon associated with aging, as well as how those living in different parts of Canada experience disability. The authors consider critical appraisals of the disability adjusted life years (DALYs) measurement concept, which is compared with statistical analyses of people's experiences of disability or illness. They also consider some ethical and legal issues related to disability and examine the role played by the *Canadian Charter of Rights and Freedoms* in ensuring the equality of disabled people.

In Chapter 15, Joel Lexchin examines the tensions between corporate and public health viewpoints in relation to pharmaceutical issues in Canada. He is especially concerned about the drug regulatory system in Canada and the differing priorities of those producing the drugs and those who may benefit from them. Lexchin explores the industry's promotion of medications and considers the relation of these activities to rising drug costs that threaten the viability of the healthcare system. The author also considers how the patent system influences drug spending, the interactions between Health Canada and the pharmaceutical industry, and the effects of recent trade agreements upon these issues.

In Chapter 16, Dennis Raphael and Toba Bryant examine public health approaches in Canada, the U.S., the United Kingdom, and Sweden. Despite three decades of Canadian government and public health statements on the importance of broader determinants of health, governmental and public health practice—with a few notable exceptions—is firmly focused on behavioural approaches to health promotion. In the U.S., there is virtually no management. In the U.K., the government's systematic efforts are addressing determinants of penetration of broader concepts of health into public health discourse or practice, which is firmly focused on ensuring access to health care and individual risk factor health inequalities, with early evidence of effectiveness. In Sweden, broader approaches to public health are firmly established and represent a continuation of Swedish approaches to public policy that ensure equitable distribution of resources among the population.

In the concluding chapter, Toba Bryant, Dennis Raphael, and Marcia Rioux outline future directions for health research and practice. The key themes they identify that emerge from the contributions to this volume include the definition of the field of health studies; models of understanding health, illness, and health care; power and influence; the importance of public policy; and public versus private governance, among others. Bryant, Raphael, and Rioux emphasize the importance of developing and applying innovative theoretical and conceptual approaches to the health field that draw upon principles of justice, equity, and democratic participation.

# CHAPTER 13

## Women, Health, and Care

*Pat Armstrong*

## INTRODUCTION

Health and care are profoundly gendered. Sex- and gender-based analysis, along with our experiences, provides the evidence. Sex is used primarily to refer to biological characteristics that distinguish males from females, while gender generally refers to social characteristics of feminine and masculine. However, we have become increasingly aware that not only is gender on a spectrum, with many variations in bodies, identities, and expressions of gender, but so too is sex (Oliffe & Greaves, 2012). Moreover, research has also led us to understand that sex and gender are overlapping, interpenetrating categories that cannot be clearly separated (Fausto-Sterling, 2005). Nevertheless, because many cultures view gender as a binary concept, with male and female as the only categories, because such views are real in their consequences, and because women as a group have been at the forefront of sex- and gender-based analysis, this chapter focuses on women.

Informed by feminist political economy theory, the chapter begins by explaining gender-sensitive analysis and why it is necessary. It uses the term gender-sensitive, rather than the more common sex- and gender-based analysis, to avoid the assumption that sex and gender can be separated. It then looks at women's access to care and the treatment they receive in care. It explores the ways reforms in health care are simultaneously working to provide more appropriate care and limiting women's access to care. The final sections examine women's care work, both paid and unpaid. While women have struggled hard to make healthcare work both visible and valued, their gains are rapidly being undermined by reforms that shift care to the home and redefine what constitutes work in care.

## GENDER-SENSITIVE ANALYSIS

Gender-sensitive analysis means much more than analyzing data by sex. For feminist political economists, it means recognizing how gender shapes and is shaped by conditions, practices, and relations, including relations of markets, of power, and of inequality, as well as by ideas (Armstrong & Pederson, 2015; see Box 13.1). It also means exploring how gender intersects with other social, physical, and economic locations such as age, culture, class, disability, and racialization, to name only a few. A gendered analysis focusing on women's health and health care requires the assessment of causes, processes, and consequences "taking into account the context of individual's lives" (DesMeules et al., 2003, p. 2). The impact may be contradictory for women, simultaneously or alternatively improving and challenging their health and capacity to provide care. And the impact may vary among women, depending on their location.

Such an analysis begins by identifying patterns in health and care. Bodies, and ideas about bodies, contribute to these patterns. However, neither bodies nor ideas about them can provide an adequate explanation for women's health, for the inequitable distribution of care work, or for the treatment women receive in health care. Policies, practices, and structures all contribute to these patterns that put the burden of care on women while often failing to respond to their needs or provide access to appropriate care.

These policies and practices are not simply neutral or evidence-based. For feminist political economists, profits, power, contradictions, and inequities frame the conditions for health and care, as do women's resistance and everyday practices. Contexts are critical, as are relations not only between and among women and men but also between employers and employees and among household members and racialized groups, to name only some of the many that matter.

Not surprisingly, much of the gender-sensitive research and policy in Canada has focused on women (Greaves, 2015). This is not surprising because it was the women's movement that began demonstrating how gender and assumptions about gender permeate policy and practices and do so in ways that assume male norms, standards, and subjects. The consequences of what Karen Messing (1998) has called "One-Eyed Science" are particularly harmful for women. As the authors of *The Politics of Women's Health* put it, medicine has played "an active role in perpetuating some aspects of women's oppression while helping to reduce other dimensions" (Sherwin et al., 1998, p. 6). Ideas matter in creating and perpetuating these differences. But inequalities perpetuated by such structural factors as differential access to education, income, benefits, and personal security, along with the organization of paid work and of the professions, the absence of public daycare, and limited public transit, play important roles as well. More women than men are poor, and fewer women than men have access to the kinds of resources that provide them with choices (Canadian Women's Foundation, 2017). In other words, the causes, processes, and consequences of health and care are not only different for women and men. They also contribute to inequality both between women and men and among women.

It is also not surprising that such analysis focused on health and care for women. In Canada, more than 80% of paid care providers are women, and women account for a similar proportion of those providing unpaid care in the home and community (Armstrong, 2015; Moyser, 2017). Moreover, women use the healthcare system more than men, and in different ways than men, not only because they have babies but also because they have more chronic health issues than men and are treated differently from men. Thus, health and health care have clearly emerged as women's issues, and women have played an active role in revealing how gender matters. This effort to have gender taken into account in ways that serve women has not been an easy process, however, and is far from complete.

Does this mean that gender-sensitive research is just about women and serves only their interests? Although gender-sensitive analysis emerged within and from the women's movement, it has neither excluded men nor been irrelevant to men. Indeed, much of the research intended to demonstrate the importance of gender required comparative data on women and men. Moreover, a great deal of health behaviour, of health care, and of other health processes involves relations between women and men, a fact not lost on those beginning from a women's perspective. Power relations in particular have played a major role in the analysis, with an emphasis on the subordination shared by most women. It should be noted, however, that gender-sensitive research is not necessarily comparative. It can study women or men without searching for comparisons or emphasizing gender relations. Yet even those who have been most concerned with women's issues and who see women as subordinate in terms of both health and care recognize that strategies for change cannot be developed in many areas without understanding what is happening with men. Perhaps more critically, this women's research developed many of the tools of analysis that allow us to see gendered causes, consequences, processes, and contexts for men. What works for women does not necessarily work for men, just as what works for men does not necessarily work for women. In fact, that is a major point of gender-sensitive research.

It was evidence and pressure from the women's movement that contributed to Health Canada (2018) expanding the list of social determinants of health beyond biological and genetic endowments to include gender. The inclusion of gender as a health determinant marked a major advance. The range of sex issues is now understood to be much broader, and biology is increasingly understood as influenced by social contexts. At the same time, gender is used to draw attention not only to the social construction of feminine and masculine differences but also to the spectrum that is gender. While it is important to understand gender as a determinant of health, it is equally important to examine how gender pervades all other determinants. Income and social status, employment and education, physical environments and social environments, social support networks and healthy child development, personal health practices and coping skills, culture and health services are all gendered. Too often, however, gender and sex are considered independent variables, while gender is controlled for and thus eliminated from the examination of other health determinants (Pederson & Armstrong, 2015). Equally important, the global, national, regional, and local political economies that set the conditions for care are too often ignored, as are differences linked to other social locations that pervade each of the determinants.

Pressure from the women's movement also contributed to Canada's adoption of the Beijing Declaration and Platform for Action (United Nations, 1995) on equality for women and the consequent federal plan for gender equality. This plan requires legislation and policy to include an analysis of the potential for differential impacts on women and men.

In its wake, Canada established a Women's Health Bureau within Health Canada, a Centres of Excellence Programme for Women's Health, the Canadian Women's Health Network, and the Canadian Institute of Health Research Institute of Gender and Health with a mandate "to support research to address how sex and gender interact with other factors that influence health to create conditions and problems that are unique, more prevalent, more serious or different with respect to risk factors or effective interventions for women and men" (Health Canada, 2003, p. 7). All these initiatives were based on the recognition that gender differences are critical in health and care and that women were often excluded from research and treated inappropriately in practice. All included gender-sensitive research, policy, and practice in their mandate.

Except for the Institute of Gender and Health, all of these federal programs disappeared under the Conservative government of Stephen Harper. However, the research from these federal initiatives did provide us with a wealth of information on women's health and care, as does the research funded by the Institute of Gender and Health. The Liberal government that replaced Stephen Harper has taken some steps to implement a

---

**Box 13.1:** Gender of Person

**Definition**

**Gender** refers to the gender that a person internally feels ("gender identity" along the gender spectrum) and/or the gender a person publicly expresses ("gender expression") in their daily life, including at work, while shopping or accessing other services, in their housing environment, or in the broader community. A person's current gender may differ from the sex a person was assigned at birth (male or female) and may differ from what is indicated on their current legal documents. A person's gender may change over time.

  **Person** refers to an individual and is the unit of analysis for most social statistics programs.

**Usage**

Sex and gender refer to two different concepts. Caution should be exercised when comparing counts for sex with those for gender. For example, female sex is not the same as female gender.

  The variable "gender of person" and the "classification of gender" are expected to be used by most social statistics programs. The variable "sex of person" and the "classification of sex" are to be used where information on sex at birth is needed, for example, for some demographic and health indicators.

---

*Source:* Statistics Canada. (2018). Gender of a person. Retrieved from http://www23.statcan.gc.ca/imdb/p3Var.pl?Function=DEC&Id=410445

gender-sensitive budget and to ensure that data collected by Statistics Canada capture intersectionality as well as violence against women and girls. But there are no new programs focused on women's health.

## WOMEN'S HEALTH

Not surprisingly, women's health varies significantly with age, with income, with education, and with racialization, to name only some of the relevant variables. And women's patterns of illness often differ from those of men.

The more education and income a woman has, the more likely she is to rate her health as excellent or very good (Bushnik, 2016, Table 1). A woman is also more likely to say so if she is Canadian born and thus not facing the stress of immigration (Bushnik, 2016, Table 2). At the same time, Indigenous women are less likely than other women to report excellent or very good health (Arriagada, 2016). The proportion of women reporting good or excellent health has been growing in most age categories, including women in the oldest age group. However, a smaller proportion of women between the ages of 20 and 34 reported good or excellent health in 2014 compared to 2003 (Bushnik, 2016, Chart 1). As this group ages, they may carry their poor health with them, especially as income inequalities grow. A quarter of this age group also say most days are quite a bit or extremely stressful, and are more likely to say so than men in the same age category (Bushnik, 2016, Chart 25). It is this age group of women that is most likely to have small children while also doing paid work. Women in this age group are more likely than men of the same age to report extreme or quite a bit of work stress.

Patterns differ by age. Young women are the most likely to suffer from eating disorders. Between 2012 and 2013, girls between the ages of 10 and 19 accounted for more than half of all women admitted to hospitals for eating disorders. By contrast, men of all ages accounted for just under 7% of all those admitted with such a diagnosis (Canadian Institute for Health Information, 2014). Girls are also more likely to report being depressed and suicidal (Bushnik, 2016, Chart 11). Body image, reinforced by media representations of females, is most frequently seen as a major factor in these differences, but there is research suggesting that many other factors, including physiological ones, may contribute.

Patterns also differ by social location and relations. For example, Indigenous women are more likely than other women to be diagnosed with a chronic condition (Arriagada, 2016). Those defined by Statistics Canada as visible minority women are more likely than other women to report poor mental health.

There are many other differences in patterns of male and female health. For example, women aged 45 to 64 are less likely than men to be diagnosed with diabetes or to die from a heart attack. Older women are significantly more likely than men to fall and are much more likely than men to have arthritis (Bushnik, 2016, Chart 34). Although the proportion of young women and men reporting disabilities is similar, more women than men over the age of 15 report disabilities that limit their daily activities (Burlock, 2017).

Women are also much more likely than men to experience sexual violence, and Indigenous women are particularly vulnerable (Quinlan, Quinlan, Fogel, & Taylor, 2017).

Each of these patterns deserves a particular analysis to investigate what contributes to them. Biology may well play a role, but so too do factors such as paid and unpaid work, access to supports of various kinds, colonialism, racism, social relations, physical environments, and income, to name only some. However, the examples above have been taken primarily from chapters (Arriagada, 2016; Bushnik, 2016; Burlock, 2017) in *Women in Canada: A Statistical Report* that emphasize what may be termed lifestyle choices such as exercise, nutrition, alcohol consumption, and smoking, providing virtually no references to structural factors beyond most women's immediate control.

## ACCESSIBLE, APPROPRIATE CARE

There is little dispute that men and women have different healthcare needs, at least when it comes to reproductive aspects of their health. Until relatively recently, research on women has focused primarily on breasts, babies, and vaginas, and women's health has been defined primarily in these terms. Women have too often been treated in ways that not only equate them with their reproductive capacities but that also limit their power. However, women have struggled against narrow definitions of their health concerns and challenged the treatment they receive in care at the same time as they have been identifying the non-biological structures and relations that shape their health and care.

Many of the challenges began with reproductive health. Women have struggled with some success to gain control. Midwifery provides a particularly good example. As Benoit (1991) points out, midwifery has a varied history across Canada and was never completely eliminated in Indigenous and remote communities, in spite of pressure from both nurses and doctors. The revival of midwifery in the last quarter of the 20th century was not only about women resisting the medical takeover of birth and the desire to restore women's control over the birth process. It was also about redefining midwifery to fit with current knowledge and to gain acceptance as a health profession providing women-centred care based on health rather than illness models.

After considerable effort on the part of women's organizations, midwives have been integrated into health systems in many parts of Canada and are offering women alternatives to medicalized care. Yet Prince Edward Island and the Yukon have yet to regulate midwifery, Newfoundland and Labrador along with New Brunswick only did so in 2016, and most provinces have too few midwives to serve the population seeking such care (Canadian Association of Midwives, 2018). Thus, the midwifery alternative remains beyond the reach of the many who do not have the money to pay for this care and for those in regions of the country where midwifery is not a regulated profession. As the authors in *Indigenous Experiences of Pregnancy and Birth* (2017) make clear, culturally safe midwifery is particularly important. The number of Indigenous midwives has grown with government support, but their numbers remain too small compared to the need.

**Box 13.2:** Indigenous Midwifery

There are many beneficial outcomes for having access to an Indigenous midwife and bringing birth back to communities, including:
- culturally safe and relevant care
- care to families where they live: in urban, rural, and remote communities
- reducing the number of routine evacuations from remote communities
- keeping families together during this important cultural and life event
- improving the health outcomes for parent and baby
- improved self-determination in health care

*Source:* National Aboriginal Council of Midwives. (2017). *Rooted in our past. Looking to our future.* Retrieved from https://canadianmidwives.org/wp-content/uploads/2017/03/NACM_SituationalAnalysis_2017_Low-resolution.pdf

Meanwhile, fewer family physicians now provide obstetrical care. Family physicians are more likely than specialists to know their patients and are less likely to use interventionist techniques, practices made evident in recent research showing a significant rise in the number of Caesarian births accompanying this increasing specialist care. Indeed, Caesarian births are now the most common reason for hospitalization, and while hospital birth rates are declining, Caesarian rates continue to climb (Canadian Institute for Health Information, 2018). In other words, for a growing number of women, childbirth is treated as a medical event in spite of the reintroduction of midwifery.

But the question of appropriate treatment is much larger than childbirth or reproductive matters more generally. Hospitalization rates for mental illness provide one indicator of differences. "For example, the percentages were 16% for women aged 25 to 29 and 20% for women aged 45 to 49, compared with 10% and 14% for men in these age groups, respectively" (Bushnik, 2016). At the same time, women over age 85 are more than twice as likely as men in the same age group to be hospitalized as a result of injury (Canadian Institute for Health Information, 2017a, Table 4). The use of emergency rooms varies as well. Males account for three-quarters of those who visit emergency rooms as a result of sports injury (Canadian Institute for Health Information, 2017b, Table 7).

Too often health issues have been treated as if they were the same for both sexes (Laurence & Weinhouse, 1997). Research is much more likely to be carried out on men, and the evidence thus gathered is assumed to apply to women. Searching for the same symptoms in women often means women's illnesses are treated as merely female complaints or imaginary problems, while providing the same treatment for women as for men may be harmful to their health. The consequence of leaving women out of the research and analyzing data by sex has frequently been inappropriate care for women and greater costs to the system resulting from poor diagnosis.

Gender-sensitive analysis has made a difference in some treatments for women. Cardiovascular disease (CVD) provides a good example (Abramson, 2009). A case study is developed in some detail in Health Canada's (2003) publication *Exploring Concepts of Gender and Health*, and is worth summarizing briefly here.

As this study points out, until the last decade, the overwhelming majority of research in CVD was done on men, both because it was assumed this was a men's disease and because it was assumed that what was true for men was true for women. The initial Aspirin trials, for instance, were done on men, and then Aspirin was prescribed for both women and men. Yet more recent research has demonstrated that Aspirin is not effective for this indication in women. Research has also shown that the causes and risk factors are different for women and men. For instance:

- Men suffer heart disease at an earlier age than women.
- High blood pressure is two to three times more common in women.
- While high levels of bad cholesterol are a risk factor for men, low levels of good cholesterol are a bigger risk factor for women.
- Diabetes is a greater risk factor for women than for men.
- Women and men have different smoking patterns and activity patterns.

The causes and risks differ by racialized groups, income, and culture as well. Indigenous women are more likely than their male counterparts to develop diabetes and are more likely than other women to die from heart disease.

Research has also shown that the processes of the disease and the treatment differ by gender. For instance:

- Women are more likely to have subtle symptoms of heart attack, such as indigestion, abdominal or mid-back pain, nausea, and vomiting.
- Women are less likely than men to be offered invasive procedures and clot-buster medicine.
- Women are less likely to be hospitalized, but stay longer than men when they do enter the hospital.
- Between 80% and 90% of heart transplant recipients are male.

Research indicates different consequences as well:

- Women are more likely to have a second heart attack within six months.
- Women fare less well after heart surgery.

And, finally, and at least as significantly, research indicates that the context of women's lives differs from those of men in ways that influence their likelihood of suffering from cardiovascular disease, of being treated for the disease, and of surviving the disease.

As a result of such gender-sensitive research, protocols are changing. New guidelines are developing for treatment that may well start to show up in outcomes. There is a move beyond thinking about gender differences simply in terms of reproductive issues to the inclusion of other biological processes. Some of the social factors that contribute to differences in health and care are being considered, such as the different reasons why young men and women take up smoking. These gender-sensitive strategies can mean not only more equal and appropriate treatment and outcomes; they can mean cost savings as well.

But there is still a long way to go before gender sensitivity is a feature of research, let alone practice. A 1998 article in the *Canadian Medical Association Journal* reported that "women were poorly represented in the randomized control trials" in their sample of leading medical journal articles on myocardial infarction, "regardless of whether the trials were funded by an agency with a gender-related policy" (Rochon, Clark, Binns, Patel, & Gurwitz, 1998, p. 321). A more recent article linked to CVD featured on the website for the Ontario Institute for Clinical Evaluative Sciences offers no mention of gender in the executive summary of their report on bypass surgery, although being female is mentioned along with a list of other factors as linked to lower survival rates (Institute for Clinical Evaluative Sciences and the Cardiacare Network of Ontario, 2008). "Although progress has been made in bringing attention to sex and gender in scientific research methodologies, some peer-reviewed health journals continue to lag behind in implementing editorial policies on sex and gender reporting" (Gahagan, Gray, & Whynacht, 2015).

Moreover, the emphasis remains on biology, albeit an expanded notion of biology. Significant gaps remain even in CVD research, and the new emphasis on a broader notion of sex differences may be more a reflection of the growing interest in genetic research than it is of a commitment to gender-sensitive research in all aspects of policy. And research into many areas provides no analysis of the specificity of women and men's diseases or intersectional patterns.

Thus, research that recognizes not only physical differences, but also how these differences are shaped by environments and relations are characterized by inequality, is essential. So is education for practitioners on these differences. However, the move to apply managerial techniques taken from the for-profit sector can challenge this recognition. Strategies are designed to increase managerial control over providers, in large measure by standardizing treatment protocols and the timing of care. For example, care pathways that set out to describe and prescribe the trajectory for an illness imply sameness rather than difference. Indeed, the intent is to make the treatment of each person and the timing of the care as similar as possible. The same can be said about the idea of best practices, given that it implies one right way. As feminists have long pointed out, same treatment does not necessarily mean equitable treatment because it fails to take into account both differences among groups of people in different social locations and the specificity of individual lives.

These examples of research and practice are concerned with appropriate care. But even appropriate care needs to be accessible. The introduction of universal public health care in Canada for hospital and doctor services made a tremendous difference in access for marginalized groups. The *Canada Health Act* clearly states that provinces and territories must work to eliminate financial or other barriers to such care, and these governments initially did make significant progress in this direction. The number of doctors and hospitals grew, and fees for these medically necessary services were virtually eliminated. Obviously, these developments were important for women given that they use the system more than men and that they are responsible for taking care of children and many of the elderly. Equally important, many more women than men lack the resources with which to purchase care or the workplace health coverage that could pay for their care.

The public healthcare system has also helped reduce inequitable access among women. For example, "women aged 65 and older in the lowest income quintile were almost as likely as those in the highest to report having a doctor (94% and 96%). Similarly, household income was not strongly associated with contact with a family doctor or general practitioner in the previous 12 months (87% of those in the lowest quintile and 89% in the highest), however, an income disparity existed in contact with a dentist (38% versus 76%)" (Bushnik, 2016).

Of course, barriers remain and marginalized groups are still at a disadvantage, especially in terms of services and treatments, such as medications and home care, not covered by the *Canada Health Act*. Moreover, reforms over the last two decades have shown increasing inequities (Armstrong et al., 2002). Patients are sent home from hospital quicker and sicker, or they never stay at all because they have day surgery and out-patient care. The *Canada Health Act* ensures that all necessary drugs, tests, treatments, and personnel are provided without fees within hospitals, but as soon as patients leave the hospital, fees can be charged. And as soon as fees are charged, there are two kinds of services and significant differences in access to care. Money then plays an important role in both access and quality. Those who are marginalized often end up with poorer care, less care, or no care at all. Provinces and territories have also been delisting services, treatments, and drugs. Removing them from coverage under the public plan has even greater consequences for those who are marginalized, because then the entire costs must be assumed by individuals or families. As Guruge, Donner, and Morrison (2000, p. 235) point out about immigrant families, paying for rent and food must take priority over paying for prescriptions, tests, therapy, or long-term institutional care.

Following a for-profit business model, governments across Canada have also been consolidating services into giant hospitals and closing small community ones (Armstrong et al., 2000). Many more women than men rely on public transport. And many more women than men have limited mobility because they have to care for children and others at home. Centralized services take people out of their social support networks, placing them far from those who provide daily connections. With centralization, then, women in particular have difficulty travelling to these centres to get care or provide care for friends and relatives, but the consequences are felt by both women and men.

In short, women's access to care has improved with public hospital and doctor care and more recently with midwifery services, reducing inequities among women in the process. However, some aspects of health services have never been part of public care and others inequities are returning as a result of reforms. While research and women's resistance have contributed to practices that recognize differences between women and men, we still have a long way to go before research and treatment recognize the specificity of individual women's lives.

## HEALTHCARE WORK IS WOMEN'S WORK

Women have long been the majority of those who do the paid and unpaid care work. Among paid workers, women make up 80.2% of those counted as part of the healthcare industry (Statistics Canada, 2018a). Women still make up the overwhelming majority of nurses, care aides, and therapists. The biggest changes have come among doctors, with women now nearly half of the family doctors and close to 40% of the specialists (Statistics Canada, 2018b), a change that reflects the successful demands from the women's movement to remove the quotas on women entering these programs. Women also provide the majority of the unpaid care work at home (Statistics Canada, 2012), providing most of the daily personal care increasingly required because of the cutbacks in hospital and long-term care. While this care work can bring many rewards to women, it can also be hazardous to their health. Without a gender-sensitive analysis, however, these hazards are often difficult to see.

The *Report of the Royal Commission on the Future of Health Care in Canada* (Romanow, 2002), more popularly known as the *Romanow Report*, provides an example of the need for such an analysis. This report was prepared after the federal policy requiring a gender-sensitive analysis was in place and remains the most recent national investigation into health services. Although several presentations at the commission's public hearings stressed the importance of providing such an analysis, the report considers gender only in relation to home care, and even then, the excessive burdens on women are mentioned, but not addressed in the recommendations (Armstrong et al., 2002).

Yet the report stresses the very high illness and injury rate among healthcare providers and the "decline in morale" apparent in health services (Romanow, 2002, p. 96). Indeed, there is growing evidence of the risks in healthcare work, and nursing has emerged as a hazardous occupation (Canadian Institute for Health Information, 2001; Shields & Wilkins, 2009). The report considers this issue without mentioning that more than 9 out of 10 registered nurses are women and this is the case for more than 80% of other categories of nurses. Why is this relevant?

Because most nurses are women, we now have a majority who are over age 40 (Statistics Canada, 2018c). This is a relatively new development. Until this generation of nurses, women were forced to leave when they got married, and somewhat later they were allowed to stay in their jobs after marriage, but had to leave when they became pregnant. As a result, nurses in the past were either young or single and senior, with the senior nurses much less likely to undertake regular bedside care. Nevertheless, nursing work organization often still assumes that young women are doing the bedside care. Indeed, the workload in this very physically demanding job has increased along with the age of the nurses as each patient requires more intense care.

Because nurses are women, we have not understood the work as physically demanding in the same way as we see much of men's labour as physically demanding. This, too, contributes to the failure to develop policies that adequately take these demands into account. Women have often been loath to stress the physical demands because they were trying to establish nursing as a profession and because they did not want to appear as weak females. They have also hesitated to report violence (Armstrong et al., 2009).

Because nurses are women, they feel responsible and are held responsible for care. New managerial strategies designed to shorten patient hospital stays and provide more care on an out-patient basis have dramatically increased the pace of nursing work. The result is not only a speed-up in the work but also a severe reduction in the time available to provide the kind of care nurses have learned to provide. Nurses tell us they still scramble to make up for the care deficit, and they are expected to do so. The expectations they have of themselves and that others have of them are directly linked to gendered assumptions of nursing work (Armstrong et al., 2000).

Because most nurses are women, many of the skills are assumed to come naturally. In practice, although nurses have years of formal education, many of the skills are learned informally from other women in the process of doing the work. Such learning takes time as well as effort, but the time for continual learning interchange is disappearing as the focus on measurable tasks increases.

Finally, because they are women, they are doing more than one job. When they go home at the end of their shift, they take up very similar work in the household. Increasingly, they are looking after family, friends, and relatives who need home care. The pressure to provide the care that is being sent home is particularly heavy on women with nursing experience.

In short, older nurses are working much harder at a double or triple shift in ways that make them more vulnerable to illness and injury. The high rates of illness and injury are a concern not only to nurses but also to their patients and to the system as a whole. Injury and illness cost us all. If the absenteeism rate of RNs were reduced to that of all other workers, the equivalent of almost 5,500 more would be at work full-time each year (Canadian Institute for Health Information, 2001). Gender is a critical component in understanding these increases in work hours and thus in addressing these adverse health outcomes. Indeed, gender is critical to understanding health care, reforms, and consequences.

Left out of the statistics on the paid healthcare labour force is the work of cooking, cleaning, and laundry. Like nursing, cleaning, cooking, and laundry work are female-dominated jobs long associated with skills that come with the genitalia. They seem like jobs any woman can do, with the result that the work is defined as unskilled. The *Romanow Report* separates these so-called ancillary services from direct healthcare services, suggesting that it is appropriate to contract out such services as cleaning, cooking, and laundry for delivery by for-profit companies because quality is "relatively easy to judge" and "competitors in the same business" could provide appropriate ancillary services (Romanow, 2002, p. 6). Indeed, many health services have done so. Yet no evidence is provided in the report to support the claim that quality is evident or that such work in health care is equivalent to similar work in other sectors. A gender-sensitive analysis or one that recognizes the full range of health determinants might come to different conclusions (Armstrong, Armstrong, & Scott-Dixon, 2008). The U.K. House of Commons Health Select Committee (1999) warned that "the often spurious division of staff into clinical or non-clinical groups can create an institutional apartheid which might be detrimental to staff morale and to patients" (quoted in Sachdev, 2001, p. 33).

Equally important, contracting out tends to exacerbate gender inequality. A systematic review of the research (Petersen, Hjelmar, & Vrangbæk, 2017) concluded that the negative consequences for workers outweighed positive ones. Contracting out resulted in poorer work conditions, decreased salaries, reductions in benefits and entitlements, and reduced job satisfaction for workers whose jobs have been contracted out. Case studies in the United Kingdom and Northern Ireland "found that exposure to tendering led to the, often dramatic, erosion of terms and conditions of employment. Estimates state that some 40 per cent of the NHS ancillary jobs were lost" (Sachdev, 2001, p. 5). Moreover, the impact on women was more extensive, resulting in a widening of the gender gap. According to the Equal Opportunities Commission of Northern Ireland (1996), most work contracted out was female-dominated. The rate of female job loss was more than double that of men. While both women and men experienced wage reductions, the proportionate reduction was larger for women. Some benefits disappeared, along with some entitlements.

The contribution of cleaning, cooking, and laundry to women's unpaid care work at home is also hard to see, and this work too has expanded with health services reforms (Armstrong, 2015). Although often described as sending care back home, much of the work women are expected to do at home is never done in the home. Modern technology has allowed complicated interventions involving such things as feeding tubes and oxygen tanks to be sent home. Day surgeries, shorter patient stays, and the closure of many psychiatric and other institutions all contribute to the shift. That such interventions can be done at home does not necessarily mean that women know how to do the work or that the work is done well. It is cheaper for governments to send this work home, but it is only cheaper if we ignore the costs of unpaid care work. While all women feel the pressure to do such work and are often assumed to be available to do it by the application of government policies, some women have the resources to pay others to do the work. The result is growing inequities among women (Guberman, 2001). Survey research (Turcotte, 2013) indicates that those who provide unpaid care experience elevated levels of psychological distress and other health consequences. Not surprisingly, such work also interferes with paid work and has other negative financial impacts not only while providing care but also in the future.

In sum, healthcare work has been and remains women's work. Although women have been able to make gains in terms of moving into the higher-paid and more powerful jobs, they remain those who do the overwhelming majority of the daily care, whether that care is paid or unpaid. This work takes a toll on women's health and creates inequities among women.

## CONCLUSIONS

There are moral reasons, effectiveness reasons, and financial reasons for gender-sensitive research, policy, and practice, but it is much easier in theory and even in research than in practice. Policy and practices reflect not only old ways of doing and new evidence; they also reflect power and political choices. In Canada, we have made some tentative moves toward gender-sensitive policy and practices, but we still have a very long way to go before we can claim gender-sensitive health and care policies and practices.

## CRITICAL THINKING QUESTIONS

1.  Should we be giving as much attention to men's health issues as we do to women's health issues? Why or why not?
2.  What are the limitations of simply treating gender as an "independent variable" in research?
3.  In what ways are health and healthcare issues related to gender similar to issues related to racialized groups in Canada? How are they different?
4.  What are the current dimensions of discussions of "appropriate care"? What should such discussions be about?
5.  What questions should we ask when we consider evidence that is applied in clinical practices? What might some of the limitations of such evidence be?

## FURTHER READINGS

Armstrong, P., Armstrong, H., & Scott-Dixon, K. (2008). *Critical to care: The invisible women in health services*. Toronto: University of Toronto Press.

*Critical to Care* uses a wide range of evidence to reveal the contributions that those who provide personal care, who cook, clean, keep records, and do laundry, make to health services. As a result of current reforms, these workers are increasingly treated as peripheral even though the research on what determines health demonstrates that their work is essential. Through a gendered analysis, *Critical to Care* establishes a basis for discussing research, policy, and other actions in relation to the work of thousands of marginalized women and men every day.

Billson, J. B., & Fluehr-Lobban, C. (2005). *Female-wellbeing: Toward a global theory of social change*. London: Zed Books.

The book tackles the complexities of social change at the global and local level, providing case studies of low- and high-income countries, including Canada. The comparative material is examined through a feminist lens, emphasizing power and inequalities not only between women and men, but also among women.

Grant, K., Amaratunga, C., Armstrong, P., Boscoe, M., Pederson, A., & Willson, K. (Eds.). (2004). *Caring for/caring about: Women, home care, and unpaid caregiving.* Aurora, ON: Garamond.
Women account for four out of every five caregivers. Women also do the overwhelming majority of unpaid care work. This collection of articles offers a conceptual guide to caregiving, as well as an assessment of existing research on gender and caregiving. One article focuses specifically on women with disabilities, while another focuses on Indigenous women. Additional articles develop portraits of women who give and receive care in Quebec and Ontario.

Messing, K. (1998). *One-eyed science: Occupational health and women workers.* Philadelphia: Temple University Press.
Internationally recognized as a definitive work on the importance of gender in occupational health, this book provides a comprehensive assessment of theory and research in this critical field.

Neufeld, H. T., Cidro, J. (Eds.). (2017). *Indigenous experiences of pregnancy and birth.* Bradford, ON: Demeter Press.
This collection provides invaluable insights into historical and contemporary issues around pregnancy and birth in Indigenous communities. The introduction is particularly useful in setting out a framework for policy and practices.

Quinlan, E., Quinlan, A., Fogel, C., & Taylor, G. (Eds.). (2017). *Sexual violence at Canadian universities. Activism, institutional responses and strategies for change.* Waterloo, ON: Wilfrid Laurier University Press.
Sexual violence on campus, as the editors of this collection point out, has recently received significant attention in the media. The wider-ranging articles consider the incidence and nature of violence before setting out strategies for change.

## RELEVANT WEBSITES

**Canadian Centre for Policy Alternatives**
www.policyalternatives.ca
   The Canadian Centre for Policy Alternatives is a research organization that covers multiple topics directly related to health.

**Canadian Health Coalition**
www.healthcoalition.ca
   The Canadian Health Coalition website offers analysis of current critical issues in health care and the social determinants of health. The coalition brings together community, religious, and union organizations dedicated to protecting and promoting public care.

**Canadian Institutes of Health Research, Institute of Gender and Health**

www.cihr-irsc.gc.ca/

This institute funds research on gender and health. It also publishes material on integrating gender-sensitive research.

**Canadian Women's Health Network**

www.cwhn.ca/

Although no longer up to date, the Canadian Women's Health Network website not only provides access to publications from the Centres of Excellence for Women's Health but also links directly to sources around the world on a broad range of issues related to women's health.

**World Health Organization, Department of Gender, Women, and Health**

www.who.int/gender/en/

The World Health Organization is a particularly good source for comparative information on research from countries around the world.

## GLOSSARY

**Feminist political economy:** An approach that sees political, economic, social, and ideological aspects as not only integrally linked but gendered. It focuses attention on power and inequalities, and on ideas and relations that shape and are shaped by people individually and collectively.

**Healthcare services:** The entire range of organizations and individuals who provide health care. The term is usually restricted to services that are paid for by government, insurance companies, or individuals. The term thus excludes unpaid care and often excludes what may be called alternative or complementary therapies, such as homeopathy.

**Policy and practice in health care:** Policy usually refers to the formal, explicit approach to health care, while practice refers to what people actually do. The first refers to what is supposed to happen, while practice refers to what actually happens. Policy and practice influence each other.

**Social context:** The conditions under which we live, as well as the relations we have with other people. It thus includes power and politics, income and educational opportunities, and household members and work colleagues, among other factors.

## REFERENCES

Abramson, B. (2009). Women and health: Taking the matter to heart. In P. Armstrong & J. Deadman (Eds.), *Women's health: Intersections of policy, research and practice.* Toronto: Women's Press.

Armstrong, P. (2015). Unpaid health care: An indicator of equity. In P. Armstrong & A. Pederson (Eds.), *Women's health: Intersections of policy, research, and practice* (pp. 238–258). Toronto: Women's Press.

Armstrong, P., Amaratunga, C., Bernier, J., Grant, K., Pederson, A., & Willson, K. (Eds.). (2002). *Exposing privatization: Women and health care reform in Canada.* Aurora, ON: Garamond.

Armstrong, P., Armstrong, H., Bourgeault, I., Choinière, J., Mykhalovskiy, E., & White, J. P. (2000). *"Heal thyself": Managing health care reform.* Aurora, ON: Garamond.

Armstrong, P., Armstrong, H., & Scott-Dixon, K. (2008). *Critical to care: The invisible women in health services.* Toronto: University of Toronto Press.

Armstrong, P., Banerjee, B., Szebehely, M., Armstrong, H., Daly, T., & LaFrance, S. (2009). *They deserve better: The long-term care experience in Canada and Scandinavia.* Ottawa: Canadian Centre for Policy Alternatives.

Armstrong, P., Boscoe, M., Clow, B., Grant, K., Pederson, A., & Willson, K. (2002). *Reading Romanow.* Ottawa: Canadian Women's Health Network.

Armstrong, P., & Pederson, A. (Eds.). (2015). *Women's health: Intersections of policy, research, and practice* (2nd ed.). Toronto: Women's Press.

Arriagada, P. (2016). First Nations, Métis, and Inuit Women. In *Women in Canada: A gender-based statistical report.* Statistics Canada Publication 89-503-x. Ottawa: Statistics Canada. Retrieved from https://www150.statcan.gc.ca/n1/pub/89-503-x/2015001/article/14313-eng.htm

Benoit, C. M. (1991). *Midwives in passage: The modernisation of maternity care.* St. John's: Institute of Social and Economic Research.

Burlock, A. (2017). Women with Disabilities. In *Women in Canada: A gender-based statistical report.* Statistics Canada Publication 89-503-x. Ottawa: Statistics Canada. Retrieved from https://www150.statcan.gc.ca/n1/pub/89-503-x/2015001/article/14324-eng.htm

Bushnik, T. (2016). The health of girls and women in Canada. In *Women in Canada: A gender-based statistical report.* Statistics Canada Publication 89-503-x. Ottawa: Statistics Canada. Retrieved from https://www150.statcan.gc.ca/n1/pub/89-503-x/2015001/article/14324-eng.htm

Canadian Association of Midwives. (2018). Midwifery in Canada. Retrieved from https://canadianmidwives.org/midwifery-across-canada/#1464901248022-ad64b0b3-051d

Canadian Institute for Health Information (CIHI). (2001). *Canada's health care providers.* Ottawa: Author.

Canadian Institute for Health Information (CIHI). (2003). *Workforce trends of registered nurses in Canada.* Ottawa: Registered Nurse Database.

Canadian Institute for Health Information (CIHI). (2004). Number of visits by gender and 5 year age groups. Retrieved from http://qstat.cihi.ca/discovered4i/viewe, 04-11-30

Canadian Institute for Health Information (CIHI). (2014). More young women being hospitalized for eating disorders. Ottawa: Author.

Canadian Institute for Health Information (CIHI). (2017a). Injury and trauma emergency department and hospitalization statistics. Ottawa: Author.

Canadian Institute for Health Information (CIHI). (2017b). NACRS emergency department use and length of stay. 2015–2016. Retrieved from https://www.cihi.ca/en/access-data-reports/results?f%5B0%5D=field_primary_theme%3A2050

Canadian Institute for Health Information (CIHI). (2018). C-section rates continue to increase while birth rates decline. Retrieved from https://www.cihi.ca/en/c-section-rates-continue-to-increase-while-birth-rates-decline

Canadian Women's Foundation. (2017). Fact sheet: Women and poverty in Canada. Retrieved from https://www.canadianwomen.org/wp-content/uploads/2017/09/Facts-About-Women

Cohen, M. G. (2003). Destroying pay equity: The effects of privatizing health care in British Columbia. Vancouver: Hospital Employees' Union.

DesMeules, M., Stewart, D., Kazanjian, A., McLean, H., Payne, J., & Vissandjée, B. (Eds.). (2003). *Women's health surveillance report: A multi-dimensional look at the health of Canadian women*. Ottawa: Health Canada and Canadian Institute for Health Information.

Equal Opportunities Commission of Northern Ireland. (1996). *Report on the formal investigation into competitive tendering in health and education services in Northern Ireland*. Belfast: Author.

Fausto-Sterling, A. (2005). The bare bones of sex: Part I—Sex and gender. *Signs: Journal of Women in Culture and Society, 30*(2), 1491–1527. doi:10.1086/424932

Gahagan, J., Gray, K., & Whynacht, A. (2015). Sex and gender matter in health research: Addressing health inequities in health research reporting. *International Journal for Equity in Health, 14*(12). Unpaginated. doi: 10.1186/s12939-015-0144-4

Greaves, L. (2015). Women, gender, and health research. In P. Armstrong & A Pederson (Eds.), *Women's health: Intersections of policy, research, and practice* (2nd ed., pp. 9–30). Toronto: Women's Press.

Guberman, N. (2004). Designing home and community care for the future: Who needs to care? In K. R. Grant, C. Amaratunga, P. Armstrong, M. Boscoe, A. Pederson, & K. Willson (Eds.), *Caring for/caring about: Women, home care and unpaid caregiving* (pp. 75–90). Aurora, ON: Garamond.

Guruge, S., Donner, G. J., & Morrison, L. (2000). The impact of Canadian health care reform on recent women immigrants and refugees. In D. L. Gustafson (Ed.), *Care and consequences: The impact of health care reform* (pp. 62–88). Halifax: Fernwood.

Health Canada. (2003). *Exploring concepts of gender and health*. Ottawa: Women's Health Bureau.

Health Canada. (2018). *Social determinants of health and health inequalities*. Retrieved from https://www.canada.ca/en/public-health/services/health-promotion/population-health/what-determines-health.html

Institute for Clinical Evaluative Sciences and the Cardiacare Network of Ontario. (2008). *Report on coronary artery bypass surgery in Ontario fiscal years 2005/06 and 2006/07*. Retrieved from www.ices.on.ca

Laurence, L., & Weinhouse, B. (1997). *Outrageous practice: How gender bias threatens women's health*. New Brunswick, NJ: Rutgers University Press.

Messing, K. (1998). *One-eyed science: Occupational health and women workers*. Philadelphia: Temple University Press.

Moyser, M. (2017). Women and paid work. In *Women in Canada: A gender-based statistical report*. Statistics Canada Publication 89-503-x. Ottawa: Statistics Canada. Retrieved from https://www150.statcan.gc.ca/n1/pub/89-503-x/2015001/article/14694-eng.htm

Oliffe, J. L., & Greaves, L. (Eds.). (2012). *Designing and conducting gender, sex and health research*. London: Sage.

Pederson, A., & Armstrong, P. (2015). Sex, gender and systematic reviews: The example of wait times for hip and knee replacements. In P. Armstrong & A. Pederson (Eds.), *Women's health: Intersections of policy, research, and practice* (2nd ed., pp. 56–72). Toronto: Women's Press.

Petersen, O. H., Hjelmar, U., & Vrangbæk, K. (2017). Is contracting out of public services still the great panacea? A systematic review of studies on economic and quality effects from 2000 to 2014. *Social Policy & Administration, 52*(5), 130–157. doi:10.1111/spol.12297

Quinlan, E., Quinlan, A., Fogel, C., & Taylor, G. (Eds.). (2017). *Sexual violence at Canadian universities: Activism, institutional responses, and strategies for change*. Waterloo, ON: Wilfrid Laurier University Press.

Rochon, P. A., Clark, J. P., Binns, M. A., Patel, V., & Gurwitz, J. H. (1998). Reporting of gender-related information in clinical trials of drug therapy for myocardial infarction. *Canadian Medical Association Journal, 159*(4), 321–327.

Romanow, R. J. (2002). *Building on values: The future of health care in Canada*. Saskatoon, SK: Commission on the Future of Health Care in Canada.

Sachdev, S. (2001). Contracting culture: From CCT to PPPs. In *The private provision of public services and the impact on employment relations*. London: UNISON.

Sherwin, S., et al. (1998). *The politics of women's health*. Philadelphia: Temple University Press.

Shields, M., & Wilkins, K. (2009). Factors related to on-the-job abuse of nurses by patients. *Health Reports, 20*(2), 2–14.

Statistics Canada. (2012). Population providing care to a family member or friend with a long-term illness, disability or aging needs by sex and main activity of respondent. Retrieved from https://www150.statcan.gc.ca/t1/tbl1/en/tv.action?pid=4410000301

Statistics Canada. (2018a). Industry by sex, data tables, 2016 Census. Retrieved from http://www12.statcan.gc.ca/census-recensement/2016/dp-pd/dt-td/Rp-eng.cfm?TABID=2&LANG=E&APATH=3&DETAIL=0&DIM=0&FL=A&FREE=0

Statistics Canada. (2018b). Occupation by sex, data tables, 2016 Census. Retrieved from http://www12.statcan.gc.ca/census-recensement/2016/dp-pd/dt-td/Rp-eng.cfm?TABID=2&LANG=E&APATH=3&DETAIL=0&DIM=0&FL=A&FREE=0

Statistics Canada. (2018c). Average age of registered nurses in Canada in 2017, by province. Retrieved from https://www.statista.com/statistics/497000/average-age-in-registered-nursing-canada-by-province/

Turcotte, M. (2013). Family caregiving: What are the consequences? Ottawa: Statistics Canada. Retrieved from https://www150.statcan.gc.ca/n1/en/pub/75-006-x/2013001/article/11858-eng.pdf?st=MoA9XdIL

United Nations. (1995). *Beijing Declaration and Platform for Action*. Fourth World Conference on Women. Retrieved from http://www.un.org/womenwatch/daw/beijing/platform/

# CHAPTER 14

## Constructing Disability and Illness

*Marcia Rioux and Tamara Daly*

*Normal is a lack of variation. There is no such thing as normal. Normal is set up
by a certain amount of people who have the power to decide, to define norms.*
  —Gregor Wolbring (2002)

*Bodies that depart from the norm—bodies marked by some condition of
disability—disrupt the rules. Striking their own "bond with the natural order," they
complicate the metaphors of science, infuse static notions of health with deeper,
richer meanings, and challenge law and policy-makers who seek to create conditions of justice for all.*
  —Catherine Frazee, Joan Gilmour, Roxanne Mykitiuk, & Michael Bach (2002)

## INTRODUCTION

In this chapter, we consider theoretical distinctions between the dominant discourses
of disability as an individual pathology compared with a social pathology. The former
includes biomedical and functional accounts of disability. Both of these accounts locate it
as an attribute of an individual's pathology and tend to conflate it with illness. The social
pathology perspective, by contrast, includes environmental and human rights approaches.
These approaches begin with the assumption that "disability is not the measles" (Rioux &
Bach, 1994). Scholarly work in this tradition locates disability within the context of the
broader social system at the level of societies' inability to flexibly adapt to individuals'
different needs, whether in terms of physical reconfigurations such as ramps or with workplace policies that prevent people with disabilities from holding full-time employment.
Disability is thus equated with social disadvantage. Viewed in this broader context, someone who has a disability may or may not have a medical illness, but the illness is separate
from the social disadvantage that a person experiences as a result of their physical or
mental impairment.

Second, we investigate the social constructions of disability and illness, and how the two are conflated. It is important at the outset to distinguish between the two, which are rooted in differing assumptions about where the source of disability is located. The use of measures such as the World Bank's Disability Adjusted Life Years (DALYs) measure is critically discussed in this section.

Third, we review disability rates in Canada. Results of the 2001 and 2006 Statistics Canada *Participation and Activity Limitation Survey* (PALS) and the Statistics Canada *Canadian Survey of Disability* (CSD)—2012 and 2017 are presented. The results show that there are much higher rates of disability in some provinces, experiences of disability increase with age, and that pain is most frequently reported. Overall, women experience higher rates of disability than men. Of equal importance is the impact of relationships among social inclusion, education, and healthcare services on the health status of people with disabilities. Finally, advances in human rights policy and law are briefly discussed.

# THEORETICAL MODELS OF DISABILITY

Table 14.1 summarizes the source of disability according to each of the four main approaches outlined below, and identifies the primary mode of action proponents use to change the conditions for people with disabilities.

## Individual Pathology Frameworks

Biomedical and functional models approach disability as a field of professional knowledge and expertise (Barton & Oliver, 1997; Rioux, 2001, 2003; Smart & Smart, 2006). Scholarly research in this tradition works within a positivist, scientific paradigm. It focuses on

**Table 14.1:** Approaches to Disability

| | Individual Pathology | | Social Pathology | |
| --- | --- | --- | --- | --- |
| | **Biomedical approach** | **Functional approach** | **Environmental approach** | **Rights outcome approach** |
| Source of disability | Disability is due to an individual's abnormality and the extent of their functional limitations | Disability is a pathology that is best treated with services that enable the individual to become as socially functional as possible | Disability arises from the failure of ordinary environments to accommodate peoples' differences | Disability has social causes resulting from the way in which individuals relate to how society is organized |
| Primary mode of action | Diagnosis and treatment | Service provision (e.g., rehabilitation) | Policy change (e.g., to building codes) | Human rights principles and legal challenges |

the prevention of disability resulting from biological and environmental conditions. Both approaches treat disability as pathology, focusing on individual deficits or incapacities in relation to non-disabled persons. These approaches tend to equate disability with anomaly. Disabled people may be viewed as a social burden. The inclusion of people with disabilities tends to be viewed as a private responsibility. Individuals with a disability are compared with a biomedically constructed idea of what is normal.

### Biomedical Approach

The biomedical approach emphasizes diagnosis and treatment of dysfunctions. This approach focuses research and clinical attention on the condition with an emphasis on individual abnormality and the extent of functional limitations.

The professional aim is to decrease the prevalence of the condition in the overall population. This approach highlights medical diagnosis and treatment, including medical or genetic therapeutic interventions. In conjunction with conventional medical models of care and therapy, institutions, other segregated housing, and all-encompassing service provision centres are also used. As many people with disabilities have been characterized as lacking in potential, life in institutions and other forms of segregated housing has been limited to providing for basic needs (e.g., food, shelter, and clothing).

In countries with increases to public benefits and institutional facilities, the medical profession has been put into the position of gatekeeper. In this role, access to education and training, financial benefits, mobility aids and devices, and rehabilitation is scientifically assessed to determine a person's needs based on criteria evaluating their range of disability.

### Functional Approach

Like the biomedical approach, this approach views disability as an individual condition or pathology. From a functional perspective, the pathology is best treated with services that enable the individual to become as socially functional as possible. Services, including physiotherapy, occupational therapy, nursing, and health, are more than therapeutic in nature and include the development of life skills, pre-vocational training, functional assessments, counselling, and job training and skills for independent living. Services' success is measured by the degree to which people who use the services can approximate the lives of "normal" people. Other categories of services include behaviour modification/adaptation and developmental programming. In the former, a number of positive or negative reinforcement techniques are used to elicit socially desirable behaviours and prevent undesirable ones. The latter focuses on levels of knowledge and skills that people usually acquire as they mature, identifies when and why someone is not at the "appropriate" level, and claims to intervene to assist individuals to maximize their "developmental" potential.

A primary limitation of this approach is that it fails to consider the impact of larger social, economic, and political factors that may play a significant role in preventing an individual from progressing or meeting their ambitions. This approach also makes several assumptions about a person's best interests that may deviate from what a person actually wants, as well as assuming that there are methods to determine appropriate development.

## Social Pathology Frameworks of Disability

Early analyses of the social construction of sickness and its related behaviours were rooted in the ideas of Talcott Parsons (1951). Other sociologists explored concepts including stigmatization and the way in which rehabilitation professionals socially construct dependence (Goffman, 1968; Scott, 1969). Throughout the 1970s, scholars continued to interrogate the claims of medicine with social science questions, theories, and methods. For instance, Navarro (1976) presented a class analysis of the United States' lack of a national health insurance program, Illich (1976) questioned the legitimacy of medical knowledge and pioneered research into iatrogenic (doctor-caused) disease, and Freidson (1970) examined the power of the medical profession. Starr (1989) unpacked the concept of privatization in its application to studying the state's relative power and policy-making ability. He argued that while economists see the market as part of the private sphere, sociologists and political economists see the market as part of the public sphere.

Since these earlier social critiques of medicine, materialist, feminist, legal, health, geography, and postmodern critiques have also challenged the hegemony of the biomedical and functional accounts of illness and disability and disentangled definitions from concepts of illness and impairment. This critical social scholarship identifies barriers in society as disabling. For instance, contributions investigate how people with physical and mental impairments are precluded from undertaking social activities as a consequence of the erection of physical and attitudinal barriers by those who are not disabled (Thomas, 2002; Guerin, Payne, Roy, & McPherson, 2016). Likewise, Stone (1984) notes that the medical profession's accumulated power, combined with the state's need to restrict access to state-sponsored welfare, constructs disability socially (Barnes, 1997).

Within the social pathology framework, there are two models of disability: the environmental and rights-outcome approaches (Barton & Oliver, 1997; Rioux, 2001, 2003; Pothier & Devlin, 2006; Iriarte, McConkey, & Gilligan, 2015). Both approaches assume that disability is neither inherent to the individual nor independent of the social structure. In other words, these analyses critique the necessary association between disability and individual impairment. The unit of analysis is the social system, meaning that the political, social, and built environments are important factors in constructing disability. Unlike the biomedical and functional models, critical social science frameworks view disability as difference, not deviance. Similar to feminist critiques of the "gendered" body, more scholars are recognizing that the body is "infused with 'able-bodied' notions" (Barnes, Mercer, & Shakespeare, 1999, p. 65). The term disability is often used to refer to a type of social oppression, much in the way that sexism and racism are characterized (Thomas, 2002).

*Environmental Approach*

An environmental approach sees personal abilities and limitations as resulting from an individual's characteristics interacting with their environment. Disability arises from the failure of ordinary environments to accommodate people's differences. The manner in which environments are arranged and ordered constructs disability. For instance, a building lacking wheelchair access creates an employment handicap for someone reliant on a wheelchair. Impairment can also be the result when workplace policies are insufficiently flexible to allow people who require time during the day to rest in order to continue to function, while making up for work later in the day.

Policy research demonstrates that an individual's physical or mental limitation can be lessened when environments are appropriately adapted to enable participation. For instance, changes to building codes, employing principles of barrier free-design, adapted curricula, and targeted policy and funding commitments have been usefully employed. When modifications and supports are used in homes, school, work, and leisure environments, people with disabilities are able to participate. This approach is grounded in disability discrimination, while the rights-outcome approach is grounded in fundamental human rights and freedoms.

*Rights-Outcome Approach*

The second of the social pathology approaches builds on the environmental approach's recognition that supports such as personal services, aids, and devices are required by some people to enable them to gain access to, participate in, and exercise self-determination as equal members of society. However, the rights outcome approach moves beyond calls for adaptations to environments, reflecting a shift that has taken place over the past 20 years in the paradigm of disability from a medical welfare model to a human rights model.

The rights-outcome approach is premised on the recognition that disability has social causes resulting from the way in which individuals relate to how society is organized (International Classification of Impairments, Disabilities, and Handicaps, 1981; Oliver, 1990; Rioux & Bach, 1994; Iriarte et al., 2015). The end goals of the latter model are non-discrimination and equality for people with disabilities (Rioux, 2001). While the approach is multi-disciplinary, the primary lens of analysis is human rights principles. These principles aim to reduce civic inequalities to address social and economic disadvantage for people with disabilities in Canada and across the world. This approach is macro-level in orientation. Its focus is on broad, systemic factors that prevent disabled people from fully participating as equals in society. In addition to legal cases that uphold the principles of non-discrimination and equity in Canada, these goals are also upheld in the United Nations *Convention on the Rights of Persons with Disabilities* and its Optional Protocol, which came into force on May 3, 2008.

Minow (1990) focuses on the ways in which difference is used in law to create exclusion and disadvantage. She locates difference not in the individual but in the limitations of society to accommodate multiple individuals' needs. In other words, society marginalizes people with disabilities, even though it is possible to incorporate people's different needs. This approach critiques inflexibility in society for creating and constructing disabilities, while recognizing the need for supporting diversity and to empower marginalized individuals.

## CONSTRUCTING DISABILITY AND ILLNESS

This section explores inherent problems from the conflation of disability with illness. A biomedical reading of the disabled body as ill and impaired focuses on a narrow individualistic approach to health. By contrast, the World Health Organization (WHO) defines health as "… a state of complete physical, mental and social well-being and not merely the absence of disease or infirmity" (WHO, 1946). This definition broadly locates health not only within each individual but also within social conditions or determinants. It acknowledges that individuals' health relies also on social well-being, which cannot be guaranteed when systemic discrimination and policies of inequity persist. The use of health as the absence of disease and disability results in a perception of health as limited to medical health. This broader view of health incorporates both medical and social health within its framework.

Health and social policy, grounded in medical assumptions, conflate disability with illness. In other words, a person with a disability is treated as if ill. In reality, people with disabilities experience periods of ill health and health in the same way as do all people. Reinforcing these inaccurate notions of disability as illness are health measures such as DALYs. We investigate from a critical perspective the use of the Disability Adjusted Life Years to measure how many years a person or population loses as a result of ill health compared with an idealized and normalized perspective of health equated with freedom from disability.

### Disability as Illness

Critical social science scholarship investigates how disability and illness are constructed, and the complex links between sites of care, power relations, the body, and identity (Dyck, 1998). The conflation of disability with ill health is grounded in a narrow definition of health based on the presence of disease or infirmity, the use of medical practitioners as gatekeepers to disability benefits, and an inability to acknowledge the multiple ways in which disabilities are often created by societal norms that inflexibly accommodate multiple needs. First, different assumptions underlie how disability is approached. Social pathology perspectives highlight how tying benefits to medical certification conflates disability with illness and constructs various disabilities as conditions requiring medical intervention. Grounded in the dominance of a biomedical view of disability as individual pathology, access to welfare state disability benefits, including non-medical benefit programs, is contingent upon medical certification of disability by physicians (or other legitimized) gatekeepers (Stone, 1984; Claussen, 1999).

Second, making medical practitioners gatekeepers to disability benefits privileges bio-medical and functional approaches to disability in the policy, program, and service realm. These approaches do not sufficiently acknowledge that the organization of society can often create disabilities. As well, human rights provisions stipulate that individuals should be treated not just equally, but also without discrimination. The premise of non-discrimination acknowledges that people need to be treated differently in order to access services and have equal rights. The case of *Eldridge v. B.C.* outlined in Chapter 4 of this volume is illustrative.

The question of equitable access to benefits is key in a political climate of welfare state restructuring, which has legitimated distinctions between categories of worthy and unworthy poor, and returned us to a "poor laws" position, escaped briefly with policies of universalism. People with able bodies and minds unwilling to work are defined as unworthy poor. By contrast, people with disabilities, those who are aging, and those who are infirm are all classed as worthy poor (Rioux & Prince, 2002). Worthy poor are accommodated from within the public sphere, whereas policies have marginalized unworthy poor to seek to accommodate their needs from within the realm of the private sphere. In terms of the funding of social welfare, the role of the state is alternately expansive or restrictive in response to pressures from the internationalized global capital system (Rioux, 2002; Iriarte et al., 2015) and the state's priority placed on efficiency and effectiveness (Stein, 2001).

At a policy-making level, neo-liberal policies associated with fiscal conservatism and neo-conservative policies that marry fiscal conservatism with moral conservatism have dominated the public agenda since just prior to 1980 (Hall, 1992). The result is a change in the role of the state, with significant implications for addressing equity policy goals. This neo-liberal discourse emphasizes individual responsibility and private action, debt and deficit reduction over social expenditure, and rights and responsibilities to accommodate citizens who form the majority or constitute the norm. It also emphasizes a shift from universal provision based on shared rights and pooled risk to the provision of services based on individual needs, with implications for concepts of citizenship and entitlement. It is also important in a political climate that privileges a role for the state in health care, while withdrawing the state role in social care for both elderly and people with disabilities, as these roles are being recast as part of private responsibility (Daly, 2007). The WHO definition of health (also used in the 1978 Alma Ata declaration and the 1968 Ottawa Charter of the first global health promotion conference) allows the identification of non-medical needs.

## Illness as Disability

The inverse—the construction of illness as disability—is also true; policies and practices reconstruct illness as disability, particularly in terms of measurement of the health status of countries with instruments such as the DALYs, which are used to measure a country's health status. The World Bank's use of DALYs to measure a country's level of ill health reconstructs illness as disability by turning all illnesses into measures of disability.

DALYs are used both as a measure of health status and as an instrument of health policy. Designed by researchers at the Harvard School of Public Health, Disability Adjusted Life Years were introduced by the World Bank in 1993 to measure the Global Burden of Disease (Metts, 2001). A basic assumption built into the use of the DALYs is that there is a "reduced value" to a life lived with a disability (Groce, Chamie, & Me, 1999), given the foci on burden and loss. Since then, DALYs have come under increasing criticism, resulting from the built-in assumptions and policy implications of using these measures.

DALYs were ostensibly designed to measure the years of life lost resulting from disease and ill health. Unlike earlier measures, such as the Quality-Adjusted Life Years (QALYs), in which groups of citizens were consulted, the DALYs relied on input and analysis from an internationally representative group of medical professionals. Twenty-two "indicator disabling conditions" were selected and evaluated by professionals from the list of diseases contained in the World Health Organization's International Classification of Disease (ICD). The participants assigned a severity weight from zero—denoting perfect health—to one—denoting death. Conditions were then grouped into disability classes. Disabilities were calculated by multiplying the age-adjusted severity weights for each condition by expected duration, calculated based on an amalgamation of community-based epidemiological research, information from health facilities, and expert judgments (Metts, 2001, p. 451).

Critical scholarship has pointed out that the calculation of DALYs falsely assumes that all conditions or disabilities result in ill health of various severities. This treats these conditions as physical disablements instead of situating disability in broader social, political, environmental, and economic factors. In other words, DALYs locate disabilities within the individual and not within the broader conditions and barriers that create a disability. The calculation of DALYs also assumes that the only way to ameliorate disability is to intervene medically (Metts, 2001), but not socially or politically. Others argue that the DALYs is a flawed tool to set priorities in health policy (Lyttkens, 2003). DALYs does not account for healthcare costs or other costs resulting from paid and unpaid care provision. Furthermore, the method of determining DALYs equates longevity with health and disability with ill health, but this correlation between the two does not necessarily exist in real life. Finally, there are ethical issues inherent in policy driven by outcomes of a measure of longevity (Lyttkens, 2003).

## HOW CANADA ACCOUNTS FOR DISABILITY

In this section, we present disability prevalence through self-reported aggregated data from the 2001 and 2006 Statistics Canada *Participation and Activity Limitation Survey* (PALS) and the 2012 and 2017 Statistics Canada *Canadian Survey of Disability* (CSD). We also consider the status of disability equality rights in Canada through analysis of several key legal challenges.

## Prevalence of Disability in Canada

Tracking self-reported disability over time in Canada involves multiple data sources. Figures 14.1–14.6 compile data from PALS and CSD. PALS is a post-censual survey of adults and children whose everyday activities are limited because of a condition or health problem. The survey works in the following way: A sample of those persons who answered "Yes" to the 2006 Census disability filter questions were chosen to participate in PALS. Approximately 39,000 adults and 9,000 children living in private, and some collective, households in the 10 provinces and 3 territories were selected to participate in the survey. PALS focuses on the relationship between functional status, daily living activities, and social participation by collecting data on the nature and severity of the activity limitations, and on the needs for assistive technology, social support, and accommodation in all spheres of life. The survey covers themes such as activity limitations, help with everyday activities, education, employment status, social participation, and economic characteristics.

The CSD is also a post-censual survey and includes all adults aged 15 and over (as of Census day) who had an activity limitation or a participation restriction associated with a physical or mental condition or health problem, who were living in private dwellings in the 10 provinces and 3 territories of Canada. This survey uses the Disability Screening Questions (DSQ), which are premised on the social model of disability. These screening questions first assess the degree of difficulty the person experiences across 10 functional domains. The survey then asks how often someone experiences limitations to their daily activities. The data reflect those with a disability as defined by having a limitation in a functional domain.

It is important to remember that post-census data excludes those living on First Nations reserves (about 300,000 people) or those living in collective health and social care dwellings. Both groups may live with disabilities of various types, and therefore these numbers likely under-represent the true proportion of people living with a disability in Canada.

Despite any limitations, we can make some broad generalizations: The prevalence of people living with a disability is increasing; disability disproportionately affects those over the age of 65 as well as women across all age categories; the rate of disability varies widely across Canada; and pain is the most frequently cited type of disability.

### (a) The Prevalence of Living with a Disability Is Increasing

More people living in Canada are currently living with a disability. In 2001, a total of 3.6 million Canadians over 15 living in private households reported activity limitations. By 2006, the number for the same group had risen to 4.4 million Canadians, representing an increase of just over 22% from 2001. By 2017, 22.3% of Canadians reported having at least one disability that limited their everyday activities, equalling about 6.25 million people (Morris, Fawcett, Brisebois, & Hughes, 2018) and representing a phenomenal growth rate of 73.6% since 2001.

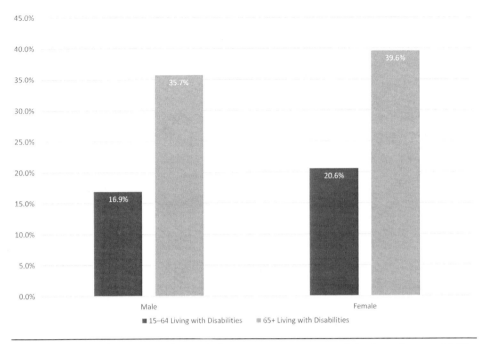

**Figure 14.1:** People Living with Disabilities as a Proportion of the Population, 2017

*Source:* Statistics Canada. (2017). Persons with and without disabilities aged 15 years and over, by age group and sex, Canada, provinces and territories. Table 13-10-0374-01.

### (b) Living with a Disability Is Associated with Sex Differences

Disability differs for women and men. Overall, more women (24%) than men (20%) over the age of 15 report living with at least one disability (Statistics Canada, 2017a). Rates have climbed since 2001, when 13.3% of women and 11.5% of men reported a disability (Statistics Canada, 2002), or since 2006, when over one-sixth of women (15.2%) experienced a disability, compared with 13.4% of men (Statistics Canada, 2006). As Figure 14.1 shows, sex and gender differences also persist as people age, with more women reporting disability in all age groups.

### (c) Living with a Disability Increases with Age

As Figure 14.1 also demonstrates, Canadians also acquire disability as they age. While 13.1% of youth (15–24) reported at least one disability, 20% of adults aged 25–64 and 38% of seniors 65 and older reported the same (Statistics Canada, 2017a, 2018).

### (d) Experiences of Disability Depend on Where You Live

Disability rates differ widely across Canada. For instance, the percentage of Canada's population who report living with a disability rose to 22.3% (2017b) from 12.4% (2001), with Nunavut reporting the lowest and Ontario reporting the highest proportions in the country.

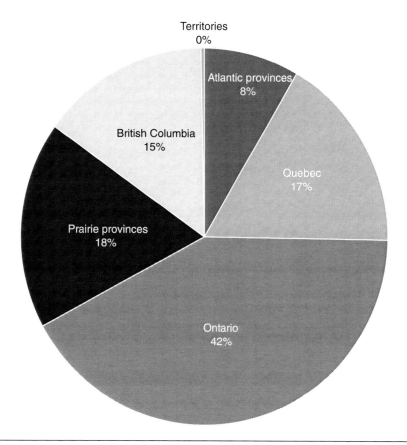

**Figure 14.2:** Persons living with disabilities aged 15 and older, in Canada by geography, 2017

*Source:* Statistics Canada. (2017). Persons with and without disabilities aged 15 years and over, by age group and sex, Canada, provinces and territories. Table 13-10-0374-01.

### (e) Disability Is Associated with Lower Rates of Employment

The labour force participation rate of people with disabilities is 53.6%, compared with a 76.9% rate across the total population of Canada (Statistics Canada, 2012). There is an age-standardized unemployment rate of 14.3%, compared with 7.8% across the country (Statistics Canada, 2012). In other words, there is lower rate of employment participation, and the unemployment experienced by people living with disabilities is nearly double that of the total population.

### (f) Days Off Required for Illness and Disability

These figures need to be viewed cautiously as the underlying reasons for days off for illness and for disability would be quite distinct. These figures may also reflect the lack of accommodation in the labour force to the needs of persons with disabilities. Across Canada,

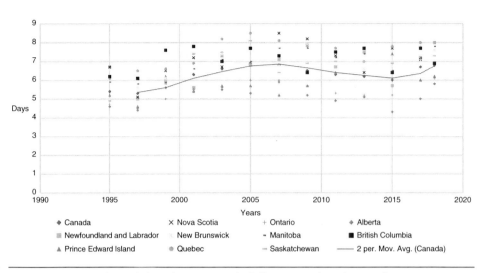

**Figure 14.3:** Number of days lost per male full-time worker due to illness or disability, Canada and provinces, 1995–2018

*Source:* Statistics Canada. Work absence due to illness or disability of full-time employees by geography, annual. Table 14-10-0190-01.

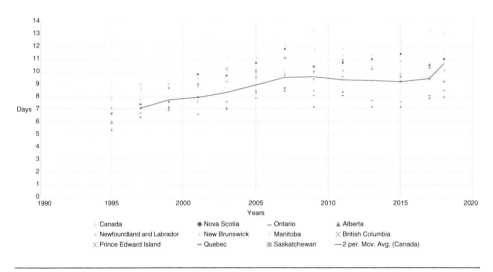

**Figure 14.4:** Number of days lost per female full-time worker due to illness or disability, Canada and provinces, 1995–2018

*Source:* Statistics Canada. Work absence due to illness or disability of full-time employees by geography, annual. Table 14-10-0190-01.

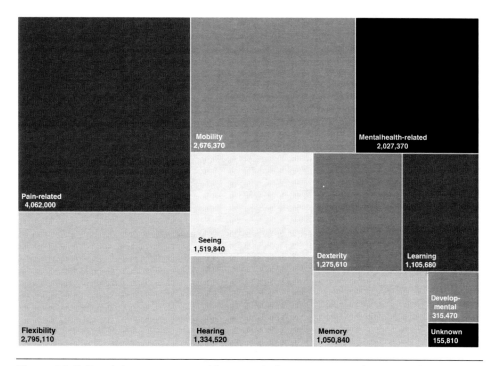

**Figure 14.5:** Disability experienced by people by type, Canadians aged 15 years and over, 2017

*Source:* Statistics Canada. (2017a). Canadian Survey on Disability.

days off among males due to disability or illness have started to increase following a period of decline from 2007–2009. For females, the average began to increase in 2017, following many years of nine days off per year.

### (g) Pain, Flexibility, and Mobility Disabilities Are the Top Reported Experiences among Adults

In 2006, most adults (81.7%) with a disability reported more than one type of disability, with pain, mobility, and agility being the most commonly reported (Statistics Canada, 2006). Of those who reported having a pain- and discomfort-related activity limitation, nearly 8 in 10 were working-aged women and just under 7 in 10 (69.3%) were working-aged men. Extrapolated to the Canadian population, almost 1 in 10 (9.5%) working-age women and just under 1 in 10 (7.6%) working-age men limited their activity due to restrictions caused by pain. By 2017, pain remained the top concern, but definitional changes resulted in flexibility and mobility affecting the most people.

### (h) A Higher Proportion of Women than Men Experience Most Types of Disabilities

As Figure 14.6 demonstrates, women experience higher rates of most types of disabilities, including those classified as memory, learning, dexterity, seeing, mental-health related,

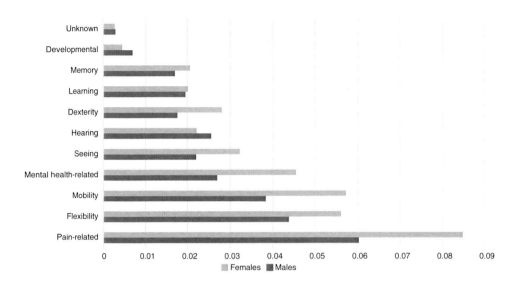

**Figure 14.6:** Types of disability among adults by sex and as a % of the Canadian population, 2018

*Source:* Statistics Canada. (2018). Type of disability for persons with disabilities aged 15 years and over, by age group and sex, Canada, provinces and territories. Table 13-10-0376-01.

mobility, flexibility, and pain-related. In contrast, men experience slightly more unknown disabilities, as well as developmental and hearing disabilities.

### (i) Disability and Non-Discrimination Accessing Health Services

Principles of non-discrimination, equality, empowerment, freedom, agency, and full participation are enshrined in Section 15 of the *Canadian Charter of Rights and Freedoms* (1985) for people with "mental and physical disabilities" in Canada (Rioux, 2001; Rioux, Pinto, & Parekh, 2015). This constitutional guarantee is applicable at every level of legal authority in Canada (i.e., municipal, provincial, and federal). This section includes both substantive and procedural rights (15(1)), and includes the option of affirmative action (15(2)). It was included to reflect social and political reality and ensures that disadvantaged groups can participate in society equally and fully. *Andrews v. Law Society* (1989) was the first legal case to address a Section 15 challenge; the Supreme Court of Canada recognized "disadvantage as central to the analysis of discrimination" (Rioux 2001; Rioux et al., 2015).

Cases since *Andrews* have continued to ensure that the equality principles are met. The courts rejected an equity model based on equal treatment in favour of a model that recognizes that equality may require different treatment (Rioux 1994, 2001). The Court has taken the position that Section 15 was intended to remedy inequality and disadvantage experienced by people with disabilities. It requires the "spending of public money and the extension of benefits to previously excluded disadvantaged groups" (Lepofsky, 1997).

Because there are legislative bans on discrimination, society is obligated to make accommodations to meet the needs of groups that are discriminated against. In terms of non-discriminatory access to health services, *Eldridge v. British Columbia* (1997) involved three deaf applicants who successfully challenged the legislation governing hospital services, because of a failure to provide sign language interpreter services as an insured service or a requirement for hospitals to provide such in delivery of healthcare services. First, the Supreme Court found the province was acting in a discriminatory manner, and more importantly, that the province failed to take action, as opposed to imposing a burden. Second, failure to accommodate was found by the Court to result in discrimination. Third, governments cannot evade responsibility by delegating implementation to private entities (i.e., hospitals). Fourth, the Supreme Court identified communication as an important part of the delivery of medical services.

While these court decisions are very important milestones and enable us to move beyond a mindset of accommodation to one of non-discrimination, they have not eliminated the persistent social and legal exclusion of disabled people. Rioux (2003; Rioux et al., 2015) argues that both the content of agreements and the ways in which countries meet their commitments to the agreements' terms perpetuates the social and legal exclusion of disabled peoples. In sum, disabled people's human rights are still under threat. Despite these agreements, people with disabilities are still not treated equally, and equality is only achieved when difference is accommodated.

## CONCLUSIONS

In this chapter, we explored how disability is structurally equated with illness, owing to the predominance of biomedical and functional approaches to disability. These approaches tend to individualize disability through medical determinants or interventions, and thereby privatize the responsibility and limit the focus of responsibility. By contrast, social, political, and rights approaches focus on social determinants of disability and interventions. These models investigate the ways in which social and political structures create disability through societies' inability to accommodate difference. In this framework, disability is equated with social disadvantage and is not simply focused on individual impairment. It requires a rights- and social justice–based response that mandates the recognition of all social determinants of health, including education, housing, social inclusion, and healthcare services, as central to health.

We have also explored the prevalence of disability in Canada and discussed some of the major legal milestones in removing discrimination of Canadians with disabilities. Some of the main ideas include:

- Biomedical and functional accounts of disability equate it with illness. These accounts focus on individuals. Broader critical, social, political, and legal approaches investigate how social structures create disability through societies' inability to accommodate difference.
- Doctors and other medical personnel often serve as gatekeepers to disability benefits, which unnecessarily perpetuates the conception of disability as illness.
- Social pathology accounts equate disability with social disadvantage, not illness.

- Disability is experienced differentially by gender, by immigrant status, by age, and by geographic region in Canada.
- The outcome of equality rights for people with disabilities involves more than the removal of physical barriers and adaptation of current structures. It is about achieving a society in which disabled people are free to fully and equally participate and be included.

In 2001, nearly 4 million Canadians self-reported having at least one disability. By 2017, about one-fifth of Canadians reported having at least one disability that limited their everyday activities, totalling 6.25 million people (Statistics Canada, 2018) and representing a rate of growth of 73.6% since 2001. Statistics Canada data show that disability is most frequently experienced by women. It is also more prevalent as people age. Pain continues to be the most prevalent disability. As well, differences in rates of disability are affected by where one lives.

Policy-making that incorporates a rights outcome approach is slowly happening through court challenges. Since the adoption of the *Charter of Rights and Freedoms*, the courts have upheld equality rights for disabled people. These rights encompass more than the removal of physical barriers and the adaptation of current structures. The courts have determined that discrimination is based on imposing a burden and failing to take action to accommodate. This distinction is important because it challenges governments and policy-makers to be proactive in eliminating the discrimination that challenges disabled people's ability to fully, equally, and freely participate in society.

Research and education in the humanities, social, and medical sciences must consider human rights issues that identify not only how society constructs barriers, but also the flaw in locating disability solely in the individual. These approaches must separate disability from illness by recognizing that people with disabilities, like other people, have periods of health and ill health. Ameliorating disability is not simply a matter of intervening medically. It is about addressing the physical, social, civic, economic, and cultural barriers experienced by people with disabilities.

## CRITICAL THINKING QUESTIONS

1. In what ways do biomedical and functional accounts of disability equate it with illness?
2. In what ways do social pathology accounts equate disability with social disadvantage rather than illness?
3. What issues are associated with doctors and other medical personnel serving as gatekeepers to disability benefits?
4. How do different groups (e.g., gender, age, geographic location) experience disability?
5. In what ways do the outcomes of equality rights for people with disabilities involve more than the removal of physical barriers and adaptation of current structures?

## FURTHER READINGS

Barnes, C., Mercer, G., & Shakespeare, T. (1999). *Exploring disability: A sociological introduction*. Cambridge: Polity Press.
This book explores how concepts of disability have changed since the 1970s by addressing both traditional and new theoretical approaches to the field. It also focuses on the social model of disability and relates scholarship to other areas such as social policy, medical sociology, politics, and cultural studies.

Metts, R. (2001). The fatal flaw in the Disability Adjusted Life Year. *Disability and Society, 16*(3), 449–452.
This article argues that the Disability Adjusted Life Year, which was developed to measure different countries' health status and to gauge the effectiveness of different health interventions, is flawed. The measure incorrectly assumes that any disabling condition always results in disability regardless of the social and political context.

Minow, M. (1990). *Making all the difference: Inclusion, exclusion and American law*. Ithaca, NY: Cornell University Press.
This book explores how difference in the law is attributed to the individual as opposed to being located in limitations in the organization of the world. It argues that the concept of difference is used in law to create disadvantage and exclusion.

Rioux, M. (2003). On second thought: Constructing knowledge, law, disability and inequality. In S. Herr, L. Gostin, & H. H. Koh (Eds.), *The human rights of persons with intellectual disabilities*. Oxford: Oxford University Press.
This chapter explores treatments of disability as individual or social pathology. It places disability policy within a human rights and social justice framework.

Zubrow, E., et al. (2009). *Landscape of literacy and disability*. Toronto: Canadian Abilities Foundation.
This atlas of maps shows, at a glance, the spatial relationships between literacy and disability across Canada. Mapping disability and literacy variables, both on their own and in combination, allowed the researchers to see the issues in inventive ways.

## RELEVANT WEBSITES

**United Nations: Enable Rights and Dignity of Persons with Disabilities**
https://www.un.org/development/desa/disabilities/
A subsection of the United Nations website dedicated to international development of disability rights. It includes information related to the UN *Convention on the Rights of Persons with Disabilities*, the latest developments, and updates.

# REFERENCES

Barnes, C. (1997). A legacy of oppression: A history of disability in Western culture. In L. Barton & M. Oliver (Eds.), *Disability studies: Past, present and future* (pp. 3–24). Leeds, U.K.: The Disability Press.

Barnes, C., Mercer, G., & Shakespeare, T. (1999). *Exploring disability: A sociological introduction.* Cambridge: Polity Press.

Barton, L., & Oliver, M. (Eds.). (1997). *Disability studies: Past, present and future.* Leeds, U.K.: The Disability Press.

Claussen, B. (1999). Physicians as gatekeepers: Will they contribute to restrict disability benefits? *Scandinavian Journal of Primary Health Care, 16*(4), 199–203. doi:10.1080/028134398750002954

Daly, T. (2007). Out of place: Mediating health and social care in Ontario's long-term care sector. *Canadian Journal on Aging, 26*(Suppl.1), 63–75. doi:10.3138/cja.26.suppl_1.063

Dyck, I. (1998). Women with disabilities and everyday geographies: Home space and the contested body. In R. Kearns & W. Gesler (Eds.)., *Putting health into place: Landscape, identity, and well-being* (pp. 102–119). Syracuse, NY: Syracuse University Press.

Frazee, C., Gilmour, J., Mykitiuk, R., & Bach, M. (2002). The legal regulation and construction of the gendered body and of disability in Canadian health law and policy. Retrieved April 3, 2005,

Freidson, E. (1970). *Profession of medicine: A study of the sociology of applied knowledge.* New York: Dodd, Mead and Company.

Goffman, E. (1968). *Stigma: Notes on the management of spoiled identity.* Harmondsworth, U.K.: Penguin Books.

Groce, N. E., Chamie, M., & Me, A. (1999). Measuring the quality of life: Rethinking the World Bank's Disability Adjusted Life Years. *International Rehabilitation Review, 49*(12), 12–15.

Guerin, B. M., Payne, D. A., Roy, D. E., & McPherson, K. M. (2017). "It's just so bloody hard": Recommendations for improving health interventions and maternity support services for disabled women. *Disability and Rehabilitation, 39*(23), 2995–2403. doi:10.1080/09638288.2016.1226971

Hall, P. A. (1992). The movement from Keynesianism to monetarism: Institutional analysis and British economic policy in the 1970s. In S. Steinmo, K. Thalen, & F. Longstreth (Eds.), *Structuring politics: Historical institutionalism in comparative analysis* (pp. 90–113). Cambridge: Cambridge University Press.

International Classificiation of Impairments, Disabilities, and Handicaps. (1981). The handicap creation process. *ICIDH International Network, 4*(1–2).

Illich, I. (1976). *Limits to medicine: Medical nemesis: The expropriation of health.* New York: Pantheon.

Iriarte, E. G., McConkey, R., & Gilligan, R. (Eds.). (2015). *Disability and human rights: Global perspectives.* London: Palgrave.

Lepofsky, D. (1997). A report card on the *Charter's* guarantee of equality to persons with disabilities after 10 years—What progress? What prospects? *National Journal of Constitutional Law, 7*(3), 263–431.

Lyttkens, C. H. (2003). Time to disable DALYs? On the use of Disability-Adjusted Life Years in health policy. *European Journal of Health Economics, 4*(3), 195–202. doi:10.1007/s10198-003-0169-2

Metts, R. L. (2001). The fatal flaw in the Disability Adjusted Life Year. *Disability and Society, 16*(3), 449–452.

Minow, M. (1990). *Making all the difference: Inclusion, exclusion and American law.* Ithaca, NY: Cornell University Press.

Morris, S., Fawcett, G., Brisebois, L., & Hughes, J. (2018). *A demographic, employment and income profile of Canadians with disabilities aged 15 years and over, 2017.* Ottawa: Statistics Canada. Retrieved from https://www150.statcan.gc.ca/n1/pub/89-654-x/89-654-x2018002-eng.htm

Navarro, V. (1976). *Medicine under capitalism.* New York: Neale Watson.

Oliver, M. (1990). *The politics of disablement.* Basingstoke, U.K.: Macmillan.

Parsons, T. (1951). *The social system.* Glencoe, IL: The Free Press.

Pothier, D., & Devlin, R. (Eds.). (2006). *Critical disability theory: Essays in philosophy, politics, policy, and law.* Vancouver: UBC Press.

Rioux, M. (1994). Towards a concept of equality of well-being: Overcoming the socio-legal construction of inequality. *Canadian Journal of Law and Jurisprudence, 7*(1), 127–147. doi:10.1017/S0841820900002605

Rioux, M. (2001). Bending towards justice. In L. Barton (Ed.), *Disability, politics & the struggle for change* (pp. 34–47). London: David Fulton Publishers.

Rioux, M. (2002). Social disability and the public good. *Man and Development, 24*(4), 179–198.

Rioux, M. (2003). On second thought: Constructing knowledge, law, disability and inequality. In S. Herr, L. Gostin, & H. H. Koh (Eds.), *The human rights of persons with intellectual disabilities: Different but equal* (pp. 287–318). Oxford: Oxford University Press.

Rioux, M., & Bach, M. (Eds.). (1994). *Disability is not measles: New research paradigms in disability.* North York, ON: Roeher Institute.

Rioux, M., & Prince, M. J. (2002). The Canadian political landscape of disability: Policy perspectives, social status, interest groups and the rights movement. In A. Puttee (Ed.), *Federalism, democracy and disability policy in Canada* (pp. 11–28). Montreal: McGill-Queen's University Press.

Rioux, M. H., Pinto, P. C., & Parekh, G. (Eds.). (2015). *Disability, Rights monitoring, and social change.* Toronto: Canadian Scholars' Press.

Scott, R. A. (1969). *The making of blind men: A study of adult socialization.* London: Sage.

Smart, J. F., & Smart, D. W. (2006). Models of disability: Implications for the counseling profession. *Journal of Counseling & Development, 84*(1), 29–40. doi:10.1002/j.1556-6678.2006.tb00377.x

Starr, P. (1989). The meaning of privatization. In S. Kamerman & A. Kahn (Eds.), *Privatization and the welfare state* (pp. 12–48). Princeton, NJ: Princeton University Press.

Statistics Canada. (2002). *A Profile of Disability in Canada, 2001.* Retrieved from http://publications.gc.ca/Collection/Statcan/89-577-X/89-577-XIE2001001.pdf

Statistics Canada. (2006). *Participation and Activity Limitation Survey 2006: Analytical report.* Ottawa: Statistics Canada.

Statistics Canada. (2012). *A profile of persons with disabilities among Canadians aged 15 years or older, 2012.* Retrieved from https://www150.statcan.gc.ca/n1/pub/89-654-x/89-654-x2015001-eng.htm.

Statistics Canada. (2012). Labour force status for adults with disabilities by disability type. Table 13-10-0348-01.

Statistics Canada. (2017a). *Canadian Survey on Disability reports: A demographic, employment and income profile of Canadians with disabilities aged 15 years and over.* Retrieved from https://www150.statcan.gc.ca/n1/pub/89-654-x/89-654-x2018002-eng.htm

Statistics Canada. (2017b). New data on disability in Canada, 2017. Retrieved from https://www150.statcan.gc.ca/n1/pub/11-627-m/11-627-m2018035-eng.htm

Stein, J. G. (2001). *The cult of efficiency.* Etobicoke, ON: House of Anansi Press.

Stone, D. A. (1984). *The disabled state.* London: MacMillan.

Thomas, C. (2002). Disability theory: Key ideas, issues and thinkers. In M. Oliver, C. Barnes, & L. Barton (Eds.), *Disability studies today.* Cambridge: Blackwell Publishers.

Tindale, J. A., & MacLachlan, E. (2001). VON "doing commercial": The experience of executive directors with related business development. In. K. L. Brock & K. G. Banting (Eds.), *The nonprofit sector and government in a new century* (pp. 189–213). Montreal: McGill-Queen's University Press.

World Health Organization. (1946). Preamble to the Constitution of the World Health Organization as adopted by the International Health Conference (pp. 19–22). New York: Author.

# CHAPTER 15

## Pharmaceutical Policy: The Dance between Industry, Government, and the Medical Profession

*Joel Lexchin*

## INTRODUCTION

Since the late 1990s, spending on prescription medicines has outstripped spending on doctors in Canada and is second only to hospital expenditures. In 2014, the bill for prescription drugs was $29.4 billion (Canadian Institute for Health Information, 2016b). Between 2005 and 2010, costs were rising by an average of 7.6% per year, although in the past few years, the average rate of rise has slowed to 1.6% annually (see Figure 15.1). How much Canadians spend and how much value, in terms of improvements in health outcomes, we

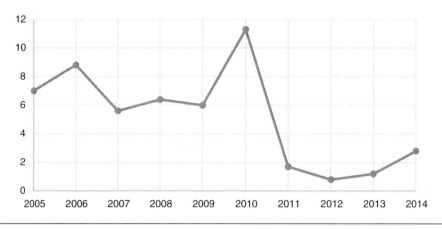

**Figure 15.1:** Percent change in retail prescription drug expenditures in Canada, 2005–2014

*Source:* Data from Canadian Institute for Health Information. (2016a). National health expenditure trends, 1975 to 2016: Data tables.

receive are determined by a series of policy decisions surrounding how drugs are approved and monitored once they are on the market, industrial policy, intellectual property rights, and how doctors are educated about medications. This chapter explores the background to these issues, how decisions about them are made, and the interplay between the main actors: the state, the pharmaceutical industry, and the medical profession.

## THE DRUG REGULATORY SYSTEM

The pharmaceutical industry and the Canadian government have long had a close relationship based on a form of interaction known as clientele pluralism (Atkinson & Coleman, 1985). This situation occurs where the state has a high degree of concentration of power in one agency (in this case, the Therapeutic Products Directorate [TPD],[1] a branch of Health Canada), but a low degree of autonomy. With respect to pharmaceuticals in Canada, government regulation of drug safety, quality, and efficacy is almost solely the responsibility of the TPD, but the state does not possess the wherewithal to undertake the elaborate clinical and pre-clinical trials required to meet the objective of providing safe and effective medications. Nor is the state willing or able to mobilize the resources that would be necessary to undertake these tasks. Therefore, a tacit political decision is made to relinquish some authority to the drug manufacturers, especially with respect to information that forms the basis on which regulatory decisions are made.

Clientele pluralism is "located in a broader political context" (Davis & Abraham, 2013, p. 11) as one expression of corporate bias theory. This theory "allows for the possibility of a relatively strong, pro-active state, which may encourage pro-business (de)regulation in collaboration with industry" (Davis & Abraham, 2013, p. 12). It contends that industry can drive regulation by influencing not just the regulatory agencies, in this case Health Canada, but also the broader government directly through lobbying and donations and through other activities, such as direct participation by having representatives appointed to task forces that help form overall government policy. The ultimate result is that the state actively supports the broad regulatory goals of industry.

The implications of a clientele pluralist type of relationship take on increasing importance when seen in light of competing visions of what the prime function of a drug regulatory authority should be. One put forward by the pharmaceutical industry holds that the main function is to facilitate the industry's efforts to develop new products and to approve them as quickly as possible. In this view, medications are commodities and the regulatory authority exists to provide a service to the industry. The second view espoused by consumer groups and public health activists sees the primary purpose as appropriately evaluating products to ensure a high standard of effectiveness and safety. Here medications are seen as an essential element of the healthcare system, and the regulatory authority exists to provide a service to the public.

# THE THERAPEUTIC PRODUCTS DIRECTORATE: CHANGING PRIORITIES?

In the Canadian context, the Therapeutic Products Directorate would nominally seem to side with consumer groups. The website that describes how drugs are reviewed contains the following statement: "Throughout the process, the safety and well-being of Canadians is the paramount concern" (Government of Canada, 2015).

Since 1994, financing for the TPD has shifted from coming entirely from government appropriations to about 60% now coming from government and the rest from pharmaceutical companies' user fees, and Health Canada is pushing for the latter to go up to 70% of the cost of running the drug regulatory system (Senate of Canada, 2017). This shift in financing of the regulatory body has raised concerns about whether the TPD's primary commitment is still to public health.

The apparent reorientation of the TPD in favour of business interests is reflected in its Business Transformation Strategy (BTS). The BTS was introduced in early 2003 and "builds on the commitments made by the Government of Canada to 'speed up the regulatory process for drug approvals,' to move forward with a smart regulations strategy to accelerate reforms in key areas to promote health and sustainability, to contribute to innovation and economic growth, and to reduce the administrative burden on business" (Therapeutic Products Directorate, n.d.).

One of the key phrases in the BTS is "smart regulation." Smart regulation means that Canada should "regulate in a way that enhances the climate for investment and trust in the markets" and "accelerate reforms in key areas to promote health and sustainability, to contribute to innovation and economic growth, and to reduce the administrative burden on business" (Government of Canada, 2003). While health is not ignored, the emphasis is clearly on creating a business-friendly environment. The federal External Advisory Committee on Smart Regulation (2004) explicitly states that risk management has an essential role in building public trust and business confidence in the Canadian market and regulatory system. Once again, the business agenda takes a prominent position.

When applied to drug regulation, risk management would mean weighing potential negative effects against potential advantages. Potential negative effects would be adverse health effects that could occur under reasonably foreseeable conditions (Health Canada, 2003a). The shift from the precautionary principle to risk management is subtle but unmistakable. The precautionary principle says that if products cannot be shown to be safe, then they should not be marketed; risk management allows products on the market unless they are shown to be harmful. Realigning regulation to conform to the principles of smart regulation would not totally abandon the concept of precaution, but it seems to imply that there would have to be a threat of serious or irreversible damage before it would come into play.

## Timeliness of Drug Approvals

The TPD is devoting significant organizational resources toward the goal of speeding up the drug approval process. Although Health Canada has explicitly denied any relationship

**Table 15.1:** Allocation of $40 million dollars for improvements in drug regulatory system, fiscal 2003–2004

| Program Area | Percent of Money | Dollars (millions) |
|---|---|---|
| Improved regulatory performance | 78.0 | 31.2 |
| Enhanced post-marketing safety | 6.5 | 2.6 |
| Optimal drug therapy | 6.0 | 2.4 |
| Price review capacity | 1.25 | 0.5 |
| Therapeutic access strategy | 8.25 | 3.3 |

*Source:* Health Canada. (2003b). *Improving Canada's regulatory process for therapeutic products: Building the action plan.* Ottawa: Public Policy Forum, slide 16.

between performance targets and user fees (The Public Policy Forum, 2003), Health Canada documents have commented on connecting performance and user fees: "A formal link between fees and review performance, recommended at the July 1995 workshop, was not included in the approved fee regulations ... However, it was agreed that the fee regulations would be amended to make this link as soon as possible after the government determines the best way to proceed" (Health Canada, 1998, p. 2). In the budget speech outlining government spending for the 2003 session of the federal Parliament, $190 million was allocated over a five-year period, mostly to improving "the timeliness of Health Canada's regulatory processes with respect to human drugs" (Department of Finance Canada, 2003). Forty million out of the $190 million was allocated for fiscal 2003–2004. Out of that amount, 78% ($31.2 million) went toward "improved regulatory performance," mainly an effort to eliminate the backlog in drug approvals and to ensure timeliness in getting drugs onto the market (Health Canada, 2003b; see Table 15.1). The TPD justifies spending the bulk of the money on improving the speed at which it approves new drugs largely because this is an area where it received intense criticism.

Who is criticizing the TPD, and why is timeliness so important that it reaches the throne speech? Patient groups are naturally concerned if effective treatments are being delayed, and Canada lags behind other countries in the speed at which it approves drugs given priority status (Rawson, 2001). However, only slightly more than 10% of the new drugs marketed in Canada qualify as either breakthrough products or significant therapeutic improvements (see Table 15.2). The loudest and most influential voice calling for faster drug approvals comes from the brand-name industry. In a 2007 document, Rx&D (now Innovative Medicines Canada) emphasized how pleased it was with the progress that Health Canada made in reducing the time it took to get a drug approved (Rx&D, 2007). From the point of view of returns on investment, industry's preoccupation with timeliness makes perfect sense. For instance, in 2009–2010, sales of Lipitor (atorvastatin) in Ontario

**Table 15.2:** Therapeutic value of new drugs

| Year | Total Number of New Drugs Approved in Canada | Total Number Evaluated for Therapeutic Value (%) | Number (%) with Major Therapeutic Value |
|------|------|------|------|
| 2005 | 23 | 21 (91.3) | 3 (14.3) |
| 2006 | 23 | 21 (91.3) | 3 (14.3) |
| 2007 | 24 | 22 (91.7) | 3 (13.6) |
| 2008 | 17 | 15 (88.2) | 2 (13.3) |
| 2009 | 27 | 26 (96.3) | 0 (0.0) |
| 2010 | 22 | 19 (86.4) | 3 (15.8) |
| 2011 | 27 | 23 (85.2) | 2 (8.7) |
| 2012 | 22 | 21 (95.5) | 3 (14.3) |
| 2013 | 40 | 37 (92.5) | 6 (16.2) |
| 2014 | 25 | 18 (72.0) | 2 (11.1) |
| 2015 | 36 | 25 (69.4) | 3 (12.0) |
| Total | 286 | 248 (86.7) | 30 (12.1) |

*Source:* Patented Medicine Prices Review Board. *Annual Reports* (Ottawa: PMPRB); Prescrire International, product reviews.

alone were $316 million, meaning that a marketing delay of just one day would have cost its maker, Pfizer, $870,000 (Ontario Ministry of Health and Long-Term Care, 2011). But whether that applies when a public health point of view is adopted is questionable.

Timeliness in the approval process has taken on even greater importance. As a result of changes to the way that user fees are collected from pharmaceutical companies' revenue, the TPD will suffer if service standards (completion of reviews of new drug applications within the targeted time) are not met. If actual performance in a given fiscal year is more than 110% of the target for a particular fee category (different types of approval applications are subject to different fees), penalties apply for the amount in excess. Fees are then to be reduced for the next reporting year by a percentage equivalent to the performance not achieved, up to a maximum of 50%. If approvals are 20%, overtime fees will drop by 20% (Health Products and Food Branch, 2007).

If services are not adequate, government departments stand to forfeit part of the user fees. As a result of missed review standards, Health Canada suffered a loss of $1.9 million in 2013–2014 and $2.7 million in 2014–2015 (Health Products and Food Branch, 2014). In order to avoid financial penalties, Health Canada may direct even more resources into ensuring that drug approval times are met at the expense of its other responsibilities, including monitoring drugs for safety, a function that is already being neglected. Health Canada is not nearly as conscientious about setting standards for drug safety and sticking to them. The 2011 Auditor General's (AG) report found that it took Health Canada at least one year to complete 34 assessments and more than two years for five medium-priority assessments. (A medium-priority assessment is one for which a labelling change will likely be necessary.) In 11 of 24 cases where it was necessary to issue risk communications to the public, it took Health Canada more than two years to assess the potential safety issue, update the drug's label (where necessary), and issue the risk communication (Auditor General of Canada, 2011).

## Drug Safety

In contrast to the $31.2 million given over to faster approvals, only $2.5 million of the $40 million was allocated for the Marketed Health Products Directorate (MHPD), which is charged with monitoring the safety and performance of drugs already approved (see Table 15.1). This discrepancy in the allocation of money came at a time when the MHPD was already under-resourced compared to the TPD. As of May 2017, the TPD had an annual allocation of $84.5 million and 833 full-time equivalent employees, compared to $23.4 million and 218 employees for the MHPD (Health Canada, personal communication, August 1, 2017). Due to a lack of resources, the MHPD has had to stop trying to assign causality when evaluating adverse drug reaction reports. Information from each adverse drug reaction report that is received is entered into a number of fields in the Canada Vigilance Adverse Drug Reaction Database. Now, because of increased workload and funding constraints, the number of essential fields in the database has been reduced, such that the "causality" field is no longer being systematically used.

Shorter approval times might adversely affect safety standards. The U.S. Food and Drug Administration (FDA) has a statutory requirement to complete its review of 90% of new drug applications within specific periods of time depending on whether it is a standard or priority review. If it fails to meet that obligation, then renewal of legislation that allows it to collect user fees from industry may be endangered. Carpenter and colleagues (2008) analyzed drugs approved in the U.S. between 1993 and 2004 and concluded that when drugs were approved in the immediate pre-deadline period, there was a substantially higher rate of withdrawals and/or safety labelling changes compared to drugs approved after the deadline. In other words, it appears that if the deadline is imminent, the FDA does a less thorough job of reviewing drugs in order to avoid missing the deadline. Drugs can be approved in Canada through the standard 300-day pathway or a 180-day priority pathway for drugs that may have offer significant therapeutic gain. Very few of the drugs approved through the latter route actually are major advances (Lexchin, 2015), but one in three of these drugs will eventually be found to have major safety issues compared to one in five drugs approved through the longer standard process (Lexchin, 2013).

Pharmaceutical companies place a premium on rapid drug approvals in order to start recouping their investment in their products. Their interest in post-marketing surveillance is decidedly secondary. When companies in the U.S. agreed to supplement the FDA budget with user fees, they stipulated that the fees could only be used to hire new reviewers; none of the money went to post-marketing surveillance.[2]

## Transparency in the Regulatory Process

Another manifestation of the clientele pluralist relationship between the state and the pharmaceutical industry is the agreement between the industry and the TPD that all of the information that companies submit as part of the regulatory approval process is deemed confidential and will not be released without the express consent of the company involved. As a result, all of the information that industry submits, including clinical trial data on safety and efficacy, is deemed confidential and can be released only with the permission of the company, even with an Access to Information request.

This approach to releasing the clinical information that companies submit reflects a common understanding between officials in Health Canada and the pharmaceutical industry that medical information is a commodity with commercial value that must be protected. Such information can be "loaned" to the government for purposes of review, but the companies do so with the expectation that the review will produce material gains through marketing of their products. This market-based view stands in marked contrast to a view that data on health and safety are something that should be shared directly with the people most affected: those who prescribe and use the products. What we have instead is information filtered through, and protected by, the officials in Health Canada.

There is no good evidence to show that companies' interests would be harmed by the disclosure of information about safety and effectiveness (McGarity & Shapiro, 1980). On the other hand, nondisclosure has serious disadvantages for the TPD, health professionals, and the public. If information submitted to regulatory agencies is never disclosed, then these data will never enter the normal peer-review channels and are therefore not subject to scrutiny by independent scientists. Without this type of feedback, TPD reviewers may be more prone to misjudge the accuracy or usefulness of the data submitted, the scientific atmosphere in the agency may be stifled, and the professional growth of its staff severely inhibited (McGarity & Shapiro, 1980). Deprived of any independent access to information, health professionals have to accept the TPD's judgment about the safety and effectiveness of products. In the case of well-established drugs, this is probably not much of a concern, but it may be different with new drugs, where experience is limited.

Finally, the public may be denied knowledge of the full health effects of products so that they can decide for themselves whether or not to use them. Even if most consumers would never take the time to read health and safety data, consumer-oriented media, in consultation with scientific experts, could use some of this information to inform the public of the risks and benefits of products (McGarity & Shapiro, 1980).

In response to calls for greater transparency, the TPD announced in 2004 that when new drugs and devices are approved, it would publish a document entitled the "Summary Basis of Decision" (SBD). The SBD would outline the scientific and benefit/risk-based reasons for the TPD's decision to grant market authorization for a product (Progestic International Inc., 2004). The key part of the SBD of importance to prescribers and consumers is the clinical information on drug effectiveness and safety. Is enough information provided to allow for safe and rational use of new medications or the extended indications for previously approved drugs?

An analysis of all 161 SBDs (containing the results of 456 clinical trials) released from the beginning of the project until the end of April 2012 showed that clinical trial information was presented haphazardly, with no apparent method. In the majority of SBDs (126 of 161), at least one-third of the potential information about patient trial characteristics (e.g., age, sex, whether they were in-patients or out-patients) and the benefits and risks of tested treatments is missing. Although basic details of clinical trials were more frequently described, any omissions or ambiguities were especially troubling given the straightforward nature of the information, for example, the number of patients per trial arm, whether the trial took place at a single or at multiple sites, and whether a unique trial identifier was included (Habibi & Lexchin, 2014).

The good news is that Health Canada finally seems to be committed to taking a significant step in the amount of clinical information that it will be willing to release. In November 2014, Parliament passed the *Protecting Canadians Against Unsafe Drugs Act*, also known as Vanessa's Law, that gives Health Canada significantly expanded powers. Once the regulations that implement the Act have been passed, Health Canada will prospectively release nearly all of the clinical trial information that companies submit to get a new drug approved (Health Products and Food Branch, 2017). Unfortunately, at the time that this chapter is being written (March 2019), more than four years after the passage of Vanessa's Law, those regulations have still not been finalized.

## Regulation of Promotion

In 2016, drug companies in Canada spent over $560 million on journal advertising and the expenses related to sales representatives, the people who visit doctors' offices to promote their companies' products (IMS Brogan, 2016). This total does not include the spending on meals, trips, free samples provided to doctors, company-sponsored continuing medical education events, and a myriad of other types of promotion. From the perspective of the companies, this process makes good economic sense as it generates large early returns on investment. However, from a public health point of view, prescribing that is driven by promotion should be avoided as there is an abundant body of literature that consistently shows an association between use of promotion and inappropriate prescribing (Spurling et al., 2010).

As of 2015, almost two-thirds of doctors were seeing sales representatives (Leslie, 2015) and 88% of those were doing so for the information that they provided

(Chalkley, 2009). One example of the biased information that doctors receive from sales representatives comes from questionnaires that family doctors in Montreal and Vancouver filled out after seeing these people. "Minimally adequate safety information" was provided in 5 out of 412 promotions (1.2%) in Vancouver and 7 out of 423 (1.7%) in Montreal. Representatives did not provide any information about harms (a serious adverse event, a common adverse event, or a contraindication) in two-thirds of interactions (Mintzes et al., 2013).

Finally, when drugs reach the market, they have been tested only on a relatively small number of highly selected patients. Consequently, no one has any idea how most people who will be getting the drug will react to it. Prescribing based on promotion therefore essentially means that many people are unwittingly participating in an experiment.

Given these negatives associated with promotion, it would seem sensible for governments to keep a tight rein on promotion and strictly control it. The *Food and Drugs Act* does give the Canadian government this power, but the government has chosen to turn over its regulatory authority to two bodies: the Pharmaceutical Advertising Advisory Board (PAAB), which controls print advertising, and the pharmaceutical industry, which regulates the behaviour of its sales representatives and how company-sponsored continuing medical education is run.

Voluntary self-regulation seems an attractive option because, lacking government–industry conflict, it is a more flexible and cost-effective option. Government regulators also reason that in a highly competitive industry, individual companies' desire to prevent competitors from gaining an edge can be harnessed to serve the public interest through a regime of voluntary self-regulation run by a trade association (Ayres & Braithwaite, 1992). The problem with the foregoing analysis is that industry will always be tempted to exploit the privilege of self-regulation by producing a socially suboptimal level of compliance with regulatory goals. Experience has repeatedly shown this to be the case in the marketing of pharmaceutical products (Kawachi, 1992).

In these circumstances, few trade associations have made systematic efforts to either monitor the advertising practices of their members or to enforce compliance. The problem is that governments and pharmaceutical manufacturers' associations have different missions and goals. The government's mission is to protect public health by encouraging rational prescribing. The trade associations' mission is primarily to increase sales and profit. From the business perspective, self-regulation is mostly concerned with the control of anti-competitive practices. Therefore, when industrial associations draw up their codes of practice, they deliberately make them vague or do not cover certain features of promotion to allow companies a wide latitude. Self-regulation works well when anti-competitive promotional practices happen to coincide perfectly with government regulators' notions of misleading advertising. Most often, however, the fit is far from perfect because, far from being anti-competitive, many misleading advertising tactics are good for business. Therefore, from the public health perspective, the results of voluntary self-regulation are suboptimal (Lexchin & Kawachi, 1996).

Certainly this is the case with the codes promulgated by the PAAB (2007, 2013) and Innovative Medicines Canada (2016). Both codes operate under a reactive as opposed to proactive style of regulation; that is, action is generally taken only upon receipt of complaints, rather than preventing breaches from occurring in the first place. Neither code has effective sanctions where breaches have occurred. PAAB has no authority to levy monetary sanctions, although it can require companies to pull offending advertisements, but by the time a complaint has been made and a ruling taken, the ad may be near to completing its run in any case. The penalty after a fourth violation of the Innovative Medicines Canada code in a single year is a $100,000 fine that, for large drug companies spending more than $30 million a year on promotion (IMS Brogan, 2016), is the equivalent of "lunch money." The PAAB code does not have any specific provision about the type size for safety information; the Innovative Medicines Canada code does not require sales representatives to provide doctors with specific information about risks, contraindications, and warnings, and they do not have to leave a copy of the government-approved Official Product Monograph, which provides detailed information about the drug.

An example of how Health Canada has abdicated its responsibilities in the area of controlling promotion is the case of direct-to-consumer promotion of prescription drugs. Regulations issued under the *Food and Drugs Act* allow companies to advertise prescription drugs only to the extent that the name, quantity, and price of the product can be displayed. Policy statements in 1996 and 2000 reinterpreted this regulation to mean that companies were allowed to run "disease awareness" ads as long as the name of a product was not mentioned, or firms could name a medication as long as its use was not discussed. The only type of advertising that remained prohibited was one where both product was named and its use was given (Michols, 1996; Rowsell, 2000).

Health Canada has been reluctant to enforce even this loose reinterpretation of its own regulations. Lexchin and Mintzes (2014) examined 10 cases where complaints had been filed about direct-to-consumer advertising in Canada. The case studies showed that broad concerns such as off-label promotion, targeting of vulnerable groups, and poor safety profile of products were ignored. Only one enforcement tool is used: negotiation with the company. Fines, sanctions, requirements for remedial action, or prosecutions were not considered.

## INTELLECTUAL PROPERTY RIGHTS AND PATENT ISSUES

Intellectual property rights (IPRs) and patent issues are key factors in determining how much individual drugs cost and the overall level of expenditure on drugs. Patent life in Canada—for all products and not just pharmaceuticals—lasts for 20 years from the date that the patent is filed. The 20-year period is dictated by the Trade Related Aspects of Intellectual Property Rights (TRIPS) Agreement, which Canada is a signatory to as a consequence of its membership in the World Trade Organization (WTO; see Box 15.1).

**Box 15.1:** Effective Monopoly Time for Patented Drugs

Typically, companies take out patents on their drugs once they have synthesized the molecule. At that time, it undergoes a variety of testing for things like chemical purity and manufacturing quality. The next step is testing in laboratory animals followed by human testing. Once all of these tests are completed, the company submits files to the Therapeutic Products Directorate to get the drug approved. By the time the drug has received marketing approval, about 12–13 years of patent life are left.

The crux of the industry's argument for strong intellectual property rights protection is that it needs a prolonged monopoly time to sell its products in order to be able to afford the costs entailed in the research and development of new drugs, drugs that may be more expensive than existing ones, but that are also more effective and/or safer.

## Profit Levels

Relative to all non-financial companies, profits in the pharmaceutical industry have been falling recently (see Table 15.3), but it is difficult to know what these numbers mean as firms may employ what is known as transfer pricing to shift profits to jurisdictions with lower tax margins. Under transfer pricing, if a local subsidiary of a multinational imports products into Canada, then there is a price that the subsidiary pays its parent for those goods. If the multinational wants to move profits out of Canada, it can increase the "transfer price" that it charges its own subsidiary (Statistics Canada, 2014). Moreover, the profit figures from Statistics Canada do not distinguish between brand-name and generic companies, so it is impossible to know exactly how profitable the brand-name subsidiaries operating in Canada actually are. Pharmaceutical companies are also not plowing their

**Table 15.3:** Profits as a percent of capital employed,* 2008–2012

|                               | 2008 | 2009 | 2010 | 2011 | 2012 |
|-------------------------------|------|------|------|------|------|
| **Pharmaceutical Industry**   | 6.2  | 5.2  | 7.6  | 6.6  | 6.1  |
| **Total Non-financial Industries** | 7.0  | 6.0  | 7.2  | 7.8  | 7.3  |

*Note:* * Capital employed is the capital investment necessary for a business to function.

*Source:* Statistics Canada. (2014). Financial and taxation statistics for enterprises, by North American Industry Classification System (NAICS), annual (dollars unless otherwise noted), Table 180-0003. Retrieved October 2, 2014, from http://www5.statcan.gc.ca/cansim/a26?lang=eng&retrLang=eng&id=1800003&paSer= &pattern=&stByVal=1&p1=1&p2=31&tabMode=dataTable&csid= - customizeTab

profits back into research and development to produce newer and better drugs. More money goes into paying out dividends and buying back corporate stock. Between 2006 and 2015, the 18 American companies listed in the S&P 500 Index spent $465 billion on R&D but $261 billion on stock buybacks and paid out $255 billion in dividends (Lazonick, Hopkins, Jacobson, Sakinç, & Tulum, 2017).

## The Cost of Developing New Drugs

PhRMA, the organization representing the large multinational companies in the U.S., cites a figure of $2.6 billion, in 2013 dollars, to research and develop a new drug (PhRMA, 2015). This figure comes from a study from the Tufts Center for the Study of Drug Development of 106 randomly selected new drugs obtained from a survey of 10 pharmaceutical firms (DiMasi, Grabowski, & Hansen, 2016). However, this estimate is highly contested (Avorn, 2015). To begin with, the names of the drugs and all the development costs associated with them are confidential so that the authors' work cannot be independently verified. The drugs analyzed exclude any products that were co-developed with or licensed-in from another company. Almost half of the amount cited is opportunity costs, that is, not money that was actually spent, but rather the "lost earnings" due to the fact that the money invested in R&D was not invested elsewhere (the opportunity cost of the investment). In a critique of an earlier estimate by the same authors, Light and Warburton (2005) raised a number of other issues about the methodology that was used, including: the inherent comparability and reliability of the survey data due to variations in internal company cost allocation methods over time and across companies; the clear interest of pharmaceutical companies in higher (rather than lower) estimates of drug development costs, and the sampled firms' likely awareness of the intended use of the survey data; the non-random sample of firms contributing research and development data; and the fact that the cost estimates were not adjusted for large public subsidies in the form of tax deductions and credits.

## Comprehensive Economic Trade Agreement (CETA) between Canada and the European Union

CETA was finalized in September 2014 and provisionally entered into force in September 2017. As with all trade deals, there were multiple elements affecting a wide variety of industries up for negotiation, and in the view of the government the concessions that Canada was willing to make about IPRs were offset by the gains that Canada would get. According to the government, "the agreement will [bring] ... a $12-billion annual increase to Canada's economy ... this is the economic equivalent of adding $1,000 to the average Canadian family's income or almost 80,000 new jobs to the Canadian economy" (Foreign Affairs Trade and Development Canada, 2014).

Canadian negotiators made unilateral concessions in the CETA that will only affect Canada and will not require changes to the intellectual property rights regime for pharmaceuticals in the European Union (EU; Sinclair, Gagnon, & Lexchin, 2014). The EU and particularly Innovative Medicines Canada were pushing Canada to extend patents for up to five years. Innovative Medicines Canada's position was that longer patent life would be good for investment and employment in the pharmaceutical industry (Rx&D, 2011). Canada rejected this demand but agreed to an extension of up to two years. This extension is designed to compensate brand-name drug manufacturers for the time between the filing for patent protection and the granting of market authorization by Health Canada, based on the assumption that the entire responsibility for the delay rests with Health Canada. However, patents can still be extended even if the patent holder itself is responsible for the delay, for example, by filing an incomplete new drug submission. Moreover, brand-name companies will be able to choose the most favourable patent for extension, that is, the one that they feel will give them the longest period of monopoly marketing.

Canada rejected the EU's push for a 10-year period of data protection,[3] but agreed to lock in its current 8–8.5-year term, making it virtually impossible for any future government to shorten this time period since amending CETA requires the agreement of all parties. The eventual effect of the IPR provisions in the CETA on overall drug expenditures in Canada could be $795 million annually or 6.2% of spending on patented drugs (Lexchin & Gagnon, 2014).

## How Intellectual Property Rights Distort the Pharmaceutical Marketplace

As we saw earlier, the large majority of drugs produced through research led by the patent incentive do not represent any significant therapeutic advances. Industry largely engages in R&D of products that are aimed at carving out a share of a lucrative market. The result is drugs that are essentially minor variations on existing medications—for example, additions to the statin group of drugs for lowering cholesterol. Since most drugs offer little or no therapeutic advantage over existing remedies, then it stands to reason that most of the money spent on R&D is going into products that will build market share, not products that will necessarily result in significantly better health outcomes.

Baker and Chatani (2002) itemize an additional five ways that patent protection leads to wasteful rent-seeking behaviour by pharmaceutical companies, that is, behaviour that seeks to increase companies' share of existing wealth without creating new wealth. The huge costs associated with promotion that were documented earlier are one element of the excess costs.

Gaining a competitive edge on rival firms leads to a restriction in sharing of research results and delays in publication of findings because of commercial concerns. Twenty-seven percent of faculty in university life science academic departments who received industry support delayed publication of their results for more than six months compared to 17% without such support. Eighty-one percent of life science companies with relationships with academic institutions reported keeping results secret for longer than was necessary to obtain a patent (Blumenthal, Campbell, Anderson, Causino, & Louis, 1997).

Communication is the lifeblood of science, and if it is impeded, so is scientific research. Without knowing what others are doing, scientists may be needlessly repeating work.

There are the direct legal costs associated with filing and protecting patents and the indirect costs that result from successful efforts such as "evergreening," which stall the marketing of generic drugs. When the Canadian Coordinating Office for Health Technology Assessment (CCOHTA; now the Canadian Agency for Drugs and Technology in Health) was about to release a report saying that the different drugs in the statin group were equivalent, Bristol-Myers Squibb (BMS), makers of one of these drugs, objected to the release of the report and went to court to block its publication. The case was eventually thrown out, but not before CCOHTA spent 13% of its annual budget defending itself (Hemminki, Hailey, & Koivusalo, 1999).

### The Cost of Prescription Medications in Canada

Publications from Innovative Medicines Canada, the organization representing the brand-name companies in Canada, invariably point out that the yearly increase in the price of individual drugs is almost always less than the rate of inflation and cite this finding as an indication that drugs are not too expensive (Rx&D, 2014). This statement is not only true but also a truism. Prices for patented drugs in Canada are set in such a way that they can never go up faster than the rate of inflation (Patented Medicine Prices Review Board, 2014). Furthermore, prices, while important, are only one component in determining how much is spent on medications. That's why, despite the stability of prices of individual drugs, overall spending on prescription drugs in Canada has gone up from $11.7 billion in 2000 to $29.4 billion in 2014, an increase of 151% in 14 years.

At over $700 per person per year, Canada spends more per capita on pharmaceuticals than any other country in the world, except the U.S., Japan, and Greece (OECD, 2015). Similarly, when measured against comparator countries in the Organisation for Economic Co-operation and Development (OECD), Canada's growth in drug spending per capita (in real terms) between 2000 to 2009 was 4.3% per year, compared to the OECD average of 3.5%. Although this rate fell to -0.3% per year from 2009–2011, the OECD average fell even further to -0.9% (OECD, 2013). The high per capita expenditure, despite the fact that Canada controls the introductory prices for new patented drugs and limits the rate of rise of their price, emphasizes the fact that controlling the price of individual drugs does not control how much overall we as a country pay for prescription medicines.

## DOCTORS AND THE PHARMACEUTICAL INDUSTRY

Probably the most significant interaction between the majority of doctors and the pharmaceutical industry comes through continuing medical education (CME). CME is the general term used for medical education that takes place after physicians start to practice. Although it can take many forms, meetings and conferences are the mainstays of CME. Studies from Canada and the United States show that 60%–70% of all monies invested in running CME come from commercial sources—mostly companies that make and sell prescription medications (Marlow, 2007b; Steinbrook, 2008). Many doctors recognize the potential bias in this situation, but only a relatively small proportion believe it affects them personally. A survey of Scottish hospital doctors and general practitioners revealed that 40% felt that industry sponsorship created a conflict of interest, but only 14% thought that attending such events would bias the way they prescribed (Rutledge, Crookes, McKinstry, & Maxwell, 2003). Only 1% of medical house staff felt that they personally would be heavily influenced by interactions with the pharmaceutical industry versus 38% who said they would be influenced a little, and 61% who denied they could be influenced at all. Interestingly, however, the same physicians were not so sure of their colleagues: 33% thought their colleagues could be influenced a lot, 51% a little, and only 16% believed that other physicians would not be affected at all (Steinman, Shlipak, & McPhee, 2001).

Nowadays, most industry sponsorship for CME comes in the form of unrestricted grants that the organizers can use as they see fit. According to Bernard Marlow (2007a), the then-director of continuing professional development for the College of Family Physicians of Canada, this and other measures ensure that "all CME … programs accredited by the College are unquestionably balanced, free of bias and not being used by pharmaceutical companies to market their products." Statements such as these can only be viewed as naïve as they ignore the many subtle ways in which companies can bias CME even when there are strict rules in place (Steinman & Baron, 2007).

Bowman and Pearle (1988) analyzed the content of two CME courses in relation to their source of funding. Both were given at a university whose policy guidelines stipulated that all course content be controlled by the institution. Nevertheless, both courses favoured the drug produced by the sponsoring company relative to other, equally effective drugs produced by other companies.

When you rely on drug companies to support CME, you are also limiting the range of topics that will be presented. Katz, Goldfinger, and Fletcher (2002) compared CME courses organized by Harvard Medical School that were independent of any commercial influence with symposia funded by pharmaceutical companies. The 221 talks offered during the Harvard courses covered 133 topics, whereas the 103 symposia focused on 30 topics, most of which were linked to new, recently approved therapeutic agents sold by the funders. Drug therapy was the central topic in 27% of the Harvard talks compared to 66% of the symposia.

## CONCLUSIONS

What pill people eventually put into their mouths is the product of a complex series of decisions that start long before the doctor reaches for his or her prescription pad. This chapter has discussed how these decisions involve economic and political factors at the national and international level and reflect the tensions between private profit and public health. Companies are interested in making as much money as possible for their shareholders and develop drugs with the largest markets, but these products usually do not offer any significant advantages over existing therapies. Hundreds of millions of research dollars rest on the decision about which drugs to develop, and because such large sums of money are involved, the companies want strong intellectual property rights to protect their investments for the longest time. Once the drug is developed, it still has to get through the regulatory process and then be prescribed by doctors. While government should be looking out for the interests of the public in all of these areas, there is increasing concern that government priorities have become reoriented to more closely reflect those of industry. Finally, how doctors prescribe is significantly determined by how they are educated, and this process has, by default, been turned over to the pharmaceutical industry, which uses it to advance its own interests.

A basic understanding of these complex issues is necessary in order to be able to formulate public policy so that Canadian society can decide how to deal with all of the questions around prescription drugs and their rapidly escalating costs.

## CRITICAL THINKING QUESTIONS

1. How can the contradictions between the profit motive and the public interest be reconciled in the area of research and development?
2. What are the ethical implications when the interests of the public and private corporations are in competition, as may be the case when it comes to new drug approvals?
3. Assuming the pharmaceutical promotion will continue to exist, what mechanisms could be used to ensure that it is accurate and unbiased?
4. What can be done to control the increasing expenditure on pharmaceuticals in Canada? How would controls affect economic activity associated with the pharmaceutical industry?
5. Should the pharmaceutical industry be held to higher moral standards than other industries? If so, how could this be accomplished?

## FURTHER READINGS

Angell, M. (2004). *The truth about the drug companies: How they deceive us and what to do about it.* New York: Random House.
Angell is a former editor of the world's most prestigious medical journal, *The New England Journal of Medicine*, and uses the knowledge that she gained in that position to present a highly critical viewpoint about the pharmaceutical industry.

Boothe, K. (2015). *Ideas and the pace of change: National pharmaceutical insurance in Canada, Australia and the United Kingdom.* Toronto: University of Toronto Press.
This book explores the reasons why Canada has universal insurance for services from doctors and hospitals but lacks a similar program for prescription drugs.

Forman, L., & Kohler, J. (Eds.). (2012). *Access to medicines as a human right: Implications for pharmaceutical industry responsibility.* Toronto: University of Toronto Press.
Chapters in this book explore a wide range of pharmaceutical issues, including access, promotion, and prices, using a human rights lens.

Lexchin, J. (2016). *Private profits vs public policy: The pharmaceutical industry and the Canadian state.* Toronto: University of Toronto Press.
The first section examines how the neo-liberal agenda has changed the Canadian drug regulatory system to favour the interests of the pharmaceutical industry, while the second section explores how neo-liberalism has shaped the economic policies of the Canadian government when it comes to pharmaceuticals.

Lexchin, J. (2017). *Doctors in denial: Why big pharma and the Canadian medical profession are too close for comfort.* Toronto: Lorimer.
Individual doctors and the societies and organizations representing the Canadian medical profession have a 60-year history of interacting with the pharmaceutical industry. The consequences of these interactions for patients are explored in this book.

Sinclair, S., & Stuart, T. (Eds.). (2016). *The Trans-Pacific Partnership and Canada: A citizen's guide.* Toronto: Lorimer.
The Trans-Pacific Partnership, although now dormant, is just one of many trade deals with the potential to affect the prices that Canadians pay for medicines and how medicines are regulated.

## RELEVANT WEBSITES

**Drug Products (Canada)**

https://www.canada.ca/en/health-canada/services/drugs-health-products/drug-products.html

This website contains pages describing the Canadian drug regulatory system, including information about how drugs are approved and monitored for safety.

**Health Action International**

http://haiweb.org

This website has an extensive listing of reports about drug pricing, access to medicines, intellectual property rights, and drug regulation both in the developed and the developing world.

**Innovative Medicines Canada**

http://innovativemedicines.ca

Presents the viewpoint of the brand-name pharmaceutical companies on a wide range of issues, including the drug approval system and patent issues.

**Pharmacare 2020**

http://pharmacare2020.ca

Pharmacare 2020 is a research-based report that presents a clear and coherent vision of Pharmacare for Canada: a public drug plan that is universal, comprehensive, evidence-based, and sustainable.

**PharmedOut**

http://www.pharmedout.org

PharmedOut advances evidence-based prescribing and educates healthcare professionals about pharmaceutical marketing practices.

## GLOSSARY

**Clientele pluralism:** A situation where the state has a high degree of concentration of power in one agency, but a low degree of autonomy, whereas in the private sector an organization has significant resources and the ability to act on behalf of its member firms.

**Cost recovery:** Companies now pay an annual fee to the Therapeutic Products Directorate for each drug that they market and a fee for the evaluation of new drug submissions. This money is used to fund the majority of the operating costs of the TPD.

**Generic competition:** Generic drugs compete with brand-name products, but are usually priced at least 25% lower. They are identical to brand-name products and in Canada are usually produced by Canadian-owned companies.

**Patent protection:** Once an invention is patented, the individual or company making the discovery is protected from competition for a period of 20 years from the date that the patent was filed.

**Research and development:** The process of discovering a new drug and doing the testing necessary to bring it to market.

## NOTES

1.  The Therapeutic Products Directorate (TPD) only approves and monitors prescription and non-prescription drugs derived from chemical manufacturing and medical devices; the Biologics and Genetic Therapies Directorate is responsible for biological and radiopharmaceutical products, including blood and blood products, viral and bacterial vaccines, genetic therapeutic products, tissues, organs, and xenografts. While responsible for different types of products, both directorates function in an almost identical manner, and for purposes of this chapter, the term "TPD" will be used for both.

2.  The U.S. legislation that initially authorized the collection of user fees was passed in 1992 and subsequently reauthorized in 1997, 2002, 2007, and 2012. In the latter three reauthorizations, some money was allocated for safety issues.

3. In order to get new drugs onto the market, companies run clinical trials that generate information about how well the drug works and how safe the drug is. Generic companies are not allowed to use this data for the first eight years after a new drug is marketed.

## REFERENCES

Atkinson, M. M., & Coleman, W. D. (1985). Corporatism and industry policy. In A. Cawson (Ed.), *Organized interests and the state* (pp. 22–44). London: Sage.

Auditor General of Canada. (2011). Chapter 4: Regulating pharmaceutical drugs—Health Canada. In *Report of the Standing Committee on Public Accounts*. Ottawa: Author.

Avorn, J. (2015). The $2.6 billion pill—Methodologic and policy considerations. *New England Journal of Medicine, 372*(20), 1877–1879. doi:10.1056/NEJMp1500848

Ayres, I., & Braithwaite, J. (1992). *Responsive regulation: Transcending the deregulation debate.* New York: Oxford University Press.

Baker, D., & Chatani, N. (2002). *Promoting good ideas on drugs: Are patents the best way? The relative efficiency of patent and public support for biomedical research* (Briefing Paper). Washington, DC: Center for Economic and Policy Research.

Blumenthal, D., Campbell, E. G., Anderson, M. S., Causino, N., & Louis, K. S. (1997). Withholding research results in academic life science. Evidence from a national survey of faculty. *JAMA, 277*(15), 1224–1228. doi:10.1001/jama.1997.03540390054035

Bowman, M. A., & Pearle, D. L. (1988). Changes in drug prescribing patterns related to commercial company funding of continuing medical education. *Journal of Continuing Education in the Health Professions, 8*(1), 13–20. doi:10.1002/chp.4750080104

Canadian Institute for Health Information. (2016a). National health expenditure trends, 1975 to 2016: Data tables. Retrieved July 26, 2017, from https://www.cihi.ca/en/access-data-reports/results?f[0]=field_primary_theme%3A2058

Canadian Institute for Health Information. (2016b). Prescribed drug spending in Canada, 2016: A focus on public drug programs. Ottawa: Author.

Carpenter, D., Zucker, E. J., & Avorn, J. (2008). Drug-review deadlines and safety problems. *New England Journal of Medicine, 358*(13), 1354–1361. doi:10.1056/NEJMsa0706341

Chalkley, P. (2009). Targeting accessible physicians. *Canadian Pharmaceutical Marketing,* 29–30.

Davis, C., & Abraham, J. (2013). *Unhealthy pharmaceutical regulation: Innovation, politics and promissory science.* Basingstoke, U.K.: Palgrave Macmillan.

Department of Finance Canada. (2003). Building the Canada we want. The budget speech 2003. Ottawa: Government Services Canada.

DiMasi, J. A., Grabowski, H. G., & Hansen, R. W. (2016). Innovation in the pharmaceutical industry: New estimates of R&D costs. *Journal of Health Economics, 47,* 20–33. doi:10.1016/j.jhealeco.2016.01.012

External Advisory Committee on Smart Regulation. (2004). Smart regulation: A regulatory strategy for Canada. Ottawa: Privy Council Office. Retrieved from http://publications.gc.ca/pub?id=9.649410&sl=0

Foreign Affairs Trade and Development Canada. (2014). Canada-European Union: Comprehensive Economic and Trade Agreement (CETA). Retrieved February 22, 2015, from http://international.gc.ca/trade-agreements-accords-commerciaux/agr-acc/ceta-aecg/understanding-comprendre/brief-bref.aspx?lang=eng

Government of Canada. (2003). The Canada we want: Speech from the Throne to open the Second Session of the Thirty-Seventh Parliament of Canada. Ottawa: Author.

Government of Canada. (2015). How drugs are reviewed in Canada. Retrieved July 26, 2017, from https://www.canada.ca/en/health-canada/services/drugs-health-products/drug-products/fact-sheets/drugs-reviewed-canada.html

Habibi, R., & Lexchin, J. (2014). Quality and quantity of information in Summary Basis of Decision documents issued by Health Canada. *PLoS One, 9*(3),), e92038. doi:10.1371/journal.pone.0092038

Health Canada. (1998). *Cost recovery*. Ottawa: Author.

Health Canada. (2003a). Health protection legislative renewal: Detailed legislative proposal. Ottawa: Author. Retrieved from http://publications.gc.ca/pub?id=9.686533&sl=0

Health Canada. (2003b). *Improving Canada's regulatory process for therapeutic products: Building the action plan*. Ottawa: Public Policy Forum.

Health Products and Food Branch. (2007). *Cost recovery framework: Official notice of fee proposal for human drugs and medical devices*. Ottawa: Health Canada.

Health Products and Food Branch. (2014). 2014 review of the fees in respect of drugs and medical devices regulations. Ottawa: Health Canada. Retrieved July 26, 2017, from http://www.hc-sc.gc.ca/dhp-mps/alt_formats/pdf/finance/cost-recovery-review-examen-prix-revu-eng_V2.pdf

Health Products and Food Branch. (2017). *Public release of clinical informaiton in drug submissions and medical device applications*. Ottawa: Government of Canada.

Hemminki, E., Hailey, D., & Koivusalo, M. (1999). The courts—A challenge to health technology assessment. *Science, 285*(5425), 203–204. doi:10.1126/science.285.5425.203

IMS Brogan. (2016). Canadian pharmaceutical industry review 2015. Retrieved October 10, 2016, from http://imsbrogancapabilities.com/YIR_2015_FINAL

Innovative Medicines Canada. (2016). Code of Ethical Practices. Retrieved October 18, 2016, from http://innovativemedicines.ca/wp-content/uploads/2015/06/IMC_Code_EN.pdf

Katz, H. P., Goldfinger, S. E., & Fletcher, S. W. (2002). Academia-industry collaboration in continuing medical education: Description of two approaches. *Journal of Continuing Educucation in the Health Professions, 22*(1), 43–54. doi:10.1002/chp.1340220106

Kawachi, I. (1992). Six case studies of the voluntary regulation of pharmaceutical advertising and promotion. In P. Davis (Ed.), *For health or for profit? Medicine, the pharmaceutical industry, and the state in New Zealand* (pp. 269–287). Auckland: Oxford University Press.

Lazonick, W., Hopkins, M., Jacobson, K., Sakinç, M. E., & Tulum, Ö. (2017). *US pharma's financialized business model*. New York: Institute for New Economic Thinking.

Leslie, C. (2015, September 15). Relationship between MDs and pharma changing. *Medical Post*, p. 45.

Lexchin, J. (2013). How safe are new drugs? Market withdrawal of drugs approved in Canada between 1990 and 2009. *Open Medicine, 8*, e14-e19.

Lexchin, J. (2015). Health Canada's use of its priority review process for new drugs: A cohort study. *British Medical Journal Open, 5,* e006816. doi:10.1136/bmjopen-2014-006816

Lexchin, J., & Gagnon, M.-A. (2014). CETA and pharmaceuticals: Impact of the trade agreement between Europe and Canada on the costs of prescription drugs. *Globalization and Health, 10,* 30. doi:10.1186/1744-8603-10-30.

Lexchin, J., & Kawachi, I. (1996).The self-regulation of pharmaceutical marketing: Initiatives for reform. In P. Davis (Ed.), *Contested ground: Public purpose and private interest in the regulation of prescription drugs* (pp. 221–235). New York: Oxford University Press.

Lexchin, J., & Mintzes, B. (2014). A compromise too far: A review of Canadian cases of direct-to-consumer advertising regulation. *International Journal of Risk & Safety in Medicine, 26*(4), 213–225. doi:10.3233/JRS-140635

Light, D. W., & Warburton, R. N. (2005). Extraordinary claims require extraordinary evidence. *Journal of Health Economics, 24*(5), 1030–1033. doi:10.1016/j.jhealeco.2005.07.001

Marlow, B. (2007a). Is continuing medical education a drug-promotion tool? *Canadian Family Physician, 53*(10), 1650–1653.

Marlow, B. (2007b). Rebuttal: Is CME a drug-promotion tool? *Canadian Family Physician, 53,* 1877, 1878–1879.

McGarity, T. O., & Shapiro, S. A. (1980). The trade secret status of health and safety testing information: Reforming agency disclosure policies. *Harvard Law Review, 93*(5), 837–888. doi:10.2307/1340420

Michols, D. (1996). *The distinction between advertising and other activities.* Ottawa: Health Canada, Therapeutics Products Programme.

Mintzes, B., Lexchin, J., Sutherland, J. M., Beaulieu, M.-D., Wilkes, M., Durrieu, G., & Reynolds, E. (2013). Pharmaceutical sales representatives and patient safety: A comparative prospective study of information quality in Canada, France and the United States. *Journal of General Internal Medicine, 28*(10), 1368–1375. doi:10.1007/s11606-013-2411-7

Ontario Ministry of Health and Long-Term Care. (2011). 2009/10 report card for the Ontario Drug Benefit Program. Retrieved June 29, 2013, from http://www.health.gov.on.ca/en/public/programs/drugs/publications/opdp/docs/odb_report_09.pdf

Organisation for Economic Co-operation and Development (OECD). (2013). *Health at a glance 2013: OECD indicators.* Paris: Author. doi:10.1787/health_glance-2013-en

Organisation for Economic Co-operation and Development (OECD). (2015). *Health at a glance 2015: OECD indicators.* Paris: Author. doi:10.1787/health_glance-2015-en

Patented Medicine Prices Review Board. (2014). Compendium of policies, guidelines and procedures—Updated June 2014. Retrieved October 6, 2014, from http://www.pmprb-cepmb.gc.ca/view.asp?ccid=492

Pharmaceutical Advertising Advisory Board. (2007). *Code of advertising acceptance.* Pickering: PAAB Code Books.

Pharmaceutical Advertising Advisory Board. (2013). *Code of advertising acceptance.* Retrieved September 13, 2014, from http://www.paab.ca/paab-code.htm

PhRMA. (2015). *2015 profile biopharmaceutical research industry.* Washington: Author.

Progestic International Inc. (2004). *Final report for the financial models project.* Ottawa: Health Canada.

The Public Policy Forum. (2003). *Improving Canada's regulatory process for therapeutic products.* Ottawa: Author.

Rawson, N. S. (2001). Timeliness of review and approval of new drugs in Canada from 1999 through 2001: Is progress being made? *Clinical Therapeutics, 25*(4), 1230–1247. doi:10.1016/S0149-2918(03)80080-2

Rowsell, L. (2000). *Advertising campaigns of branded and unbranded messages.* Ottawa: Health Canada, Therapeutic Products Directorate.

Rutledge, P., Crookes, D., McKinstry, B., & Maxwell, S. R. J. (2003). Do doctors rely on pharmaceutical industry funding to attend conferences and do they perceive that this creates a bias in their drug selection? Results from a questionnaire survey. *Pharmacoepidemiology and Drug Safety, 12*(8), 663–667. doi:10.1002/pds.884

Rx&D. (2007). *A vision for a healthier tomorrow.* Ottawa: Author.

Rx&D. (2011). *Reality check: Analysis of the CGPA's economic impact assessment of proposed pharmaceutical IP provisions.* Ottawa: Author.

Rx&D. (2014, March 10). Letters to the editor. Retrieved October 6, 2014, from http://www.canadapharma.org/editorletters.asp?a=view&id=68

Senate of Canada. (2017). The Standing Senate Committee on Social Affairs, Science and Technology: Evidence. Retrieved July 26, 2017, from https://sencanada.ca/en/Content/Sen/Committee/421/SOCI/53348-e

Sinclair, S., Gagnon, M.-A., & Lexchin, J. (2014). Intellectual property rights: Pharmaceuticals. In S. Sinclair, S. Trew & H. Mertins-Kirkwood (Eds.), *Making sense of the CETA: An analysis of the final text of the Canada-European Union comprehensive economic and trade agreement* (pp. 56–61). Ottawa: Canadian Centre for Policy Alternatives.

Spurling, G. K., Mansfield, P. R., Montgomery, B. D., Lexchin, J., Doust, J., Othman, N., & Vitry, A. I. (2010). Information from pharmaceutical companies and the quality, quantity, and cost of physicians' prescribing: A systematic review. *PLoS Medicine, 7*(10), e1000352. doi:10.1371/journal.pmed.1000352

Statistics Canada. (2014). Financial and taxation statistics for enterprises, by North American Industry Classification System (NAICS), annual (dollars unless otherwise noted). Table 180-0003. Retrieved October 2, 2014, from http://www5.statcan.gc.ca/cansim/a26?lang=eng&retrLang=eng&id=1800003&paSer=&pattern=&stByVal=1&p1=1&p2=31&tabMode=dataTable&csid= - customizeTab

Steinbrook, R. (2008). Financial support of continuing medical education. *JAMA, 299*(9), 1060–1062. doi:10.1001/jama.299.9.1060

Steinman, M. A., & Baron, R. B. (2007). Rebuttal: Is CME a drug-promotion tool? YES. *Canadian Family Physician, 53*(11), 1877.

Steinman, M. A., Shlipak, M. G., & McPhee, S. J. (2001). Of principles and pens: Attitudes and practices of medicine housestaff toward pharmaceutical industry promotions. *American Journal of Medicine, 110*(7), 551–557. doi:10.1016/S0002-9343(01)00660-X

Therapeutic Products Directorate. (n.d.). *Business transformation progress report.* Ottawa: Health Canada.

Wiktorowicz, M. E., Lexchin, J., Moscou, K., Silversides, A., & Eggertson, L. (2010). *Keeping an eye on prescription drugs, keeping Canadians safe: Active monitoring systems for drug safety and effectiveness in Canada and internationally.* Toronto: Health Council of Canada.

# CHAPTER 16

## The Political Economy of Public Health: Public Health Concerns in Canada, the U.S., U.K., Norway, and Sweden

*Dennis Raphael and Toba Bryant*

## INTRODUCTION

Promoting health by governmental authorities comprises three distinct, though potentially related, sets of activities: (1) the activities carried out by federal, provincial, and municipal public health agencies and units; (2) governments developing health-related public policy that improves the quality and equitable distribution of the social determinants of health; and (3) health care that delivers healthcare services. Public health activities and health-related public policy—our focus in this chapter—are *primarily* concerned with maintaining and promoting the health of the population, while healthcare services are *primarily* concerned with providing treatments to individuals who are ill or at risk of falling ill. In Canada, these components generally operate independently. With few exceptions, Canadian public health agencies carry out disease- and injury-prevention activities, governmental ministries and departments design public policy in their designated spheres of responsibility, and healthcare institutions deliver health services. While there is increasing recognition among Canadian public health agencies and organizations of the importance of integrating these activities, actual success in integrating these endeavours has been sporadic.

The extent to which integration of public health and health-related public policy, as well as health care, activities is possible depends upon a variety of factors. An important determinant of integration is the model of health that is dominant within each jurisdiction. If health is seen as a highly individualized matter that reflects biological dispositions and risk behaviours, healthcare policy will dominate and public health approaches will primarily focus on managing biomedical and behavioural risk factors (Raphael, 2000). The emphasis will be on managing hypertension, cholesterol levels, weight, tobacco use, and diet through medically oriented healthcare system interventions such as screening and testing, physician directives, and pharmaceutical intervention. Public health will be limited to promoting access to health care and developing so-called healthy lifestyles.

There will be an emphasis on information dissemination and social marketing of lifestyle messages, and public policy development focused on modifying individual risk behaviours such as the imposition of sin taxes, promoting bicycle use, and limiting advertising of sweets to children. There will be little focus on improving the quality of the social determinants of health and making their distribution more equitable through public policy action.

In contrast, if health is understood as being shaped by structural factors (e.g., how a society organizes and distributes economic and social resources), public health approaches will focus on strengthening professional and public understandings of the social determinants of health and developing health-supportive public policy that promotes employment, income, housing, and food security; provides employment training and improves workplace quality; and guarantees accessible and responsive program and service provision. The distinction between these two kinds of activities is important as evidence has accumulated that structural approaches to promoting health are not only more likely to address the most important determinants of health, but are also more likely to achieve better health outcomes (Scott-Samuel & Smith, 2015). Additionally, the behavioural risk factors that are the focus of so much Canadian public health activity are themselves shaped in large part by structural factors that form the basis of a broader approach to promoting health (see Chapter 6, this volume).

In the previous editions of *Staying Alive*, we found Canada to be somewhat more advanced than the U.S. in awareness of the importance of addressing the social determinants of health, but both Canada and the U.S. lagged well behind the U.K., Norway, and Sweden in adopting and implementing a structural approach to public health. We concluded that public health activities and governmental approaches to health-related public policy were profoundly shaped by the political economy of each nation.

Norway and Sweden's long-standing and advanced commitments to a structural approach to public health issues were a direct result of decades of social democratic party rule. The U.K.'s attention to a structural analysis of health issues was a result of the 1997 election of a Labour government after decades of conservative rule. Canada's and the U.S.'s undeveloped approaches were driven by a neo-liberal resurgence in governmental approach that emphasized the marketplace as the primary arbiter of how economic and other resources should be distributed among the population. Related to this were systematic efforts in Canada and the U.S. to reduce governmental interventions in the workings of the economy in efforts to promote the equitable distribution of economic and social resources.

In this chapter, we update our examination of governmental statements about health, the structure and activities of public health agencies, and the relationship of public health to other arms of government activity in the nations. By identifying the principles and concepts that direct public health activities in each nation, we ascertain the extent to which public health preoccupations reflect emerging theory and research findings concerning the social determinants of health. We also consider how these principles and concepts appear to be directly tied to the form of each nation's political economy.

# CANADA

Canada had been seen as a leader in developing innovative approaches to public health (Restrepo, 1996). Canadians were strong contributors to health-promotion principles of equity and participation and health-promoting public policy (Raphael, 2012). However, many public health units in Canada are only just now raising these issues, and there has been little application of these concepts to developing health-promoting public policy at any level of government (Raphael & Sayani, 2017). Canada is now well behind other nations in applying its own concepts to promoting health (Hancock, 2011).

## Canadian Approaches as Presented in Statements, Documents, and Reports

Canada provides a fascinating example by which at first glance it appears to be a "health equity powerhouse" but is actually a "health equity laggard" (Bryant, Raphael, Schrecker, & Labonte, 2011). For decades, Canadian governmental and professional associations have discussed the role of "the determinants of health and healthy public policy" with little to show for it in terms of public policy activity (see Chapter 9, this volume).

The federal government's *A New Vision of Health for Canadians* identified four fields shaping health: human biology, lifestyles, environment, and health care (Lalonde, 1974). The identification of the environment field signalled the beginning of a broader health promotion era that saw its realization in the *Ottawa Charter*'s definition of health promotion as "the process of enabling people to increase control over their health and its determinants, and thereby improve their health" (World Health Organization, 1986). But in Canada, governments and public health officials seized upon the lifestyle field—tobacco use, activity level, healthy diet, etc.—to exclude the role played by social conditions (Legowski & McKay, 2000). The lifestyle emphasis was again challenged by the federal document *Achieving Health for All*, which emphasized structural aspects of society as shaping health (Epp, 1986). The implementation of this vision, however, was also not realized (Legowski & McKay, 2000).

The Canadian Public Health Association (CPHA) produced numerous reports that drew attention to homelessness, employment security, food insecurity, poverty, and other broader determinants of health (Manzano & Raphael, 2010). The CPHA's *Action Statement on Health Promotion*, for example, states that since "policies shape how money, power and material resources flow through society and therefore affect the determinants of health .... advocating for healthy public policies is the single most important strategy for improving health" (Canadian Public Health Association, 1996).

Since then, Canada has contributed to the Commission on Social Determinants of Health, managing two of its Knowledge Hubs: Early Child Development and Globalization and Health, and contributing to the Employment and Health hub (World Health Organization, 2008). The Public Health Agency of Canada has created a slew of documents stating its commitment to addressing the social determinants of Canadians' health and summarizing what it sees as efforts in this direction (Public Health Agency of

Canada, 2007, 2011b, 2015). Canada's Chief Health Officer has reported on the importance of addressing health inequalities (Butler-Jones, 2008, 2010).

Canada has also created a Canadian Council on the Social Determinants of Health and a number of Collaborating Centres charged with furthering action on the social determinants of health (Canadian Council on the Social Determinants of Health, 2018; National Collaborating Centre for Determinants of Health, 2015; National Coordinating Centre for Healthy Public Policy, 2014). These agencies have produced several reports and documents on why addressing these issues is important and how to go about doing so. Finally, the Canadian Institute for Health Information, the Canadian Population Health Initiative, and Statistics Canada have also produced reports stressing the need to promote health equity by reducing health inequalities (Canadian Institute for Health Information, 2018; Canadian Population Health Initiative, 2008; Tjepkema, Wilkins, & Long, 2013).

At the federal level, these commitments have been associated with recent efforts to address Indigenous issues in Canada but have not been made an explicit part of the federal government's broad public policy agenda (Indigenous Services Canada, 2018). Canada's official public health goals say nothing about addressing these issues (Public Health Agency of Canada, 2011a). Box 16.1 summarizes these developments.

Provincial authorities have produced statements and reports on the importance of achieving health equity by reducing inequalities in health. As just three examples, Quebec's Ministry of Health has produced a report about the importance of addressing health inequalities through public policy action (Lambert et al., 2014), Ontario's Medical Officers of Health have released a series of reports calling for action to promote health equity through action on the social determinants of health (King, 2010, 2011; Williams, 2018), and New Brunswick's Medical Officer of Health has also reported on health inequities (Muecke, 2016).

Locally, municipal health authorities in Saskatoon, Sudbury, and Vancouver Coastal Health have provided exemplary approaches to addressing health equity issues (National Collaborating Centre for the Determinants of Health, 2012; Sudbury and District Health Unit, 2012; Vancouver Coastal Health, 2011). In Ontario, a majority of local health units are undertaking activities to address health equity through action on the social determinants of health (Raphael & Sayani, 2017). These latter activities have been supported by funding by the Ontario Ministry of Health and Long-Term Care, which allows two health nurses for each local health unit to focus on the social determinants of health (Raphael & Brassolotto, 2015).

## Canadian Public Policy to Promote Health Equity

Despite concepts of health equity and the social determinants of health being widespread in federal, provincial, and in some cases, municipal public health statements, for the most part, federal and provincial ministries of health continue to focus on disease and infection control and programs promoting healthy lifestyles. Public policy at the federal, provincial,

**Box 16.1:** Canadian Developments in Developing a Structural Approach to Public Health

---

- Alberta Public Health Units collaborate to create a Health Equity Network
- Canadian Population Health Initiative publishes numerous reports addressing social determinants of health
- Chief Public Health Officer of Canada issues a report on inequalities in health
- Conference Board of Canada establishes a round table on socio-economic determinants of health
- Health-related organizations address the social determinants of health:
  - Association of Ontario Health Centres
  - Canadian Medical Association
  - Canadian Nurses Association
- *Ideas* program on CBC devotes a two-hour series to the social determinants of health
- WHO Commission on the Social Determinants of Health places two learning hubs— early childhood and globalization—in Canada
- National Collaborating Centre for Determinants of Health is established at St. Francis Xavier University in Antigonish, Nova Scotia
- Senate Sub-committee on Population Health addresses the social determinants of health and issues a series of reports
- Health Council of Canada publishes *Stepping It Up: Moving the Focus from Health Care in Canada to a Healthier Canada*
- Sudbury Health Unit publishes a framework to incorporate social and economic determinants of health into the Ontario public health mandate
- *Social Determinants of Health: The Canadian Facts* is published
- Public Health Agency of Canada establishes the Canadian Council on the Social Determinants of Health
- Upstream established by Saskatchewan physician Ryan Meili to educate the public about the social determinants of health
- Video on health equity produced by Sudbury and District Health Unit adopted by majority of Ontario Public Health Units

and even the municipal level does not explicitly aim to improve the quality and equitable distribution of the social determinants of health. Promoting health equity and reducing health inequalities is totally absent from the public policy agenda of any level of government across Canada (Raphael, 2015b; see Chapter 9, this volume). When there are policy initiatives that address issues of poverty, housing, employment, or early child development, they are not linked to these health-related concepts, and even then are very modest in their scope, with little effect on the quality and distribution of the social determinants of health (Raphael, 2011). Income inequality is increasing and poverty is deepening (Curry-Stevens, 2016). None of the social determinants of health are being distributed more equitably (Raphael, 2016).

Scholarship has considered some of the reasons for this yawning gap between knowledge and action. These include the narrow purview of traditional health sciences research, emphasis upon individualistic conceptions of health, and increasing reluctance of governments to implement public policy in the service of strengthening the social determinants of health (Collins & Hayes, 2007; Lavis, 2002; Raphael, Curry-Stevens, & Bryant, 2008).

A strong argument has been made that Canadian public policy continues to be made in the service of powerful economic sectors of society that actually profit from inequality (Langille, 2016; Raphael, 2015a; see Chapter 3, this volume). Canada's history as a liberal welfare state places the business and corporate sector in a dominant position in shaping public policy. To maximize profits, this sector calls for reducing the role of government in managing the economy. The result is increasing inequity in the distribution of the social determinants of health. Wages lag behind the rise in living costs, governments do little to equitably distribute resources by providing affordable housing, making taxation fairer by increasing taxes on corporations and the wealthy, or improving benefits and services to the least well-off (Raphael, 2015a).

Any government attempt to address these issues sparks a string of backlash from the business community (Raphael, 2015a). Governments ignore their own documents, statements, and reports on the importance of promoting health equity by improving the quality and equitable distribution of the social determinants of health. As noted, income inequality continues to increase, poverty is deepening, and governmental concern with reducing inequality is declining (Banting & Myles, 2013).

## Toward the Future

There is continuing and even increasing interest in the importance of promoting health equity through public policy action on the social determinants of health among the public health community. As just a few examples, the Canadian Medical Association produced a report concerned with these issues (Canadian Medical Association, 2013), a monograph entitled *Social Determinants of Health: The Canadian Facts* has been downloaded over 800,000 times (Mikkonen & Raphael, 2010), and the organization Upstream is specifically focused on educating the public on the importance of addressing the social determinants of health (Upstream, 2013).

In Saskatchewan, family doctor Ryan Meili first wrote a book entitled *A Healthy Society: How a Focus on Health Can Revive Canadian Democracy* (Meili, 2017); went on to found Upstream, an organization dedicated to publicizing the importance of the social determinants of health; and then became provincial leader of the Saskatchewan New

Democratic Party on a platform of making all public policy take cognizance of their effects on the social determinants of health (CBC News, 2018).

However, these developments have done little to shift the portrait we presented in the first and second editions of *Staying Alive*. The failure of broader determinants-related knowledge to be translated into public policy activity in support of the social determinants of health continues to constitute the primary dilemma facing the public health community in Canada. A research agenda for identifying means of improving the situation calls for studying Canadians' understandings of these broader health issues, why policy-makers will not address these issues, means of redressing power imbalances between the corporate and business and the labour sector, and how developments in other nations can be applied to the Canadian scene (Raphael, 2015b).

## UNITED STATES

The U.S. has one of the worst health profiles of modern industrialized nations and one of the least developed welfare states (see Chapter 9, this volume). It is the only modern industrialized nation that does not provide health care for all citizens as a matter of course.

Nevertheless, broader population health concepts have penetrated into government and health agency documents, and these same documents are now raising broader issues concerning the determinants of health. This concern with broader determinants of health has traditionally been focused on racial and ethnic disparities with rather less attention given to how public policy causes these differences. However, there has been an expansion of interest in the social determinants of health and the importance of promoting health equity, albeit through local action rather than through broader public policy-making.

Interestingly, the U.S. continues, for the most part, to use the term "health disparity" rather than "health inequalities" or "health inequities." This reflects a continuing focus on epidemiologically based issues of disease prevention rather than a social justice health equity orientation. However, some agencies and organizations have adopted a health inequalities/health equity approach to these issues.

However, as is the situation in Canada, there continues to be a wide gap between knowledge concerning the social determinants of health and public policy action to address the inequitable distribution of these social determinants. Despite very promising local actions instituted by some states and cities, the deteriorating public policy environment in the U.S. has led to actual declines in life expectancy across wide areas of the nation (Bezruchka, 2012).

### National Policy Documents and Reports

The Centers for Disease Control and Prevention (CDC) is the national agency in the U.S. responsible for addressing public health issues. For many years, the CDC has been producing reports on the social determinants of health. Also joining the act has been the

National Academy of Sciences, which produced a lengthy report entitled *Communities in Action: Pathways to Health Equity* (National Academies of Sciences, Engineering, & Medicine, 2017). Other agencies and associations, such as the National Association of County and City Health Officials (NACCHO), have also been raising the issue of promoting health equity and reducing health inequities.

## Centers for Disease Control and Prevention

The CDC website has an entire portal devoted to the social determinants of health (CDC, 2019b). It provides section links of: Sources for Data on SDOH; CDC Research on SDOH; Tools for Putting SDOH into Action; CDC Programs Addressing SDOH; and Policy Resources to Support SDOH. The CDC provides these definitions of health equity and health inequities (Brennan Ramirez, Baker, & Metzler, 2008, p. 6):

> Health equity is achieved when every person has the opportunity to "attain his or her full health potential" and no one is "disadvantaged from achieving this potential because of social position or other socially determined circumstances." Health disparities or inequities, are types of unfair health differences closely linked with social, economic or environmental disadvantages that adversely affect groups of people.

Currently, the CDC speaks of the social determinants of health as follows: "Conditions in the places where people live, learn, work, and play affect a wide range of health risks and outcomes. These conditions are known as social determinants of health" (CDC, 2019b). Initially, the CDC listed these social determinants of health: how a person develops during the first few years of life (early childhood development); how much education a person obtains; being able to get and keep a job; what kind of work a person does; having food or being able to get food (food security); having access to health services and the quality of those services; housing status; how much money a person earns; and discrimination and social support. As part of their efforts, the CDC hosts the National Center for Chronic Disease Prevention and Health Promotion (NCCDPHP; CDC, 2019a). However, in direct contrast to the CDC position on social determinants of health, the Center demonstrates a pervasive lifestyle drift by stating that most chronic diseases are caused by a short list of risk behaviours:

- Tobacco use and exposure to second-hand smoke;
- Poor nutrition, including diets low in fruits and vegetables and high in sodium and saturated fats;
- Lack of physical activity; and
- Excessive alcohol use.

The CDC has produced numerous reports focusing on the role that addressing the social determinants of health could play in improving health (CDC, 2016). However, these reports and projects are rather narrowly defined, focusing on health issues such as asthma, diabetes, hepatitis A, colorectal screening, and HIV, among others. These initiatives are for the most part community-based and do not delve into broader issues of resource distribution across the population.

*Healthy People 2020* is the national plan for public health and contains a large number of health objectives (Office of Disease Prevention and Health Promotion, 2014). It has four overarching goals:

1. Attain high-quality, longer lives free of preventable disease, disability, injury, and premature death;
2. Achieve health equity, eliminate disparities, and improve the health of all groups;
3. Create social and physical environments that promote good health for all; and
4. Promote quality of life, healthy development, and healthy behaviours across all life stages.

It identifies 42 topics and objectives, which are presented in Box 16.2. Interestingly, *Healthy People 2020* "developed a 'place-based' organizing framework, reflecting five key areas of SDOH" that are assumed to reflect each of these objectives:

1. Economic Stability
2. Education
3. Social and Community Context
4. Health and Health Care; and
5. Neighbourhood and Built Environment

It recognizes developments in theory and findings concerning the broader determinants of health. However, in many cases the social determinants are placed in a somewhat background role. For example, consider the section on heart disease and stroke. The section states:

The leading modifiable (controllable) risk factors for heart disease and stroke are: High blood pressure; High cholesterol; Cigarette smoking; Diabetes; Unhealthy diet and physical inactivity; and Overweight and obesity.

 Over time, these risk factors cause changes in the heart and blood vessels that can lead to heart attacks, heart failure, and strokes. It is critical to address risk factors early in life to prevent these devastating events and other potential complications of chronic cardiovascular disease. (Office of Disease Prevention and Health Promotion, 2014)

**Box 16.2:** Topic Areas for *Healthy People 2020*

| | |
|---|---|
| Access to Health Services | Heart Disease and Stroke |
| Adolescent Health | HIV |
| Arthritis, Osteoporosis, and Chronic Back Conditions | Immunization and Infectious Diseases |
| | Injury and Violence Prevention |
| Blood Disorders and Blood Safety | Lesbian, Gay, Bisexual, and Transgender Health |
| Cancer | |
| Chronic Kidney Disease | Maternal, Infant, and Child Health |
| Dementias, Including Alzheimer's Disease | Medical Product Safety |
| Diabetes | Mental Health and Mental Disorders |
| Disability and Health | Nutrition and Weight Status |
| Early and Middle Childhood | Occupational Safety and Health |
| Educational and Community-Based Programs | Older Adults |
| | Oral Health |
| Environmental Health | Physical Activity |
| Family Planning | Preparedness |
| Food Safety | Public Health Infrastructure |
| Genomics | Respiratory Diseases |
| Global Health | Sexually Transmitted Diseases |
| Health Communication and Health Information Technology | Sleep Health |
| | Social Determinants of Health |
| Health-Related Quality of Life & Well-Being | Substance Abuse |
| | Tobacco Use |
| Healthcare-Associated Infections | Vision |
| Hearing and Other Sensory or Communication Disorders | |

*Source:* Office of Disease Prevention and Health Promotion. (2014). *Healthy people 2020.* Washington, DC: Author.

It is not until a later section that the document states:

Disease does not occur in isolation, and cardiovascular disease is no exception. Cardiovascular health is significantly influenced by the physical, social, and political environment, including:

Maternal and child health; Access to educational opportunities; Availability of healthy foods, physical education, and extracurricular activities in schools; Opportunities for physical activity, including access to safe and walkable communities; Access to healthy foods; Quality of working conditions and worksite health; Availability of community support and resources; and Access to affordable, quality health care. (Office of Disease Prevention and Health Promotion, 2014)

Yet no information is provided on the direct links of these factors to cardiovascular health, nor are there any recommendations on how to improve the quality of these background factors. The other topic sections are similar. The diabetes section makes no mention of the broader factors that shape type 2 diabetes such as poverty, stress, and food insecurity. Emphasis is on medical care and lifestyle change.

## National Academies of Sciences, Engineering, and Medicine

In 2002, the Institute of Medicine—a unit of the National Academies—published *The Future of the Public's Health*, which provided an accurate presentation of developments in the field of population health by calling for "adopting a population health approach that considers the multiple determinants of health" (Institute of Medicine, 2002). At that time, however, virtually all examples of issues to be addressed were health care–related or behaviourally focused on poor diet, tobacco use, or physical inactivity. Policy was conceived narrowly: legislative activities related to risk behaviours and health protection.

A more recent report by the National Academies entitled *Communities in Action: Pathways to Health Equity* is a 550-page compendium of locally based activities working to provide health equity (National Academies of Sciences, Engineering, & Medicine, 2017). It provides up-to-date information on concepts of health equity and inequity, the social determinants of health, and the mechanisms by which these shape health. It provides voluminous examples of local activity that aims to reduce health inequities. Box 16.3 provides a summary of its key aspects.

In addition to providing numerous examples of local and state action to address health equities and the inequitable distribution of the social determinants of health, the report details how public policy changes have exacerbated these conditions. The report could serve as a handbook for public policy action if the political will was present to promote health equity through public policy action. However, it is well documented that the current political environment and long-standing economic and political traditions make such efforts unlikely in the present or near future.

## The American Public Health Association

The American Public Health Association (APHA) has also engaged in promoting health equity through action on the social determinants of health (American Public Health Association, 2019). It states:

Creating *health equity* is a guiding priority and core value of APHA. By health equity, we mean everyone has the opportunity to reach their highest attainable level of health.

**Box 16.3:** Key Aspects of *Communities in Action:*
*Pathways to Health Equity*

The Report in Brief:

A. Health equity is crucial for the well-being and vibrancy of communities. The United States pays the high price of health inequity in lost lives, potential, and resources (Chapters 1 and 2).

B. Health is a product of multiple determinants. Social, economic, environmental, and structural factors and their unequal distribution matter more than health care in shaping health disparities (Chapter 3).

C. Health inequities are in large part a result of poverty, structural racism, and discrimination (Chapter 3).

D. Communities have agency to promote health equity. However, community-based solutions are necessary but not sufficient (Chapters 4 and 5).

E. Supportive public and private policies at all levels and programs facilitate community action (infrastructure of policies, funding, political will, etc.) (Chapter 6).

F. The collaboration and engagement of new and diverse (multi-sector) partners is essential to promoting health equity (Chapter 7).

G. Tools and other resources exist to translate knowledge into action to promote health equity (Chapter 8).

H. Conclusion (Chapter 9).

*Source:* National Academies of Sciences, Engineering, & Medicine. (2017). *Communities in action: Pathways to health equity.* Washington, DC: National Academies Press.

*Inequities* are created when barriers prevent individuals and communities from accessing these conditions and reaching their full potential. Inequities differ from *health disparities*, which are differences in health status between people related to social or demographic factors such as race, gender, income or geographic region. Health disparities are one way we can measure our progress toward achieving health equity.

*How do we achieve health equity?* We optimize the conditions in which people are born, grow, live, work, learn and age. We work with other sectors to address the factors that influence health, including employment, housing, education, health care, public safety and food access. We name racism as a force in determining how these social determinants are distributed.

A special issue of APHA's journal *The Nation's Health* highlights *Addressing Health Equity through State, Regional Partnerships* (American Public Health Association, 2018). It discusses state, regional, and municipal actions to promote health equity through action on the social determinants of health. The APHA website provides further resources (American Public Health Association, 2019).

## National Association of County and City Health Officials (NACCHO)

NACCHO has provided both conceptual and practical leadership for public health units across the U.S. aiming to promote health equity. NACCHO links health equity directly to social justice through its Health Equity and Social Justice program (NACCHO, 2019a).

> The goal of NACCHO's Health Equity and Social Justice program is to advance the capacity of local health departments to confront the root causes of inequities in the distribution of disease and illness through public health practice and their organizational structure. The program's initiatives explore why certain populations bear a disproportionate burden of disease and mortality and what social arrangements and institutions generate those inequities, in order to design strategy to eliminate them.

NACCHO provides support to health units across the U.S. through numerous initiatives. These include *The Roots of Health Inequity: A Web-Based Course for the Public Health Workforce* (NACCHO, 2019c). This course allows health department staff to investigate the relationship between social injustice—the fundamental cause of health inequities—and everyday public health practice.

*The Building Networks Project: Aligning Public Health and Community Organizing* shows how public health can link with the discipline and strategies of community organizing in five states in the Midwest: Michigan, Minnesota, Missouri, Ohio, and Wisconsin (NACCHO, 2014). It aims to create strong, flexible, and durable statewide teams that can realize structural reforms.

The *Health Equity and Social Justice Toolkit* is a database of health equity tools, publications, and resources, available in NACCHO's Toolbox (NACCHO, 2019b). These publications include the anthologies *Expanding the Boundaries: Health Equity and Public Health Practice* and *Exploring the Roots of Health Inequity: Essays for Reflection.*

NACCHO recently released *Advancing Public Narrative for Health Equity and Social Justice* (NACCHO, 2018). It provides guidance in identifying, examining, and countering dominant public narratives and the systems that support them. The volume contains exercises and questions for reflection and dialogue that allow public health practitioners and their allies to use effective narrative strategies to achieve health equity. It promotes a social justice–based public narrative to engage people in collective action to build a just society.

## Unnatural Causes: Is Inequality Making Us Sick?

California Newsreel undertook a project of providing a documentary series that would serve as the basis for establishing a new approach to public health in the U.S. (Adelman, 2008). Through funding from a variety of sources, it produced the four-hour documentary *Unnatural Causes: Is Inequality Making Us Sick?* and expended significant efforts to support those attempting to implement its message that Americans' health is profoundly affected by the social determinants of health and the public policies that determine their quality. The website provides a model that could be applied in Canada to build awareness of and support for a broader approach to public health (www.unnaturalcauses.org).

In summary, public health activity in the U.S. that addresses broader determinants of population health has expanded over the past 10 years. While a focus on behavioural risk factors remains, as does emphasis on examining and responding to racial and ethnic health differences (National Center for Health Statistics, 2016), in relation to the CDC, National Academies, and NACCHO work, there is increased activity in support of adopting a broader public health approach to promoting health equity.

The hope is this will lead to increased attention to how public policy change can be an appropriate focus of public health action. The harsh public policy environment in the U.S. associated with the Donald Trump era makes shifts in the public policy environment unlikely. Indeed, the U.S. is the only developed nation experiencing a decline in overall life expectancy (Muennig, Reynolds, Fink, Zafari, & Geronimus, 2018). Similarly, health inequalities appear to be on the rise despite the increased public health attention to the promotion of health equity (Bor, Cohen, & Galea, 2017).

# UNITED KINGDOM

The U.K. has a long-standing intellectual and academic concern with inequalities in health. In 1980, the *Black Report* revealed that despite a generation of accessible health care, class-related health inequalities had not only been maintained but in many instances had increased (Black & Smith, 1992). The report appeared at the onset of the conservative Thatcher era, and its content and recommendations were ignored for two decades. During that period, numerous public policies widened income and health inequalities. The election of a Labour government in 1997 saw the ongoing academic and policy concern with health inequalities translated into a government-wide effort to address health inequalities through the development of public policy. Careful documentation and analysis of these efforts were carried out. These reviews illustrate how evidence, combined with the political will to address broader determinants of health, can translate into effective policy development and action.

However, recent events show that the initial successes of this program in England are now being reversed by a Conservative national government that came to power in 2010

(Barr, Higgerson, & Whitehead, 2017). With devolution, other members of the United Kingdom (Scotland, Wales, and Northern Ireland) have taken different public policy paths toward promoting health equity (Smith & Bambra, 2012). In all cases, however, health inequalities continue to be the subject of reports and documents, although broader public policies that would reduce them appear to be in rather short supply.

## The Black Report and Health Divide Inquiries

The 1980 *Black Report* and the 1992 *Health Divide* (Townsend, Davidson, & Whitehead, 1992) described how lowest employment-level groups showed a greater likelihood of suffering from a wide range of diseases and dying prematurely from illness or injury at every stage of the life cycle. Among various interpretations available, it concluded that the material conditions under which people live—availability of income, working conditions, and quality of available food and housing, etc.—were the primary determinants of these findings. As noted, the implications of these findings were ignored by the U.K. government until 1997 and its loss of power.

## The Election of 1997

Upon its election in 1997, the Labour government created the Acheson Commission into Inequalities in Health. The commission considered a wide range of evidence and concluded that:

> The weight of scientific evidence supports a socioeconomic explanation of health inequalities. This traces the roots of ill health to such determinants as income, education and employment as well as to the material environment and lifestyle. (Acheson, 1998)

It offered recommendations across a wide range of health determinants: poverty, income, tax, and benefits; education; employment; housing and environment; mobility, transport, and pollution; nutrition and agriculture policy; mothers, children, and families; young people and adults of working age; older people; ethnicity; gender; and the National Health Service (NHS). The most important were: (1) all policies likely to have an impact on health should be evaluated in terms of their impact on health inequalities; (2) high priority should be given to the health of families with children; and (3) further steps should be taken to reduce income inequalities and improve the living standards of poor households.

The Labour government of the U.K. developed and implemented policies for addressing inequalities in health by addressing the broader determinants of health. The efforts expended to achieve a reduction in health inequalities were significant and associated with extensive public and media debate and formed the basis of ongoing evaluations of effectiveness.

## Government Action Plans

The government responded quickly to these recommendations. Among the major English policy initiatives was the document *Reducing Health Inequalities: An Action Report* (Department of Health, 1999). The action areas are outlined in Box 16.4.

At the same time, the U.K. government began to devolve responsibility for health to the nation members of the U.K.: England, Scotland, Wales, and Northern Ireland. Each began to address health inequalities in their own way. Table 16.1 gives examples of how each U.K. nation placed an emphasis on the broader determinants of health during the early 2000s.

---

**Box 16.4:** Reducing Health Inequalities: The U.K. Agenda for Action

---

Upon election in 1997, the U.K. Labour government organized a strategy based on nine themes. Specific policies are listed to illustrate its action approach.

- *Raising living standards and tackling low income* by introducing a minimum wage and a range of tax credits and increasing benefit levels
- *Improving education and early years* by introducing policies to improve educational standards and creating "Sure Start," preschool services in disadvantaged areas, free to those on low incomes
- *Increasing employment* by creating a range of welfare-to-work schemes for different priority groups
- *Improving transport and mobility* by setting targets to reduce road traffic accidents, develop safe walking and cycling routes, and standardize concessionary fares for older people
- *Issues for the NHS* include working in partnership with local authorities to tackle the wider determinants of health, reviewing the resource allocation formula to local healthcare agencies, developing frameworks to standardize care across the country for particular conditions, and broadening the NHS's performance framework to include fair access and improving health
- *Building healthy communities* by investing in a range of regeneration initiatives in disadvantaged areas, including Health Action Zones
- *Improving housing* by changing capital financial rules to promote investment in social housing and introducing special initiatives to tackle homelessness
- *Reducing crime* by investing in a range of community-led crime-prevention schemes and tackling drug misuse
- *Addressing public health issues*—the first-ever minister for public health oversaw a range of initiatives to encourage healthy lifestyles, strengthen the public health workforce, and tackle specific problems such as fluoridation of water supplies

---

*Source:* Adapted from Benzeval, M. (2002). "England." In J. Mackenbach & M. Bakker (Eds.), *Reducing inequalities in health: European perspectives* (p. 207, Box 12.3). London: Routledge.

**Table 16.1:** Illustrative Examples of the Universal Emphasis Placed on Social and Economic Determinants of Health in the Early Post-Devolution Years

| U.K. Region | Illustrative Extract |
|---|---|
| England | *From Vision to Reality* (Department of Health, 2001, p. 1): "The worst health problems in the country will not be tackled without dealing with their fundamental causes—poverty, lack of education, poor housing, unemployment, discrimination and social exclusion." |
| Northern Ireland | *Investing for Health* (Department of Health, Social Services and Public Safety, 2002, p. 3): "A large proportion of this unnecessary premature death and disease is determined by social and economic inequalities. The evidence is clear—there is a direct correlation between poverty, social disadvantage and your health." |
| Scotland | *Our National Health* (Scottish Executive, 2000, p. 7): "Poverty, poor housing, homelessness and the lack of educational and economic opportunity are the root causes of major inequalities in health in Scotland. We must fight the causes of illness as well as illness itself." |
| Wales | *Well Being in Wales* (Public Health Strategy Division, 2002, p. 5): "The mix of social, economic, environmental and cultural factors that affect individuals' lives determines their health and well being. We can only improve well being in the long term by addressing these factors." |

*Source:* Smith, K. E., & Hellowell, M. (2012). Beyond rhetorical differences: A cohesive account of post-devolution developments in UK health policy. *Social Policy and Administration, 46*(2), 178–198.

## Reviews of These Initiatives

A 2003 evaluation concluded that significant progress had been made in tackling health inequalities (Exworthy, Stuart, Blane, & Marmot, 2003). Evidence concerning health inequalities had been gathered, health inequalities had been placed on the policy agenda, and a diverse range of activities had been developed. Indicators of outcomes and policy implementation were emerging, though impacts upon health status were not yet apparent. The authors concluded: "Many challenges remain but the prospects for tackling inequalities are good" (Exworthy et al., 2003, p. 52).

A 2005 evaluation concluded the Labour government had taken seriously the issues of poverty and social exclusion (Hills & Stewart, 2005). Evaluations of these initiatives were positive, though effects were modest. There was success in reducing child poverty as a result of the government's tax and benefit reforms. But while overall poverty rates declined, rates for working-age adults without children had reached all-time high levels by 2002–2003. By 2008, an evaluation concluded that the government had begun to downplay its emphasis on reducing health inequalities (Hills, Sefton, & Stewart, 2009a, 2009b). In addition, specific results concerned with reducing health inequalities were disappointing.

Since then, a study found that the efforts to reduce health inequalities during the 1997–2010 period had been somewhat successful (Barr et al., 2017). Geographical health inequalities in relative and absolute differences in male and female life expectancy at birth between the most deprived local authorities in England and the rest of the country were reduced during this period. In addition, since the disbandment of the program in 2010 by the incoming Conservative government, these inequalities have begun to increase.

## Developments Since the 2010 Electoral Loss by Labour

In 2010, the Labour government was defeated by the Conservatives. The sustained initiatives of the Labour government to address health inequalities came to an end in England. But like the situation in Canada, the issue remains prominent in English public policy documents. There are reports on the extent of health inequalities in England, and the National Health Service (NHS) has been given responsibility for addressing these.

One example is the report about northern England entitled *Due North: Report of the Inquiry on Health Equity for North* (Whitehead, 2014). It is an excellent overview of the extent of health inequalities in the North of England, the factors driving these inequalities, and recommendations for reducing them. Box 16.5 provides the four key recommendations from the inquiry, which have relevance everywhere.

Public Health England issues annual reports containing data and insights from other sources to give a broad picture of the health of people in England. Its acts as an independent agency whose aim is to advise and support government, local authorities, and the NHS. Its 2018 report contains chapters on inequalities in health and wider determinants of health (Public Health England, 2018). These chapters are very detailed and give an excellent picture of the situation in England. The determinants chapter provides details on (1) the built and natural environment, (2) education, (3) income, (4) work and the labour market, (5) crime, and (6) social capital.

NHS documents have been released that also contain data on the extent of health inequalities and means by which the NHS can reduce these (Public Health England, 2017; National Health Service England, 2018). These recommendations certainly cover all of

---

**Box 16.5:** Recommendations from the *Inquiry on Health Equity for the North*

1. Tackle poverty and economic inequality within the North and between the North and the rest of England
2. Promote healthy development in early childhood
3. Share power over resources and increase the influence that the public has on how resources are used to improve the determinants of health
4. Strengthen the role of the health sector in promoting health equity

*Source:* Whitehead, M. (2014). *Due north: Report of the inquiry on health equity for the North.* Prepared by the Inquiry Panel on Health Equity for the North of England.

the different levels in which interventions can take place: physiological risks, behavioural risks, and psychosocial risks. It also identifies the risk conditions that cause these issues, such as poverty, unemployment, discrimination, and gaps in government services and supports. Clearly, these recommendations are being hindered by the broader social policies in England that are reducing programs and services and increasing income and wealth inequalities. The NHS as an agency is not able to shape broader public policy issues related to the distribution of economic and social resources.

In the other nations of the U.K., the issue of health equity remains prominent. In Scotland, the national government commissioned a number of reports that detail and stress the importance of addressing health inequalities (NHS Health Scotland, 2018a). The Scottish government has stated that: "Reducing inequalities in health is critical to achieving the Scottish Government's aim of making Scotland a better, healthier place for everyone, no matter where they live" (Scottish Government, 2018).

A 2013 report entitled *Health Inequalities Policy Review for the Scottish Ministerial Task Force on Health Inequalities* made these recommendations (NHS Health Scotland, 2018b):

1.  Health inequalities policy should be at the heart of the Scottish Government's drive for social justice, a key plank of the Single Outcome Agreements and central to the preventive spend agenda. Priority must be given to addressing the upstream fundamental causes of health inequalities which include poverty and income, as well as the wider environmental factors such as housing and education, over the downstream consequences like smoking and alcohol abuse.

2.  The Scottish Government and COSLA should regularly review the balance of policy and resources directed to actions aimed at tackling the fundamental causes of health inequalities rather than individual lifestyle interventions, which do not, on their own, deliver the changes required.

    a)  A future inequalities strategy should consider actions at all levels of the social determinants of health—the economic and social conditions in our society and how they are distributed.

    b)  A life course approach is helpful particularly if actions and resources are targeted at early years which offers the best opportunity of preventing future health inequalities.

    c)  Central and local government need to focus on the implementation of the measures which are most likely to be effective and to discontinue those which widen inequalities.

3.  While action will be taken at a national level, a significant contribution needs to take place locally, connecting with communities and building the hopes of people that face the greatest challenges. The National Community Planning Group should advocate that those CPP areas that contribute most to health inequalities in Scotland should prioritise their actions in a drive to

narrow health inequalities. The focus for spending needs to shift away from meeting the cost of dealing with health and social problems after they have developed, to prevention and early intervention.

4.   There is a continuing role for national and local government, meeting regularly, to ensure the political focus on cross-government and cross-agency work to address the fundamental causes and social determinants of health inequalities, with linkage to equality. There is also a key role for a national agency, such as NHS Health Scotland, with a remit to drive forward the necessary changes in policy, practice and, ultimately, outcomes.

Despite these excellent analyses of the sources of health inequalities in Scotland, the health equity situation is deteriorating as a result of imposed austerity by the U.K. government. *The Guardian* reports: "One million Scots are now living in poverty as the impact of austerity cuts in recent years bites, official figures have revealed. The incomes of poorer households fell further behind those of middle earners, pushing more people into poverty. Poorer households with children have been worse hit, falling further behind those on middle incomes" (McNab, 2018). The Scottish government responded to this by stating: "We know that in the face of UK Government cuts and continuing austerity, which are having a damaging impact on thousands of Scottish households, our actions mean we are fighting poverty with one hand tied behind our back" (McNab, 2018).

In Wales, there is also an apparent commitment to tackling health inequalities. The Wales government website states why it is a priority (Public Health Wales, 2019):

Health inequality refers to differences in health outcomes between groups; for example, a higher rate of lung cancer incidence in more deprived areas compared to less deprived areas. The term health inequities relates to perceived unfair differences in health outcomes between groups that are potentially avoidable.

Poor social and economic circumstances affect health and well-being throughout life. Disadvantage has many forms and can include: having few family assets; a poorer education; a lower paid job or insecure employment; living in poor housing and trying to bring up a family in difficult circumstances.

Numerous reports are available that document the extent of health inequalities in Wales, identify means of addressing them, and report on progress. The Public Health Wales Observatory website provide links to the latest relevant publications from the Public Health Observatory and key data sources and key evidence sources on health inequalities in Wales.

Like Scotland, Wales is subject to the austerity measures emanating from the U.K. government. The government states (Welsh Government, 2018):

Any suggestion this Conservative government's failed policy of austerity is over—as the Prime Minister claimed just a few weeks ago—on the evidence of this budget, is wrong. There is little else in the UK Budget for Wales, besides confirmation of the 70th anniversary NHS funding consequential which we were already expecting and a few other crumbs from the table.

At the very best this is a "treading-water budget" while we await the outcome of Brexit negotiations. It's very disappointing as far as Wales is concerned.

Finally, in Northern Ireland, the government publishes annual reports that present a comprehensive analysis of regional health inequality gaps (Northern Ireland Department of Health, 2018). Its most recent report documents health inequalities between the most and least deprived areas of NI and sub-regional gaps across a range of health indicators.

However, like the situation in Scotland and Wales, Northern Ireland is seen as suffering from the austerity agenda emanating from the central U.K. government. The Opposition Party in Northern Ireland states: "Yet public services across Northern Ireland remain in crisis, and there was little in this budget to suggest that things will improve here anytime soon" (BBC Northern Ireland, 2018).

## Pronouncements versus Public Policy Reality

Despite these stated commitments to addressing health inequalities, the general public policy environment in the U.K. related to the promotion of health equity has darkened. Indeed, a recent report from the Special Rapporteur on Poverty from the United Nations concluded that "UK austerity policies have plunged people into despair" (*The Irish Times*, 2018).

The U.K. situation illustrates that even when there appears to be an explicit concern with addressing health inequalities, the ability to do so is limited by the broader public policy environment. The present government is doing little to improve the quality and equitable distribution of the social determinants of health. Indeed, by any indicator the situation is growing much worse in terms of the social inequalities that lead to health inequalities.

In summary, public health and health policy attention in the U.K. has been, during the Labour-led government, directed to addressing inequalities in health. Compared to Canada and the U.S., there has been a strong public policy concern with addressing the basic determinants of health. The present commitment to addressing these issues remains in government documents, yet the public policy situation makes these goals extremely difficult to achieve.

# NORWAY

Norway provides an example of a nation where a long-standing commitment to a well-developed welfare state was well positioned to incorporate a concern with inequalities in health (Fosse, 2009). A structural approach to public health shares many of the same concerns that shape public policy in well-developed welfare states: provision of citizen security, reduction of social inequalities, assurance of universal and response health and social services, and promotion of employment and reducing social exclusion. The most important recent development has been the national government providing funding and support for hiring of a health equity co-ordinator for every single municipality in Norway and mandating various health-equity promoting activities at the municipal level (Hagen, Øvergård, Helgesen, Fosse, & Torp, 2018).

## History of Concern with Health Inequalities

Fosse (2012) summarizes the evolution of Norway's structural approach to public health until 2010. In 1984, a Norwegian government White Paper adopted the World Health Organization's *Health for All 2000 Strategy*. There was a specific commitment to reduce social inequalities identified as the causes of health inequalities: "With the adoption of the WHO targets for all in 2000, Norway has made a commitment to reduce social differences by improving health conditions for the most vulnerable" (Fosse, 2008, p. 242). Though there was certainly emphasis upon improving health services and risks for the most vulnerable, there was also a strong emphasis on increasing focus on health in all public sectors. Since then, a series of documents (see Box 16.6) has further developed Norway's approach.

In 2003, another government White Paper, entitled *Prescriptions for a Healthier Norway*, outlined a balance placed between individual responsibility for health and societal responsibility. Vulnerable groups were identified and even though there was an emphasis on behavioural risk factors, there was recognition of the broader social context:

> Risk factors are often particularly concentrated in vulnerable parts of the population. There is a need to shed more light on the special health problems of the immigrant population. In general there is a need for improved adjustment of interventions to the needs of groups at risk for developing health problems. (Fosse, 2008, pp. 242–243)

More importantly, the government's goals were sensitive to the issues of social inequalities and the societal structures that shape them. The government's goals in the 2003 document involved the following:

- Interventions to influence lifestyles will be assessed in terms of their consequences for social inequalities in health.
- New actions aimed at vulnerable groups or geographic areas will be assessed in terms of the target of reducing social inequalities in health.
- Social inequalities in health will be introduced as an element in health impact assessment.
- Competence in this policy area will be set up.

## Box 16.6: Developments in Norway's Approach to Public Health

1984: Norway accepts the WHO's strategy for "Health for All 2000."

1987: The government White Paper is published as a follow-up to the adoption of the 1984 WHO's strategy *Health for All 2000*. It pledges: "With the adoption of the WHO targets for Health for all in 2000, Norway has made a commitment to reduce social differences by improving health conditions for the most vulnerable."

1999: The *Equitable Redistribution White Paper* identifies nine target groups for public intervention: (1) households with long-term low income, (2) disadvantaged immigrants, (3) disadvantaged families with small children, (4) people with psychiatric illness, (5) people with long-term illness, (6) the long-term unemployed and occupationally impaired, (7) disadvantaged pensioners, (8) the disabled, and (9) drug addicts and homeless people.

2003: The government White Paper on Public Health, *Prescriptions for a Healthier Norway*, outlined Norway's public health policy for the next decade. In this White Paper the balance between individual responsibility and society's responsibility for health is underlined.

2005: Directorate of Health and Social Affairs publishes the *Challenge of the Gradient*, which contains an action plan to address inequalities in health across the entire socio-economic distribution.

2007: The government White Paper *National Strategy to Reduce Social Differences in Health* has a 10-year perspective for developing policies and strategies to reduce health inequities. The overall strategy covers four areas:
- Reduce social inequalities that contribute to health differences
- Reduce social inequalities in health behaviour and use of health services
- Target efforts for social inclusion
- Develop increased knowledge and tools for cross-sectoral collaboration and planning

2012: The 2012 *Public Health Act* calls for co-ordinating health equity across local, regional, and national levels of government. Each of the 428 municipalities in Norway is provided with a mandate and tools for promoting health equity amongst its residents.

*Source:* Adapted from Fosse, E. (2008). Norway. In C. Hogstedt, H. Moberg, B. Lundgren, & B. Backhans (Eds.), *Health for all? A critical analysis of public health policies in eight European countries* (pp. 241–266). Stockholm: Swedish National Institute for Public Health.

- A plan of action will be developed to combat social inequalities in health. (Fosse, 2008, p. 51)

The focus of these public health activities was on the most vulnerable. However, the action plan that was developed to follow up began to shift focus to health differences across the entire socio-economic/educational distribution of citizens. *The Challenge of the Gradient*

(Fosse, 2008) now concerned itself with health inequalities right across the entire population. Fosse (2008) notes that the plan took a much more developed approach toward health policy:

> Working to reduce social inequalities in health means making efforts to ensure that all social groups can achieve the same life expectancy and be equally healthy. Differences in health not only affect specific occupational groups or the poorest people or those with least education. On the contrary, research indicates that we will not address the relation between socioeconomic position and health if we base our activities on strategies that focus on "the poor" as an isolated target group. (p. 243)

## The 2007 *National Strategy to Reduce Social Inequalities in Health*

At the time, this document represented a high point in Norway's—and probably elsewhere—public health analysis of health inequalities and their structural determinants. It begins with the basic premise that: "A fair distribution is good public health policy" (Norwegian Ministry of Health and Care Services, 2007).

The report comes down squarely on the side of a structural analysis of health determinants and explicitly outlines the role that governments can play in promoting health through public policy action:

> The Government believes that public health work needs to be based on society assuming greater responsibility for the population's health. Each individual is responsible for their own health, and it is important to respect the right of the individual to have authority and influence over their own life. However, the individual's sphere of action is limited by factors outside the individual's control. Even lifestyle choices such as smoking, physical activity and diet are greatly influenced by socioeconomic background factors not chosen by the individual. As long as systematic inequalities in health are due to inequalities in the way society distributes resources, then it is the community's responsibility to take steps to make the distribution fairer. (Norwegian Ministry of Health and Care Services, 2007)

Four sets of public health objectives are outlined with the key priority being *reduce social inequalities in health by levelling up*. The four priority areas for achieving are:

- Reduce social inequalities that contribute to inequalities in health
- Reduce social inequalities in health behaviour and use of the health services
- Targeted initiatives to promote social inclusion
- Develop knowledge and cross-sectoral tools (Norwegian Ministry of Health and Care Services, 2007, p. 7)

Further details concerning these initiatives can be found in the second edition of *Staying Alive*.

### The 2012 *Public Health Act*

This Act took the promoting of health equity to a new level (literally and figuratively) in Norway (CHRODIS, 2018). It calls for co-ordinating health equity both horizontally across various sectors and vertically between government at local, regional, and national levels. Each of the 428 municipalities in Norway is provided with a mandate and tools for promoting health equity among its residents.

Each municipality is provided with (a) a health profile of the jurisdiction by the Norwegian Public Health Institute, (b) Regulations and Guidelines from the Ministry of Health and Care, and (c) Guidelines from the Norwegian Directorate of Health (Hagen, Torp, Helgesen, & Fosse, 2016). They are required to hire a Public Health Coordinator, whose role it is to co-ordinate activities across the various components of municipal governance in collaboration with other local groups.

The Coordinator works with these sectors and groups to produce an overview of health, including the positive and negative factors shaping health across the overall population and sub-populations (Hagen et al., 2018). Some of the areas that have been focused upon include (a) green and recreational areas, (b) universal design, (c) housing, (d) physical activity, and (e) kindergartens (Fosse & Helgesen, 2015).

Evaluations of these activities have indicated that municipalities report these supports have strengthened their abilities to promote health, and increased collaboration with voluntary organizations and with actors external to municipal government. These collaborations have included cross-sectorial strategic working groups (Hagen et al., 2018). These activities are unique among developed nations.

But there continue to be challenges (Bekken, Dahl, & van Der Wel, 2017). Smaller municipalities report more challenges in addressing living and working conditions than larger municipalities. In addition, at the national level, a drift toward more conservative public policies under a centre-right government has made the health promotion efforts of local municipalities more difficult. These include changes to tax policies and social programs that are increasing income inequality (Bekken et al., 2017). Nevertheless, this is a profoundly important development with implications for all those seeking to promote health equity.

## SWEDEN

In Sweden, long-standing concern with guaranteeing citizen security has melded well with increasing knowledge and evidence concerning the importance of strengthening the social determinants of health. Public health activities in Sweden were among the first to focus on strengthening democratic participation, promoting security and well-being of families, and reducing health inequalities. At one time, Sweden provided the most developed example of a progressive public health vision that strives to support health through health-related public policy.

However, there was evidence of a drift away from these principles during the eight-year reign of a centre-right government from 2006 to 2014. During that time, public policies led to increases in poverty rates and income inequality levels and a decline in supports and benefits that had been the hallmark of the Swedish social democratic welfare state (Raphael, 2014). However, the election of a centre-left government in 2014 saw the establishment of a Commission on Social Determinants of Health, offering the prospects of a renewed emphasis on promoting health equity through public policy action on the social determinants of health.

## The 2001 Health Equity Statement and Policy

The 2001 Swedish Ministry of Health and Social Affairs document *Towards Public Health on Equal Terms* illustrated long-standing government understandings of the nature of health:

> The health of the population is affected by a range of what are known as determinants. These are factors that in part relate to the structure of society and in part to people's lifestyles and habits. The Government's work in the public health field extends to both these types of factors. (Swedish Ministry of Health and Social Affairs, 2001)

The 2001 document proposed an explicit role for public health policy in reducing health inequalities between various groups in society. Policy areas identified include employment, education, agriculture, culture, transport, and housing. The January 2003 report emphasized promoting health and closing the major health gaps in society (Swedish Ministry of Health and Social Affairs, 2003). The National Committee for Public Health's 2000 report to the government proposed national public health objectives: "To ensure that society: reinforces and enhances social capital; promotes favourable conditions for child development; improves conditions in working life; creates a good physical environment; encourages health promoting lifestyles and habits; and develops good public health infrastructures" (Swedish Ministry of Health and Social Affairs, 2001, p. 2).

The 2002/2003 Public Health report outlined plans for promoting these objectives. Municipalities and county councils were to draw up and evaluate targets and report on these activities. National co-ordination of these was led by the minister for Public Health and Social Services and carried out by the National Institute of Public Health. The institute drew up a plan for skills development in public health work for those already working in relevant professions. It wrote, in co-operation with the Swedish Council for Working Life and Social Research, a status report aimed at strengthening research in the field of public health. Regional centres were developed with the National Board of Health and Welfare, the Swedish Federation of County Councils, and the Swedish Association of Local Authorities to facilitate these activities.

**Box 16.7:** The 11 Target Areas of the New Swedish Public Health Policy

The Swedish government defined 11 target areas for all who work in the field of public health:
- involvement in and influence on society
- economic and social security
- secure and healthy conditions for growing up
- better health in working life
- healthy, safe environments and products
- health and medical care that more actively promotes good health
- effective prevention of the spread of infections
- secure and safe sexuality and good reproductive health
- increased physical activity
- good eating habits and safe foodstuffs
- reduced use of tobacco and alcohol, a drug- and doping-free society and a reduction in the harmful effects of excessive gambling

*Source:* Swedish National Institute for Public Health. (2003). *Sweden's new public health policy* (p. 6). Stockholm: Author. Retrieved from www.fhi.se/upload/PDF/2004/English/newpublic0401.pdf

The Swedish National Institute of Public Health objectives directed these activities and focused on the "factors in society or in our living conditions" that influence health (Box 16.7). The first six objectives "relate to what are normally considered to be structural factors, i.e., conditions in society and our surroundings that can be influenced primarily by moulding public opinion and by taking political decisions on different levels." The last five "concern lifestyles which an individual can influence him/herself, but where the social environment normally plays a very important part" (Swedish National Institute for Public Health, 2003, pp. 5–6).

## Developments from 2005 to 2012

The 2005 Public Health Policy Report provided a set of indicators for implementation of public health policy at the national, regional, and local level during phase 1 (2003–2005). As a result of extensive consultations, 42 priority proposals were presented. Twenty-nine dealt with how inequitable living conditions contributed to mental health, working life, air pollution and accidents, communicable diseases, overweight and physical inactivity, tobacco, alcohol, violence against women, and inequalities in health. Thirteen dealt with policy and included increasing capacity for public health promotion involving more active engagement, co-ordinated regional public health promotion, and support for more

**Table 16.2:** Swedish Public Health Goals Domains and Indicators

| Objective Domain | Health Determinants—Principal Indicators |
| --- | --- |
| 1. Participation and influence in society | Democratic participation, gender equality |
| 2. Economic and social security | Economic conditions, labour market status |
| 3. Secure and favourable conditions environment during childhood and adolescence | Domestic environment, preschool environment during childhood and adolescence School environment, children's and young people's skills |
| 4. Healthier working life | Work environment factors |
| 5. Healthy and safe environments and products | Air pollution, persistent organic substances, noise |
| 6. A more health-promoting health service | |
| 7. Effective protection against communicable diseases | Prevalence of infectious matter, prevalence of immunity, prevalence of drug-resistant infectious matter |
| 8. Safe sexuality and good reproductive health | Unprotected sex |
| 9. Increased physical activity | Physical activity |
| 10. Good eating habits and safe food | Good eating habits, energy balance, breastfeeding, food safety |
| 11. Reduced use of tobacco and alcohol, a society free from illicit drugs and doping, and a reduction in the harmful effects of excessive gambling | Tobacco use, harmful alcohol consumption, illicit drug use, excessive gambling (gambling addiction) |

*Source:* Backhans, M., & Moberg, H. (2008). Sweden. In C. Hogstedt, H. Moberg, B. Lundgren, & B. Backhans (Eds.), *Health for all? A Critical analysis of public health policies in eight European countries* (pp. 292–331). Stockholm: Swedish National Institute of Health.

competence in public health matters among municipalities (Swedish National Institute for Public Health, 2005). Table 16.2 provides the indicators associated with each objective.

These public health plans were passed by a social democratic government that was supported by the left and the green parties. In 2006, a four-party centre-right alliance took control of government and adopted a renewed public health policy that was approved by Parliament in 2008. Its key aspects appeared to be unchanged (see Chapter 16 in the second edition of this volume):

• The overall national public health aim remains "create social conditions that will ensure good health on equal terms for the entire population."

- Under the policy, equity in health has an overall priority (socio-economic, education, profession, age, gender, ethnicity, or sexual orientation), and many sectors and players are thus responsible.
- The overall aim shall be achieved by implementing initiatives in 31 public policy areas related to 11 domains of objectives.

Nonetheless, there is a suggestion that the change in political power in 2006 saw a shift from a clearly societal approach to health to one more focused on individual responsibility for health. In this latter approach, this shift toward strengthening the role of families and civic society was seen as potentially problematic (Pettersson, 2007). Others feel that the general thrust of the policy did not change. What did change, however, was the central government's general approach to health-related public policy.

During the period of 2006 to 2014, Swedish public policy in general was shifted toward a more conservative approach. Poverty levels increased rapidly, and many aspects of the Swedish welfare state, such as social benefits and supports, withered (Raphael, 2014). There was also increased privatization of the healthcare system. Indeed, these changes led to a backlash such that the 2014 election saw a centre-left coalition return to power.

The importance of these national changes is seen in an extensive study that examined whether the 2003 national public health policy influenced efforts amongst Swedish county councils/regions and municipalities during the period 2004–2013. This is important since in Sweden the 21 county councils and regions are responsible for regional economic growth and development, healthcare services, and strategic planning in the region.

The study found that 89% of respondents from county councils and regions and 74% of respondents from the municipalities felt that the national public health policy has assisted public health efforts. The areas that were most focused on were conditions during childhood and adolescence, where 89% of county councils and regions had done so, as had 82% of municipalities. Of less focus was economic and social conditions, where only 21% of county councils and regions and 16% of municipalities had done so. The lower figures for economic and social conditions are important as these were the areas where the central government began to take a more conservative approach. Local authorities seem to be unable to take on these issues in light of these developments.

## Developments since 2014

One of the changes wrought by this return to power of the centre-left was the establishment in 2015 of a Swedish Commission on Equity in Health (Lundberg, 2018a). The Commission called for focus on seven central areas of life to reduce the social inequalities that lead to health inequalities: early life development; knowledge, skills, and education; work, working conditions, and working environment; incomes and economic resources; housing and neighbourhood conditions; health factors; and control, influence, and participation (Lundberg, 2018b).

The Government of Sweden quickly followed up on these recommendations and presented in mid-2018 a new public health bill entitled *Good and Equitable Public Health—An Advanced Public Health Policy* (Government Offices of Sweden, 2018), in which it stated, "The overarching objective of public health policy will be reworded, with a clearer focus on equitable health throughout the population, and the goal of reducing avoidable health inequalities within a generation." It has eight action areas:

1. Conditions in early life
2. Knowledge, skills, and education/training
3. Work, working conditions, and work environment
4. Income and opportunities to earn a living
5. Accommodation and neighbourhood
6. Living habits
7. Control, influence, and participation
8. Equitable and health-promoting health and medical services

The Public Health Agency of Sweden is being tasked with co-ordinating activities across governmental departments and identifying methods and procedures for regional governments to work with the national government on these eight areas. A Council for Equitable Health has also been established to include representatives from local authorities, academia, business, and civil society to work together on promoting health equity (Government Offices of Sweden, 2018). Whether the new government and its public health bill will be able to reverse some of the increases in economic and social insecurity brought on by the previous government and reduce health inequalities remains an open question.

In summary, it is apparent that a public health approach, based on the broader determinants of health, is consistent with long-standing Swedish approaches to public policy (see Chapter 8, this volume). Sweden implemented social welfare policies during the 1920s, and the long tradition of establishing and maintaining a strong welfare state makes Swedish public health officials receptive to new developments in health promotion, population health, and the broader determinants of health. While public health policy may have been consistent across centre-left and centre-right governments, broader health-related public policy has not been. It appears that while explicit support for promoting health equity is important, developing broader public policies that reduce social inequalities is also required. This is more likely to occur when political parties of the left, rather than the right, are in power.

## CONCLUSIONS

Approaches to public health appear to be driven by dominant political ideologies within jurisdictions. The accumulating evidence concerning the impact upon health and well-being of broader determinants of health is available to policy-makers in Canada, the U.S., the U.K., Norway, and Sweden. What is striking is the degree of variation in commitment to applying these findings across these nations.

In Canada and the U.S., progressive concepts associated with health promotion and population health are inconsistent with nascent neo-liberal approaches to governance that emphasize individualist, rather than communal, approaches to resource allocation. Concern with newly emerging infections such as SARS and the avian flu virus has reinforced biomedical, epidemiological-oriented approaches upon the concrete and observable rather than the social and conceptual. Canadian and American public health, health policy, and healthcare communities rarely discuss the reasons for the contradiction between theory and knowledge with practice. There are some positive developments in these nations, especially in the U.S.

We conclude that leaving the promotion of population health to health professionals—which occurs when government policy-makers show little commitment to promoting equity in health outcomes—allows prevailing epidemiological, class, and professional biases to dominate public discourse. As an analysis showed, the majority of empirical research in Canada is focused on individual approaches to health risk (Raphael et al., 2004). If we allow the dominant perspectives of the professional health communities (e.g., medicine, nursing, nutritionists, health promoters, etc.), reinforced by the beliefs and paradigmatic views of the average health researcher and service worker, to determine the health approach, attention to broader determinants of health will always take a back seat.

Stated another way, evidence follows policy, rather than the reverse. That is, governments direct attention to evidence that is consistent with their beliefs about society and health. Despite the accumulating evidence concerning the broader determinants of health—such as the profound, health-threatening effects of poverty—such evidence will not appear on the radar screen of governments whose policy approaches are not consistent with the implications of such evidence (see Chapter 9, this volume).

In situations, however, where public policy directions are uncertain, the influence of population health perspectives that stress broader determinants of health may be crucial. In the U.K., Sweden, and Norway, we see that ideological commitments to health equity provide fertile soil in which policy can be developed from empirical research findings concerning broader determinants of health. In Canada and the U.S., the public health community can profoundly influence the public policy environment, and there are many supports for a progressive public health agenda. There is some evidence that the public health community is becoming more receptive to joining these debates in a serious way. Developments in Sweden and Norway show how fruitful such an approach can be.

## CRITICAL THINKING QUESTIONS

1.  What might be some of the reasons that Canadian public health officials resist integrating findings about the broader determinants of health into their mandates? What would need to change for them to apply these concepts in their practice?

2. What is the likelihood of U.S. cities and states being able to reduce health inequalities in light of the very regressive pubic policies that increase inequality and economic and social insecurity? Why is this the case?

3. What does it say that it was the election of a social democratic Labour government in the U.K. that led to a concern with inequalities in health? What lessons are there for Canada?

4. What lessons could North American policy-makers and elected representatives learn from Norwegian and Swedish approaches to public health?

5. How do public health approaches to the determinants of health shape public understandings of the causes of disease and illness? How could public health agencies educate the public about the sources of health and causes of disease and illness?

## FURTHER READINGS

The King's Fund. (2018). *A vision for population health: Towards a healthier future.* London: Author. Retrieved from https://www.kingsfund.org.uk/sites/default/files /2018-11/A%20vision%20for%20population%20health%20online%20version.pdf
This report sets out a vision for population health that can be used to inform and influence the debate about the future of population health in the U.K.

National Academies of Sciences, Engineering, & Medicine. (2017). *Communities in action: Pathways to health equity.* Washington, DC: National Academies Press. Retrieved from https://www.nap.edu/catalog/24624/communities-in-action-pathways-to-health-equity
This text examines how cities and states can support community action in support of health equity in the U.S.

Public Health Agency of Canada. (2018). *Key health inequalities in Canada: A national portrait.* Retrieved from https://www.canada.ca/content/dam/phac-aspc/documents/ services/publications/science-research/hir-full-report-eng_Original_version.pdf
A detailed report of the extent of health inequalities in numerous areas across Canada. It uses various measures of social inequalities, such as income, education, and employment status, to identify the sources of health inequalities across groups in Canada.

Swedish Commission on Equity in Health. (2017). *The next step towards more equity in health in Sweden—How can we close the gap in a generation?* Stockholm: Author. Retrieved from http://kommissionjamlikhalsa.se/en/
After a decade of conservative party rule that saw income inequality and poverty increase, the Swedish government is recommitting to promoting health equity and reducing health inequalities. This document contains the new health objectives and provides background information about this recommitment.

van der Wel, K. A., Dahl, E., & Bergsli, H. (2016). The Norwegian policy to reduce health inequalities: Key challenges. *Nordic Welfare Research, 1*(1), 19–29.
This article presents the main features of the Norwegian health equity strategy and discusses possible obstacles to a successful implementation and a prolonged commitment to reducing health inequalities in Norway.

## RELEVANT WEBSITES

**Public Health Agency of Canada—Understanding the Report on Key Health Inequalities in Canada.**
https://www.canada.ca/en/public-health/services/publications/science-research-data/understanding-report-key-health-inequalities-canada.html
This website provides means of accessing and understanding recent research on health inequalities in Canada.

***Healthy People 2020***
https://www.healthypeople.gov/
This interactive data tool allows users to explore data and technical information related to the *Healthy People 2020* objectives.

**The King's Fund—Health Inequalities**
https://www.kingsfund.org.uk/topics/health-inequalities?gclid=EAIaIQobCh-MIkr6Zh9fj3wIVCcRkCh159QRmEAAYASAAEgLfVvD_BwE
This website brings together recent developments and reports in the United Kingdom related to health equity and health inequalities.

**Norwegian Institute of Public Health—Social Inequalities in Health**
https://www.fhi.no/en/hn/social-inequalities-in-health/
This government website provides details and publications about the Norwegian approach to public health and public policy.

**Public Health Agency of Sweden**
https://www.folkhalsomyndigheten.se/the-public-health-agency-of-sweden/
This Swedish government website provides details and publications about the Swedish approach to public health and public policy.

## GLOSSARY

**Health impact assessment (HIA):** The estimation of the effects of a specified action on the health of a defined population. The actions concerned may range from projects (for instance, a housing development or a leisure centre) to programs (such as an urban regeneration or a public safety program) to policies (like the integrated transport strategy, the introduction of water metering, or the imposition of value-added tax on domestic fuel). HIA builds on the understanding that a community's health is determined not only by its health services but also by a range of economic, social, psychological, and environmental influences (Scott-Samuel, Birley, & Ardern, 2001).

**Health promotion:** A comprehensive social and political process of enabling people to increase control over the determinants of health and thereby improve their health. It embraces not only actions directed at strengthening the skills and capabilities of individuals, but also action directed toward changing social, environmental, and economic conditions so as to improve health. Participation is essential to sustain health promotion action (Nutbeam, 1998).

**Healthy public policy (HPP):** An explicit concern for health and equity in all areas of policy and accountability for health impact. The aim of HPP is to create a supportive environment to enable people to lead healthy lives. Such a policy makes healthy choices possible or easier for citizens and social and physical environments more health enhancing. In pursuit of HPP, government sectors concerned with agriculture, trade, education, industry, and communications need to take into account health as an essential factor when formulating policy and be accountable for the health consequences of their policy decisions. They should pay as much attention to health as to economics (ACT Health Promotion, 2004).

**Population health:** Focuses on improving the health status of the population rather than individuals. Focusing on the health of populations also requires reducing health inequalities between groups. One assumption of a population health approach is that reductions in health inequities require reductions in material and social inequities (Health Canada, 2004).

**Public health:** The organized efforts of society to protect, promote, and restore people's health. It is the combination of science, skills, and beliefs directed to the maintenance and improvement of the health of all people through collective or social actions. Public health activities change with variations in technology and social values, but the goals remain the same: to reduce the amount of disease, premature death, and disease-produced discomfort and disability in the population. Public health is thus a social institution, a discipline, and a practice (Institute for Medical Education, 2004).

## REFERENCES

Acheson, D. (1998). *Independent inquiry into inequalities in health report.* Retrieved from https://assets.publishing.service.gov.uk/government/uploads/system/uploads/attachment_data/file/265503/ih.pdf

ACT Health Promotion. (2004). *History of health promotion.* Retrieved June 3, 2004, from http://www.healthpromotion.act.gov.au/whatis/history/default.htm

Adelman, L. (2008). *Unnatural causes: Is inequality making us sick?* San Francisco: California Newsreel with Vital Pictures, Inc.

American Public Health Association. (2018). *The nation's health: Addressing health equity through state, regional partnerships.* Retrieved January 2, 2019, from http://thenationshealth. aphapublications.org/content/special-section-addressing-health-equity-through-state-regional-partnerships

American Public Health Association. (2019). *Health equity.* Retrieved January 2, 2019, from https://www.apha.org/topics-and-issues/health-equity

Banting, K., & Myles, J. (Eds.). (2013). *Inequality and the fading of redistributive politics.* Vancouver: UBC Press.

Barr, B., Higgerson, J., & Whitehead, M. (2017). Investigating the impact of the English health inequalities strategy: Time trend analysis. *British Medical Journal, 358,* j3310. doi:10.1136/bmj.j3310

BBC Northern Ireland. (2018). *Budget 2018: Mixed political reaction to NI spending plans.* Retrieved January 3, 2019, from https://www.bbc.com/news/uk-northern-ireland-46026719

Bekken, W., Dahl, E., & van Der Wel, K. (2017). Tackling health inequality at the local level: Some critical reflections on the future of Norwegian policies. *Scandinavian Journal of Public Health, 45*(18 Suppl.), 56–61. doi:10.1177/1403494817701012.

Bezruchka, S. (2012). American experiences. In D. Raphael (Ed.), *Tackling inequalities in health: Lessons from international experiences* (pp. 33–62). Toronto: Canadian Scholars' Press.

Black, D., & Smith, C. (1992). The Black Report. In P. Townsend, N. Davidson & M. Whitehead (Eds.), *Inequalities in health: The Black Report and the Health Divide.* New York: Penguin Books.

Bor, J., Cohen, G. H., & Galea, S. (2017). Population health in an era of rising income inequality: USA, 1980–2015. *The Lancet, 389*(10077), 1475–1490. doi:10.1016/S0140-6736(17)30571-8

Brennan Ramirez, L. K., Baker, E. A., & Metzler, M. (2008). *Promoting health equity: A resource to help communities address social determinants of health.* Washington, DC: Centers for Disease Control and Prevention. Retrieved January 8, 2019, from https://www.cdc.gov/nccdphp/dch/programs/healthycommunitiesprogram/tools/pdf/sdoh-workbook.pdf

Bryant, T., Raphael, D., Schrecker, T., & Labonte, R. (2011). Canada: A land of missed opportunity for addressing the social determinants of health. *Health Policy, 101*(1), 44–58. doi:10.1016/j.healthpol.2010.08.022

Butler-Jones, D. (2008). *Report on the state of public health in Canada 2008: Addressing health inequalities.* Ottawa: Public Health Agency of Canada.

Butler-Jones, D. (2010). *Report on the state of public health in Canada 2009: Growing up well— Priorities for a healthy future.* Ottawa: Public Health Agency of Canada.

Canadian Council on the Social Determinants of Health. (2018). *About CCSDH.* Retrieved October 15, 2018, from http://ccsdh.ca/

Canadian Institute for Health Information. (2018). *Health inequalities.* Retrieved January 25, 2018, from https://www.cihi.ca/en/health-inequalities

Canadian Medical Association. (2013). *What makes us sick?* Ottawa: Author.

Canadian Population Health Initiative. (2008). *Reducing gaps in health: A focus on socio-economic status in urban Canada.* Ottawa: Author.

Canadian Public Health Association. (1996). *Action statement for health promotion in Canada*. Retrieved July, 2002, from http://www.cpha/cpha.docs/ActionStatement.eng.html

*CBC News*. (2018). "Winds of change": Ryan Meili wins Sask. NDP leadership. Retrieved October 24, 2018, from https://www.cbc.ca/news/canada/saskatchewan/saskatchewan-ndp-leadership-ryan-meili-trent-wotherspoon-1.4560240

Centers for Disease Control and Prevention. (2016). Strategies for reducing health disparities— Selected CDC-sponsored interventions, United States, 2016. *Morbidity and Mortality Weekly Report, 65*(Suppl. 1).

Centers for Disease Control and Prevention. (2019a). *Promoting Physical activity: Physical activity prevents chronic disease*. Retrieved January 2, 2019, from https://www.cdc.gov/chronicdisease/index.htm

Centers for Disease Control and Prevention. (2019b). *Social determinants of health: Know what affects health*. Retrieved January 2, 2019, from https://www.cdc.gov/socialdeterminants/

CHRODIS. (2018). *Norwegian Public Health Act*. Retrieved November 8, 2018, from http://chrodis.eu/wp-content/uploads/2017/03/norwegian-public-health-act.pdf

Collins, P. A., & Hayes, M. V. (2007). Twenty years since Ottawa and Epp: Researchers' reflections on challenges, gains, and future prospects for reducing health inequities in Canada. *Health Promotion International, 22*(4), 337–345. doi:10.1093/heapro/dam031

Curry-Stevens, A. (2016). Precarious changes: A generational exploration of canadian incomes and wealth. In D. Raphael (Ed.), *Social determinants of health: Canadian perspectives* (3rd ed., pp. 60–89). Toronto: Canadian Scholars' Press.

Department of Health. (1999). *Reducing health inequalities: An action report*. London: Author.

Epp, J. (1986). *Achieving health for all: A framework for health promotion*. Ottawa: Health and Welfare Canada.

Exworthy, M., Stuart, M., Blane, D., & Marmot, M. (2003). *Tackling health inequalities since the Acheson Inquiry*. Bristol, U.K.: Policy Press.

Fosse, E. (2008). Norway. In C. Hogstedt, H. Moberg, B. Lundgren & B. Backhans (Eds.), *Health for all? A critical analysis of public health policies in eight European countries*. (pp. 241–266). Östersund: Swedish National Institute for Public Health.

Fosse, E. (2009). Norwegian public health policy: Revitalization of the social democratic welfare state? *International Journal of Health Services, 39*(2), 287–300. doi:10.2190/HS.39.2.d

Fosse, E. (2012). Norwegian experiences. In D. Raphael (Ed.), *Tackling health inequalities: Lessons from international experience* (pp. 185–208). Toronto: Canadian Scholars' Press.

Fosse, E., & Helgesen, M. K. (2015). How can local governments level the social gradient in health among families with children? The case of Norway. *International Journal of Child, Youth and Family Studies, 6*(2), 328–346.

Government Offices of Sweden. (2018). *Public health policy to be more equitable*. Retrieved November 7, 2018, from https://www.government.se/articles/2018/05/public-health-policy-to-be-more-equitable/

Hagen, S., Øvergård, K. I., Helgesen, M., Fosse, E., & Torp, S. (2018). Health promotion at local level in Norway: The use of public health coordinators and health overviews to promote fair distribution among social groups. *International Journal of Health Policy Management, 7*(9), 807–817. doi:10.15171/IJHPM.2018.22

Hagen, S., Torp, S., Helgesen, M., & Fosse, E. (2016). Promoting health by addressing living conditions in Norwegian municipalities. *Health Promotion International, 32*(6), 977–987. doi:10.1093/heapro/daw052

Hancock, T. (2011). Health promotion in Canada: 25 years of unfulfilled promise. *Health Promotion International, 26*(Suppl. 2), ii263–ii267. doi:10.1093/heapro/dar061

Health Canada. (2004). *Population Health Approach*. Retrieved Jnauary 30, 2005, from http://www.phac-aspc.gc.ca/ph-sp/phdd/approach/approach.html

Hills, J., Sefton, T., & Stewart, K. (Eds.). (2009a). *Towards a more equal society? Poverty, inequality and policy since 1997.* Bristol, U.K.: Policy Press.

Hills, J., Sefton, T., & Stewart, K. (Eds.). (2009b). *Poverty, inequality and policy since 1997.* Joseph Rowntree Foundation. Retrieved June 22, 2009, from http://www.jrf.org.uk/publications/poverty-inequality-and-policy-1997

Hills, J., & Stewart, K. (Eds.). (2005). *A more equal society? New labour, poverty, inequality and exclusion.* Bristol, U.K.: Policy Press.

Indigenous Services Canada. (2018). *Government of Canada, with First Nations, Inuit and Métis Nation leaders, announce co-developed legislation will be introduced on Indigenous child and family services in early 2019.* Retrieved December 3, 2018, from https://www.newswire.ca/news-releases/government-of-canada-with-first-nations-inuit-and-metis-nation-leaders-announce-co-developed-legislation-will-be-introduced-on-indigenous-child-and-family-services-in-early-2019-701636712.html

Institute for Medical Education. (2004). *Glossary of medical education terms.* Retrieved January 30, 2005, from http://www.iime.org/glossary.htm#P

Institute of Medicine. (2002). *The future of the public's health in the 21st century.* Washington, DC: National Academies Press.

*The Irish Times.* (2018). UK austerity policies have "plunged people into despair," says UN envoy. Retrieved January 3, 2019, from https://www.irishtimes.com/news/world/uk/uk-austerity-policies-have-plunged-people-into-despair-says-un-envoy-1.3700511

King, A. (2010). *Public health—Everybody's business.* Toronto: Ontario Ministry of Health and Long-Term Care.

King, A. (2011). *Health, not health care—Changing the conversation.* Toronto: Ontario Ministry of Health and Long-Term Care.

Lalonde, M. (1974). *A New perspective on the health of Canadians: A working document.* Ottawa: Health and Welfare Canada.

Lambert, R., St-Pierre, J., Lemieux, L., Chapados, M., Lapointe, G., Bergeron, P., … Trudel, G. (2014). *Policy avenues: Interventions to reduce social inequalities in health.* Quebec: Institut National de Santé Publique du Québec Retrieved August 24, 2018, from https://www.inspq.qc.ca/pdf/publications/1830_Policy_Reduce_Social_Inequalities_Synthesis.pdf

Langille, D. (2016). Follow the money: How business and politics define our health. In D. Raphael (Ed.), *Social determinants of health: Canadian perspectives* (3rd ed., pp. 470–490). Toronto: Canadian Scholars' Press.

Lavis, J. (2002). Ideas at the margin or marginalized ideas? Nonmedical determinants of health in Canada. *Health Affairs, 21*(2), 107–112. doi:10.1377/hlthaff.21.2.107

Legowski, B., & McKay, L. (2000, October). *Health beyond health care: Twenty-five years of federal health policy development.* Ottawa, Canada: Canadian Policy Research Networks (CPRN).

Lundberg, O. (2018a). The next step towards more equity in health in Sweden: How can we close the gap in a generation? *Scandinavian Journal of Public Health, 46*(22 Suppl.), 19–27. doi:10.1177/1403494818765702

Lundberg, O. (2018b). *The next step towards more equity in health in Sweden—How can we close the gap in a generation?* Stockholm: Swedish Commission on Equity in Health. Retrieved January 3, 2019, from http://kommissionjamlikhalsa.se/en/

Manzano, A., & Raphael, D. (2010). CPHA and the social determinants of health: An analysis of policy documents and recommendations for future action. *Canadian Journal of Public Health, 101*(5), 399–404. doi:10.1007/BF03404861

McNab, S. (2018). One million Scots now living in poverty as austerity bites. *The Scotsman.*

Meili, R. (2017). *A healthy society: How a focus on health can revive Canadian democracy*: Vancouver: UBC Press.

Mikkonen, J., & Raphael, D. (2010). *Social determinants of health: The Canadian facts.* Retrieved November 1, 2010, from http:/thecanadianfacts.org

Muecke, C. (2016). *Health Inequities in New Brunswick.* Fredericton: New Brunswick Department of Health.

Muennig, P. A., Reynolds, M., Fink, D. S., Zafari, Z., & Geronimus, A. T. (2018). America's declining well-being, health, and life expectancy: Not just a white problem. *American Journal of Public Health, 108*(12), 1626–1631. doi:10.2105/AJPH.2018.304585

National Academies of Sciences, Engineering, & Medicine. (2017). *Communities in action: Pathways to health equity.* Washington, DC: National Academies Press.

National Association of County and City Health Officials. (2014). Building networks project: Aligning public health and community organizing. *Health Equity, 13*(1). Retrieved January 2, 2019, from http://cookcountypublichealth.org/files/weplan-2020/january-2016/naccho-exchange-healthy-equity-articles.pdf

National Association of County and City Health Officials. (2018). *Advancing public narrative for health equity & social justice.* Retrieved January 2, 2019, from http://eweb.naccho.org/eweb/DynamicPage.aspx?WebCode=proddetailadd&ivd_qty=1&ivd_prc_prd_key=68df828b-ce9e-4834-8e3f-a60d478cb559&Action=Add&site=naccho&ObjectKeyFrom=1A83491A-9853-4C87-86A4-F7D95601C2E2&DoNotSave=yes&ParentObject=CentralizedOrderEntry&ParentDataObject=Invoice%20Detail

National Association of County and City Health Officials. (2019a). Health equity and social justice. Retrieved January 2, 2019, from https://www.naccho.org/programs/public-health-infrastructure/health-equity

National Association of County and City Health Officials. (2019b). Health equity and social justice toolkit. Retrieved January 2, 2019, from http://toolbox.naccho.org/pages/index.html?id=&userToken=051f13e2-4404-468c-8e21-1779ac104569&Site=NACCHO

National Association of County and City Health Officials. (2019c). The roots of health inequity. Retrieved January 2, 2019, from http://www.rootsofhealthinequity.org/

National Center for Health Statistics. (2016). *Health, United States 2015: With special feature on racial and ethnic health disparities*. Hyattsville, MD: CDC. Retrieved January 2, 2019, from https://www.cdc.gov/nchs/data/hus/hus15.pdf

National Collaborating Centre for Determinants of Health. (2012). *Bridging the gap between research and practice: Improving health equity in saskatoon: From data to action*. Antigonish, NS: Author. Retrieved October 24, 2018, from http://nccdh.ca/images/uploads/Saskatoon_EN.pdf

National Collaborating Centre for Determinants of Health. (2015). *Social determinants of health*. Antigonish, NS: Author. Retrieved April 1, 2012, from http://nccdh.ca/resources/type/category/social-determinants-of-health

National Coordinating Centre for Healthy Public Policy. (2014). What we do. Retrieved May 22, 2014, from http://www.ncchpp.ca/62/What_We_Do.ccnpps

National Health Service England. (2018). *NHS England—Board paper: "Scene setter" on current trends in health inequalities*. Retrieved January 2, 2019, from https://www.england.nhs.uk/wp-content/uploads/2018/03/09-pb-29-03-2018-scene-setter-on-current-trends-health-inequalities.pdf

NHS Health Scotland. (2018a). Health inequalities. Retrieved January2, 2019, from http://www.healthscotland.scot/health-inequalities

NHS Health Scotland. (2018b). *Health inequalities policy review for the Scottish Ministerial Task Force on health inequalities*. Retrieved January 2, 2019, from http://www.healthscotland.scot/media/1053/1-healthinequalitiespolicyreview.pdf

Northern Ireland Department of Health. (2018). Health inequalities—Annual report 2018. Retrieved January 3, 2019, from https://www.health-ni.gov.uk/news/health-inequalities-annual-report-2018

Norwegian Ministry of Health and Care Services. (2007). *National strategy to reduce social inequalities in health*. Oslo: Norwegian Ministry of Health and Care Services.

Nutbeam, D. (1998). *Health Promotion Glossary*. Geneva: World Health Organization.

Office of Disease Prevention and Health Promotion. (2014). *Healthy people 2020*. Washington, DC: Author.

Pettersson, B. (2007, December 1). Transforming Ottawa Charter health promotion concepts into Swedish public health policy. *Global Health Promotion, 14*(4), 244–249. doi:10.1177/1025 3823070140041201

Public Health Agency of Canada. (2007). Background: Canada's response to WHO Commission on Social Determinants of Health. Retrieved March 1, 2008, from http://www.phac-aspc.gc.ca/sdh-dss/bg-eng.php

Public Health Agency of Canada. (2011a). *Health goals for Canada*. Retrieved October 15, 2018, from https://www.med.uottawa.ca/sim/data/assets/documents/Health%20Goals%20for%20Canada%202005.pdf

Public Health Agency of Canada. (2011b). *Reducing health inequalities: A challenge for our times*. Retrieved October 15, 2018, from http://publications.gc.ca/collections/collection_2012/aspc-phac/HP35-22-2011-eng.pdf

Public Health Agency of Canada. (2015). *Rio political declaration on social determinants of health: A snapshot of Canadian actions 2015*. Retrieved October 15, 2018, from http://healthycanadians. gc.ca/publications/science-research-sciences-recherches/rio/alt/rio2015-eng.pdf

Public Health England. (2017). *Reducing health inequalities: System, scale and sustainability*. Retrieved January 2, 2019, from https://assets.publishing.service.gov.uk/government/ uploads/system/uploads/attachment_data/file/731682/Reducing_health_inequalities_ system_scale_and_sustainability.pdf

Public Health England. (2018). *Health profile for England: 2018*. Retrieved January 2, 2019, from https://www.gov.uk/government/publications/health-profile-for-england-2018

Public Health Wales. (2019). North Wales public health priorities: Health inequalities. Retrieved January 3, 2019, from http://www.wales.nhs.uk/sitesplus/888/page/87546

Raphael, D. (2000). Health inequalities in Canada: Current discourses and implications for public health action. *Critical Public Health, 10*(2), 193–216.

Raphael, D. (2011). Anti-poverty strategies and programs. In D. Raphael (Ed.), *Poverty in Canada: Implications for health and quality of life* (2nd ed., pp. 406–437). Toronto: Canadian Scholars' Press.

Raphael, D. (2012). Canadian experiences. In D. Raphael (Ed.), *Tackling health inequalities: Lessons from international experiences* (pp. 124–153). Toronto: Canadian Scholars' Press.

Raphael, D. (2014). Challenges to promoting health in the modern welfare state: The case of the Nordic nations. *Scandinavian journal of public health, 42*(1), 7-17.

Raphael, D. (2015a). Beyond policy analysis: The raw politics behind opposition to healthy public policy. *Health Promotion International, 30*(2), 380–396. doi:10.1093/heapro/dau044

Raphael, D. (2015b). The political economy of health: A research agenda for addressing health inequalities in Canada. *Canadian Public Policy, 41*(Suppl. 2), S17–S25.

Raphael, D. (Ed.). (2016). *Social determinants of health: Canadian perspectives* (3rd ed.). Toronto: Canadian Scholars' Press.

Raphael, D., & Brassolotto, J. (2015). Understanding action on the social determinants of health: A critical realist analysis of in-depth interviews with staff of nine Ontario public health units. *BMC Research Notes, 8*(1), 105. doi:10.1186/s13104-015-1064-5

Raphael, D., Curry-Stevens, A., & Bryant, T. (2008). Barriers to addressing the social determinants of health: Insights from the Canadian experience. *Health Policy, 88*(2–3), 222-235. doi:10.1016/j.healthpol.2008.03.015

Raphael, D., Macdonald, J., Labonte, R., Colman, R., Hayward, K., & Torgerson, R. (2004). Researching income and income distribution as a determinant of health in Canada: Gaps between theoretical knowledge, research practice, and policy implementation. *Health Policy, 72*(2), 217–232. doi:10.1016/j.healthpol.2004.08.001

Raphael, D., & Sayani, A. (2017). Assuming policy responsibility for health equity: Local public health action in Ontario, Canada. *Health Promotion International, 34*(2), 215–226 doi:10.1093/heapro/dax073

Restrepo, H. E. (1996). Introduction. In *Health promotion: An anthology* (pp. ix–xi). Washington, DC: Pan American Health Organization.

Scott-Samuel, A., Birley, M., & Ardern, K. (2001). *The Merseyside guidelines for health impact assessment* (2nd ed.). Liverpool, U.K.: International Health Impact Assessment Consortium.

Scott-Samuel, A., & Smith, K. E. (2015). Fantasy paradigms of health inequalities: Utopian thinking? *Social Theory & Health, 13*(3–4), 418–436. doi:10.1057/sth.2015.12

Scottish Government. (2018). Health inequalities. Retrieved January 2, 2019, from https://www2. gov.scot/Topics/Health/Healthy-Living/Health-Inequalities

Smith, K., & Bambra, C. (2012). British and Northern Irish Experiences. In D. Raphael (Ed.), *Tackling health inequalities: Lessons from international experiences* (pp. 93–121). Toronto: Canadian Scholars' Press.

Sudbury and District Health Unit. (2012). *10 Promising Practices Fact Sheets*. Retrieved December 1, 2012, from http://www.sdhu.com/content/healthy_living/doc. asp?folder=22203&parent=3225&doc=13088&lang=0

Swedish Ministry of Health and Social Affairs. (2001). *Towards public health on equal terms*. Stockholm: Swedish Ministry of Health and Social Affairs.

Swedish Ministry of Health and Social Affairs. (2003). *Public health objectives*. Stockholm: Swedish Ministry of Health and Social Affairs.

Swedish National Institute for Public Health. (2003). *Sweden's new public-health policy*. Stockholm: Author.

Swedish National Institute for Public Health. (2005). *The 2005 public health policy report: A summary*. Stockholm: Author.

Tjepkema, M., Wilkins, R., & Long, A. (2013). Cause-specific mortality by income adequacy in Canada: A 16-year follow-up study. *Health Reports, 24*(7), 14–22.

Townsend, P., Davidson, N., & Whitehead, M. (Eds.). (1992). *Inequalities in health: The Black Report and the Health Divide* (3rd ed.). New York: Penguin Books.

Upstream. (2013). About Upstream. Retrieved from https://www.thinkupstream.net/ about_upstream

Vancouver Coastal Health. (2011). *Population health: What makes our communities healthy?* Retrieved June 25, 2011, from http://www.vch.ca/your_health/population_health/

Welsh Government. (2018). *"UK government's Autumn Budget provides no evidence austerity is over"—Finance Secretary Mark Drakeford*. Retrieved January 3, 2019, from https://gov.wales/ uk-governments-autumn-budget-provides-no-evidence-austerity-over-finance-secretary- mark-drakeford

Whitehead, M. (2014). *Due north: Report of the inquiry on health equity for the North*. Prepared by the Inquiry Panel on Health Equity for the North of England.

Williams, D. (2018). *Improving the odds: Championing health equity in Ontario—2016 Annual Report of the Chief Medical Officer of Health of Ontario*. Toronto: Ontario Ministry of Health and Long-Term Care.

World Health Organization. (1986). *Ottawa Charter for Health Promotion*. Retrieved June 14, 2011, from http://www.who.int/hpr/NPH/docs/ottawa_charter_hp.pdf

World Health Organization. (2008). *Commission on the Social Determinants of Health*. Retrieved March 15, 2008, from http://www.who.int/social_determinants/en/

# CHAPTER 17

## Toward the Future: Current Themes in Health Research and Practice in Canada

*Toba Bryant, Dennis Raphael, and Marcia Rioux*

## INTRODUCTION

Health studies is a complex field concerned with a wide range of phenomena. It also has profoundly important consequences—often involving life and death and quality of life—for individuals, families, communities, and entire nations, as exemplified by the title of this volume, *Staying Alive*. These phenomena include the experience and understanding of illness and disability; differential access to both health and health care; the political, economic, and social forces that shape health and health care; and the intersection of social class, gender, and race with all of these issues. Despite the variety of conceptual perspectives and emerging findings available for considering these issues, most of the research and professional healthcare preoccupations remain strangely narrow, focused on the biology of disease, individual risk factors for these afflictions, and identifying and evaluating the efficacy of medical treatments. Not surprisingly, then, public understanding of key health issues—such as the causes of diseases and the organization of the healthcare system—is also narrowly focused on access to healthcare professionals, the length of wait times for treatment by specialists, and the adoption of lifestyle approaches to prevent disease. There is evidence, however, that the public is becoming increasingly aware of the broader determinants of health, the different access to health, and the importance of having governments address these issues through health-promoting public policy.

To further these developments, this volume has provided the latest conceptual developments and empirical findings concerning the status of health, illness, and health care in Canada. The contributors to Part I provided four important conceptual perspectives—epidemiological, sociological, political economy, and human rights—that assist in framing health studies questions and providing means of answering these questions. Contributors to Part II provided the latest evidence concerning the role of various social determinants of health in promoting health and explaining health inequalities. Part III focused on the Canadian healthcare system. Its history was traced and recent developments in its evolution were outlined. In Part IV, critical issues related to gender, disability, pharmaceuticals, and approaches to promoting public health were explored.

**Box 17.1:** Themes Related to Health, Illness, and Health Care in Canada

- Defining the field of health studies
- Conflict versus consensus models
- Prevention versus cure
- The public versus private debate
- Constructing illness and disability
- The role of public policy
- The future of the welfare state

In this final chapter, we identify some key themes that run through these contributions. These seven themes are presented in Box 17.1. It is our belief that these issues have historically been neglected by the dominant health sciences perspectives that are customarily applied to the promotion of health, treatment of illness, and analysis and reform of the Canadian healthcare and public health systems. Many of these concepts have their origins in the social sciences and the related areas of public policy studies and comparative politics.

## DEFINING THE FIELD OF HEALTH STUDIES

The field of health studies is moving beyond traditional concepts of risk epidemiology and healthcare treatment evaluation. The complexity of health and healthcare issues, strides in healthcare technology, growing understanding and appreciation of the influence of the societal determinants of health, and the increasing gaps in the social and health status of groups in Canada are spawning innovative approaches to research and practice. The value of these new lines of inquiry is apparent in the contributions in this volume.

Health studies are now recognizing health, illness, and health care in broader terms than has previously been the case. Health itself is more than the absence of illness and disease, but also the capacity to realize aspirations and access opportunities for human fulfillment and the highest level of health. Studies of health are increasingly concerned with how societal structures influence the opportunities for good health for the population as a whole and for specific groups. The contributors to this volume drew upon developments in the disabilities area, gender and women's studies, history of medicine, legal studies, policy studies, political economy, political science, social epidemiology, and sociology to inform their analyses. Virtually all emphasize the importance of the social determinants of health for understanding health issues. Public policy is also seen as having a key role in influencing health status and the organization of health care. Understanding the policy development and change process is important to improving the health of Canadians and improving the healthcare system through research, advocacy, and policy development.

# CONFLICT VERSUS CONSENSUS MODELS

The contributors to this book illustrate the role played by competing political, economic, and social forces in determining health and organizing and delivering health services. These presentations speak to the value of conflict and consensus models for understanding the nature and incidence of health and illness, and the organization and delivery of health care. Consensus models such as structural functionalism focus on the interrelationships between social structures and individuals and how social order is maintained. These approaches are driven by an assumption of consensus among different groups in society about the desired goals and outcomes. The stability of social, economic, and political systems is assumed, and conflict among various participants and actors in these systems is minimized. There is an assumption of common shared goals.

Conflict models, however, recognize the tensions inherent in societies and the role played by power and influence in shaping health and health care. These tensions lead to fissures in society generally along the lines of of social class, gender, disability, and race, and to considering how these fissures shape the health of different groups in society. Conflict models consider how such tensions influence societal organization—such as the balance between the marketplace and publicly controlled structures—which determines the experience of health and health care. Political and economic forces are key contributors to these tensions.

Virtually all contributors to this volume drew upon concepts associated with conflict theory, such as the way in which political ideology and power relations within society are the sources of social class, gender, and racial differences in health outcomes. Political ideology and power relations make explicit how competing political and economic visions shape public policy, thereby influencing the quality and distribution of health. The history and evolution of the healthcare system can be interpreted through these concepts.

Increasing economic globalization and its effects upon public policy lead us to expect that conflict models will continue to be a rich source of insights for understanding the determinants of health and the organization and evolution of healthcare services. As pointed out by Bourgeault in Chapter 2, "The key approach to take is one that is critical of common and often unquestioned assumptions of how society is, and ought to be, and in doing so, focuses on the centrality of power."

# PREVENTION VERSUS CARE

There is often conflict between focusing attention on prevention (e.g., the social determinants of health, healthy public policy, and the organization of society, etc.) versus care (e.g., optimizing the quality and accessibility of healthcare services, etc.). In Canada, government focus and policy-making—mirrored by media coverage and public understandings of health—are firmly focused on the healthcare system. Not surprisingly, public operating funds and research funding are allocated overwhelmingly toward care rather than prevention. Much of this has to do with the immediacy and concrete nature of illness and disease

for individuals as opposed to the more abstract concepts associated with the social determinants of health and the development of public policy in support of these determinants.
It also reflects the continuing dominance of the medical profession in public discussions of
health and the healthcare system. Media coverage and public understandings reflect these
dominant approaches. Monitoring of health services is often reduced to focusing on the
number of services provided rather than the quality of the services and the engagement of
those receiving the services. The assumption that there is consensus about how to prioritize health services precludes the addressing of tensions about what individuals are looking
for in recognizing social determinants of health and of the meaning of health generally.
For example, immigrants and refugees are much more impacted by crowded housing conditions than the middle classes, so their determination of the priorities in health services
would be those diseases that are the result of poor nutrition and overcrowding and poverty.

In Canada, the ability to raise issues of prevention is complicated by the dominant
political economy, which is liberal (or market-oriented), and the growing influence of
neo-liberalism (even more market-oriented political ideology). Market approaches downplay collectivity and make it difficult to implement public policy in support of health and
quality of life. The individualism associated with neo-liberalism as a political and economic ideology reinforces the biomedical and lifestyle approaches to health and disability
advanced by governments, health officials, and service providers.

Even the increased concern with seemingly obvious health issues such as obesity can
be misplaced. As Feldberg, Vipond, and Bryant point out in Chapter 10:

> The new diseases, often labelled lifestyle diseases, are actually diseases of
> circumstance. They reflect living conditions, poverty, and access to housing
> and income. For historical reasons, Canada has not integrated these social and
> economic domains into the modern organization or financing of health.

An emphasis upon prevention and increasing the health status of citizens requires attention to public policies that ensure income security, employment security, housing security,
and food security, among others. As governments neglect these issues, it is not surprising
that policy-makers—reinforced by the medical profession, the media, and public understandings of health and illness—direct their attention to lifestyle approaches to prevention
and relatively narrow healthcare issues such as waiting lists. Despite the evidence provided
by most contributors to this volume of the value of looking upstream at the organization of
society and the distribution of resources as important determinants of health and healthcare organization, raising these issues remains a difficult task. Health-promoting policies
discussed by several contributors to this volume will be implemented only when the public
comes to a better understanding of these issues. As Bezruchka points out in Chapter 1:

> If Canadians want a healthier population, the government can take policy steps
> that further social and economic justice. The first step is to create awareness of
> what conditions produce health in populations, and then promote policies to
> ameliorate those conditions.

# THE PUBLIC VERSUS PRIVATE DEBATE

The public versus private debate is concerned with issues of ownership and control of both societal resources in general and the healthcare system in particular. While this issue is often framed in terms of economic efficiency, it also has strong implications for the health of the population in general and for vulnerable populations like people with chronic diseases such as HIV/AIDS, people with disabilities, Canadians of Indigenous ancestry, new Canadians, women, and people with low income.

The debate has implications for both the social determinants of health and the quality of health services. More specifically, the move to privatize areas of public activity directly affects the availability of societal resources such as income and housing, the quality and accessibility of health care, and the availability of pharmaceuticals to consumers. Concerning the social determinants of health, nations that have well-developed public services that decommodify resources—that is, that break the link between receiving a benefit and being able to pay for it—have stronger public sectors and better health indicators. As Raphael and Bryant argue in Chapter 3:

> It has long been recognized, however, that without state intervention in the operation of the market economy, the distribution of economic resources becomes skewed in favour of the wealthy and powerful ... The welfare state arose because the economic system itself is not capable of dealing with provision of basic societal resources such as education, health care, housing, and other programs and services that provide citizens with resources necessary for well-being.

Bourgeault, in Chapter 12, discusses how governments try to control costs by privatizing healthcare services. Privatization and its concomitant force, rationalization, emphasize cost containment. Rationalization leads to lowering costs so much that "the least expensive worker performs tasks at the lowest unit cost." While such reforms may seem efficient and necessary to hospital CEOs, these changes ultimately affect the quality of care that is provided and usually result in poorer-quality care and health outcomes.

As another example of how the privatization of a previously public domain can affect health, Lexchin, in Chapter 15, discusses how the regulation of the drug industry in Canada has been weakened by the devolution of these duties to the private sector. Lexchin argues that a political decision to relinquish authority for laboratory testing to the pharmaceutical industry affects the quality and safety of medications available to Canadian consumers. Indeed, Bourgeault (in Chapter 12) argued that increased privatization threatens Canadian institutions:

> Although some argue that the only conceivable solution to rising costs in health care and other public services is thought to be further market penetration and the adoption of more for-profit practices, Armstrong et al. (2003) argue that the mixing of public and private, for-profit partnerships squeezes out public

values and practices. What are left are corporate, for-profit values and methods combined with limited choice.

## CONSTRUCTING ILLNESS AND DISABILITY

Disease and disabilities are socially constructed categories that reflect societal values, dominant health paradigms, and societal willingness to adjust to meet the needs of all its members. Rioux and Daly (in Chapter 14) outline different approaches to understanding disability and illness. Biomedical and functional theoretical approaches conflate disability with illness in perceiving disability as individual pathology. In contrast, social pathology approaches, such as human rights and political economy, situate disability in broader social systems.

Disability and illness can be viewed primarily in terms of disease and variation from an accepted norm. Such a limited view places the power to influence people so defined and related policy firmly in the hands of medical professionals. The concept of Disability Adjusted Life Years (DALYs) illustrates many of these issues. Use of DALYs implies a "reduced value" of a life lived with a disability. It treats these conditions as physical disablements instead of situating disability in broader social, political, environmental, and economic factors. It also makes a second false assumption that the only way to ameliorate disability is to intervene medically. In contrast, if the limitations of those with disabilities and illness are seen as reflecting society's failures to make accommodations to meet the needs of these individuals, then the area is open to much broader concepts of societal responsibilities, rules of citizenship, and conforming to ethical principles and values. In Chapter 14, Rioux and Daly comment that:

> ... social, political, and rights approaches focus on social determinants and interventions. These models investigate the ways in which social and political structures create disability through societies' inability to accommodate difference. In this framework, disability is equated with social disadvantage and is not simply focused on individual impairment.

Leaving the field of disabilities to the medical profession has led to perceptions of illness and disability in solely functional terms. The larger point is that we measure health by morbidity and mortality rather than by the conditions that affect them. By doing so, it becomes inevitable that the money (and policy decisions) flow toward investment in medical care because that is what tells us how well we are doing.

This approach has been associated with denial of basic human rights to people with disabilities or other chronic conditions. As noted by Bryant in Chapter 9, Canadian spending on disabilities-related supports and services is among the lowest of any industrialized nation. Disability can be redefined as societies' capacity to adapt to the diverse needs of individual citizens to enable them to participate in civil society. The message that emerges is that of a need to focus on the social origins of disability. There needs to be investigations of the ways in which social structures create disability through societies' inability to accommodate difference.

These insights from the disabilities field have profound implications for the treatment of those with chronic illness who then experience some form of disability. The changed state of people that results from chronic illness requires society's attention to continuing their involvement in the activities normally expected of society's members. This opens up discussion of issues of programs, supports, and policies that will make such involvement possible.

## THE ROLE OF PUBLIC POLICY

A central aim of this volume is to understand the centrality of public policy in structuring population health and health outcomes. Public policy refers to decisions made by governments and other large organizations on how to address identified problems. Virtually every contributor considered how public policy influences the health and well-being of the population in general and certain groups in particular by shaping the quality of the social determinants of health and the organization and delivery of healthcare services. The picture that emerges from the analysis of different forms of welfare states and the public policies that each formulate is summarized by Bryant in Chapter 9:

> Differences exist among countries using Esping-Andersen's typology of liberal, social democratic, conservative, and Latin welfare states. ... Liberal welfare states (which include Canada) lag behind social democratic and conservative welfare states in instituting public policies that deliver higher-quality and equitable distribution of the social determinants of health.... As a result, there is minimal public policy activity to promote health.

Political variables such as union density, left party governance, political ideology, and the electoral system (e.g., proportional representation versus "first-past-the-post" elections) affect the quality of health and social policies that are accepted and implemented. Social democratic nations have the most progressive social and health policies, and these reflect a long-standing commitment to social equality and population health and well-being. These welfare states were established prior to the Second World War in contrast to other Western nations, such as Canada, the U.S., and the U.K., which all established their welfare states in the post-war era.

Public policy clearly determines the organization and delivery of healthcare services. All of the debates concerning privatization, competition, and financing of the healthcare system are essentially debates about public policy, yet health science professionals receive little education and training in public policy analysis. Since social reform and healthcare system evolution involves having governments and agencies develop and adopt policies, it is essential that the policy process—especially the policy change process—be understood by those researching and advocating for health.

And since public policy in general, and healthcare policy in particular, is subject to the effects of international forces related to economic globalization and the adoption of international trade agreements, the need for an understanding of the policy process is even more important. Many aspects of our society and its healthcare systems are increasingly influenced by these developments. Bryant (Chapter 9) concludes that: "Directing the health sector's gaze to broader political and economic factors may be the most effective means of improving population health and reducing inequalities in health."

## THE FUTURE OF THE WELFARE STATE

This volume has outlined several areas for reforming the organization of society, the redistribution of resources in general, and the healthcare system in particular to improve the health outcomes and well-being of Canadians. These are fundamental issues concerning the nature of the welfare state in Canada. As Raphael and Bryant argue in Chapter 3, the nature of our economic system varies from nation to nation and affects the welfare state regime that is adopted. And numerous contributors show how the political economy of a nation determines its willingness to address public policy issues supportive of population health.

The social democratic welfare regimes, as described by Raphael and Bryant in Chapter 3 and Bryant in Chapter 9, are more likely to create the conditions necessary for health than is the case for other welfare regimes. These include equitable distribution of wealth and progressive tax policies that create a large middle class; strong programs that support children, families, and women; and economies that support full employment. They do so through more generous programs and services to their citizens in the form of universal entitlements. In contrast, liberal welfare states such as Canada have means-tested assistance, modest universal transfers, and modest social-insurance plans. While Canadian public policy has been moving toward a neo-liberal model, reversals are possible. In Sweden, many of the advances in health equity put in place during the early 2000s were reversed by centre-right governments, but the recent election of a centre-left government is responding to these challenges. Ideologies are flexible and national social policies can be changed.

There are a variety of forces that shape the welfare state. These include the power of progressive political parties, the strength of labour unions, the presence of proportional representational electoral processes, and attitudes toward those who are poor and marginalized. The influence of well-organized lobby groups that are striving for increased privatization of public institutions must also be considered. History suggests that public policy in support of health frequently results from social movements that arise from expressed needs of the population. Health researchers and advocates have much to offer by identifying health issues for public discussion and appropriate policy responses.

## CONCLUSIONS

The current public policy environment in Canada is one of opportunity to effect movement toward public policies supportive of health for all people. There is also clear recognition that priorities need to be set by the general population rather than by elite groups. These elite groups involve not only those attempting to privatize the publicly organized healthcare system, but also those with specific agendas. For example, breast cancer gets priority over other forms of cancer, such as lung cancer, and special priority is given to hip and knee replacements, which benefits the middle class, while less attention is given to accessing prescription drugs by the less fortunate.

Concern about income equality and continuing high poverty rates provides a window for positive change that will be supportive of the health of the population to occur. There is renewed discussion of the need for universal child care and pharmacare programs, and the lack of affordable housing is now seen as a crisis. The importance of providing quality and equitable distribution of the social determinants of health has permeated all levels of the healthcare and public health communities, though implementation of public policies that would achieve this goal continues to be lacking.

Concerning the healthcare system, the recent Supreme Court of Canada's ruling that banning health insurance for private healthcare providers is unconstitutional has energized the debate about the organization and delivery of healthcare services. Strong economic and political forces have pushed for increased privatization of healthcare services. These forces, however, are being opposed by equally strong forces that evoke the spirit of medicare's founder, Tommy Douglas, in defence of the system. Such active policy environments require that the questions raised in this volume—and their potential solutions—receive the attention they deserve from health researchers, policy-makers, service providers, and the public.

> Medicine, as a social science, as the science of human beings, has the obligation to raise such questions and to attempt their theoretical solutions; the politician, the practical anthropologist, must find the means for their actual solution. (Virchow, 1848/1985, p. 217)

## REFERENCE

Virchow, R. (1985). Report on the typhus epidemic in Upper Silesia. In L.J. Rather (Ed.), *Collected essays by Rudolph Virchow on public health and epidemiology* (vol. 1, pp. 205–319). Canton, MA: Science History Publications. Originally published 1848.

# About the Contributors

**Pat Armstrong**, Ph.D., is Professor of Sociology at York University, Toronto. She is a Distinguished Research Professor in Sociology and a Fellow of the Royal Society of Canada. Focusing on equity in the fields of social policy, of women, work, and the health and social services, she has published widely, co-authoring more than a dozen books and co-editing another dozen, as well as many journal and technical reports. Dr. Armstrong was Chair of Women and Health Care Reform, a group funded for over a decade by Health Canada. She is principal investigator of a seven-year SSHRC-funded project on "Reimagining Long-term Residential Care: An International Study of Promising Practices." Currently, Dr. Armstrong serves as co-chair of the Canadian Association of University Teachers' Equity Committee.

**Stephen Bezruchka**, M.D. M.P.H., was raised in Toronto and received his B.Sc. in mathematics and physics from the University of Toronto and an M.A. in mathematics from Harvard University before completing medical school at Stanford University and an M.P.H. in public health from Johns Hopkins University. He worked as an emergency physician and now teaches in the School of Public Health at the University of Washington. He directs the Population Health Forum and is on the board of Washington Physicians for Social Responsibility, where he co-chairs the Economic Inequity Health Task Force.

**Ivy Lynn Bourgeault**, Ph.D., is Professor in the Telfer School of Management at the University of Ottawa. She holds the Canadian Institutes of Health Research Chair in Gender, Work and Health Human Resources. She is the lead co-ordinator of the Pan Canadian Health Workforce Network. Dr. Bourgeault was inducted into the Canadian Academy of Health Sciences in 2016 and received the 2017 University of Ottawa Award for Excellence in Research.

**Toba Bryant**, Ph.D., is Associate Professor, Faculty of Health Sciences, at the University of Ontario Institute of Technology. She is author of *Health Policy in Canada* and has published numerous book chapters and articles on policy change, housing, employment, health within a population health perspective, and community quality of life. She is editor of *Women's Health and Urban Life*, a peer-reviewed journal located at the Faculty of Health Sciences, University of Ontario Institute of Technology.

**Tamara Daly**, Ph.D., is a feminist political economist and health services researcher, Professor at York University, the Director of the York University Centre for Aging Research and Education, and the Director of the SSHRC Partnership for Age-Friendly Communities within Communities. She recently completed a CIHR Research Chair in

Gender, Work and Health. Her scholarship highlights gender and health access; advances working, living, and visiting conditions in long-term care; and promotes promising practices, principles, and policies to improve access and health equity for older adults and for those who provide their care. She has received several teaching and research awards for her work.

**Georgina Feldberg**, Ph.D., was Associate Professor of Social Science at York University and served as director of the Centre for Health Studies and co-ordinator of the Health and Society Programme. She wrote and taught on the historical foundations of health care and health policy. The Royal Society of Canada awarded her book *Disease and Class* the Hannah Medal. Dr. Feldberg passed away in 2010. The Gina Feldberg Prize at York University honours the memory of her distinguished teaching record by recognizing academic excellence in a fourth-year Health & Society Honours major.

**Joel Lexchin**, M.D., graduated from the Faculty of Medicine at the University of Toronto. He taught health policy at York University from 2001 to 2016. He currently works as an emergency physician at the University Health Network in Toronto. His research focuses on pharmaceutical policy, and he is an author or co-author on 200 peer-reviewed publications on this topic. His book *Private Profits versus Public Policy: The Pharmaceutical Industry and the Canadian State* was published by University of Toronto Press in September 2016, and *Doctors in Denial: Why Big Pharma and the Canadian Medical Profession Are Too Close for Comfort* was published by Lorimer in 2017.

**Stefanie Machado**, B.Sc., is a Master's of Public Health (Global Health) candidate in the Faculty of Health Sciences at Simon Fraser University. She received her B.Sc. Health Promotion from Dalhousie University, where she conducted her honours thesis on international university students' access to sexual health services. Currently, Stefanie works as a Research Assistant at the Centre for Gender & Sexual Health Equity (CGSHE) and supports qualitative research exploring the sexual and reproductive health access of im/migrant women in Metro Vancouver. Stefanie has completed internships in health promotion and global public health with the Island Sexual Health Society, Health Promotion Canada, CGSHE, and the University of California San Diego. Locally, she volunteers with the Pacific Immigrant Resources Society.

**Ann Pederson**, Ph.D., is the Director of Population Health Promotion at BC Women's Hospital & Health Centre in Vancouver and Adjunct Professor in the School of Population and Public Health at the University of British Columbia and the Faculty of Health Sciences at Simon Fraser University. Ann has co-edited a dozen books, notably *Health Promotion in Canada*, now in its fourth edition, and *Women's Health: Intersections of Policy, Research, and Practice*. Ann is a senior leader in the healthcare system, responsible for a portfolio of women's and maternal health initiatives. She is involved in several research collaborations in Canada and internationally on critical issues of women, gender, and health.

**Dennis Raphael**, Ph.D., is Professor at the School of Health Policy and Management at York University in Toronto. Dr. Raphael is editor of *Social Determinants of Health: Canadian Perspectives*, *Tackling Health Inequalities: Lessons from International Experiences*, and *Immigration, Public Policy, and Health: Newcomer Experiences in Developed Nations*, and author of *Poverty in Canada: Implications for Health and Quality of Life* and *About Canada: Health and Illness*.

**Marcia Rioux**, Ph.D., is Distinguished Research Professor at the School of Health Policy and Management, York University, Canada. She has published widely in the area of disability and human rights. She is the Director and Principal Investigator of Disability Rights Promotion International (DRPI), a multi-year group of projects to monitor disability rights. She has developed Indicators under the UN *Convention on the Rights of Persons with Disabilities* and the UN Sustainable Development Goals that recognize the importance of the input of grassroots voices and Global South country voices in the way we measure progressive realization. Dr. Rioux is internationally known, having taught, researched, and advised on policy issues in numerous countries in the Americas, Europe, Africa, and Asia. She was made a member of the Order of Canada in 2014.

**Ambreen Sayani**, M.D., M.Sc., Ph.D. candidate, is a surgeon by training and has worked closely with cancer patients and their families. She is committed to advocating for patients' rights and has carried out both bench and bedside cancer research to improve treatment and provide socially just care. She has held leadership roles across multiple healthcare industries and has consulted for private-sector organizations and governments. At present, Dr. Sayani's research is focused on the interface between social and health equity, and its implications for cancer risk, treatment, and survival. She has presented at numerous conferences in Canada and internationally, and has several peer-reviewed publications. Dr. Sayani is a member of the Equity Advisory Committee for the Canadian Partnership Against Cancer and is a Community Ambassador for the Region of Peel's Diversity, Equity and Inclusion Charter. Dr. Sayani has a medical degree from Dubai Medical College in the United Arab Emirates and a Master's degree in Oncology from Vrije University in Amsterdam, and is currently completing her Ph.D. in Health Policy and Equity at York University in Toronto.

**Robert Vipond**, Ph.D., is Professor in the Department of Political Science at the University of Toronto. He is interested in political development, especially in Canada and the U.S. This approach spans a variety of subject areas: federalism, constitutional politics, health care, education, and the discipline of political science. His most recent monograph is entitled *Making a Global City: How One Toronto School Embraced Diversity* (University of Toronto Press, 2017), which won the Joseph Brant Prize from the Ontario Historical Society in 2018 for the best book on the history of multiculturalism in Ontario.

**Mary E. Wiktorowicz**, Ph.D., is Professor in the School of Health Policy and Management, York University. Professor Wiktorowicz adopts a comparative lens to study transnational governance and policy focused on global health, mental health, pharmaceutical regulation, and anti-microbial resistance. She has advised the Canadian Senate Standing Committee on Social Affairs, Science and Technology, the House of Commons Standing Committee on Health, the Ontario Local Health Integration Network Collaborative on Mental Health, and the Ontario Ministry of Health and Long-Term Care, and was a CIHR Best Brain advising on mental health policy.

**Michelle Wyndham-West**, Ph.D., is Adjunct Professor at the School of Health Policy and Management at York University. Michelle is a critically applied medical anthropologist specializing in gender, health, and public policy. Michelle holds an M.A. in political anthropology from the University of Toronto and undergraduate degrees in political science and social anthropology from Western University and York University, respectively. Current research focuses upon the convergence of, and friction between, culture, power relations, and gender conceptualizations in policy processes through the case studies of dementia strategy development and policy promoting healthy aging for seniors living with HIV.

# Copyright Acknowledgements

organizational health equity intervention in primary care clinics. *International Journal for Equity in Health*, 17(1), 154. doi: 10.1186/s12939-018-0820-2. Reprinted with permission.

## CHAPTER 12

Figure 12.1: Bourgeault, I. L., Demers, C., & Bray, E. (2015). The need for a pan-Canadian health human resources strategy and coordinated action plan. In S. Carson, K. Nossal, & J. Dixon (Eds.), *Toward a healthcare strategy for Canadians*. Montreal: McGill-Queen's University Press. Reprinted with permission.

## CHAPTER 15

Figure 15.1: Source for the data from Canadian Institute for Health Information. (2016a). National health expenditure trends, 1975 to 2016: Data tables. Used with permission.

# Index

*Page numbers in italics indicate glossary definitions.*

Aboriginal peoples, *226*
    ancestry, 75
    in Canada, 203–4
    colonialism and, 213, 215–16
    cultural safety and humility, 217, 221–22
    *Declaration on the Rights of Indigenous*
        *Peoples* (UNDRIP), 88–89, 96
    determinants of health, 212–13
    diabetes, 214, 339
    disability and, 359
    educational levels, 212
    epidemic diseases, 263
    gender equality, 200
    healing tradition, 312
    health inequities, 28
    health insurance, 266
    health status, 212–15
    herbalism, and traditional
        medicines, 262
    infant mortality rates, 51, 268
    intersectionality and, 206
    life expectancy, 51, 214
    maternal mortality rates, 214, 268
    median income, 212
    midwifery, 337–38
    Missing and Murdered Indigenous
        Women, 216
    mortality rates, 28, 51
    National Household Survey (2011), 212
    as "other," 50
    race, health and, 216, 217
    racism, 213
    right to traditional medicine, 96
    smoking, 214
    social determinants of health and, 96, 141
    social exclusion of, 213
    strategies to address inequities, 217–19
    subordination of, 99

    Truth and Reconciliation Commission, 51,
        216, 217–18
    vulnerability of, 222–23
    women, 212–16, 336
abortion, 297
acceptability, 90, 95
access to care
    equity-oriented care, 220–22
    im/migrant populations, 207–8, 209, 211,
        218–19
    legal status and, 209
    Medicaid/Medicare, 293–95
    women and, 340–41
accessibility
    categories of, 90
    disability and, 93–94
    of health information, 103
    to health services, 130
    HIV/AIDS, 99, 130
    non-discrimination and, 95, 103, 104
active labour policy, *253*
acute stress response, 23
adaptive planning, 292
addiction, 141–42
*Additional Protocol to the American Convention on*
    *Human Rights in the Area of Economic, Social*
    *and Cultural Rights*, 95
adolescence
    Committee on the Rights of the Child
        (CRC), 96–97
    tobacco use and, 127
adrenaline, 23
adult mortality, 11, 22
adverse childhood experiences (ACES), 21–22
*African Charter on Human and Peoples'*
    *Rights*, 95
agriculture
    development of, impact on health, 24–25

Alberta
    Health Equity Network, 398
    midwifery, 275
Alberta Health Services (AHS), 302
alcohol use, 401
    as coping mechanism, 77, 150
    harm reduction, 222
allopathic biomedicine, 263–64
allostatic load, 23–24
alternative medical practitioners, 313
alternative service delivery, *278*
American Medical Association
    opposition to reform, 284–85
American Public Health Association (APHA),
    404–6
        *Addressing Health Equity through State,*
        *Regional Partnerships*, 405–6
        *The Nation's Health*, 405
ancillary health services, 343–44
ancillary professions, 313
*Andrews v. Law Society*, 364
antibiotics, development of, 264
Antipodean welfare state, 242
anti-racism, 39, 50–51, *55*, 221
anxiety, 209
Armstrong, Hugh, 45–46
Armstrong, Pat, 45–46
Aspirin, 339
Association of Ontario Health Centres, 398
asthma, 402
austerity policies, health inequalities and,
    245–46, 413
Australia
    infant mortality rates, 78
    as liberal welfare state, 69, 154
    parallel private health care, 289
    social expenditures as percentage GDP, 70
Austria
    infant mortality rates, 78
    social expenditures as percentage GDP, 70
autism, 261, 275
availability of services, 90, 95, 103

bacteria
    cancer and, 184

causal relationship to disease, 264
barber surgeons, 312
Barer, Morris, 315
Barer-Stoddart Report, 315, 316
Barker, David, 21
Baudrillard, Jean, 51
Bégin, Monique, 261
behavioural factors, 46
Beijing Declaration and Platform for Action
    (UN), 334–35
Belgium
    as conservative welfare state, 69, 154
    infant mortality rates, 78
    social expenditures as percentage
        GDP, 70
best practices, 340
biological embedding, 24
biological programming, 24
biomedical approach to health, 156–57
    disability, and illness, 352, 353, 356–57,
        364
    public health, 394
biomedicine, 263–64
biotechnology, *107*
*Bitter Medicine* (documentary), 311
black lung disease, 44, 47
block funding, 273
Blue Cross, 266
Bourdieu, Pierre, 173
Bowlby, John, 21
*Boys in White* (Becker), 42
breast cancer, 179–85
Bristol-Myers Squibb (BMS), 385
British Columbia
    Declaration of Commitment to Cultural
        Safety and Humility, 217
    electoral reform, 246–47
    gender-based violence online
        course, 221
*British North America (BNA) Act* (1867), 263
Bush, George W., 236
business and corporate sector
    globalization, impact of, 101
    influence on public policy, 62–65
    neo-liberal approach of, 64, 74

Canada

*Achieving Health for All*, 396

block funding, 273

*Canada Health Act* (1984), 261, 263, 269, 270, 272–73, *278*, 341

*Charter of Rights and Freedoms*, 92, 364

Commission on Social Determinants of Health, 396

Comprehensive Economic and Trade Agreement (CETA), 383–84

drug spending per capita, 385

early childhood education and care (ECEC), 248

equality rights, 85, 108n2

e-Referral platforms, 302

External Advisory Committee on Smart Regulation, 374

federal transfers, 273

federal/provincial healthcare jurisdictions, 263, 269, 275

first-past-the-post electoral system, 246

*Food and Drugs Act*, 380

government spending as function of GDP, 248

*Health Accord* (2004), 274

health insurance, 263, 265–68

health promotion, definition of, 396

health research themes, 435–43

healthcare developments, 273–74

healthcare policy, 282–83

healthcare reform, 269–73

healthcare system, origins of, 261–76

*Hospital and Diagnostic Services Act*, 263, 266

hospitals. *see* hospitals

housing policy, 247–48

im/migrant populations, 207

improved health, social determinants of, 143

income inequality, 28, 148, 151

inequality profile of, 18

infant mortality rates, 78, 148

integrated delivery networks (IDNs), 301–3

international agreements, 159–60

labour policy, 250

as liberal welfare state, 69, 154

life expectancy, 12–13, 27, 148

maternal mortality, 14, 214

*Medical Care Act* (1967), 267, 269, 270, *278*

*Medical Services Act*, 272

medicare, 143, 267

Mental Health Commission, 94

migration terminology, 205

minimum-income benefit, 148

national child care program, 248

neo-liberal policies. *see* neo-liberalism

*A New Vision of Health for Canadians*, 396

*Ottawa Charter for Health Promotion*, 141

Patented Medicines Prices Review Board, 303–4

per-capita healthcare expenditures, 13

percentage of GNP spending on health care, 268, 270

politics, and political institutions, 285–87

population health, 146, 148

poverty rates, 17, 148, 238–41

prerequisites for health, 141

primary healthcare division of labour, 316

*Protecting Canadians Against Unsafe Drugs Act* (Vanessa's Law), 379

provincial healthcare systems, regionalization of, 286

Public Health Agency of Canada, 396–97

public health approach, 396–400

public social spending, 148, 235–38

regional health authorities (RHAs), 302

*Report of the Royal Commission on the Future of Health Care in Canada*, 342, 343

right to health, 261

*Romanow Report*, 342, 343

social assistance programs, 250

social determinants of health, 140, 141–42

social expenditures, 27

social expenditures as percentage GDP, 70, 274

social welfare, residual approach to, 238

social-welfare services as government
responsibility, 28
total public social spending, comparison to
Western nations, 240–41
universal health care, 17
universal health insurance, 269
U.S. health divergence, 27–29
as welfare state, 66, 67, 241
*Canada Health Act* (1984), 261, 263, 269, 270,
272–73, *278*, 341
Canada Health and Social Transfer (CHST),
270, *278*
Canada Vigilance Adverse Drug Reaction
Database, 377
Canadian Agency for Drugs and Technology in
Health, 385
Canadian Commonwealth Federation
(CCF), 285
Canadian Coordinating Office for Health
Technology Assessment (CCOHTA), 385
Canadian Council on the Social Determinants of
Health, 397
Canadian Institute for Health Information, 397
Canadian Institute for Health Research
Institute of Gender and Health, 335
Canadian Medical Association (CMA), 285, 398
*Social Determinants of Health*, 399
"state health insurance," 266
*Canadian Medical Association Journal*, 265
control trials, representation of women
in, 340
Canadian Nurses Association, 398
Canadian Population Health Initiative, 397, 398
Canadian Public Health Association
*Action Statement on Health Promotion*, 396
Canadian Women's Health Network, 335
cancer, 271
race and, 124
social class, impact on health outcomes,
171, 177–79
survival numbers, 179
upstream, midstream, and downstream
disease management, 185–87
*See also* cancer by type

capitalism
congruence with biomedicine, 47
health effects of on labour, 44–45
influence on public policy, 62–65
and the welfare state, 65, 66, 239
capitation fees, 272, 320
carcinogens, occupational exposure
to, 184
cardiovascular disease, 23, 144–45, 153, 171,
339–40, 403–4
care, vs prevention, 437–38
care co-ordination programs, 302
caring dilemma, 49
Carnegie Foundation, 312
case control, 124
case manager, *307*
case-management programs, 302
categorical welfare state, 242
CBC, *Ideas*, 398
cellular level of health, 5–7
Centers for Disease Control and Prevention
(CDC), 294, 400, 401–4
*Healthy People 2020*, 402–4
social determinants of health, 141
*centres locaux de santé communitaire*
(CLSCs), 272
Centres of Excellence Programme for Women's
Health, 335
cervical cancer, 184, 214
*Chaoulli* case (Quebec), 286–87
chemotherapy, 179
child care, decommodification of, 71
child labour, 101
child mortality, 11
child poverty, 23, 145–46, 148, 173, 246
comparison of in wealthy nations, 149
child welfare
early childhood education and care
(ECEC), 248
public policy and, 234
childbirth
Caesarian births, 338
medicalization of, 48–49, 337–38
midwifery, 49

childhood
  adverse childhood experiences (ACES), 21–22
  basic needs, 19–20
  Committee on the Rights of the Child (CRC), 96–97
  early life, impact on adult health, 20–21, 23, 153
  non-adaptive reaction to stress, 77
chiropractic, 275
cholera, 4–5
Christian democratic welfare state, 243–44
chronic disease, 271
  acute stress response and, 23
  austerity policies, impact of, 246
  integrated delivery networks (IDNs), 301–3
  risk behaviours, 401
  root causes, and downstream effects, 7–8
chronic fatigue syndrome, 10
Cidro, J., *Indigenous Experiences of Pregnancy and Birth*, 337–38
city planning, "sanitary ideal" of, 263
civil rights, 85
civil society sector, influence on public policy, 63, 65
class/power mobilization, 71
clientele pluralism, 373, 378, *389*
clinical depression, 182
clinical epidemiology, 116
Clinton, Bill, 286
cluster analysis, 126
cohort studies, 24
College of Family Physicians of Canada, 386
Collins, Patricia Hill, 50
colonial period, healing traditions, 262–63
colonization, settler society healthcare systems, 51
colorectal screening, 402
community cohesion, 126
community health centres, 271
compensationitis, 47

complementary practitioners, 313
Conference Board of Canada, 398
confidentiality, 97, 99
conflict theory, 44, 48, 53, 56n6
  vs consensus models, 437
conflict vs consensus models, 437
congruence thesis, *56*
consent
  free and informed, 97, 103
  non-consensual medical treatment, 90
Conservative party, 285
conservative welfare state, 63, 69, *81*, 154–55, 159, 243–44
constructivism, 117
"contested illnesses," 10
controlling for a factor, *33*
Cooley, Charles, 41
co-payments, 269, 273, 275
coronary artery disease, 144–45
corporate bias theory, 373
corporate power, *81*
cortisol, 23
cost recovery, *389*
counselling services, 275
crime, 77
critical analysis approach, 128–29
  examples of, 129
  historical analysis, 129
  human rights and, 129–30, 131
critical materialist approach, 61–62
critical theory, 117–18, *133*
cross-sectional studies, 24, 124, 125
Cruz, Ted, 300
cultural acceptability, 103
cultural capital, 173
cultural factors, 46
cultural humility, 217, 221–22
cultural relativism, 51
cultural rights, 85
cultural safety, 217, 221–22
cultural-behavioural approach, 148–50
  social class, impact on health outcomes, 175–76, 180–81

cumulative effects, 153
customer choice, 322

DALYs. *See* Disability Adjusted Life Years
    (DALYs)
decommodification, 70–71, *81*
    cash nexus, 71
dengue virus, 100
Denmark
    infant mortality rates, 78
    life expectancy, 22
    as social democratic welfare state, 68, 154
    social expenditures as percentage GDP, 70
dental assistant work, 313
dental care, decommodification of, 71
dental hygiene, 313
depression, 271
    in women, 336
Depression, Great
    origins of welfare state, 67
    U.S. redistribution programs, 27
Derrida, Jacques, 51
deviance, 41
    medicalization of, 43
diabetes, 144–45, 152, 153, 214, 271, 336,
    339, 402
    stress and, 23
diphtheria, 143
disability
    access to health services, 93–94
    activity limitations, 359
    age, 360, 366
    age-adjusted severity weights, 358
    benefits, equitable access to, 356–57
    biomedical accounts of, 351
    biomedical approach to, 352, 353, 356, 364
    in Canada, 358–65
    confidentiality, 97
    *Convention on the Rights of Persons with
        Disabilities* (UN), 88, 93, 94–95
    decommodification of, 71
    denial of rights and, 440
    Disability Adjusted Life Years (DALYs),
        10, 352, 356, 357–58, 440

discrimination against, 355
    exclusion, social and legal, 355–56
    functional accounts of, 351
    gender and, 360, 363–64
    geographic location and, 360–61
    human rights approaches to, 351, 352, 354,
        355–56
    as illness, 356–57
    illness and, construction of, 351–66,
        440–41
    illness as, 357–58
    individual impairment and, 354, 355
    as individual pathology, 351, 352–54, *368*
    labour force and, 361–63
    mental illness, 94–95
    non-discrimination, 357, 364–65
    normal, concept of, 351
    "reduced value" of life with, 358, 440
    right to health and, 93–97, 108n9
    selective non-treatment, 94
    self-reported prevalence of, 358,
        359–65, 366
    as social burden, 353
    social construction of, 352
    as social determinant of health, 75, 141
    as social pathology, 351, 352, 354–56,
        364, *368*
    within society vs within individual, 358
    state role in social care of, 357
    stigmatization of, 97
    theoretical models of, 352–56
    by type, 363
    women and, 336
    women vs men and, 352, 360, 362,
        363–64, 366
    workplace policies on, 351, 355
Disability Adjusted Life Years (DALYs), 10, 356,
    *368*, 440
    as measure of health status, 357–58
Disability Rights Promotion International
    (DRPI), 103–4
Disability Screening Questions (DSQ), 359
discourse analysis, 127
discriminant analysis, 126

discrimination
    disability and, 355
    *Eldridge v. British Columbia*, 92–93,
      357, 365
    freedom from, 86
    against im/migrant populations, 207, 211
    *Moore v. British Columbia (Education)*, 92
    prohibition against, 91–92
    race/gender-based, 216–17
    subordination of vulnerable peoples,
      99, 200
    systemic, 92
disease
    Canada-U.S. comparison, 268
    "contested illnesses," 10
    domestic animals, proximity to, 25
    epidemiological approach to, 7–8
    interconnections with life experience, and
      poverty, 271
    lifestyle diseases, 276
    political aspect in defining, 10
    social production of disease hypothesis, 44,
      176–77
    upstream/root cause approach, 7–8, 10
disease management
    midstream of, 181, 182
    upstream, midstream, and downstream
      disease management, 185–87
Dominion-Provincial Conference on
    Reconstruction, 266
Douglas, Tommy, 261, 267, 443
Down syndrome, 94
downstream effects, 7–8, 11
drift hypothesis, 46
Durkheim, Émile, 38, 39
dyslexia, 92

early childhood education and care (ECEC), 248
early life
    adverse childhood experiences (ACES),
      21–22
    care, and future development, 21
    fetal origins hypothesis, 21
    Helsinki birth cohort, 21

    impact of on adult health, 20–21, 23
    as social determinant of health, 75–76,
      141–42
eating disorders, 336
economic accessibility, 103
economic collapse (2008), 27
economic justice, vs social justice, 73
economic rights, 85
economic system, market economy and, 72
education
    apprenticeship, 262
    continuing medical education sponsorship
      by pharmaceutical industry, 379, 380,
      385–86
    decommodification of, 71
    early childhood education and care
      (ECEC), 248
    as human right, 86
    income inequality and, 15
    as measure of social class, 174, 175
    medical, 42, 264–65, 312–13, 325n1
    as social determinant of health, 75–76,
      141–42
efficiency, 282–83
elderly population
    health insurance, 286
    state role in social care of, 357
*Eldridge v. British Columbia*, 92–93, 357, 365
electoral systems, 246–47
employer-based health insurance, 177
employment, and working conditions
    as social determinant of health, 75–76,
      141–42, 144
Engels, Friedrich, 138, 176–77
    *The Condition of the Working Class in
      England*, 139
environmental approach, disability and, 352, 355
environmental factors, power and inequality, 28
environmental hazards, and globalization, 101
epidemic, 4
epidemic diseases, 263
epidemiological approaches, 4–29
    cohort studies, 24
    cross-sectional studies, 24

to disease, 7–8

disease focus of research, 10

ecological fallacy of population findings, 17–18

epistemology, 119–20

examples of, 123–24

Helsinki birth cohort, 21

horizontal structures, 155

mechanisms and pathways influencing health, 156

multi-level modelling, 24

observational ecological studies, 24

ontology, 114, 118–19

positivism, 114, 115–17

quantitative methods used, 122–24

quantitative research methods, 121–26

realism, 115, 117–18

to social determinants of health, 155–56

vertical structures, 155

epidemiology, 4–29, *133*

basic terms, 123

clinical epidemiology, 116, 122

developmental origins of health and disease, 20–21

early epidemiology, 4–5

experimental research design, 122, 123–24

methods used in, 24, 122–24

ontology, and positivism, 118–19

political epidemiology and, 9

population health and, 9–11, 24–29

"shoe leather epidemiology," 9

statistical analyses, 122, 123

training, 9–10

epigenetic mechanisms, 24

epistemology, 119–20

research design, 114

equality rights

access to treatment, 85, 108n2

*Andrews v. Law Society*, 364

*Charter of Rights and Freedoms*, 92

disability and, 364, 366

to well-being, 85

Equiphealth-care.ca, 220

equity in health, *164*

erectile dysfunction, 43

e-Referral platforms, 302

estrogen-replacement therapy, 49

ethics, *107*

ethnic minority groups

social class, impact on health outcomes, 181–82

ethnicity. *See* race

ethnographies, 126

ethnography, institutional, 48

*European Social Charter*, 95

European Union

Comprehensive Economic and Trade Agreement (CETA), 383–84

excluded professions, 313

experimental research design, 122–24, 125

extra billing, 269, 275

factor analysis, 126

familial health determinants, 76–77

family, decommodification of, 71

family health determinants, 63

family physicians, 315–16, 325n3

obstetrical care by, 338

family policy, *253*

Farr, William, 5

feminism, 39, 47–50

postmodernism and, 52

symbolic interactionism and, 48

feminist political economy, *347*

feminist political economy theory, 332

fibromyalgia, 10

fight-or-flight response, 23, 150

Finland

infant mortality rates (IMR), 78

smoking, 26

as social democratic welfare state, 68, 154

social expenditures as percentage GDP, 70

First Nations peoples. *See* Aboriginal peoples

Flexner, Abraham, 265

Flexner Report, 312, 325n1

focus groups, 127

Foege, William, *The Fears of the Rich, the Needs of the Poor*, 5

Food and Drug Administration, U.S. (FDA)
    drug approval process, 377

food security
    as human right, 86
    as social determinant of health, 75–76, 141–42

for-profit healthcare, 311, 320

for-profit/non-profit programs, 248

Foucault, Michel, 51–52
    *The Birth of the Clinic*, 51, 52
    *Discipline and Punish*, 51
    *The History of Sexuality*, 51
    *Madness and Civilization*, 51

France
    as conservative welfare state, 69, 154
    health insurance, 289
    infant mortality rates, 78
    social expenditures as percentage GDP, 70

free market
    government intervention and, 284
    vs planned economy, 282–83

functionalism. *See* structural functionalism

gender, *226, 335*
    critical analysis and, 128
    as exclusionary criterion, 312, 325n2
    healthcare professions, stratification of by, 264–65
    intersectionality and, 204, 206
    power dynamics, 218
    premature mortality and, 144–45
    segregation by, 49, 183
    social class, impact on health outcomes, 181–82
    as social construct, 202–3
    as social determinant of health, 75, 141–42, 199–200, 211–12, 219, 334
    stereotypes, 210, 211, 218
    vs sex, 202–3, 332, 335

gender equality, 200, 222–23, 334–35

gender inequality
    institutional apartheid and, 344

patriarchy and, 47–49

gender relations, 202–3

gender wage gap, 219

gender-based violence, 209–11, 217, 221

gender-sensitive analysis, 332–36, 343–44

gender-transformative interventions, 200, 219

generic competition, *389*

geography, as social determinant of health, 75, 141–42

George, Lloyd, 263, 265

Germany
    as conservative welfare state, 69, 154
    infant mortality rates, 78
    private insurance (sickness funds), 288–89
    social expenditures as percentage GDP, 70

Global Burden of Disease, 358

global health law, 101

globalization, *107*
    class structure, and health status, 47
    health impacts of, 159
    migrant/refugee crisis, 29
    right to health and, 101, 104

glucose, 6

Goffman, Erving
    *Asylums*, 41
    *Stigma*, 41

governance, *56*

government
    role of in health care, 282–83
    role of in political economy perspective, 63, 64

governmentality, 52

Greece
    austerity policies, 245–46
    infant mortality rates, 78
    as Latin welfare state, 69
    social expenditures as percentage GDP, 70

gross domestic product (GDP), *253*
    life expectancy and, 19–20

gynecologists, 316

Haas, Jack, 42

harm reduction, 222

Harper, Stephen, 274, 335

Harris, Mike, 270

Harvard Community Health Plan, 272

Harvard Medical School, 386

Harvard School of Public Health, 358

healing traditions, pre-colonial/colonial periods, 262–63

health, *107, 368*

    basic needs, 19–20

    cellular level of, 5–7

    definitions of, 11

    determinants of, 90

    differential access to, 90–93

    early life, 20–22

    links with human rights, 85–86

    population level of, 5–7

    prehistoric to present timeline, 11

    trends in selected countries, 12–13

    vs health care, 14, 27

Health Canada

    direct-to-consumer promotion and, 381

    drug safety standards, 377

    *Exploring Concepts of Gender and Health,* 339–40

    gender as health determinant, 334

    missed review standards, financial penalties, 376–77

    Therapeutic Products Directorate (TPD), 373, 374–81, 389n1

    Women's Health Bureau, 335

health care

    delisting of services, 341

    developments in, 273–74

    equitable health services, 220–22

    federal/provincial jurisdictions, 263

    for-profit/not-for-profit programs, 290–92

    freedom from non-consensual medical treatment, 90

    gender-sensitive analysis, 332–36

    gender-transformative health promotion, 219

    harm reduction, 222

    "model" family, 201

    origins of, 261–76

    private practice–public payment, 267, 275

    regionalization of, 302

    trauma- and violence-informed care, 220–21

    two-tiered systems, 274

    vs health, 14, 27

Health Council of Canada, *Stepping It Up,* 398

health data, on populations, 11–24

health equity, *107,* 160

health good practice, vs right to health good practices, 102–3

health human resource issues, 314–15, 318

    conceptual framework for, 318

health impact assessment (HIA), *426*

health inequality, 63, 77, 129, 139

    cancer, and social class, 177–79

    cultural-behavioural model, 175–76, 178, 180–81

    life-course choices, 175–76, 177, 178, 184–85

    materialist model, 176–77, 178, 182–84

    neo-liberalism, and austerity, 245–46

    psychosocial model, 176, 178, 181–82

    social class and, 171–87

    social determinants of health and, 143–46

    upstream, midstream, and downstream disease management, 185–87

    vs inequity, 9

health inequities. *See* inequities

health insurance

    Blue Cross, 266

    drug insurance coverage, 303

    early attempts, 263

    employer-based health insurance, 305

    employer-sponsored, 285

    employment-based, 266

    fee-for-service model, 267

    integrated delivery networks (IDNs) and, 301–3

    liberalism vs socialism, 282–83

    Medicare/Medicaid (US), 236, 263, 267, 269, 282, 293–95

    *The Patient Protection and Affordable Care Act* (2010), 236, 273–74, 281, 295–301, 305

health insurance (*continued*)
> private, 236, 286
> private vs public, 282–83
> public vs. private healthcare systems, 287–90
> as right of citizenship, 267
> veterans' plans, 266, 282

health maintenance organizations (HMOs), 271–72, *307*
> integrated delivery networks (IDNs) and, 301–3

health outcomes, 63
> inequality of biology, 22–24

health professions
> reforms in who provides care, 314–18
> regulation of, 314–15

health promotion, *427*

health service organizations (HSOs), 271–72

health services, public policy and, 76

health status
> of im/migrant populations, 208–10
> social class differences and, 46–47
> social spending and, 272

health studies, field of, 436

healthcare costs
> cancer treatment, 179
> cost controls, 311
> workforce planning, 314–18

healthcare policy: evolution of, 281–305
> allocation, 287
> delivery of healthcare services, 287, 290–93
> diverging premises for, 281–93
> financing, 287–90
> ideological perspective on, 282–83
> information technology (IT), 302
> integrated health systems, policy convergence, 301–3
> interest groups and, 286
> organizational design, 287–93
> pharmaceuticals, 303–5
> political institutions and, 283–87
> recent reforms, 293–301
> recentralization, 302
> regionalization, 302

healthcare professions, stratification of, 264–65

healthcare providers
> caring dilemma, 49
> cultural humility training, 217
> gendered division of labour, 49, 183, 312–13, 325n2, 342
> im/migrant populations, negative interactions with, 209, 211
> medical socialization, 42
> physical/mental demands of, 342–43
> racism against immigrant providers, 51
> trauma- and violence-informed care, 220–21
> types of, 313
> work intensification, 45–46
> workload, and burnout, 318

healthcare provision
> public vs private, 321–22
> reforms in managing care, 319–21
> reforms in who provides care, 313–18

healthcare reform, 269–73, 283–87
> management reform, 319–21
> mosaic model, guiding "principles," 296–97
> *The Patient Protection and Affordable Care Act* (2010), 295–301
> provincial healthcare systems, regionalization of, 286
> United States, 283–87

healthcare services, *347*
> im/migrant women and, 211
> non-discrimination within, 86
> private non-profit, 290–93
> public financing, 290–93
> public social spending, 235–38
> right to health freedoms, 90
> role of in producing health, 18–19
> as social determinant of health, 141–42

healthcare spending, funding formulas, 273

healthcare systems
> international, comparison of financing/ delivery, 288–89
> privatization of, 70
> two-tiered, 70
> US/Canada comparison, 265–76

"Healthy Immigrant Effect," 208

healthy public policy (HPP), *427*

heart attack, 336

heart disease, 6, 13, 144–45, 152, 271, 339, 402–3

hegemony, *368*

helicobacter pylori, 184

hepatitis A, 402

hepatitis B/C, 184, 214

hepatocellular carcinoma, 184

herbalism, 262

herbalists, 313

historical materialism, *81*

HIV/AIDS, 99–100, 104, 145, 214, 402

    gender-transformative interventions, 219

    pharmaceutical access, 130

    XIIIth International AIDS Conference, 218

holistic monitoring approach, 103–4

homelessness, 248, 271

homeopathic therapy, 275, 313

homosexuality. *See* LGBT people

hospitals

    community hospitals, consequences of closing, 341

    growth of, 266

    integrated delivery networks (IDNs) and, 301–3

    out-patient services, 319

    reforms in managing care, 319–21

    standardization of care protocols, 319

housing

    affordable, lack of, 443

    Canadian housing policy, 247–48

    social assistance and, 75

    as social determinant of health, 75–76, 141–42, 144

    social rental housing, 248

Hughes, Everett, 42

human papilloma virus, 184

human rights

    as indicator of well-being, 103

    international agreements, 85, 86–89, 94–95, 96, 99, 108nn2–5, 108–9n10

    principles, 85

    respect for diversity, 104

    right to health, key aspects, 89, 95

    well-being and, 104

human rights approaches, 84–105, *133*

    critical analysis and, 129–30

    disability and, 93–97, 352, 354, 355–56

    methodology, 120

    realism, 118–19

    reproductive health, 97–99

    social determinants of health, 159–60

    social imperative of, 86–90

Hunt, Paul, 102–3

hydrotherapy, 276

iatrogenic disease, 354

idealism, 113, 114–15, 117, 130

    methodology, 120

    *See also* interpretivism

ideological system

    dichotomies within, 73–74

    state distribution of resources, 73–74

Illich, Ivan, 354

illness

    as biographical disruption, 42

    as disability, 357–58

    disability and, construction of, 440–41

    disability as, 356–57

    doctor-patient models, 40

    reconstitution of the self, 42

    the sick role and, 39–40

illness career, 42

im/migrant populations

    access to care, 207–8, 209, 211, 218–19

    defined, 204

    diversity among, 208

    educational attainment of, 207–8

    eligibility for healthcare benefits, 271

    health status of, 208–10

    intersectionality, 210–12

    language barriers, 211

    legal status, and access to care, 209

    marginalization of, 207

    negative interactions with healthcare providers, 209, 211

im/migrant populations (*continued*)
  overrepresentation of in lower status
    occupations, 207–8
  political empowerment of, 200
  population profile, 206–8
  reproductive health care, 209–10, 211,
    222–23
  social determinants of health and, 209, 211–12
  vulnerability of, 222–23
immigrant status, 75, 141–42
imprisonment rates, income inequality and, 15
incidence, 123
income distribution
  geographic level of, 17–18
  impact on health, 20, 64, 138
  as measure of social class, 174
  as social determinant of health, 75–76,
    141–42, 151
income inequality, 129, 399
  access to care and, 341
  austerity and, 16
  Canada-U.S. comparison, 28
  health and social problems related to, 16
  impact on health, 15–18
  male vs female differences, 129
  neo-liberalism and, 64–65
  premature mortality and, 144–45
  social class and, 173
  Soviet Union, 26
  wage gap between men and women, 207–8
  women and, 144, 336
Indigenous Cultural Safety program, 221
Indigenous peoples. *See* Aboriginal peoples
individual pathology, disability and, 351
inequality
  biology of, 22–24
  health and, 19–20, 139
  measures of, 16–17
  population health and, 26
  power relationships and, 28
  racialization and, 50
  vs inequities, 9
  *See also* health inequalities; income
    inequality

inequities
  Canadian documents on, 396–97
  public health concerns, 394–427
  reproductive health, 98–99
  stratification and, 71
  vs health disparities, 405
  vs inequalities, 9
infant mortality rates (IMR), 11, 26, *33*, 77, 243
  Aboriginal peoples, 51
  among OECD nations, 78
  black infant mortality, 28
  Canada-U.S. comparison, 268
  income inequality and, 15
inflammation, 21
inflammatory response markers, 23–24
influenza, 143
information technology (IT), 302
  electronic medical records (EMRs), 302
  e-Referral platforms, 302
Innovative Medicines Canada, 381, 384
Institute for Health Metrics and Evaluation, 10
Institute of Medicine
  *The Future of the Public's Health*, 404
  *U.S. Health in International Perspective*, 14
institutional ethnography, 48
institutional settings, marginalized groups in, 91
institutional welfare state, 242
integrated delivery networks (IDNs), 301–3
integrated delivery systems, *308*
integrated health systems, 301–3
integration, 302
intellectual property rights, 383–85, 390n3
  Trade Related Aspects of Intellectual
    Property Rights (TRIPS) Agreement,
    381–82
international human rights agreements, 85,
  86–89, 94–95, 96, 99, 108nn2–5, 108–9n10
International Organization for Migration, 204
Internet pharmacies, 304
internists, 316
interpretivism, 117, 119
  *See also* idealism
intersectionality, 204, 206–16
  examples of, 206

im/migrant populations, 206–12

intimate partner violence

> against Aboriginal women, 214–15
>
> against im/migrant women, 208, 210–11

Ireland

> infant mortality rates, 78
>
> as liberal welfare state, 154
>
> social expenditures as percentage GDP, 70

Italy

> infant mortality rates, 78
>
> as Latin welfare state, 69
>
> social expenditures as percentage GDP, 70

Japan

> at end of Second World War, 25–26
>
> health of population, 7
>
> inequality profile of, 18
>
> life expectancy, 12–15
>
> smoking, prevalence of, 7, 26
>
> *wa* (culture of), 26

Johnson, Lyndon B., 267

Johnson, Terence, 52

King, Martin Luther, Jr., 104–5

Kinney, Eleanor, 87

knowledge perspectives, 113–31

> components of, 118–20
>
> usefulness of, 120–21

Koch, Robert, 263, 264

labelling theory, 41

labour force

> disability and, 361–63
>
> institutional apartheid and, 344
>
> sex segregation of, 312–13, 325n2
>
> workforce planning, 314–18

labour movement

> health insurance and, 285
>
> welfare reform and, 67

labour policy

> active labour policy, *253*
>
> unemployment, and job security, 75–76, 250

labour sector

> child labour, 101
>
> influence on public policy, 63, 65–66
>
> organized labour, 65

labour unions

> power and influence of, 63, 65–66
>
> union density, 65–66, 158, 247

latent effects, 153

Latin welfare state, 69, 242

Lean healthcare model, 319

left political parties, *253*

LGBT people

> homosexuality as disease, 10, 52
>
> discrimination against, 99
>
> violence against im/migrant populations, 209–10

Liberal party, 285

liberal welfare state, 63, 69–70, *81*, 154–55, 159, 177, 243–44

> infant mortality rates (IMR), 77, 78
>
> means-tested social assistance, 241–42

liberalism vs socialism, 73

life expectancy (LE), 11–15, 22, *33*, 268

> Aboriginal peoples, 51
>
> Canada-U.S. comparison, 27
>
> discrepancies between countries, 139
>
> gross domestic product (GDP) and, 19–20
>
> income distribution and, 15–16
>
> reductions in early life mortality, 25

life-course choices

> impact of on adult health, 20–21, 145–46
>
> social class, impact on health outcomes, 175–76, 177, 184–85
>
> social determinants of health and, 152–53

lifestyle diseases, 276

> prevention vs care, 437–38

lifestyle risk factors, 77, 142, 143, 145, 401

Lillie, Frank Rattray, 265

limited professions, 313

Lipitor (atorvastatin), 375–76

logistic regression, 123

longitudinal studies, 124, 125

lung cancer, 21, 123, 175, 179

> Danish women, 22

Luxembourg
    infant mortality rates, 78
    social expenditures as percentage GDP, 70
Luxembourg Income Study (LIS), 238, 246

MacArthur, Douglas, 25
Machado, Stefanie, 200–201
Mackenzie King, William Lyon, 266
mammography, 180
managed care, *325*
    definition of, 320
    as means of rationing care, 320–21
managed care plans, 290–91, 295
managed healthcare plan, *308*
marginal professions, 313
marginalization
    of disabled, 355–56
    of im/migrant populations, 207
    of vulnerable populations, 200
marginalized people
    access to care and, 341
    compromised health and well-being of,
        91, 100
    discrimination against, 91
market economy, 72
Marketed Health Products Directorate (MHPD),
    377–78
marketing, of harmful substances, 101
Marx, Karl, 38, 44, 172
Marxism, 44, 46–47
material circumstances, 76–77
material conditions of life, 150
    improvements in, 143
materialism, 44–47, 53, 56n6, 117–18
materialist model
    social class, impact on health outcomes,
        176–77, 182–84
materialist-structuralist approach to social
    determinants of health, 148–50
maternal mortality rates
    Aboriginal women, 214
    black women, 28
    Canada-U.S. comparison, 268, 269–70
    ratio, 11

United States, 14, 28
maternity benefits, 203, 249
McCain, John, 300
McCrea, Frances, 48–49
McGill College, 262, 312
McKeown, Thomas, *The Role of Medicine*, 272
Mead, George Herbert, 41
measles, 143
measurement artifact, 46
media
    social determinants of health,
        representation of, 160–61
medical dominance, decline of, 313
medical interventions, measuring impacts
    of, 268
medical practice, stratification of healthcare
    professions, 264–65
medical profession
    clinical autonomy of, 286
    as dominant health occupation, 312
    as gatekeepers, 353, 356, 364
    gendered division of labour, 312–13,
        325n2
    sponsorship of, 312, 325n1
    support occupations of women, 313
medical socialization, 42
medical sociology, 38, 53
    feminist perspective of, 47–50
    Foucault and, 52
medical training, 262, 264–65
    cloak of competence, 42
medicalization, *56*
    of childbirth, 48–49, 337–38
    of daily living, 43, 56n5
    of deviance, 43
    of menopause, 48–49
    of pregnancy, 48–49
    of women's bodies, 48–49, 52
Medicare, *278*
medicine
    clinical gaze of, 52
    as institution of social control, 46–47
Meili, Ryan, 398
    *A Healthy Society*, 399

men
> gender vs sex, 202–3
> gender-sensitive analysis and, 333–34
> health-related differences between women and, 333–34, 336–40
> masculinity, gender norms of, 203, 218, 219

menopause
> medical definitions of, 49
> medicalization of, 48–49

mental health care
> among im/migrant populations, 209
> austerity policies, impact of, 246
> underfunding of, 287, 305

mental health needs, 171
> among im/migrant populations, 211

mental illness, 52, 336
> access to care post-migration, 209
> hospitalization of women, 338
> income inequality and, 15
> right to health, 94–95, 108n7

Merton, Robert, *The Student Physician*, 42

Messing, Karen, 333

methodology, research design, 114, 120

midstream interventions, 181, 182, 185–86

midwifery, 49, 262, 275, 312, 313, 337–38

migrant/refugee crisis, 204
> global inequality and, 29

migration, subordination of vulnerable peoples, 200

migration patterns, 207
> high-income vs low-income countries, 51

migration terminology, 205

Mills, C. Wright, 122

Missing and Murdered Indigenous Women, 216

monopsony, 288–89, 293

*Moore v. British Columbia (Education)*, 92

morbidity, 77, 123, 268

mortality, 123

mortality measures, 11, 77
> infant mortality rates (IMR), 11
> relationship to income inequality, 17

mortality rates
> Aboriginal peoples, 51
> among older people, 126
> breast cancer, 179–80

Canada-U.S. comparison, 27, 268

multi-level modelling, 24

multiple regression, 126

multivariate analyses, 123, 126

National Academies of Sciences, Engineering, and Medicine
> *Communities in Action*, 401, 404, 405

National Association of County and City Health Officials (NACCHO), 401
> *Advancing Public Narrative for Health Equity and Social Justice*, 408
> *The Building Networks Project*, 406
> *Expanding the Boundaries*, 406
> *Health Equity and Social Justice Toolkit*, 406
> *The Roots of Health Inequity*, 406

National Center for Chronic Disease Prevention and Health Promotion, 401

National Collaborating Centre for Aboriginal Health, 204, 218

National Film Board, *Bitter Medicine*, 311

National Indigenous Cultural Safety Learning Series, 221

National Tuberculosis Association, 265

Native Women's Association of Canada, 216

naturalistic inquiry, *133*

naturopathic therapy, 275

Navarro, Vicente, 44–45, 46–47, 354
> *Medicine Under Capitalism*, 47

"neglected diseases," 100, 109n11

neighbourhood, and built environments, 141–42

neo-liberalism
> austerity, and health inequalities, 245–46
> Canada-U.S. comparison, 28
> defined, 245
> disability and, 357
> free market approach of, 64
> key tenets of, 74
> political, economic, and social forces shaping, 244–45
> prevention vs care, 437–38
> public health and, 424
> public policy and, 158
> relationship to health outcomes, 22, 177

neo-materialist approach to social determinants
of health, 150–51

nervous system, plasticity of, 24

Nestel, Sheryl, 50

Netherlands

as conservative welfare state, 69, 154

infant mortality rates, 78

private insurance (sickness funds), 288–89

social expenditures as percentage GDP, 70

Neufeld, H.T., *Indigenous Experiences of Pregnancy
and Birth*, 337–38

New Brunswick

drug benefit programs, subsidized, 303

electoral reform, 246–47

midwifery, 337

recentralization of health authorities, 302

New Democratic Party (NDP), 285, 400

New Zealand

cultural safety, 221

infant mortality rates, 78

as liberal welfare state, 154

social expenditures as percentage GDP, 70

Newfoundland and Labrador

midwifery, 337

non-discrimination, *108*

accessibility and, 90

of human rights policy, 85

non-governmental organizations, 160

normative judgments, 116

Northern Ireland, 414

ancillary health services, 344

Norway

*The Challenge of the Gradient*, 416–17

*Equitable Redistribution* White Paper, 416

health inequalities, concern with, 415–17

health status of Norwegians, 141

income inequality, 148, 151

infant mortality rates (IMR), 78, 148

labour policy, 250

life expectancy, 148

minimum-income benefit, 148

*National Strategy to Reduce Social Differences
in Health*, 416, 417

population health, 146, 148

poverty rates, 148, 237–39

*Prescriptions for a Healthier Norway*,
415–16

*Public Health Act* (2012), 416, 418

public health approach, developments
in, 416

public social spending, 148, 235–38

as social democratic welfare state, 68,
154, 238

social expenditures as percentage GDP, 70

nostalgia, as constructed memory, 261

Nunavut

disability rates, 360

nurse practitioners, 315–17

scope of practice, 314–15

nurse-midwives, 314–15

nursing, 312

care deficit, 343

caring dilemma, 49

devaluation of nursing work, 317

as extension of caring services, 317

negative impact of reforms on, 319–20

physical/mental demands of, 342–43

RNs, replacement of, 317

subordination of, 49, 313

nutrition, 401

Obama, Barack, 236, 273–74

obesity, 15, 77

stress and, 23

observational ecological studies, 24

occupation, as indicator of social class, 174

old age pensions, 236–37

"One-Eyed Science," 333

Ontario

disability rates, 360

electoral reform, 246–47

Health Professions Legislation Review
(HPLR), 314–15

Indigenous Cultural Safety program, 221

Local Health Integration Networks
(LHINs), 302

midwifery, 275

reports on health equity, 397

Ontario Committee of the Healing Arts, 314

Ontario Institute for Clinical Evaluative Sciences, 340

ontology, 114, 118–19

open-ended interviews, 127

opioid use/abuse, stress of inequality and, 16

oral health, 171

organ transplants, 94

Osler, William, 265

oxygen, 6

paid parental leave, 21

pandemics, 101

parametric statistics, 125

parental benefits, 203, 249

Parsons, Talcott, 53, 354

  *The Social System*, 39

participant observation, 126–27

participatory monitoring, 104

patent protection, 383–85, *389*

Patented Medicines Prices Review Board, 303–4

pathway effects, 153

patient-centred medical home (PCMH) model, 302

patriarchy, *56*

  gender inequality and, 47–49

Pederson, Ann, 201–2

pediatricians, 316

per-capita healthcare expenditures, 13–14

personal support workers (PSWs), 317

Pfizer, 375–76

pharmacare programs, 443

Pharmaceutical Advertising Advisory Board (PAAB), 380, 381

pharmaceutical industry, 439–40

  Comprehensive Economic and Trade Agreement (CETA), 383–84

  continuing medical education sponsorship by, 379, 380, 385–86

  drug approval process, 374–77

  drug regulatory system, 373

  intellectual property rights, 381–85, 390n3

  lobby, and price regulation, 304–5

physicians and, 385–86

post-marketing surveillance, 378, 389n2

profit levels, 382–83

regulation of, 373–74

relationship with Canadian government, 373

self-regulation of, 380–81

timeliness of approvals, and returns on investment, 375–76

trade associations, 380

transfer pricing, 382–83

transparency and, 378–79

user fees, 374, 375

pharmaceutical policy, 372–87

pharmaceuticals

  access to, 130, 303–5

  adverse events, 374, 380

  adverse reactions reports, 377

  breakthrough products, 375–76

  development costs, 383

  direct-to-consumer promotion and, 381

  disclosure of information, transparency in, 378–79

  drug benefit programs, subsidized, 303

  drug insurance coverage, 303

  drug regulatory system, 373

  drug safety, 377–78

  efficacy of, 373, 379–80

  "evergreening," 385

  generic drugs, 385

  intellectual property rights, 381–85, 390n3

  Internet pharmacies, 304

  off-label promotion, 381

  patent issues, 381–85

  price regulation, 303–5

  promotion of, 379–81

  research and development, 383, *389*

  risk management vs precautionary principle, 374

  significant therapeutic improvements, 375–76

philanthropic associations, 265

PhRMA, development costs, 383

physical accessibility, 103

physical activity, 401

physician assistants, 316

physicians

    complementary role with patients, 39

    continuing medical education sponsorship, 379, 380

    inappropriate prescribing, 379–80

Pickett, Kate, *The Spirit Level*, 15

Piketty, Thomas, *Capital in the Twenty-First Century*, 18, 25

planned market initiatives, 291–92

Plato, 138

policy and practice in health care, *347*

polio, 143

polis vs market, 73–74

political determinants of health, 8, 9

political economy perspective, 61–79

    critical, 61–62

    critical analysis and, 128

    epistemology, 119–20

    familial health determinants, 76–77

    feminist, 332

    methodology, 120

    positivism and, 116–17

    public policy, 75, 78–79, 234, 250

    realism, 117–19

    role of government, 63, 64

    social class, impact on health outcomes, 176–77

    social determinants of health and, 157–59

    social expenditures as percentage GDP, 70

    stratification, 70–71

    welfare state, 65, 66–70

political empowerment

    of vulnerable populations, 199–200

political ideology

    electoral systems, 246–47

    and the "left," 157–58, 234, 246–47, *253*

    public policy and, 61–62, 237, 243–44

    social determinants of health and, 154–55

political parties

    "left," 246–47, *253*

    types of, 243–44, 246–47

    United States, 284

political policies, income inequality and, 29

political power

    inequality and, 28

    influence on public policy, 62, 157–58

political rights, 85

political system, 72–73

poor people

    health insurance, 286

    worthy vs unworthy poor, 357

population health, *33, 427*

    epidemiology and, 24–29

    health data, 11–24

    materialist/structuralist factors in social determinants of health, 148–50

    promotion of, 424

    public policy and, 234

    public social spending, 235–38

    upstream determinants of health and, 29

Portugal

    infant mortality rates, 78

    as Latin welfare state, 69

    social expenditures as percentage GDP, 70

positivism, 113, 114, 115–17, 130, *133*

    epistemology, 119–20

post-colonialism, 50–51

post-marketing surveillance, 378, 389n2

postmodernism, 27, 39, 51–52, 53

postpartum depression, 209

post-structuralism, 51–52

post-traumatic stress disorder (PTSD), 209

poverty, *164*, 173, 399

    among Aboriginal peoples, 51

    among immigrants of colour, 129

    austerity policies, impact of, 246

    as brain toxin, 23

    child poverty in wealthy nations, comparison, 149

    as determinant of health, 5

    as illness, 5

    impact on health, 5, 15–18, 21

    interconnections with life experience, and disease, 271

powerlessness and, 9

public social spending and, 237, 238

rates of, and taxes/transfers, 17

rates of as indicator of progressive public
    policy, 238–41

rates of by age groups, 239

power relations

gender inequality and, 47–49, 218

inequality and, 28

influence on health, 157–58

influence on public policy, 62–66, 78–79

between men and women, 91

*pouvoir/savoir*, 52

of social class, 172–73

subordination of women, 334

pre-existing illnesses, coverage of, 288

pregnancy

gender-based violence, 221

medicalization of, 48–49

reproductive rights, 97–98

stress during, 21, 23

teenage births, 15

premature mortality, 144–45

prescription medicine

accessibility, and income, 143, 183

cost of, 385

delisting of, 273

drug spending per capita (Canada), 385

generic drugs, 385

spending on, 372

*See also* pharmaceuticals

prevalence, 123

prevention vs care, 437–38

primary care, 27

primary care nurse practitioners, 315–17

primary care specialists, 316

primary health care, 315–16, 325n3

Prince Edward Island

midwifery, 337

private practice–public payment, 267, 275, 311

privatization, *325*

privatization of health care, 70, 354

case against, 322

vs public care, 321–22, 439–40

profitization, 321, *325*

proportional representation, 247, *253–54*

prospective studies, 124

prostate cancer, 124

psychiatry, 42

psychosocial model

social class, impact on health outcomes,
    176, 181–82

public health, *427*

Canadian approaches to, 396–400

health equity promotion, 397–99

health promotion and, 394–95

integration with public policy, 394–95

medical sociology and, 38

Norwegian approaches to, 414–18

pharmaceuticals and, 377–81

political economy of, 394–424

political ideologies and, 423–24

structural approach, Canadian
    developments, 398

structural approaches to, 395

Swedish approach to, 418–23

UK approaches to, 407–14

US approaches to, 400–407

public health agencies, 394

public health care

vs private profit, 386–87

vs privatization, 321–22

public health law, coercive use of, 99

public health policy

sociology of health and, 38

public health units, 160

public pension programs, 236–37

public policy, *164*

action/inaction, 161

definition of, 233–34

disability and, 357

factors influencing development of, 62–65,
    234, 237

health equity promotion, 397–99

neo-liberalism, and austerity,
    245–46

political, economic, and social forces
    shaping, 244–45

public policy (*continued*)
  political economy perspective, 75, 78–79, 234, 250
  population health profiles, 243–44
  prescription medicines and, 387
  progressive, poverty rates as indicator of, 238–41
  relationship to economic sectors, 399
  role of, 441–42
  role of government, 63, 64
  social determinants of health and, 75–76, 78–79, 153–54, 443
  welfare states and, 241–43
public social spending, 235–38
  means-tested social assistance, 241–42
  poverty and, 238–41
public vs. private health care, 287–90, 439–40
public–private partnerships (P3s), 273

qualitative data analysis, 127
qualitative research methods, 117, 126–27
quality of care, 95, 103
quality of life study, 127
quantitative research methods, 115, 121–26, 130
Quebec, 278n1
  Bill 33, 286–87
  *Chaoulli* case, 286–87
  community health centres, 271
  drug benefit programs, subsidized, 303
  Ministry of Health report on health inequalities, 397
  *Quebec Charter of Human Rights and Freedoms*, 286

race, 75, 141
  anti-racism and, 50–51
  critical analysis and, 128
  ethnicity and, 203
  historical mortality indicators and, 268
  intersectionality and, 204, 206
  as social determinant of health, 199–200
  strategies to address inequities, 217–19
racialization
  anti-racism and, 50–51

of im/migrant populations, 207–8, 216–17
  as social construct, 203
  of vulnerable populations, 200
racialized groups
  overrepresentation of in lower status occupations, 207–8
racism, *226*
  anti-racism programs, 221
  as barrier to health, 28, 201
  against im/migrant populations, 211
Radcliffe-Brown, A.R., 39
rage, psychosocial impacts of stress, 16
rationalization, *325*
  cost containment and, 439–40
  of healthcare resources, 313–14, 319–21
rationing, *325*
Rawls, J., *A Theory of Justice*, 283
realism, 113, 115, 117–18, 131
  critical analysis and, 128
  methodology, 120
redistribution of healthcare costs, 282–83
regionalization of health care, 302
registered practical nurses (RPNs), 317
regulated markets, 292
rehabilitation services, 94, 160
religious orders, 312
reproduction
  patriarchal control over, 49
reproductive health
  access to by im/migrant women, 209–10, 211, 222–23
  culturally appropriate, access to, 217, 337–42
  right to health and, 97–99, 218
research
  approaches to, 113–15
  disease focus of, 10
  epidemiological approaches, 122–24
  epistemology, 119–20
  gender-sensitive analysis and, 338–40
  human rights approaches, 129–30
  methodology, 120
  ontology, 118–19
  parametric statistics, 125

quantitative methods, social science, 125–26

quantitative research methods, 115, 121–26

socio-economic status, controlling for, 10

research and development, *389*

research design, 114–15

research paradigms

upstream/root cause approach, 7–8

residual welfare state, 242

resilience

theoretical foundations, 204–6

vulnerability and, 199–200

respiratory disease, 145

Reverby, Susan, 49

right to health

differential access to, 90–93

entitlements, 90

freedom from non-consensual medical
treatment, 90

globalization and, 101

health good practice vs right to health
good practice, 102–3

health research, 100–101

HIV/AIDS, 99–100

international agreements, 85, 86–89,
94–95, 96, 99, 108nn2–5, 108–9n10

key aspects, 89, 95

monitoring, 102–3

outcome indicators, 102

process indicators, 102

reproductive health, 97–99

rights-based monitoring, 103–4

social justice and, 84–86

structural indicators, 102

taxonomy of, 103

rights

civil, 85

cultural, 85

economic, 85

human rights, 84–105

of nations, 85

political, 85

social, 85

rights outcome approach

disability and, 352, 354, 355–56

rights-based monitoring, 103–4

risk-related behaviours

as coping mechanism, 77, 150

lifestyle risk factors, 142, 184–85

Rockefeller Foundation, 265

Romania

austerity policies, 245–46

root cause approach to disease, 7–8

Rose, Geoffrey, 9

Russia

life expectancy, 26

population health and, 26

Ryan, Paul, 299

Sanders, Bernie, *Medicare for All* bill, 300

San'yas Indigenous Cultural Safety Training, 221

SARS (severe acute respiratory syndrome),
101, 424

Saskatchewan

doctors' strike, 263, 267

medicare, 263, 267, 285–86

Sauvé, Jeanne, 219

Scandinavia, *Scandinavian Common Sense*, 68

scarlet fever, 143

scholarship, gap between knowledge and action,
397–99

scientific method, and positivism, 115–17

Scotland

*Health Inequalities Policy Review for the
Scottish Ministerial Task Force on Health
Inequalities*, 412–13

screening, access to, 211

Second World War, and the welfare state, 67

securitization, and neo-liberalism, 247–48

self-assessed health (SAH), 11

self-provision of care, 312

severe acute respiratory syndrome (SARS),
101, 424

sex, *227*, 335

vs gender, 202–3, 332

sexism, *227*

sexual health, 97–98

sexually transmitted disease, 97, 98, 210

Shaffir, William, 42

Sherwin, S., *The Politics of Women's Health*, 333

"shoe leather epidemiology," 9

sick leave, 249

sick role, 39–40

sildenafil, 43

sin taxes, 395

Sinclair, Upton, 10

Slovenia

    austerity policies, 245–46

smart regulations strategy, 374

Smith, Barbara Ellen, 44

Smith, Dorothy, 48

smoking, 7, 14–15, 214, 219, 339, 340, 401

    as coping mechanism, 77, 150

    in Japan, 7, 26

    lung cancer, 123

Snow, John, 4–5, 9

social assistance, 75, 250

social capital, 173

social class

    cancer and, 177–79

    critical analysis and, 128

    cultural-behavioural model, 175–76, 178

    definitions of, 172–73

    differences in health status, 46–47

    health and, 175–77

    health inequality and, 171–87

    historical mortality indicators and, 268

    income inequality and, 173

    life-course choices, 175–76, 177, 178

    materialist model, 176–77, 178, 182–84

    measurement of, 173–75

    psychosocial model, 176, 178, 181–82

    as social determinant of health, 141–42

social comparison approach to social
    determinants of health, 151–52

social conditions, relationship to health, 140–41

social constructionism, 41–44

    disease as political accomplishment, 42–43

    postmodernism and, 51

social context, *347*

social democratic welfare state, 63, 68–69, *81*,
    154–55, 158–59, 243–44

social determinants of health, *33*, 138–61, *164*

Aboriginal peoples and, 141, 144

areas of needed inquiry, 160–61

differences between nations, 146–48

evidence concerning, 142–48

familial health determinants, 76–77

gender, ethnicity/race and, 199–200,
    211–12

health inequalities and, 143–46

health perspectives on, 155–61

health-related organizations
    addressing, 398

im/migrant populations and, 209, 211–12

improved health and, 143

mechanisms and pathways influencing
    health, 148–52, 156

media coverage, 128

political economy approach to, 63, 73

politics, political ideology and, 154–55

poverty, 5, 145–46, 148

prevention vs care, 437–38

public policy and, 75–76, 78–79,
    153–54, 233

public vs. private health care, 439–40

right to health and, 94–95

social epidemiology and, 9

strategies to address inequities, 217–22

vs lifestyle choices, 142, 143, 147, 152–53

social epidemiology, 9, 116, 155

social exclusion, 75, 141–42, 144

social expenditures

    Canada-U.S. comparison, 27

    as percentage GDP, 70

social gradient, *189*

social inequalities, 15–18

social inequality, *189*

    stratification and, 70–71

social infrastructure, public social spending,
    235–38

social insurance plans

    conservative welfare state, 69

social isolation, 126

social justice

    critical analysis and, 128

    health equity and, 160

links between health and human rights,
84–86, 139–40
public needs and, 283
vs economic justice, 73
social location, *189*
social pathology, disability and, 351, 354–56, 364
social policy, 75
social position, *81*
social production of disease hypothesis, 44
social protection, 282–83
social rights, 85
social safety net, 75–76, 141, 144
social science
examples of qualitative approaches, 127–28
historical analysis, 129
key questions, 122
qualitative approaches, 126–28
quantitative methods in, 125–26
research design, 125
statistics, and statistical analysis, 125–26
social selection, 46
social stratification, 69, 70–71, *189*
social support, 141–42, 182
socialism vs liberalism, 73
society, concepts of
market vs. polis, 73–74
socio-economic status, *189*
controlling for in research studies, 10
health and, 15–18, 22–24
health-related behaviours and, 26
income inequality and, 15–16
intersectionality of im/migrant
populations, 210–12
sociological perspectives, 38–53
disciplinary approaches, professions,
156–57
epistemology, 119–20
evolution of, 39–52
idealism, 117
institutional mandates, and political
issues, 157
key questions, 122
psychological constructs, 156
realism, 117–18, 119
social determinants of health and, 156–57

sociology
definition of, 38
of health, 38–53
institutionalization of, 38
medical sociology, 38
in medicine vs of medicine, 38
Soviet Union (former)
population health, 26
Spain
infant mortality rates, 78
as Latin welfare state, 69
social expenditures as percentage GDP, 70
Sri Lanka, female adult mortality, 14
St. Francis Xavier University, 398
state, role of in welfare state, 70–71
statistical analyses, 122–23, 125–26
Statistics Canada, 397
*Canadian Survey of Disability* (CSD), 352,
358, 359
*Participation and Activity Limitation Survey*
(PALS), 352, 358, 359
Stewart, Isabel Maitland, 265
stigma, Goffman's conceptualization of, 41
stigmatization, 354
of im/migrant populations, 208
Stoddart, Greg, 315
stomach cancer, 184
Stowe, Emily, 265
stratification, 69, 70–71
Straus, Robert, 38
Strauss, Anselm, 42
stress
acute stress response, 23
chronic stress, impact of, 23–24
impact on immune system, 181
non-adaptive reaction to, 77
during pregnancy, 21, 23
psychosocial impacts of, 16
as social determinant of health, 141–42, 150
stroke, 152, 402–3
structural functionalism, 39–41, 53
conflict vs consensus models, 437
disability and, 352, 353–54
public health and, 395
public health, Canadian developments, 398

structuralism, 117–18

subjectivism, 51

substance use/abuse, harm reduction, 222

Sudbury Health Unit, 398

surrogate markers, 21

Sustainable Development Goals

pillars of sustainability, 218

Sweden

Commission on Equity in Health (2015), 422–23

Commission on Social Determinants of Health, 419

Council for Equitable Health, 423

*Good and Equitable Public Health*, 238, 423

health equity statement and policy (2001), 419–20

health-related public policy, 418–23

income inequality, 419

infant mortality rates, 78

labour policy, 250

National Institute of Public Health objectives, 420

poverty rates, 17, 237–39, 419, 422

privatization of health care, 422

Public Health Policy Report (2005), 420–22

public social spending, 25, 235–38

as social democratic welfare state, 68, 154, 238

social expenditures as percentage GDP, 70

Switzerland

infant mortality rates, 78

social expenditures as percentage GDP, 70

symbolic interactionism, 41–44

feminism and, 48

postmodernism and, 51

systemic monitoring, 103–4

teenagers, 127

Thatcher, Margaret, 407

Therapeutic Products Directorate (TPD), 373, 374–81, 389n1

cost recovery, *389*

disclosure of information, transparency in, 378–79

financing for, 374, 377

smart regulations strategy, 374

Summary Basis of Decision (SBD), 379

tobacco use. *See* smoking

Todd, Emmanual, 26

trade agreements, health impacts of, 159

transport, 141–42

trauma, patient safety and, 220–21

Triple Negative Breast Cancer, 185

Trudeau, Justin, 246

Truman, Harry S., 266

Trump, Donald, 237, 282, 299–300, 407

Truth and Reconciliation Commission, 216, 217–18

tuberculosis, 263, 264, 271, 272

Tunisia, child mortality, 14

Turner, Bryan, 52

Two Spirit people. *See* LGBT people

typhoid, 143

under-5 mortality, 11

unemployment, 141–42

employment insecurity, 75–76

unemployment benefits, 65, 71

union density, 65–66, 158, 247

unions, power and influence of, 63, 65–66, 157–58, 247

United Kingdom

Acheson Commission into Inequalities in Health, 408

austerity policies, 245–46, 413

*Black Report*, 46, 148–49, 407, 408

child poverty, 410

Clinical Commissioning Groups (CCGs), 291

developments post-2010 election, 411–14

*Due North*, 411

for-profit healthcare, 236

government action plans, 409–11

green space exposure, 28

*Health Act 2009*, 290

*Health and Social Care Act 2012*, 290, 291
Health and Wellbeing Boards
   (HWBs), 291
*Health Divide*, 148–49, 408
Health Select Committee, 344
income inequality, 408
infant mortality rates, 78
*Inquiry on Health Equity for the North*, 411
*Insurance Act*, 263, 265
labour policy, 250
as liberal welfare state, 69, 154
life expectancy, 411
National Health Service, 292, 408,
   409, 411
parallel private health care, 289
planned market initiatives, 291–92
poverty, 237, 410
public policy reality, 414
public social spending, 235–38
*Reducing Health Inequalities*, 409–10
social determinants of health, 141–42
social exclusion, 410
social expenditures as percentage
   GDP, 70
United Nations
   Commission on Human Rights, 87, 95
   Committee on Economic, Social, and
      Cultural Rights (CESCR), 90, 94
   Committee on the Rights of the Child
      (CRC), 96–97
   *Convention on the Elimination of All
      Forms of Discrimination against Women*
      (CEDAW), 87, 96, 97–98
   *Convention on the Protection of the Rights of
      All Migrant Workers and Members of Their
      Families*, 88
   *Convention on the Right of the Child*, 88
   *Convention on the Rights of Persons with
      Disabilities*, 88, 93, 94–95, 355
   *Declaration of the High-level Dialogue
      on International Migration and
      Development*, 89
   *Declaration of the International Summit for
      Social Development*, 159

*Declaration on HIV/AIDS*, 99,
   108–9n10
*Declaration on the Elimination of the Violence
   against Women*, 91
*Declaration on the Rights of Indigenous
   Peoples* (UNDRIP), 88–89, 96
Economic and Social Council
   (ECOSOC), 94
General Comment, 86–87, 108n5
*Human Development Report*, 12
International Conference on Population
   and Development, 98
International Conference on Women, 98
*International Convention on the Elimination
   of All Forms of Racial Discrimination*, 87
*International Covenant on Civil and Political
   Rights*, 108n4
*International Covenant on Economic, Social,
   and Cultural Rights*, 86, 87, 94–95,
   108n4
*Principles for the Protection of Persons with
   Mental Illness and the Improvement of
   Mental Health Care*, 94
Special Rapporteur on the Right to
   Health, 102–3
Special Rapporteur reports, 95
*Universal Declaration of Human Rights*,
   87, 159
*Vienna Declaration and Programme of
   Action*, 95
United States
   access to care, 269–70, 305
   Accountable Care Organizations
      (ACOs), 302
   *Affordable Care Act* (ACA). *See* United
      States, *The Patient Protection and
      Affordable Care Act* (2010)
   *American Health Care Act* (2017), 299
   *Better Care Reconciliation Act of 2017*, 300
   Canada health divergence, 27–29
   Children's Health Insurance Program
      (CHIP), 293
   drug benefit programs, subsidized, 303
   drug insurance coverage, 303–4

United States (*continued*)

*Ensuring Enforcement and Implementation of Abortion Restrictions in the Patient and Affordable Care Act* (2010), 297

Family Medical Leave Act, 249

family policy in, 249

*Health Care Freedom Act*, 300

"health disparity," 9, 400

health insurance, 263, 265–68, 269

health policy reforms, 284–85

health profile, 400–407

health status of Americans, 141

healthcare management, 320–21

healthcare policy, 282–83

healthcare system, origins of, 261–76

Hyde Amendment, 297

income inequality, 148, 151

*Individual Tax Reform and Alternative Minimum Tax Act*, 300–301

inequality profile of, 18

infant mortality rates, 78, 141, 148

integrated delivery networks (IDNs), 301–3

labour policy, 250

as liberal welfare state, 69, 154, 237

life expectancy, 12–15, 22, 27, 141, 148, 407

managed care plans, 290–91, 295

maternal mortality, 14

Medicaid, 236, 263, 267, 269, 282, 293–95

Medicare, 237, 263, 267, 269, 282, 293–95

*Medicare Prescription Drug, Improvement, and Modernization Act* (2003), 294

Medicare Shared Savings Program (MSSP), 302

*Migrant Health Act* (1962), 267

minimum-income benefit, 148

National Longitudinal Survey, 152

national policy documents and reports, 400–401

*ObamaCare Repeal Reconciliation Act* (2017), 300

paid parental leave, 21

*The Patient Protection and Affordable Care Act* (2010), 236, 273–74, 281, 295–301, 305

per-capita healthcare expenditures, 13–14

percentage of GDP spending on health care, 274

percentage of GNP spending on health care, 268, 270

population health, 146, 148

post-marketing surveillance, 378, 389n2

poverty rates, 17, 148, 237, 238–40

primary healthcare division of labour, 316

private for-profit care, 311

privatization of social programs, 236–37

public social spending, 25, 148, 235–38

"section 1115" waivers, 294

smoking, 26

social determinants of health, and public policy, 400

social expenditures as percentage GDP, 70, 274

Social Security, 236–37

*Social Security Act* (1965), 267

social welfare, residual approach to, 238

state-based health insurance exchanges, 295–96

universal health insurance, 266

"War on Poverty," 267

*The Work, Family and Equity Index*, 249

univariate analyses, 123, 125–26

universal health care, 236

Canadian development of, 265–68, 275

role of in producing health, 18–19

as social service, 17

universal health insurance, 269

universalism, 244, 357

*Unnatural Causes* (documentary), 407

Upstream, 398, 399

upstream approach to disease management, 185–86

upstream/root cause approach, 7–8, 10

urban-rural disparities in health insurance, 266

user fees, 245–46, 273

utilization review, *308*, 322

vaccines, 143

Vanessa's Law, 379

*Vienna Declaration and Programme of Action*
 (UN), 95
violence
        against Aboriginal women, 214–15
        gender-based violence, 209–11, 221
        healthcare response to, 221
        im/migrant populations, experience of
            violence, 209–11
        intimate partner violence against im/
            migrant women, 208
        sexual, 337
        trauma- and violence-informed care,
            220–21
        against women and children, 86, 91
Virchow, Rudolph, 176–77
        *Report on the Typhus Epidemic in Upper
            Silesia*, 138–39, 140–41
viruses, cancer and, 184
vulnerability
        Aboriginal women, 222–23
        groups excluded from health
            insurance, 305
        im/migrant women, 222–23
        political empowerment and, 199–200
        resilience and, 199–200
        social determinants of, 99
        theoretical foundations, 204–6

*wa* (culture of), 26
waiting lists, 292
Wales
        Public Health Wales Observatory, 413–14
Weber, Max, 38, 41, 56n6, 172
welfare
        child and family policy, 75
        housing policy, 75
        social assistance, 75
welfare state, 66–70, *81*, *164*
        Antipodean welfare state, 242
        benefits and supports by, 65
        categorical welfare state, 242
        central features of, 68
        Christian democratic, 243–44
        conservative, 63, 69, 154–55, 159, 243–44

defined, 66, 67
electoral systems, 246–47
forms of, 154–55
future of, 442
healthcare systems, 68–69
infant mortality rates (IMR), 77, 78
influence on public policy, 63
institutional welfare state, 242
Latin welfare state, 69, 242
liberal, 63, 69–70, 154–55, 159, 243–44
political, economic, and social forces
    shaping, 244–45
population health and, 126, 243–44
programs and services, provision of, 67
public policy and, 241–43, 441–42
public social spending, 235–38
redistribution of economic resources, 67–68
residual welfare state, 242
social class, impact on health outcomes, 177
social democratic, 63, 68–69, 154–55,
    158–59, 243–44
social determinants of health and, 154–55
social expenditures as percentage GDP, 70
well-being
        Aboriginal dimensions of, 212–13
        differential access to, 90–93
West of Scotland Collaborative Study, 152
Wilkinson, Richard, *The Spirit Level*, 15
Witz, Anne, *Professions and Patriarchy*, 49
women
        Aboriginal, 212–16, 336
        accessible and appropriate care, 337–42
        in ancillary health services, 343–44
        body image, 336
        childbirth, medicalization of, 48–49,
            337–38
        division of labour and, 342
        early exclusion from medical practice, 265
        eating disorders, 336
        exclusion from medical schools, 312,
            325n2
        gender vs sex, 202–3
        health-related differences between men
            and, 333–34, 336–40

women (*continued*)
in im/migrant population, 207–8
income inequality, 144, 336
paid vs unpaid labour, 333, 337, 342
poverty and, 333
research, gender-sensitive analysis and, 338–40
"semi-professional" status of, 313
stereotypes, 218, 219
subordination of, 334
support occupations, 313
*See also* violence
*Women in Canada*, 337
Women's Health Bureau, 335
women's movement
gender-sensitive analysis and, 333–34
working conditions
as social determinant of health, 141–42
workplace discrimination, 100

World Health Organization (WHO)
*Closing the Gap in a Generation*, 139–40
Commission on Social Determinants of Health, 139–40, 199, 398
*Declaration of Alma Atal*, 86, 108n3
definition of health, 11, 356
health, and disease, 272
*Health Systems Financing*, 95
International Classification of Disease (ICD), 358
"neglected diseases," 100, 109n11
Wright, Erik Olin, 172–73

Yukon
midwifery, 337

Zola, Irving
medicalization of daily living, 43, 56n5